Mosby's 1994 Nursing Drug Cards

Joseph A. Albanese, R.Ph., Ph.D.

Professor Emeritus,
College of Staten Island,
City University of New York,
Staten Island, New York

Patricia A. Nutz, R.N., M.S.N., M.Ed.

Instructor,
School of Nursing, St. Francis Hospital,
New Castle, Pennsylvania

Mosby

St. Louis Baltimore Boston Chicago London Madrid Philadelphia Sydney Toronto

Mosby
Dedicated to Publishing Excellence

Sr. Vice President and Publisher: Alison Miller
Editor-in-Chief: Nancy Coon
Editor: Robin Carter
Developmental Editor: Gina Gay Chan
Project Manager: Patricia Tannian
Production Editor: Suzanne C. Fannin
Designer: Gail Morey Hudson
Manufacturing Supervisor: Pat Stinecipher

Fourth Edition

International Standard Book Number ISBN 0-8016-7897-8

93 94 95 96 97 / 9 8 7 6 5 4 3 2 1

Printed in the United States of America
Composition by Mosby Electronic Production, St. Louis
Printing/binding by Banta

Mosby-Year Book, Inc.
11830 Westline Industrial Drive
St. Louis, Missouri 63146

A NOTE TO THE READER: The authors and publisher have made every attempt to check dosages and nursing content for accuracy. Because the science of pharmacology is continually advancing, our knowledge base continues to expand. We therefore recommend that the reader always check product information for changes in dosage or administration before administering any medication. This is particularly important with new or rarely used drugs.

Mosby's 1994 Nursing Drug Cards include over 500 generic and 900 trade drugs. All drugs have been thoroughly updated to provide the latest content for nurses and nursing students administering these drugs in the clinical setting. A unique **new feature** is the inclusion of dosages for over 100 OTC preparations arranged by brand name. Also **new** is the placement of an IV compatibility chart inside the box cover for easy referral. In addition, 24 **new drugs** have been added, and in response to our polling a number of faculty at various associate degree, baccalaureate, and diploma nursing programs across the country, the package has been improved to provide the student with the greatest convenience at an affordable price.

DRUG CARD EXPLANATION

CATEGORY: Classifies the drug by using pharmacologic and/or therapeutic descriptors. **Rx:** Any drug that contains on the package the label: "Caution: Federal law prohibits dispensing without prescription." **OTC:** Any drug that can be sold legally over the counter (OTC) without a prescription. **Schedule Drug:** Controlled substance; any drug that is listed in Schedule C-II, C-III, C-IV, or C-V of the Comprehensive Drug Abuse Prevention and Control Act of 1970. Schedule C-II drugs have the greatest potential for misuse and addiction, whereas Schedule C-V drugs exhibit the least potential for misuse and addiction. Schedule C-I drugs have no accepted medical use and are illegal. Examples include diacetylmorphine (heroin), LSD, and mescaline. **Pregnancy Categories:** The purpose of the pregnancy categories is to establish a reasonable presumption for the possibility of drug-induced fetal harm and/or teratogenic effects. The categories established by the FDA are A,B,C,D, and X (NA indicates that an FDA category has not been assigned). Category A drugs represent relatively no risk; Category B, relatively no risk but not confirmed; Category C, potential risk, conclusive studies not available; Category D, therapeutic benefits must outweigh potential risks; and Category X, contraindicated during pregnancy. No drug was assigned a pregnancy category unless it was listed on the FDA labeling for the drug. ***New!* Nursing Management** has been expanded in the drug category section to include the full nursing process format. Patient education, dietary management, lab test evaluation, and geriatric (G)/pediatric (P)/obstetric (OB) special considerations are included when appropriate.

BRAND NAMES: Lists the proprietary (brand) name and manufacturer for the drug. Most cards present a complete list of brand name preparations. Abridged listings were used when the available proprietary preparations were too numerous to list. Drugs available only in Canada are marked with an asterisk (*). A footnote to this effect appears on all cards. Drugs not available in proprietary preparations are listed as available dosage forms without manufacturer identification.

COMBINATION PRODUCTS: Lists the formula(s) of the product(s), the manufacturer(s), and the available dosage form(s).

ACTION: Gives a brief description of the action(s) and effect(s) of the drug.

USE: Lists and describes the current medical use(s) of the drug. Nonlabeled use(s) of the drug (not approved by the FDA on the current labeling for the drug) or experimental use(s) are listed for selected drugs.

PHARMACOKINETICS: Lists the available data as stated by the company that developed the drug, whenever possible. **Absorption:** Passage of drug molecules from the site of administration into the circulating body fluids. **Duration:** Total time of clinical drug activity obtained after administration. **Excretion:** Removal of the drug or its metabolites from the body. **Half-life:** Time required to reduce the concentration of unchanged drug by 50% in the body. **Onset:** Time required to produce a measurable clinical drug effect after administration. **Peak:** Time required to produce the maximum clinical drug effect after administration. **Protein Binding:** Occurs when the drug combines with a body protein (usually plasma albumin) to form a reversible drug-protein complex. Protein-bound drug molecules must dissociate to produce therapeutic activity.

DOSAGE: Gives the recommended oral and parenteral dose ranges, including elderly and pediatric dosages when appropriate. Whenever discrepancies existed in the literature, the FDA labeling for the specific drug was used as the final authority. Routes include IA, intraarticular; IM, intramuscular; IV, intravenous; IVPB, intravenous piggyback; PO, oral; RC, rectal; SC, subcutaneous; SL, sublingual; and TOP, topical.

CONTRAINDICATIONS: Cites specific patient conditions that preclude use of the drug.

SIDE/ADVERSE EFFECTS: Undesired effects produced by the drug. Those listed are condensed. Common side effects appear in *italics*; serious adverse effects appear in ***boldface italics.*** Abbreviations for side/adverse effects include CNS, central nervous system; CV, cardiovascular; EENT, eye, ear, nose, and throat; END, endocrine;

GI, gastrointestinal; GU, genitourinary; HEM, hematological; HEP, hepatic; INT, integumentary; MET, metabolic; MS, musculoskeletal; PSYCH, psychiatric, and RESP, respiratory.

DRUG INTERACTIONS: Drug interactions listed are limited to the more serious reactions.

NURSING MANAGEMENT: Nursing responsibilities associated with each drug are summarized under the following categories. **Administration:** Major nursing responsibilities related to preparation, administration, and storage. **Evaluation:** Major nursing responsibilities related to monitoring the specific drug's effects on the patient following administration. **Education:** Major nursing responsibilities related to considerations for patient education, including discharge teaching, patient teaching in the hospital, or ambulatory care setting.

For category cards the nursing management also includes:

POTENTIAL NURSING DIAGNOSES ndx: Any NANDA nursing diagnoses that could be associated with drug administration. These are subdivided into **Therapeutic Effects:** Nursing diagnoses that may require use of a drug within the specific drug category (drug indications) and **Adverse Effects:** Nursing diagnoses that may result from the administration of a drug within the specific drug category (drug side effects).

OVERDOSE MANAGEMENT: Describes the recommended antidotal treatment for the drug.

The authors with to thank the following people who reviewed portions of previous editions of *Mosby's 1994 Nursing Drug Cards:* June M. Chandler, RN, EdD; Bruce Clayton, BS, PharmD; Pat Howard, RPh; Donna M. Kauffman, RN, MSN; Marlene Lindeman, RN, MSN; Linda T. Meyers, RN, MSN, CCRN; Jacqueline Murphy, BSc, MSc; Judith L. Meyers, RN, MSN; Keith M. Olsen, PharmD; Lisa Pope, PharmD; Michele Poradzisz, RN, MS; Donna Rios, RN, MSEd; Mildred Russin, RN, MSN; Roberta J. Secrest, PhD, PharmD, RPh; Linda Strand, PhD; and Richard E. Watters, BSc, RN, BEd. We welcome comments from users so that we may continue to provide nursing-oriented drug information in as useful a manner as possible.

Joseph A. Albanese
Patricia A. Nutz

Selected Manufacturer Abbreviations

A-H	Allen & Hanburys
A-U	American-Urological
B-I	Boehringer Ingelheim
BM-ONC	Bristol-Myers Oncology
B-W	Burroughs Wellcome
H-R	Hoechst-Roussel
MMD	Marion Merrell Dow
MJP	Mead Johnson Pharmaceutical
MSD	Merck Sharp & Dohme
P-D	Parke-Davis
P-G	Procter & Gamble Pharmaceuticals
P-F	Purdue Frederick
R-C	Reed & Carnrick
RPR	Rhone-Poulenc Rorer
R-R	Reid-Rowell
S-W	Sanofi Winthrop
S-S	Schiapparelli Searle
SKB	SmithKline Beecham
W-C	Warner Chilcott
W-A	Wyeth-Ayerst

Abbreviations

Symbols

α, β	Alpha, beta
↑, ↓	Increase(d), decrease(d)
2°	Secondary; second-degree
1°	Primary; first degree
▲, △, ◆	Alternate salt(s) of drug

Time

ac	Before meals
bid	Twice/day
d	Day
h	Hour
hs	Bedtime
m	Minute, meter
mo	Month
pc	After meals
prn	As needed
q	Every
qd	Daily
qid	Four times/day
qod	Every other day
tid	Three times/day
wk(s)	Week(s)
y/o	Years old
yr(s)	Year(s)

Miscellaneous

ABG	Arterial blood gas
ACE	Angiotensin-converting enzyme
ALT	Alanine aminotransferase
APTT	Activated partial thromboplastin time
ARC	AIDS-related complex
AST	Aspartate aminotransferase
BM	Bowel movement
BP	Blood pressure
BUN	Blood urea nitrogen
$\bar{c}$	With
cAMP	Cyclic adenosine monophosphate
CBC	Complete blood cell count
CHF	Congestive heart failure
CN	Cranial nerve
CO_2	Carbon dioxide
COPD	Chronic obstructive pulmonary disease
CR	Controlled-release
C&S	Culture and sensitivity
CSF	Cerebrospinal fluid
CVP	Central venous pressure
D/C	Discontinue
dig	Digitalis/digitalized
DS	Double strength
D_5W	5% dextrose in water

dx	Diagnosis	P	Pediatrics
ECG	Electrocardiogram	PDA	Patent ductus arteriosus
EEG	Electroencephalogram	PPD	Purified protein derivative
esp	Especially	ppt	Precipitate
FBS	Fasting blood sugar	pt(s)	Patient(s)
F/E	Fluid/electrolye	PT	Prothrombin time
G	Geriatrics	PTT	Partial thromboplastin time
H&H	Hemoglobin and hematocrit	PVC	Premature ventricular contraction; polyvinyl chloride
hx	History		
incl	Including	RBC	Red blood cell
I&O	Intake and output	REM	Rapid eye movement (sleep)
ICP	Intracranial pressure	ROM	Range of motion
IOP	Intraocular pressure	Rx	Prescription
IPPB	Intermittent positive-pressure breathing	rx	Reaction
LA	Long acting	SA	Sinoatrial
LDH	Lactate dehydrogenase	SLE	Systemic lupus erythematosus
LDL	Low-density lipoprotein	SR	Sustained release
LE	Lupus erythematosus	T_3, T_4	Triiodothyronine, thyroxine
LOC	Level of consciousness	TCA	Tricyclic antidepressant
µg	Microgram	TSH	Thyroid-stimulating hormone
MAO-I	Monoamine oxidase inhibitors	U	Unit
MI	Myocardial infarction	UA	Urinalysis
MIC	Minimum inhibitory concentration	UOQ	Upper outer quadrant
NG	Nasogastric	URI	Upper respiratory (tract) infection
NPN	Nonprotein nitrogen	UTI	Urinary tract infection
NSAIA	Nonsteroidal antiinflammatory agents	VS	Vital signs
N/V/D	Nausea/vomiting/diarrhea	WBC	White blood cell
OB	Obstetrics	w/in, w/out	Within, without
OD	Overdose		

Bibliography

American Society of Hospital Pharmacists: AHFS drug information 1993, Bethesda, Md, 1993.

Clark W, Brater C, Johnson AR: *Medical pharmacology,* ed 13, St Louis, 1991, Mosby.

Clayton BD, Stock Y: *Basic pharmacology for nurses,* ed 10, St Louis, 1993, Mosby.

Drug interaction viewer, Nutley, NJ, Roche Laboratories.

Gahart B: *Intravenous medications,* ed 6, St Louis, 1992, Mosby.

Goodman LS, Gilman A, editors: *The pharmacological basis of therapeutics,* ed 8, New York, 1990, Macmillan.

Kastrup E, editor: *Facts and comparisons,* St Louis, current, Facts and Comparisons.

Kim MJ: *Pocket guide to nursing diagnoses,* ed 5, St Louis, 1992, Mosby.

Pharmaceutical manufacturers' current catalogs.

Physicians' desk reference, ed 46, Oradell, NJ, 1993, Medical Economics.

Professional drug package inserts from various pharmaceutical manufacturers.

Remington's pharmaceutical sciences, ed 18, Easton, Pa, 1990, Mack.

Shannon MT, Wilson BA: *Drugs and nursing implications,* ed 7, Norwalk, Conn, 1992, Appleton & Lange.

Skidmore-Roth L: *Mosby's 1993 nursing drug reference,* St Louis, 1993, Mosby.

USP DI, ed 13, United States Pharmacopeial Convention, Rockville, Md, 1993.

Contents

acebutolol hcl • (a-se-byoo-toe-lole)

CATEGORY: *Beta-adrenergic blocker:* antiarrhythmic, antihypertensive Rx; Preg Cat B

BRAND NAME
Sectral (W-A)

DOSAGE FORMS
Capsule: 200, 400mg

ACTION: Blocks access of catecholamine neurotransmitters to $beta_1$ receptors located in heart; antihypertensive effect not determined. **USE:** Treatment of hypertension as sole agent or in combination c̄ other antihypertensives (esp thiazide diuretic) ▪ Treatment of ventricular premature beats.

PHARMACOKINETICS

PO absorption	Peak	Half-life	Protein binding	Excretion
90%	2.5h	3-4h	26%	30%-40% via urine, 50%-60% nonrenal

CONTRAINDICATIONS: Hypersensitivity, severe bradycardia, heart block >1st°, overt cardiac failure, cardiogenic shock.

DOSAGE
Adult PO Individualized dose starting c̄ 400mg/d. Usual range 400-800mg/d divided. Dose range for ventricular arrhythmia 600-1200mg/d divided

SIDE/ADVERSE EFFECTS: CNS: *fatigue, headache,* dizziness, insomnia, depression ▪ CV: bradycardia, ***heart failure,*** hypotension, chest pain ▪ EENT: abnormal vision ▪ GI: constipation, diarrhea, dyspepsia, flatulence, nausea ▪ GU: urinary frequency ▪ MS: arthraglia ▪ RESP: dyspnea.

DRUG INTERACTIONS: Use c̄ reserpine, other catecholamine-depleting drugs can result in serious adrenergic blockage ▪ Nonselective beta-adrenergics antagonize therapeutic response ▪ Use c̄ Ca blockers may prolong AV conduction ▪ Diabetics may require adjustment of antidiabetic agent(s).

NURSING MANAGEMENT
ADMINISTRATION: Assess for hx of beta blocker hypersensitivity ▪ Assess BP, apical pulse; if <60/m hold drug,

notify physician ▪ Assess hepatic function, I&O; may require ↓ dosage if impaired ▪ Do *not* administer in presence of respiratory distress (asthma, CHF, COPD) ▪ Avoid exposure to heat/moisture in storage ▪ Avoid abrupt withdrawal; D/C gradually ▪ Elderly may require ↓ dosage.

EVALUATION: Monitor hepatic, renal, respiratory status ▪ Monitor BP, pulse ▪ Monitor CBC, FBS (diabetics) ▪Assess for CHF (dyspnea, peripheral edema, ↑ weight); notify physician ▪ Assess for depression ▪ May produce alteration in blood glucose levels; may mask signs of hypoglycemia.

EDUCATION: Take as directed by physician; do *not* skip doses ▪ May take w/out regard to food ▪ Procedure for checking radial pulse ▪ Check pulse before taking; if <60/m do *not* take drug, notify physician ▪ Do *not* D/C w/out notifying physician ▪ Check c̄ physician/pharmacist before taking OTC/Rx preparations ▪ Drowsiness/dizziness may occur; use caution when engaging in potentially hazardous activities ▪ Avoid changing positions (lying/sitting/standing) rapidly ▪ Diabetics: carefully monitor blood/urine glucose; observe for symptoms of hypoglycemia (headache, ↑ sweating, hunger, weakness) ▪ May experience ↑ sensitivity to cold ▪ Notify physician of respiratory distress or leg edema ▪ Notify physician/dentist of beta blocker use before treatment ▪ Maintain optimum weight; follow low-Na^+ diet ▪ Keep scheduled appointments c̄ physician ▪ Store in well-closed container ▪ Avoid ↑ exercise, temperature extremes, smoking ▪ Women: avoid breastfeeding.

NOTES:

acetaminophen • (a-seat-a-<u>mee</u>-noe-fen)

CATEGORY: *Analgesic: p*-aminophenol, nonsalicylate analgesic — OTC

BRAND NAMES
Anacin-3 (Whitehall)
**Atasol (Horner)*
**Campain (Winthrop)*
Dapa (Ferndale)
Datril (Bristol-Myers)
Dolanex (Lannett)
**Exdol (Frosst)*
Liquiprim (Norcliff-Thayer)
Panadol (Glenbrook) Sterling [Canada]
Panex (Hauck)
**Raunox (Rougier)*
**Robigesic (Robins)*
Tempra (MJP)
Tylenol (McNeil)

COMBINATION PRODUCTS
Rx-C111-Preg Cat C
Anexia 7.5/650 (Beecham)
Capital c̄ Codeine (Carnick)
Phenaphen c̄ Codeine (Robins) #2, #3, #4
Tylenol c̄ Codeine (McNeil) #1, #2, #3, #4

DOSAGE FORMS
Caplet, capsule, chewable tablet, drops, elixir, liquid, suspension, suppository, tablet, wafer

ACTION: ↑ Pain threshold; affects hypothalamic heat-regulating center, resulting in analgesia/antipyresis about equal to aspirin; exerts no antiinflammatory or uricosuric activity. **USE:** Analgesic for mild to moderate pain as sole agent or in combination c̄ other analgesics or narcotics ▪ Antipyretic for febrile states ▪ ↓ Pain and fever associated c̄ DPT inoculations.

PHARMACOKINETICS

PO absorption	Peak	Half-life	Protein binding	Excretion
Almost complete	0.5-1.5h	1.5-3h	25%	80% excreted as conjugates in complete urine

CONTRAINDICATIONS: Hypersensitivity, known glucose-6-phosphate dehydrogenase deficiency.

Note: Side/adverse effects: common in *italic;* serious in ***boldface italic.***

*Available in Canada only.

DOSAGE

Pediatric	0-3 mo 40mg	4-5y/o 240mg
PO/Rectal q4-6h	4-11 mo 80mg	6-8y/o 320mg
	1-2y/o 120mg	9-10y/o 400mg
	2-3y/o 160mg	11-12y/o 480mg
Adult	325-650mg; do *not* exceed 4g/d, 2.6g/d c̄ long-term use	

SIDE/ADVERSE EFFECTS: HEM: anemia, leukopenia, neutropenia, pancytopenia; ***hemolytic anemia,*** methemoglobinemia (rare) ▪ HEP: jaundice ▪ INT: erythematous reactions, urticaria.

DRUG INTERACTIONS: PO anticoagulants can be displaced from protein storage sites; excessive use can enhance bleeding tendencies ▪ Use c̄ phenothiazines may produce hypothermia.

NURSING MANAGEMENT

ADMINISTRATION: Assess for hx of hypersensitivity ▪ Shake suspensions well before administering ▪ Administer c̄ food if GI irritation occurs ▪ Store suppositories in refrigerator.

EVALUATION: Assess hepatic, renal status during long-term therapy ▪ Assess for bleeding (GI, GU, skin/mucous membrane) c̄ long-term high-dose therapy.

EDUCATION: Notify physician if rash develops; D/C drug ▪ *Not* effective as antiinflammatory agent ▪ Avoid use c̄ alcohol ▪ Compliance c̄ prescribed dosage regimen.

OVERDOSE MANAGEMENT: Principal symptoms: sweating, gastric irritation, chills, cyanosis, oliguria, jaundice, coma, convulsions, death from respiratory failure ▪ Treatment: removal of drug by emesis or gastric lavage followed by acetylcysteine to ⬇ liver toxicity.

NOTES:

acetazolamide/acetazolamide sodium ▲ • (a-seet-a-zole-a-mide)

CATEGORY: *Carbonic anhydrase inhibitor: diuretic* RX; Preg Cat NA

BRAND NAMES
Diamox (Lederle)
**Acetazolam (ICN)*

DOSAGE FORMS
Tablet: 250 mg
Injection (IM/IV) ▲: 500 mg/vial
Sustained-release capsules
Sequels: 500mg
Tablet: 125, 250mg

ACTION: Diuretic effect due to inhibition of carbonic anhydrase in renal tubules; results in moderate diuresis c̄ alkaline urine, which leads to systemic acidosis; in addition, reduction in aqueous humor of eye; anticonvulsant activity. **USE:** Adjunct for open-angle, secondary glaucoma ▪ Adjunct anticonvulsant and in treating of edema due to CHF ▪ Pre-op reduction of pressure in acute-angle glaucoma ▪ Acute mountain sickness.

CONTRAINDICATIONS: Hypersensitivity, marked kidney/liver disease, low serum Na^+/K^+, hyperchloremic acidosis, adrenal gland failure.

DOSAGE

Glaucoma
Pediatric *PO* 8-30mg/kg/d divided
5-10 mg/kg q6h
IM/IV 250mg-1g/d divided
Adult *PO/IM/IV* 500mg repeated in 2-4h prn

Epilepsy
Pediatric/Adult *PO* 8-30 mg/kg/d; usual range 375mg-1g/d

Edema
Pediatric *PO* 5mg/kg/d
Adult *PO* 250-375mg/d (5mg/kg) on alternate days or for 2 days with day of rest
500-100mg/d divided

Mountain sickness
Adult *PO* 0.5-1g/d in divided doses prn

PHARMACOKINETICS

PO absorption	Tablet Onset	Tablet Peak	Tablet Duration	Sequel Onset	Sequel Peak	Sequel Duration	Excretion
Good	1h	2-4h	8-12h	2h	8-18h	18-24h	Unchanged via urine

Note: Side/adverse effects: common in *italic;* serious in ***boldface italic.*** *Available in Canada only.

SIDE/ADVERSE EFFECTS: CNS: drowsiness, confusion, *paresthesias, convulsions* ▪ EENT: transient myopia ▪ GI: anorexia, melena ▪ GU: polyuria, hematuria, glycosuria ▪ INT: urticaria, photosensitivity (rare) ▪ MET: acidotic states (long-term therapy).

DRUG INTERACTIONS: ↑ Dig toxicity due to hypokalemia; quinidine toxicity due to ↓ renal excretion ▪ Severe hypokalemia c̄ corticosteroids ▪ PO hypoglycemics may require dosage adjustment c̄ concurrent therapy.

NURSING MANAGEMENT

ADMINISTRATION: Assess for hx of sulfonamide-derivative hypersensitivity ▪ Diuretic: administer single PO dose in AM c̄ food ▪ Parenteral: reconstitute contents of vial (500mg) c̄ 5ml sterile H_2O for injection; use w/in 24h ▪ IM: painful; direct IV recommended ▪ Assess serum electrolytes ▪ Institute seizure precautions (epileptic) ▪ Maintain hydration ▪ Avoid abrupt withdrawal (anticonvulsant) ▪ Avoid exposure to heat/moisture during storage.

EVALUATION: Monitor F/E, hepatic, renal status ▪ Assess for fluid retention (I&O, daily weight) ▪ Assess for signs of sulfonamide toxicity (fever, rash, crystalluria, renal calculus) ▪ Assess for hyperglycemia (diabetics) ▪ Monitor IOP.

EDUCATION: Take as directed by physician; do *not* omit dose ▪ Take c̄ food; swallow SR capsules whole ▪ Drowsiness may occur; use caution in potentially hazardous activities ▪ Avoid changing positions (lying/sitting/standing) rapidly ▪ Eat foods high in K^+ (bananas, citrus fruits, raisins); avoid black licorice ▪ Symptoms of hypokalemia (anorexia, nausea, lethargy, muscle weakness, mental confusion, hypotension); D/C, notify physician of hypokalemia, tingling/tremors, sore throat, fever, skin rash, unusual bleeding/bruising ▪ May cause temporary visual disturbances (esp far vision) ▪ ↑ Fluid intake (8-10 glasses/d) ▪ Diabetics: carefully monitor blood/urine glucose ▪ Maintain optimum weight; avoid high Na^+ substances ▪ Store in tightly closed container ▪ Avoid changing brand-name preparations ▪ Carry identification (MedicAlert) if epileptic.

NOTES:

acetohexamide/chlorpropamide • (a-seet-oh-hex-a-mide/ klor-proe-pa-mide)

CATEGORY: *Oral hypoglycemic:* antidiabetic sulfonylurea Rx; Preg Cat C

BRAND NAMES	**DOSAGE FORMS**
acetohexamide	
Dymelor (Lilly)	Tablet: 250, 500mg
chlorpropamide	
Diabinese (Pfizer)	Tablet: 100, 250mg
**Novopropamide (Novopharm)*	Tablet: 250mg

ACTION: Antidiabetic activity due to stimulation of insulin release from functioning beta cells of pancreas. **USE:** Management of type II (non-insulin-dependent) diabetes that cannot be controlled by diet alone.

PHARMACOKINETICS

PO absorption	Onset	Peak	Duration	Half-life	Excretion
Acetohexamide					
Rapid	1h	3h	12-24h	1.3h	80%-90% via urine
Chlorpropamide					
Rapid	1h	2-4h	24h or more	36h	80%-90% via urine

CONTRAINDICATIONS: Hypersensitivity, diabetic ketoacidosis c̄ or w/out coma.

DOSAGE	Must be individualized
Adult *PO* acetohexamide	Usual maintenance range 250mg-1.5g/d
chlorpropamide	Usual maintenance range 100-500mg/d

SIDE/ADVERSE EFFECTS: GI: *nausea, epigastric fullness,* heartburn ▪ HEM: ***aplastic anemia, agranulocytosis leukopenia, hemolytic anemia,*** pancytopenia, ***thrombocytopenia*** ▪ INT: erythema, morbilliform/maculopapular eruptions, photosensitivity ▪ MET: hypoglycemia.

DRUG INTERACTIONS: Use c̄ alcohol, MAO-I phenylbutazones, beta blockers can significantly ↑ hypoglycemic effects ▪ Use c̄ anabolic steroids, chloramphenicol, guanethidine, PO anticoagulants, probenecid, salicylates, sulfinpyrazones, sulfonamides ↑ hypoglycemic effects ▪ Use c̄ adrenergics, corticosteroids,

Note: Side/adverse effects: common in *italic;* serious in ***boldface italic.***

*Available in Canada only.

phenytoin, thiazides, thyroid preparations ↓ hypoglycemic effects ▪ Use c̄ NSAIAs can ↑ hypoglycemic effects.

NURSING MANAGEMENT

ADMINISTRATION: Assess for hx of hypersensitivity ▪ Maintenance dose <1g/d, administer as single AM dose c̄ breakfast; >1g, administer in AM & PM c̄ meals ▪ Avoid exposure to moisture in storage ▪ Elderly may require ↓ dosage.

EVALUATION: Monitor hepatic, renal, hematologic status ▪ Monitor FBS ▪ Evaluate pt closely during 1st wk to assess effectiveness ▪ Monitor for signs of hypo/hyperglycemia.

EDUCATION: Compliance c̄ special diet therapy ▪ Blood/urine glucose/ketone testing procedure ▪ Symptoms of hypoglycemia (anxiety, headache, fatigue, nausea, sweating); notify physician immediately ▪ Always carry lump of sugar/candy for quick use if hypoglycemia occurs ▪ Avoid alcoholic beverages ▪ Check c̄ physician before taking OTC preparations ▪ Symptoms of hyperglycemia (excessive hunger, thirst, urination, rapid pulse, sweet-smelling breath, weight loss); notify physician immediately ▪ Need for good personal hygiene ▪ Carry medical identification (MedicAlert) ▪ Store in tightly closed containers ▪ Keep scheduled appointments c̄ physician/for blood glucose determinations ▪ Schedule periodic eye exams ▪ Maintain optimum body weight ▪ Avoid prolonged exposure to sunlight; use sunscreen, protective clothing ▪ Women: avoid breastfeeding ▪ PO hypoglycemic needs may change c̄ ↑ stress, ↑ exercise, ↓ appetite; notify physician.

NOTES:

acyclovir/acyclovir sodium▲ • (ay-sye-kloe-veer)

CATEGORY: *Antiviral*: purine nucleoside analog

Rx; Preg Cat C

BRAND NAME

Zovirax (B-W)

DOSAGE FORMS

Capsule: 200mg
Powder for injection (IV)▲: 500mg/vial
Ointment: 5%
Suspension: 200mg/5ml
Tablet: 800mg

ACTION: Antiviral activity due to interference c̄ virus DNA polymerase, and DNA replication in virus-infected host cells; selective for herpesvirus (HSV-1, HSV-2), varicella-zoster (VZV). **USE:** Management of herpes genitalis (HSV-2), mucocutaneous herpes simplex (HSV-1) in immunocompromised pts ▪ Acute treatment of herpes zoster ▪ Treatment of chickenpox.

PHARMACOKINETICS

Half-life	Protein binding	Excretion
2-3.5h	9%-33%	Urine via tubular secretion, glomerular filtration primarily as unchanged drug

CONTRAINDICATIONS: Hypersensitivity.

DOSAGE

Topical	Apply ointment q3h 6 times/d for 7d
Pediatric *IV*	250 mg/m^2 administered at constant rate for 1h q8h for 7d for HSV-1 and HSV-2. For encephalitis and varicella zoster 500mg/m^2 q8h for 10d
PO	Chickenpox: 20mg/kg (do *not* exceed 800mg) 4 times/d. Initiate at earliest symptoms
Adult *IV*	5mg/kg administered at constant rate for 1h q8h for 7d for HSV-1 and HSV-2. For encephalitis and herpes zoster 10mg/kg q8h for 10d
PO	Initial genital herpes: 200mg q4h 5 times/d for 10d Long-term suppression/recurrent disease: 400mg bid for up to 12mo, or 200mg tid or 5 times/d Intermittent treatment: 200mg q4h 5 times/d for 5d Herpes zoster: 800mg q4h 5 times/d for 7-10d

SIDE/ADVERSE EFFECTS: CNS: agitation, confusion, hallucinations, lethargy, tremors, seizures/coma (all systemic) ▪ CV: *inflammation* or *phlebitis* at infusion site, hypotension ▪ INT: *burning/stinging* at application site (topical), rash, hives, pruritus.

DRUG INTERACTIONS: Probenecid will ↓ urinary excretion of acyclovir, causing accumulation c̄ potential toxicity ▪ Use c̄ caution c̄ interferon/methotrexate; neurologic rxs may occur.

NURSING MANAGEMENT

ADMINISTRATION: Parenteral: administer only by IV infusion over 1h; use infusion control device; avoid rapid/bolus dose; dilute 500mg vial c̄ 10ml sterile H_2O for injection (50mg/ml); shake vial well until solution is clear, stable for 12h (room temperature); further dilute c̄ dextrose/electrolyte solutions to ≥70mg (7mg/ml), use w/in 24h (room temperature); precipitate occurs c̄ refrigeration, will redissolve at room temperature ▪ PO suspension: shake well before pouring ▪ Topical: use glove to prevent herpes transmission ▪ Maintain hydration ▪ Avoid exposure to heat/moisture in storage ▪ Administer at *end* of hemodialysis.

EVALUATION: Monitor F/E, hepatic, renal status ▪ Assess for ↑ BUN, serum creatinine (IV).

EDUCATION: Take exactly as directed by physician ▪ Take PO form c̄ food; shake suspension well before use ▪ Dizziness may occur; use caution when engaging in potentially hazardous activities ▪ ↑ Fluid intake (8-10 glasses/d) ▪ Use condoms if sexually active ▪ Information on herpes (symptoms, hygiene, transmission) ▪ Women: avoid breastfeeding ▪ Store in tightly closed container ▪ Procedure for topical application.

NOTES:

allopurinol • (al-oh-pure-i-nole)

CATEGORY: *Antigout:* xanthine oxidase inhibitor   Rx; Preg Cat C

BRAND NAMES	DOSAGE FORMS
**Alloprin (ICN)*	Tablet: 100, 200, 300mg
**Novopurinol (Novopharm)*	Tablet: 100, 200, 300mg
**Purinol (Horner)*	Tablet: 100, 200, 300mg
**Roucal (Rougier)*	Tablet: 100, 200, 300mg
Zyloprim (B-W)	Tablet: 100, 300mg

ACTION: Antigout effect due to inhibition of xanthine oxidase, which converts purines into uric acid.

USE: Treatment of gout, uric acid neuropathy, recurrent uric acid stone formation ▪ Prevention of tissue urate deposition, renal calculi, uric acid nephropathy in pts c̄ leukemia, lymphomas, malignancies receiving chemotherapy ▪ Management of recurrent calcium oxalate calculi in pts c̄ daily uric acid excretion rates of over 800mg/d (males) and 750mg/d (females).

PHARMACOKINETICS

PO absorption	Peak	Half-life	Excretion
90%	1.5h	1-2h	80% via urine, 20% via feces

CONTRAINDICATIONS: Hypersensitivity.

DOSAGE

Adult *PO*   200-600mg/d c̄ maximum 800mg/d

SIDE/ADVERSE EFFECTS: CNS: peripheral neuritis ▪ EENT: cataracts ▪ GI: N/V/D ▪ HEM: ***agranulocytosis,*** anemia, ***aplastic anemia***, bone marrow depression ▪ HEP: vasculitis or necrotizing angiitis leading to irreversible hepatotoxicity/death ▪ INT: *rash*, ***exfoliative dermatitis***, urticaria, ***Stevens-Johnson syndrome, toxic epidermal necrolysis***.

DRUG INTERACTIONS: Use c̄ azathioprine/mercaptopurine will significantly alter their biotransformation; dosage adjustment required ▪ ↑ PO absorption of iron preparations ▪ Use c̄ dicumarol may ↑ bleeding time.

NURSING MANAGEMENT

ADMINISTRATION: Assess CBC, hepatic, renal function; may require ↓ dosage if impaired ▪ Administer >300mg in divided doses ▪ Administer pc ▪ ↑ Fluid intake (3000ml/d).

Note: Side/adverse effects: common in *italic;* serious in ***boldface italic.***   *Available in Canada only.

EVALUATION: Monitor hepatic, renal status ▪ Monitor CBC, serum uric acid, I&O ▪ May produce ↓ serum glucose ▪ Normal serum uric acid: 2.5-6mg/100ml.

EDUCATION: Drowsiness may occur; use caution when engaging in potentially hazardous activities ▪ Take as directed by physician ▪ Take after meals ▪ D/C, notify physician of rash/flu-like symptoms ▪ Used to prevent, *not* relieve, gout attacks ▪ Avoid alcohol intake ▪ ↑ Fluid intake (10-12 glasses/d) ▪ Do *not* take c̄ iron preparations ▪ Store in tightly closed container ▪ Keep scheduled appointments for serum uric acid determinations ▪ Women: avoid breastfeeding ▪ Check c̄ physician before taking vitamin C preparations (↑ kidney stone formation) ▪ Maintain optimum weight ▪ ↓ Intake of high purine foods (organ meats, legumes) ▪ Full drug effects may require several months of therapy.

NOTES:

alprazolam/halazepam • (al-praz-oh-lam/hal-az-e-pam)

CATEGORY: *Benzodiazepine*: antianxiety agent, anxiolytic Rx C-IV; Preg Cat D

BRAND NAMES	DOSAGE FORMS
alprazolam	
Xanax (Upjohn)	Tablet: 0.25, 0.5, 1mg
halazepam	
Paxipam (Schering)	Tablet: 20, 40mg

ACTION: Anxiolytic activity due to depression of CNS at brainstem reticular formation, limbic, thalamic areas.
USE: Short-term treatment of anxiety.

PHARMACOKINETICS

PO absorption	Peak	Half-life	Protein binding	Excretion
alprazolam				
Very good	1-2h	12-15h	80%	Via urine as unchanged drug, metabolites
halazepam				
Rapid	1-3h	14h	—	Via urine as metabolites (99%)

CONTRAINDICATIONS: Hypersensitivity, narrow-angle glaucoma.

DOSAGE

alprazolam	
Adult *PO*	0.25-0.5mg tid. Do *not* exceed 4mg/d
Geriatric *PO*	0.25 mg bid or tid or higher if needed and tolerated
halazepam	
Adult *PO*	20-40mg , 3-4 times/d
Geriatric *PO*	20mg, 1-2 times/d

SIDE/ADVERSE EFFECTS: CNS: *drowsiness, fatigue, ataxia*, paradoxical anxiety, hallucinations, hyperexcitation ▪ CV: hypotension ▪ HEM: neutropenia (rare).

DRUG INTERACTIONS: Use c̄ other CNS depressants produces additive effects ▪ Use c̄ MAO-I can produce serious toxic effects.

NURSING MANAGEMENT
ADMINISTRATION: Assess for hx of benzodiazepine hypersensitivity ▪ Avoid exposure to heat, moisture, light

during storage ▪ Avoid abrupt withdrawal ▪ Have emergency support measures available ▪ Elderly may require ↓ dosage ▪ Ventilation of feelings, sympathetic listening contribute to relief of anxiety.

EVALUATION: Monitor renal, hepatic status ▪ Assess for symptoms of abrupt withdrawal (tremor, abdominal/muscle cramps, convulsions) c̄ prolonged use ▪ Check for signs of dependence c̄ prolonged therapy (↑ drug request) ▪ Monitor activity status (safety precautions) ▪ Assess for tolerance to therapeutic dose ▪ Assess for paradoxic rxs (CNS stimulation), esp elderly ▪ Check for depression; suicide precautions prn.

EDUCATION: Drowsiness may occur; use caution when engaging in potentially hazardous activities ▪ Avoid use c̄ alcohol, other CNS depressants ▪ Indiscriminate use may lead to dependence ▪ Do *not* keep at bedside ▪ Take as ordered by physician; do *not* ↑ dose ▪ Check c̄ physician/pharmacist before taking any OTC drugs ▪ Women: avoid breastfeeding ▪ Use alternate methods (relaxation exercises, ventilation of feelings) to ↓ anxiety.

NOTES:

aluminum hydroxide • (a-loom-in-um hye-drox-ide)

CATEGORY: *Antacid* OTC

BRAND NAMES	DOSAGE FORMS
Amphojel (W-A)	PO suspension: 320mg/5ml Tablet: 300, 600mg
ALternaGEL (J&J-Merck)	Liquid: 600mg/5ml
AluCap (Riker)	Capsule: 475mg
Alu-Tab (Riker)	Tablet: 600mg
Dialume (Armour)	Capsule: 500mg

ACTION: Chemical neutralization of gastric acidity. **USE:** Treatment of hyperacidity associated c̄ gastritis, gastric hyperacidity, peptic esophagitis, peptic ulcer, hiatal hernia ▪ Treatment of hyperphosphatemia.

PHARMACOKINETICS: Not applicable.

DOSAGE

Pediatric/Adult *PO*	300-1800mg 3-6 times/d; pediatric dose for hyperphosphatemia 50-150mg/kg/d divided

SIDE/ADVERSE EFFECTS: CNS: possible aluminum accumulation leading to intoxication ▪ GI: *constipation* ▪ MET: body phosphorus depletion.

DRUG INTERACTIONS: Avoid taking c̄ antibiotics (esp tetracyclines).

NURSING MANAGEMENT

ADMINISTRATION: Assess for CHF, hypertension, fluid retention; avoid Na^+- containing preparations if present ▪ Shake PO suspensions well before pouring; follow c̄ H_2O to ensure reaching stomach ▪ Avoid concurrent administration c̄ any drug.

EVALUATION: Monitor GI status ▪ Assess dietary patterns ▪ Observe for abdominal pain, GI discomfort, neurotoxicity/encephalopathy; notify physician ▪ Normal serum phosphorus: 4-7mg/L.

EDUCATION: ANTACID: take 1-3h pc, also hs/prn; followed c̄ H_2O ▪ Check c̄ physician if GI discomfort recurs or if taking >2 wks ▪ Check c̄ physician before taking c̄ Na^+-restricted diet ▪ Do *not* give to children <6y/o ▪ Do *not* take w/in 2h of other drugs ▪ Chew tablets well before swallowing ▪ Shake PO suspension well before taking ▪ Notify physician of constipation ▪ Store in tightly closed container ▪ Avoid spicy/irritating foods.

Note: Side/adverse effects: common in *italic;* serious in ***boldface italic.*** *Available in Canada only.

NOTES:

amantadine hcl • (a-man-ta-deen)

CATEGORY: *Anti-Parkinson agent, antiviral* Rx; Preg Cat C

BRAND NAME
Symmetrel (Du Pont)

DOSAGE FORMS
Capsule: 100mg
Syrup: 50mg/5ml

ACTION: Anti-Parkinson activity may be due to increase in dopamine release in brain; antiviral activity appears related to prevention of release of viral nuclei into host cell. **USE:** Treatment of Parkinson disease, drug-induced extrapyramidal rxs, CO-induced Parkinson disease ▪ Prevention, treatment of influenza A virus respiratory tract infections.

PHARMACOKINETICS

PO absorption	Peak	Half-life	Excretion
Good	4h	15h	Via urine as unchanged drug

CONTRAINDICATIONS: Hypersensitivity.

DOSAGE

Pediatric *PO*	Influenza: 1-9y/o 2-4mg/kg/d. Do *not* exceed 150mg/d 9-12y/o 100mg bid
Adult *PO*	Parkinson disease: usual range 100-200mg divided. 400mg/d may be necessary Influenza: 100-300mg/d divided

SIDE/ADVERSE EFFECTS: CNS: *depression,* dizziness, headache ▪ CV: ***CHF,*** *orthostatic hypotensive episodes,* peripheral edema ▪ GI: anorexia, nausea, constipation, vomiting, dry mouth ▪ GU: *urinary retention* ▪ HEM: leukopenia, neutropenia ▪ INT: skin rash, eczematoid dermatitis ▪ PSYCH: *psychosis,* confusion, anxiety.

DRUG INTERACTIONS: Use c̄ anticholinergics will produce additive anticholinergic effects ▪ Use c̄ CNS stimulants is best avoided because of CNS additive effects.

NURSING MANAGEMENT
ADMINISTRATION: Assess for hx of hypersensitivity ▪ Assess for CHF, fluid retention, renal impairment;

requires ↓ dosage ▪ Administer pc; do *not* administer hs (insomnia) ▪ Avoid abrupt withdrawal (may induce parkinsonian crisis); D/C drug gradually.

EVALUATION: Monitor CV, GI, GU, hepatic, neurologic, renal status ▪ Monitor VS ▪ Monitor I&O ▪ Assess for muscle weakness ▪ Observe for exaggerated anticholinergic effects (dry mouth, urinary retention) ▪ Observe for CNS stimulation/psychiatric manifestations; notify physician.

EDUCATION: Dizziness may occur; avoid engaging in potentially hazardous activities ▪ Avoid changing positions (lying/sitting/standing) rapidly ▪ Take as directed by physician ▪ Take pc ▪ Do *not* D/C w/out notifying physician ▪ May cause blurred vision ▪ Redness/mottling of skin may occur; will disappear after several wks of therapy ▪ Use sugarless gum/hard candy to diminish dry mouth ▪ Use calibrated measuring device for PO liquid forms ▪ Avoid alcohol intake ▪ Women: avoid breastfeeding ▪ Store in tightly closed container ▪ Safety precautions c̄ ↑ activity ▪ Notify physician if Parkinson symptoms reappear (trembling, shuffling gait, rigidity) ▪ Full drug effects may require several days of therapy.

NOTES:

amikacin sulfate • (am-i-kay-sin)

CATEGORY: *Aminoglycoside*: antibiotic

Rx; Preg Cat D

BRAND NAME	**DOSAGE FORMS**
Amikin (Apothecon)	Injection (IM/IV): 50, 250mg/ml

ACTION: Bactericidal activity due to inhibition of ribosomal protein synthesis in susceptible organisms. **USE:** Treatment of infections caused by susceptible strains of *Enterobacter aerogenes, Escherichia coli, Klebsiella pneumoniae, Mima-Herellea (Acinetobacter), Proteus* spp, *Providencia* spp, *Pseudomonas* spp, *Serratia* spp ▪ Alternate for resistant *Staphylococcus* infections, gentamicin/tobramycin-resistant gram(-) infections ▪ In combination c̄ penicillin for neonatal sepsis.

PHARMACOKINETICS

IM peak	Half-life	Protein binding	Excretion
1h	2h	0%-11%	92% excreted unchanged in urine in 8h

CONTRAINDICATIONS: Hypersensitivity, previous hx of serious aminoglycoside toxicity.

DOSAGE: *IM/IV* for pts c̄ normal renal function, usually 7-10d

Neonatal	Loading dose 10mg/kg, then 7.5 mg/kg q12h
Pediatric/Adult	15mg/kg/d in 2-3 equal doses. Do *not* exceed 1.5g/d

SIDE/ADVERSE EFFECTS: CNS: headache, paresthesia ▪ EENT: ***ototoxicity*** (both auditory and vestibular damage: dizziness, vertigo, tinnitus, roaring in ears, hearing loss) ▪ GU: ***nephrotoxicity*** (casts, proteinuria, ↑ in BUN, NPN, serum creatinine) ▪ INT: rash ▪ Other: fever.

DRUG INTERACTIONS: Avoid use c̄ neurotoxic or nephrotoxic drugs such as other aminoglycosides, colistin, ethacrynic acid, furosemide, polymyxin B, vancomycin, viomycin ▪ Dimenhydrinate can mask aminoglycoside ototoxicity ▪ ↑ Activity of succinylcholine or tubocurarine; Ca^{++} salts can reverse blockage ▪ PO anticoagulant activity may ↑ due to ↓ intestinal vitamin K synthesis.

Note: Side/adverse effects: common in *italic;* serious in ***boldface italic.***

*Available in Canada only.

NURSING MANAGEMENT

ADMINISTRATION: Assess for hx of aminoglycoside hypersensitivity ▪ Obtain C&S before therapy ▪ Obtain pt weight for dosage calculation ▪ Determine creatinine clearance before administration ▪ IV: 500mg vial add to 200ml sterile diluent; infuse over 30-60m ▪ Do *not* mix $\bar{c}$ other drugs ▪ Do *not* administer w/in 1h of other parenteral antibiotics ▪ Original solution is stable at room temperature for 2 yrs; pale yellow color does *not* indicate ↓ potency; store in original container ▪ Diluted solution is stable for 24h ▪ IM: administer by *deep, slow* injection; rotate sites; avoid inflamed areas ▪ Maintain hydration ▪ Elderly may require ↓ dosage.

EVALUATION: Assess for hearing dysfunction ▪ Monitor hepatic, renal, VIII CN function ▪ Monitor VS, esp temperature ▪ Assess for edema in extremities ▪ Assess for neuromuscular blockade, respiratory paralysis, nephrotoxicity ▪ Observe for signs of superinfection (diarrhea, URI, coated tongue) ▪ Assess for hypersensitivity (fever, difficult breathing, rash) ▪ Assess peak (<25 μg/ml), trough (< 10 μg/ml) serum concentrations.

EDUCATION: Report hearing, balance difficulties to nurse/physician at once ▪ ↑ Fluid intake (10-12 glasses/d).

NOTES:

amiloride hcl • (a-mill-oh-ride)

CATEGORY: *Potassium-sparing diuretic* Rx; Preg Cat B

BRAND NAME
Midamor (MSD)

DOSAGE FORM
Tablet: 5mg

COMBINATION PRODUCT
Moduretic (MSD) Amiloride 5mg/hydrochlorothiazide 50mg/tablet

ACTION: Antikaliuretic mechanism not established; weak antihypertensive, diuretic, natriuretic activity. **USE**: Adjunct (antikaliuretic) c̄ thiazides/other kaliuretic diuretics in treatment of CHF, hypertension.

PHARMACOKINETICS

PO absorption	Onset	Peak	Half-life	Excretion
50%	2h	6-10h	6-9h	Unchanged via urine (50%), feces (40%) in 72h

CONTRAINDICATIONS: Hypersensitivity, hyperkalemia, impaired renal function, potassium supplements.

DOSAGE
Adult *PO* 5-10mg/d to prevent hypokalemia, c̄ 10-20mg/d for persistent cases. Moduretic dose usually 1-2 tablets/d

SIDE/ADVERSE EFFECTS: CNS: *headache*, dizziness ▪ GI: *N/V, anorexia*, abdominal pain ▪ GU: impotence, polyuria, dysuria, urinary frequency.

DRUG INTERACTIONS: Use c̄ lithium is best avoided because of ↓ renal clearance ▪ Use c̄ antikaliuretic agents/potassium supplements produces significant hyperkalemia.

NURSING MANAGEMENT
ADMINISTRATION: Assess renal function; do *not* administer if impaired ▪ Assess serum K^+ (normal: 3.5-5mEq/L); notify physician of ↑ level ▪ Administer c̄ meals/milk on arising ▪ Maintain hydration ▪ Elderly may require ↓ dosage.

Note: Side/adverse effects: common in *italic;* serious in ***boldface italic.*** *Available in Canada only.

EVALUATION: Monitor F/E, hepatic, renal status ▪ Monitor BP ▪ Monitor serum K^+; do *not* administer if hyperkalemic ▪ Monitor fluid retention (I&O, daily weight).

EDUCATION: Expect ↑ urine output; have bathroom facilities easily accessible ▪ May cause weakness, lethargy ▪ Take as directed by physician even if symptom free; do *not* skip doses ▪ Take on waking, at same time each day. ▪ Used to control, *not* cure, hypertension ▪ Notify physician of signs of hyperkalemia (difficult breathing, tingling extremities, nervousness, irregular heartbeat) ▪ Avoid changing positions (lying/sitting/standing) rapidly ▪ Avoid foods high in K^+ (bananas, citrus juices, raisins) ▪ Avoid high-Na^+ foods (canned soups, lunch meats, cheese) ▪ Notify physician of N/V/D ▪ Maintain optimum weight ▪ Store in tightly closed container ▪ Check $\bar{c}$ physician before taking OTC/Rx preparations ▪ Notify physician/dentist of use before treatment.

NOTES:

aminophylline • (am-in-off-i-lin)

CATEGORY: *Bronchodilator*: antiasthmatic, xanthine drug — Rx; Preg Cat C

BRAND NAMES

Aminophylline (various)
**Corophyllin (Beecham)*
**Palaron (Fisons)*
Phyllcontrin (P-F)

DOSAGE FORMS

Injection (IV), PO liquid, rectal solution, suppositories, tablets

ACTION: Bronchodilation due to direct relaxation of respiratory smooth muscle; in addition, drug stimulates CNS, produces diuresis, has positive chronotropic/inotropic cardiac effect. **USE:** Treatment of asthma, reversible bronchospasm associated c̄ COPD.

PHARMACOKINETICS

PO absorption	Peak	Protein binding	Excretion
Usually complete	1-2h	60%	90% as metabolites via urine

CONTRAINDICATIONS: Hypersensitivity to any xanthine bronchodilator.

DOSAGE

Pediatric *PO*	12mg/kg/24h in 4 divided doses
Parenteral	For continuous infusion, loading dose 6mg/kg, then 1.2mg/kg/h for 12h, 0.8mg/kg/h beyond 12h for 6mo-9y/o. 1mg/kg/h for 12h, 0.8mg/kg/h for children 9-16y/o & young adult smokers
Rectal	12mg/kg in 3-4 divided doses for suppositories/retention enema
Adult *PO*	600-1600mg in 3-4 divided doses
Parenteral	For continuous infusion, loading dose 0.6mg/kg, then 0.7 mg/kg/h for 12h, 0.5mg/kg/h beyond 12h for nonsmokers. 0.6mg/kg/h for 12h, 0.3mg/kg/h for older pts
Rectal	250-500mg 1-3 times/d. Retention enema 500mg 3-4 times/d

SIDE/ADVERSE EFFECTS: CNS: headache, reflex hyperexcitability, clonic/tonic generalized convulsions, insomnia, nervousness ▪ CV: hypotension, tachycardia, ***ventricular arrhythmias,*** palpitations ▪ GI: N/V/D, epigastric pain ▪ GU: albuminuria, diuresis ▪ RESP: tachypnea.

Note: Side/adverse effects: common in *italic;* serious in ***boldface italic.***

*Available in Canada only.

DRUG INTERACTIONS: ↑ Serum levels c̄ cimetidine, allopurinol, erythromycin, PO contraceptives, flu vaccine ▪ ↑ Excretion of lithium, ↓ in propranolol effects ▪ Use c̄ adrenergic drugs will ↑ CNS stimulation.

NURSING MANAGEMENT

ADMINISTRATION: Assess for hx of xanthine-derivative administration/hypersensitivity ▪ PO: administer c̄ full glass of H_2O/food ▪ Rectal: administer after evacuation ▪ IV: dilute to 25mg/ml; administer *slowly* (25mg/m); do *not* mix in syringe c̄ other medications; use infusion control device; check compatibility c̄ other drugs ▪ Do *not* administer discolored/precipitated solutions ▪ Have emergency support equipment (IV) available ▪ Maintain hydration (2000ml/d) ▪ Heavy smokers may require ↑ dosage ▪ Dosage adjustment must be made when switching from IV to PO.

EVALUATION: Monitor CV, F/E, hepatic, renal status ▪ Monitor VS, ECG (IV), I&O ▪ Monitor respiratory status, auscultate lungs, ABG ▪ Observe for signs of toxicity (nausea, CNS stimulation, headache, diarrhea, arrhythmias); stop administration if present, notify physician ▪ Monitor therapeutic blood levels: 10-20 μg/ml (adult).

EDUCATION: Take as prescribed by physician at evenly spaced intervals ▪ Dizziness may occur; avoid hazardous activities ▪ Check c̄ physician before taking any OTC preparation ▪ Avoid caffeine, charcoal-broiled foods ▪ ↑ Fluid intake (8-10 glasses/d) ▪ Avoid changing brand-name preparations ▪ Notify physician if experiencing rapid heartbeat, diarrhea, CNS stimulation ▪ Keep scheduled appointments c̄ physician/blood work ▪ Retain suppository/rectal solution 30m.

OVERDOSE MANAGEMENT: Symptoms incl anorexia, nausea, restlessness, hyperthermia, convulsions, cardiac arrhythmias ▪ Emergency treatment incl: maintaining respiration c̄ oxygen; 5% dextrose for dehydration; controlling convulsions c̄ IV diazepam for short-acting barbiturates.

NOTES:

amitriptyline hcl • (a-mee-<u>trip</u>-ti-leen)

CATEGORY: *Tricyclic antidepressant:* mood elevator   Rx; Preg Cat C

BRAND NAMES	**DOSAGE FORMS**
Elavil (Stuart)	IM injection: 10mg/ml Tablet: 10, 25, 50, 75, 100, 150mg
Endep (Roche)	Tablet: 10, 25, 50, 75, 100, 150mg
**Levate (ICN)*	
**Meraril (Medic)*	
**Novatriptyn (Novopharm)*	

COMBINATION PRODUCTS
Etrafon products (Schering)
Triavil products (MSD)
(see *Perphenazine/amitriptyline*)

ACTION: Antidepressant activity appears related to inhibition of norepinephrine reuptake in central adrenergic neurons. **USE:** Treatment of endogenous depression.

PHARMACOKINETICS

PO absorption	Peak	Half-life	Excretion
Complete	4-12h	10-50h	Up to 50% via urine as metabolites in 24h

CONTRAINDICATIONS: Hypersensitivity, MAO-I therapy, myocardial infarction (acute recovery period).

DOSAGE

Adolescent/Geriatric *PO*	10mg tid, 20mg hs
Adult *PO*	75-150mg/d divided
IM	20-30mg qid

SIDE/ADVERSE EFFECTS: CNS: *drowsiness,* dizziness, headache, extrapyramidal symptoms, paresthesia (extremities), insomnia ▪ CV: ***arrhythmias,*** hypertension, orthostatic hypotension ▪ EENT: blurred vision, tinnitus ▪ GI: anorexia, N/V, dry mouth, constipation ▪ GU: urinary hesitancy ▪ INT: skin rash, photosensitivity, alopecia, jaundice ▪ PSYCH: disorientation, hallucinations ▪ Other: parotid swelling.

DRUG INTERACTIONS: Significant depressant effects c̄ alcohol ▪ Anticholinergics, chlorpromazine produce ↑ atropine-like effects; paralytic ileus could occur ▪ Significant ↑ in activity c̄ epinephrine, levarterenol, other adrenergic agents ▪ Significant antagonism to effects of reserpine, guanethidine-type antihypertensives ▪ Use c̄ MAO-I best avoided.

Note: Side/adverse effects: common in *italic;* serious in ***boldface italic.***   *Available in Canada only.

NURSING MANAGEMENT

ADMINISTRATION: Assess for hx of tricyclic antidepressant hypersensitivity, hepatic dysfunction, glaucoma ▪ PO: administer as single dose/d hs c̄ food ▪ Institute suicide/safety precautions ▪ Parenteral: do *not* administer IV ▪ ↑ Dosage *slowly* ▪ Avoid abrupt withdrawal; D/C gradually ▪ Heavy smokers may require ↑ dosage.

EVALUATION: Monitor CV, hepatic, renal status ▪ Monitor VS (esp BP), CBC, hepatic function tests, fluid retention, constipation ▪ Assess for symptoms of abrupt withdrawal (nausea, headache, malaise).

EDUCATION: Dizziness/drowsiness may occur; use caution in potentially hazardous activities ▪ Avoid changing positions rapidly ▪ Avoid alcohol, other CNS depressants for up to 1 wk after ending therapy ▪ Take PO forms c̄ food to ↓ GI irritation ▪ Take as directed by physician ▪ Use sugarless gum/hard candy to diminish dry mouth ▪ ↑ Fluids, bulk-containing foods ▪ Check c̄ physician before taking OTC/Rx preparations ▪ May produce peculiar taste ▪ Notify physician/dentist of use before treatment ▪ Store in tightly closed container ▪ Avoid exposure to direct sunlight/UV light (sun lamps); use sunscreen, protective clothing ▪ Notify physician of fever, sore throat, malaise ▪ May turn urine blue-green ▪ Keep scheduled appointments c̄ physician ▪ Full drug effects may require several wks of therapy.

NOTES:

amoxapine • (a-mox-a-peen)

CATEGORY: *Tricyclic antidepressant*: mood elevator — Rx; Preg Cat C

BRAND NAME
Asendin (Lederle)

DOSAGE FORMS
Tablet: 25, 50, 100, 150mg

ACTION: Antidepressant activity appears related to inhibition of norepinephrine reuptake in central adrenergic neurons. **USE:** Treatment of endogenous, reactive, psychotic depression ▪ Treatment of depression accompanied by anxiety/agitation.

PHARMACOKINETICS

PO absorption	Peak	Half-life	Protein binding	Excretion
Complete	90m	8h	90%	80% via urine, 20% via feces as metabolites

CONTRAINDICATIONS: Hypersensitivity, MAO-I therapy, myocardial infarction (acute recovery period).

DOSAGE

Adult *PO*	≥50-100μg tid. Usual maintenance range 150-300mg/d
Geriatric *PO*	≥25-50mg tid. Usual maintenance range 150-300mg/d

SIDE/ADVERSE EFFECTS: CNS: *drowsiness*, dizziness, headache, incoordination, tremors, extrapyramidal symptoms, paresthesia (extremities), insomnia ▪ CV: ***arrhythmias***, myocardial infarction, stroke, ***heart block***, hypotension, orthostatic hypotension ▪ EENT: tinnitus ▪ END: testicular swelling, galactorrhea, breast enlargement ▪ GI: *dry mouth*, anorexia, N/V/D, cramps, constipation ▪ GU: urinary hesitancy ▪ HEM: ***agranulocytosis***, eosinophilia, ***thrombocytopenia*** ▪ HEP: cholestatic jaundice ▪ INT: skin rash, photosensitivity, alopecia ▪ PSYCH: disorientation, hallucinations, exacerbation of psychosis ▪ Other: parotid swelling.

DRUG INTERACTIONS: Significant depressant effects $\bar{c}$ alcohol ▪ Anticholinergics, chlorpromazine produce ↑ atropine-like effects; paralytic ileus could occur ▪

Significant ↑ in activity c̄ epinephrine, levarterenol, other adrenergic agents ▪ Significant antagonism to effects of reserpine, clonidine, guanethidine-type antihypertensives ▪ Use c̄ MAO-I best avoided.

NURSING MANAGEMENT

ADMINISTRATION: Assess for hx of tricyclic antidepressant hypersensitivity ▪ Assess for impaired hepatic, renal function; hx of glaucoma, prostatic hypertrophy; may require ↓ dosage ▪ Administer c̄ food ▪ Institute suicide/safety precautions ▪ ↑ Dosage slowly, maintenance dose lowest dose that will maintain remission of depression ▪ Avoid abrupt withdrawal; D/C gradually ▪ Heavy smokers may require ↑ dosage ▪ Elderly may require ↓ dosage.

EVALUATION: Monitor CV, hepatic, renal status ▪ Monitor VS, esp BP ▪ Monitor CBC, esp long-term ▪ Monitor fluid retention (I&O, daily weight), constipation ▪ Assess for symptoms of abrupt withdrawal (nausea, headache, malaise) ▪ Assess for actual swallowing of PO forms.

EDUCATION: Dizziness/drowsiness may occur; use caution in potentially hazardous activities ▪ Avoid changing positions (lying/sitting/standing) rapidly ▪ Avoid alcohol, other CNS depressants for up to 1 wk after therapy has ended ▪ Take c̄ food to ↓ GI irritation ▪ Take as directed by physician ▪ Use sugarless gum/hard candy to diminish dry mouth ▪ Constipation may occur; ↑ fluids, bulk-containing foods ▪ Check c̄ physician before taking OTC/Rx preparations ▪ May produce peculiar taste ▪ Notify physician/dentist of use before treatment ▪ Store in tightly closed container ▪ Avoid exposure to direct sunlight, UV light (sun lamps); use sunscreen, protective clothing ▪ Encourage recreational/diversional interests ▪ Notify physician of fever, sore throat, malaise ▪ Keep scheduled appointments c̄ physician ▪ Full drug effects may require several wks of therapy.

NOTES:

amoxicillin trihydrate • (a-mox-i-sill-in)

CATEGORY: *Aminopenicillin*: antibiotic

Rx; Preg Cat B

BRAND NAMES

Amoxil (SKB)
(Ayerst in Canada)
**Apo-Amoxi (Apotex)*
**Novamoxin (Novopharm)*
Polymox (Apothecon)
Trimox (Apothecon)
Wymox (W-A)

DOSAGE FORMS

Capsule, chewable tablet, powder for pediatric drops/PO suspension

COMBINATION PRODUCTS Rx

Augmentin (SKB)
**Clavulin (Beecham)*

Amoxicillin/clavulanate per tablet: 250mg/125mg, 500mg/125mg; per chewable tablet: 125mg/31.5mg, 250mg/62.5mg; per 5ml: 125mg/31.25mg, 250mg/62.5mg

ACTION: Bactericidal activity due to inhibition of mucopeptide cell wall synthesis in susceptible organisms; clavulanic acid, chemical similar to penicillins, added to amoxicillin (Augmentin) to block activity of penicillinase (β-lactamase) against amoxicillin, thus amoxicillin (Augmentin) can be used to treat infections caused by penicillinase-producing organisms. Dosage for Augmentin based on amoxicillin content; essentially same as for amoxicillin **USE:** Treatment of auditory, GU, respiratory, GI tract infections caused by susceptible strains of *Escherichia coli, Haemophilus influenzae, Neisseria gonorrhoeae, Proteus mirabilis* ▪ Treatment of *Streptococcus faecalis, Streptococcus pneumoniae* infections ▪ Augmentin indicated for treatment of β-lactamase (penicillinase)-producing *E. coli, Enterobacter* spp, *H. influenzae, S. aureus* infections.

PHARMACOKINETICS

PO absorption	Peak	Half-life	Protein binding	Excretion
74%-92%	1-2h	40-84m	20%	In urine in 6-8h

*Available in Canada only.

CONTRAINDICATIONS: Penicillin hypersensitivity.

DOSAGE

Pediatric *PO*	<20kg: 20-40mg/kg/d divided, q8h
Adult *PO*	250-500mg q8h. 3.5g c̄ 1g probenecid as single dose for gonorrhea

SIDE/ADVERSE EFFECTS: CV: edema ▪ GI: N/V/D, glossitis, stomatitis ▪ HEM: anemia, ***thrombocytopenia***, thrombocytopenic purpura, eosinophilia, leukopenia, ***agranulocytosis*** ▪ HEP: ↑ in serum AST ▪ INT: maculopapular rash, ***erythema multiforme, exfoliative dermatitis***, urticaria ▪ MS: arthralgia ▪ Other: fever, laryngeal edema, ***anaphylaxis***.

DRUG INTERACTIONS: Antacids, antidiarrheal suspensions, ion-exchange resins ↓ PO absorption ▪ Concurrent use of bacteriostatic antibiotics c̄ any penicillin can produce antibiotic antagonism ▪ Antibiotics that ↓ intestinal flora may ↑ activity of PO anticoagulants.

NURSING MANAGEMENT

ADMINISTRATION: Assess for hx of penicillin/cephalosporin hypersensitivity ▪ Obtain C&S before therapy ▪ Reconstitute powder for drops/PO suspension according to manufacturer's directions; use w/in 14d (room temperature or refrigerated) ▪ Shake drops/PO suspension well before using ▪ Avoid exposure to moisture in storage ▪ Have support equipment available for anaphylaxis.

EVALUATION: Monitor pts c̄ allergies/asthma (high risk for hypersensitivity) ▪ Monitor renal, hepatic, hemopoietic status ▪ Observe for signs of superinfection (diarrhea, itching, coated tongue) ▪ Monitor VS, esp temperature.

EDUCATION: Complete full course of therapy (usually 10d) even if symptoms subside ▪ Can be taken c̄ meals; *best* on empty stomach ▪ Take at equal intervals around clock to maintain blood levels ▪ Diarrhea may occur ▪ Store in dry, tightly closed container ▪ Discard outdated preparations ▪ Maintain good personal hygiene (esp perineal, oral) ▪ ↑ Fluid intake (8-10 glasses/d) ▪ Women: avoid breastfeeding ▪ Notify physician of symptoms of allergic rx (fever, difficult breathing, rash) ▪ Carry identification (MedicAlert) if penicillin allergic.

NOTES:

amphotericin B • (am-foe-ter-i-sin)

CATEGORY: *Antibiotic:* antifungal, antimonilial — Rx; Preg Cat B

BRAND NAME	DOSAGE FORMS	DOSAGE	
Fungizone (Squibb)	Cream: 3% Lotion: 3% Powder for injection (IV): 50mg/vial Ointment: 3%	Pediatric/Adult *IV*	Initial daily dose 0.25mg/kg; total daily dosage may range from 1-1.5mg/kg; do *not* exceed total daily dose 1.5mg/kg
		Topical	Apply several times/d

ACTION: Antifungal activity in susceptible fungi due to binding c̄ cell membrane sterols, resulting in leakage of vital intracellular fungal components. **USE:** Treatment of aspergillosis, coccidioidomycosis, cryptococcosis, disseminated moniliasis, histoplasmosis, mucormycosis, North American blastomycosis, sporotrichosis ▪ Topical treatment of candidiasis (moniliasis).

PHARMACOKINETICS: Administered IV because of poor PO absorption; exhibits high protein binding (90%-95%), long half-life; excreted via kidneys over period of days.

CONTRAINDICATIONS: Hypersensitivity.

SIDE/ADVERSE EFFECTS: CNS: *headache*, vertigo, peripheral neuropathy, ***convulsions*** ▪ CV: local venous pain at injection site c̄ phlebitis, ***thrombophlebitis, arrhythmias, cardiac arrest*** ▪ EENT: diplopia, hearing loss ▪ GI: *N/V/D*, dyspepsia, epigastric pain ▪ GU: azotemia, hyposthenuria, tubular acidosis ▪ HEM: ***coagulation defects, thrombocytopenia***, leukopenia, ***agranulocytosis*** ▪ HEP: ***acute liver failure*** (rare) ▪ MET: hypokalemia.

DRUG INTERACTIONS: Use c̄ decamethonium, gallamine, succinylcholine, tubocurarine, dig will ↑ their toxicity ▪ Use c̄ corticosteroids produces hypokalemia, severe superinfections ▪ Use c̄ nephrotoxic drugs produces additive toxicity.

Note: Side/adverse effects: common in *italic;* serious in ***boldface italic.***

*Available in Canada only.

NURSING MANAGEMENT

ADMINISTRATION: Assess for hx of hypersensitivity ▪ Obtain C&S before therapy ▪ Assess renal function; may require ↓ dosage if impaired ▪ IV: reconstitute c̄ 10ml sterile H_2O for injection (5mg/ml), shake until clear; further dilute c̄ 5% dextrose (pH>4.2); use strict aseptic technique; infuse *slowly* (6h), protect from light, stable in dark for 24h at room temperature, 1wk refrigerated; may use in-line membrane filter of mean pore diameter >1 µm; for hospital use only, observe pt closely ▪ Topical: rub liberal amounts on affected area; avoid occlusive dressings ▪ Do *not* administer discolored/precipitated solutions ▪ Store powder for injection in refrigerator; protect from light ▪ Avoid mixing c̄ saline solutions, antibiotics, or bacteriostatic agents.

EVALUATION: Monitor hepatic, renal status ▪ Monitor VS, esp temperature ▪ Observe injection site for signs of inflammation; rotate sites ▪ Monitor I&O ▪ D/C if BUN >40mg/100ml, serum creatinine >3mg/100ml ▪ Assess for signs of hypokalemia (anorexia, lethargy, muscle weakness, mental confusion); notify physician.

EDUCATION: Report any discomfort at infusion site *immediately* ▪ Procedure for topical application; avoid occlusive dressing ▪ Cream may discolor skin; lotion, ointment may discolor nails ▪ Discoloration of fabrics can be removed by washing c̄ soap & H_2O (cream, lotion) or standard cleaning fluid (ointment).

NOTES:

ampicillin sodium ▲ /ampicillin trihydrate • (am-pi-sill-in)

CATEGORY: *Aminopenicillin*: antibiotic — Rx; Preg Cat B

BRAND NAMES

Omnipen-N (W-A)
Polycillin-N ▲ (Squibb)
Totacillin-N ▲ (SKB)
**Ampilean (Organon)*
**Apo-Ampi (Apotex)*
Omnipen (W-A)
Polycillin (Apothecon)
Principen (Apothecon)
Totacilin (SKB)

DOSAGE FORMS

Capsule, powder for injection (IM/IV) powder for PO suspension

COMBINATION PRODUCTS — Rx

Unasyn (Roerig) — amipicillin Na/sulbactam Na per vial: 1g/0.5g, 2g/1g

ACTION: Bactericidal activity due to inhibition of mucopeptide cell wall synthesis in susceptible organisms. **USE:** Treatment of auditory, GU, respiratory, GI tract infections caused by susceptible strains of *Escherichia coli, Haemophilus influenzae, Neisseria gonorrhoeae, Neisseria meningitidis, Proteus mirabilis, Salmonella* spp, *Shigella* spp ▪ Treatment of subacute bacterial endocarditis, enterococci infections ▪ Drug of choice for treating typhoid fever (*Salmonella typhosa*) resistant to chloramphenicol.

PHARMACOKINETICS

PO absorption	Peak	Half-life	Protein binding	Excretion
30%-55%	1-2h	40-84m	20%-25%	Via urine

CONTRAINDICATIONS: Penicillin hypersensitivity.

DOSAGE

Pediatric	*PO*	<20kg: 50-100mg/kg/d divided q6-8h >20kg: 250-500mg qid
	IM/IV	25-50mg/kg divided qid Meningitis: 100-200mg/kg/d in equal doses
Adult	*PO*	250-500mg qid Gonorrhea: single dose, 3.5g c̄ 1g probenecid
	IM/IV	250-500mg q6h Meningitis: 8-14g in equal doses

SIDE/ADVERSE EFFECTS: CV: edema ▪ GI: N/V/D, glossitis, stomatitis ▪ HEM: anemia, ***thrombocytopenia,*** thrombocytopenic purpura, eosinophilia, leukopenia, ***agranulocytosis*** ▪ HEP: ↑ serum AST ▪ INT: maculopapular rash, ***erythema multiforme, exfoliative dermatitis,*** urticaria ▪ MS: arthralgia ▪ Other: fever, laryngeal edema, ***anaphylaxis.***

DRUG INTERACTIONS: Antacids, antidiarrheals, ion-exchange resins ↓ PO absorption ▪ Concurrent use of bacteriostatic antibiotics c̄ any penicillin can produce antibiotic antagonism ▪ Antibiotics that ↓ intestinal flora may ↑ activity of PO anticoagulants.

NURSING MANAGEMENT

ADMINISTRATION: Assess for hx of penicillin/cephalosporin hypersensitivity ▪ Obtain C&S before therapy ▪ Reconstitute powder for drops/PO suspension/injection according to manufacturer's directions ▪ Shake drops/PO suspension well before using; use w/in 7d at room temperature, 14d refrigerated ▪ Handle solution carefully to avoid contact dermatitis ▪ Avoid exposure to moisture in storage ▪ Administer 1h ac/2h pc ▪ Have support equipment available for anaphylaxis.

EVALUATION: Monitor pts c̄ allergies/asthma ▪ Monitor VS, esp temperature; renal, hepatic, hematologic status ▪ Observe for signs of superinfection (diarrhea, itching, coated tongue) ▪ Monitor pts receiving anticoagulant therapy; may potentiate bleeding ▪ Differentiate characteristic drug rash, hypersensitivity rx.

EDUCATION: Complete full course of therapy (usually 10d) even if symptoms subside ▪ Take on empty stomach at equal intervals ▪ Diarrhea may occur ▪ Store in dry, tightly closed container ▪ Maintain good personal hygiene (esp perineal, oral) and fluid intake (6-8 glasses/d) ▪ Use Clinistix/Tes-Tape for urine testing ▪ Women: avoid breastfeeding ▪ Notify physician of symptoms of allergic rx (fever, difficult breathing, rash) ▪ Carry identification (MedicAlert) if penicillin allergic.

NOTES:

amrinone lactate • (am-ri-none)

CATEGORY: *Cardiac inotropic agent* Rx; preg Cat C

BRAND NAME
Inocor (Winthrop)

DOSAGE FORM
Injection (IV): 5mg/ml

ACTION: Produces + inotropic effect that ↑ force/velocity of myocardial systolic contractions by inhibiting myocardial cyclic adenosine monophosphate phosphodiesterase activity, which ↑ cardiac cellular level of cAMP; does not inhibit Na-K-activated adenosine triphosphatase activity (produced by dig); produces direct relaxant effect on vascular smooth muscle. **USE:** Short-term treatment of CHF in closely monitored pts who have not responded to dig, diuretics, or vasodilators.

PHARMACOKINETICS

Onset	Peak	Duration	Half-life	Protein binding	Excretion
2-5m	10m	0.5-2h	3.6h	10%-50%	Excreted in urine, c̄ 18% in feces

CONTRAINDICATIONS: Hypersensitivity to drug or bisulfites used as stabilizers.

DOSAGE

Adult *IV* 0.75mg/kg slowly over 2-3m, then usual maintenance dose 5-10μg/kg/m

SIDE/ADVERSE EFFECTS: CV: ***arrhythmia, hypotension***, thrombocytopenia ▪ GI: N/V, abdominal pain, anorexia, ▪ HEP: cell necrosis, ↑ enzyme levels ▪ Other: chest pain, fever.

DRUG INTERACTIONS: Use c̄ disopyramide produced excessive hypotension in one pt ▪ Appears to be compatible c̄ most CV drugs, anticoagulants, insulin, diazepam.

NURSING MANAGEMENT

ADMINISTRATION: Assess for hx of hypersensitivity (incl bisulfites) ▪ Administer via infusion control device for continuous IV infusion ▪ Concurrent K^+ supplements may be ordered in hypokalemia ▪ Avoid exposure to light during storage ▪ Dilute c̄ normal saline solution; use w/in 24h ▪ Avoid mixing c̄ dextrose solutions ▪ Do *not* mix c̄ IV furosemide (precipitation occurs).

EVALUATION: Monitor serum electrolytes (hypokalemia, hypercalcemia enhance toxicity), hemodynamic parameters ▪ Assess renal status; monitor I&O, daily weight ▪ Monitor VS, esp BP, heart rate ▪ Assess platelet count qd ▪ Check cardiac monitor for arrhythmia.

EDUCATION: Notify nurse/physician of rx (abnormal heartbeat, GI distress, bleeding).

NOTES:

aspirin (acetylsalicylic acid) • (as-pir-in)

CATEGORY: *Salicylate*: analgesic, antiinflammatory, antipyretic, antiplatelet, NSAIA OTC

BRAND NAMES

**Apo-Asen (Apotex)*
ASA (Lilly)
Ascriptin (Rorer)
Bufferin (Bristol-Myers)
Ecotrin (SKB)
Empirin (B-W)
Measurin (Winthrop)
**Novasen (Novopharm)*

DOSAGE FORMS

Capsule, enteric tablets, suppository, tablet

ACTION: Produces analgesia by ↑ pain threshold, ↓ synthesis of prostaglandins; antipyresis due to effects on hypothalamic heat-regulating center; antiinflammatory effect due to ↓ in prostaglandin synthesis, release; ↓ prothrombin synthesis, platelet adhesiveness. **USE:** Analgesic for mild/moderate pain as sole agent in combination c̄ other analgesics/narcotics ▪ Antipyretic ▪ Rheumatoid/osteoarthritis, other arthritic diseases ▪ Symptomatic treatment of rheumatic fever ▪ Prophylaxis of thrombosis-related diseases, esp coronary artery disease.

PHARMACOKINETICS

Absorption PO/Rectal	Duration	Protein binding	Excretion
70%-100%	4-6h	88%	In urine as metabolites

CONTRAINDICATIONS: Hypersensitivity to any salicylate; active ulcers.

DOSAGE

Pediatric *PO/Rectal*

Analgesic	11-16mg/kg 4-6 times/d
Antirheumatic	16mg/kg 6 times/d, to 10mg/kg 6 times/d
Rheumatic fever	90-130mg/kg/d divided, q4-6h

Adult *PO/Rectal*

Analgesic	325-650mg 4-6 times/d
Antirheumatic	1g 4-6 times/d. Do *not* exceed 10g/d
Antithrombotic	325-650mg 2-4 times/d
Rheumatic fever	4-8g/d divided, q4-6h

Note: Side/adverse effects: common in *italic;* serious in ***boldface italic.***

*Available in Canada only.

SIDE/ADVERSE EFFECTS: CNS: tinnitus ▪ CV: hypoprothrombinemia ▪ GI: epigastric distress, nausea, ***bleeding ulcer*** ▪ HEP: ↑ serum AST, ALT ▪ INT: skin rash.

DRUG INTERACTIONS: Use c̄ large amounts of antacids best avoided ▪ Buffered aspirin better ▪ Use c̄ ulcerogenic drugs best avoided ▪ ↑ Activity of PO anticoagulants, antidiabetic agents ▪ ↓ Uricosuric effects of probenecid, sulfinpyrazone ▪ ↓ PO absorption, uricosuric action of indomethacin.

NURSING MANAGEMENT

ADMINISTRATION: Assess for hx of salicylate hypersensitivity ▪ Administer c̄ food if GI irritation occurs ▪ Avoid large amounts of concurrent antacid suspensions ▪ Do *not* crush enteric-coated/timed-release preparations.

EVALUATION: Assess for bleeding (GI, GU, skin, mucous membrane) ▪ Diabetics: monitor for hypoglycemia ▪ Monitor for signs of overdose (CNS disturbances, tinnitus, hyperventilation).

EDUCATION: Check c̄ physician/pharmacist before taking OTC products ▪ Notify physician if signs of bleeding occur ▪ Take c̄ food/milk/antacids to ↓ GI irritation ▪ Swallow enteric-coated/timed-release preparations whole ▪ Notify physician of constant ringing in ears; D/C drug.

OVERDOSE MANAGEMENT: Remove drug by emesis or lavage followed by activated charcoal and a saline cathartic ▪ Maintain respiration and adequate blood volume c̄ IV fluids ▪ Treat alkalosis, acidosis, hyperkalemia, etc., as they arise.

NOTES:

astemizole • (a-<u>stem</u>-uh-zole)

CATEGORY: *Antihistamine*: H_1 blocker, H_1 antihistamine Rx; Preg Cat C

BRAND NAME
Hismanal (Janssen)

DOSAGE FORM
Tablet: 10mg

ACTION: H_1 antihistamine activity due to competitive inhibition of histamine at H_1 histamine receptors on peripheral cells; drug exhibits low to no anticholinergic activity; does not readily cross blood-brain barrier. **USE:** Symptomatic treatment of seasonal allergic rhinitis and chronic idiopathic urticaria.

PHARMACOKINETICS

PO absorption	Onset	Peak	Duration	Protein binding	Excretion
Good ac	Slow	1h	Up to 24h	96.7%	In feces, primarily as metabolite

CONTRAINDICATIONS: Hypersensitivity.

DOSAGE:
Pediatric (7-12y/o)/Adult *PO* 10mg ac once/d

SIDE/ADVERSE EFFECTS: CNS: *Drowsiness, headache, fatigue,* dizziness, nervousness ▪ EENT: *dry mouth,* sore throat, conjunctivitis ▪ GI: N/D, abdominal pain ▪ Other: arthralgia, *increased appetite, weight gain.*

DRUG INTERACTIONS: Use with CNS depressants may produce additive effects.

NURSING MANAGEMENT

ADMINISTRATION: Assess for hx of antihistamine hypersensitivity ▪ Administer 1h ac/2h pc; delay food intake for 1h after dose ▪ Avoid exposure to heat, moisture, light in storage ▪ Maintain hydration.

EVALUATION: Monitor VS, esp BP ▪ Assess for tolerance to therapeutic dose ▪ Closely monitor asthmatic pts (possible anticholinergic effect).

EDUCATION: Drowsiness may occur; use caution in potentially hazardous activities ▪ Take on empty stomach; avoid food for 1h after taking drug ▪ Use sugarless gum/hard candy to diminish dry mouth ▪ ↑ Fluid intake (8-10 glasses/d) ▪ Notify physician of symptoms of allergic rx (fever, difficult breathing, rash) ▪ Carry identification (MedicAlert) if antihistamine allergic ▪ Notify physician of antihistamine use before allergy testing ▪ Expect symptom relief in 1h ▪ Store in tightly closed, light-resistant container in cool, dry area ▪ Take only as needed; do *not* exceed prescribed dose ▪ Do *not* administer to children under 12y/o ▪ Women: avoid breastfeeding.

NOTES:

atenolol • (a-ten-oh-lole)

CATEGORY: *Beta-adrenergic blocker*: antianginal, antihypertensive Rx; Preg Cat A

BRAND NAME
Tenormin (ICI Pharma)

DOSAGE FORMS
Tablet: 50, 100mg
Injection (IV): 0.5 mg/ml

COMBINATION PRODUCTS
Tenoretic (ICI Pharma) atenolol/chlorthalidone per tablet: 50mg/25mg, 100mg/25mg

ACTION: Blocks access of catecholamine neurotransmitters to $beta_1$ receptors located in heart; at higher doses, blockage of $beta_2$ receptors will occur in bronchial tree, vascular smooth muscle; antihypertensive effect not determined. **USE:** Treatment of hypertension as sole agent or $\bar{c}$ other antihypertensive agents (esp thiazide diuretic) ▪ Long-term management of angina ▪ To reduce mortality rate in stable pts after MI.

PHARMACOKINETICS

PO absorption	Peak	Half-life	Protein binding	Excretion
50%	2-4h	6-7h	6%-16%	Via urine, feces as unchanged drug

CONTRAINDICATIONS: Hypersensitivity, serious bradycardia, heart block >1st°.

DOSAGE

Adult *PO*

Hypertension	Starting dose of 50mg/d and ↑ to 100mg/d prn. Doses >100mg do not produce further results
Angina	Starting dose of 50mg/d and ↑ to 200mg/d prn
MI prevention	50mg given 10m after last IV dose followed by 50mg in 12h. Then 50-100mg/d for 6-9d or until discharge
IV	5mg over 5m followed by another 5mg in 10m for initiation of MI prevention
Tenorectic *PO*	Usual range 1-2 tablets/d

SIDE/ADVERSE EFFECTS: CNS: *dizziness, tiredness*, drowsiness, *depression* ▪ CV: *cold extremities*, bradycardia, postural hypotension ▪ GI: D/N, constipation, anorexia ▪ RESP: dyspnea, wheeziness.

DRUG INTERACTIONS: Use c̄ reserpine, other catecholamine-depleting drugs can result in serious adrenergic blockage ▪ Nonselective beta-adrenergics antagonize therapeutic response ▪ Use c̄ furazolidone, general anesthetics, MAO-I best avoided.

NURSING MANAGEMENT

ADMINISTRATION: Assess for hx of beta blocker hypersensitivity ▪ Assess BP, apical pulse; if <60/m hold drug, notify physician ▪ Assess hepatic function, I&O; may require ↓ dosage if impaired ▪ Do *not* administer in presence of respiratory distress (asthma, CHF, COPD) ▪ Avoid exposure to heat/moisture in storage ▪ Avoid abrupt withdrawal; D/C gradually ▪ Elderly may require ↓ dosage.

EVALUATION: Monitor hepatic, renal, respiratory status ▪ Monitor BP, pulse ▪ Monitor CBC, FBS (diabetics) ▪ Assess for depression ▪ May produce alteration in blood glucose levels; may mask signs of hypoglycemia.

EDUCATION: Take as directed by physician even if symptom free; do *not* skip doses ▪ May take w/out regard to food ▪ Do *not* D/C w/out notifying physician ▪ Procedure for checking radial pulse ▪ Check pulse before taking; if <60m do *not* take drug, notify physician ▪ Check c̄ physician before taking OTC/Rx preparations ▪ Drowsiness may occur; use caution when engaging in potentially hazardous activities ▪ Avoid changing positions (lying/sitting/standing) rapidly ▪ Diabetics: carefully monitor blood/urine glucose; observe for symptoms of hypoglycemia (headache, ↑ sweating, hunger, weakness) ▪ May experience ↑ sensitivity to cold ▪ Notify physician of respiratory distress, leg edema ▪ Notify physician/dentist of beta blocker use before treatment ▪ Maintain optimum weight; follow low-Na^+ diet ▪ Keep scheduled appointments c̄ physician ▪ Store in tightly closed container ▪ Avoid ↑ exercise, temperature extremes, smoking ▪ Women: avoid breastfeeding.

NOTES:

atropine sulfate • (a-troe-peen)

CATEGORY: *Anticholinergic*: antimuscarinic, parasympatholytic Rx; preg Cat C

AVAILABLE PREPARATIONS

Atropine sulfate (various)
Ophthalmic preparations; injection (IM/IV/SC), tablets

ACTION: Anticholinergic activity due to competition c̄ acetylcholine for muscarinic receptors at postganglionic fiber of parasympathetic nervous system. **USE:** Treat, manage, cause bradycardia, cardiospasm, colitis, dysmenorrhea, enuresis, GI spasm, inhibition of secretions, mydriasis/cycloplegia, pylorospasm, spastic/rigid states due to CNS injury, ureteral colic, urinary frequency ▪ Antidote for cholinergic drug overdose and systemic-type insecticide ingestion.

PHARMACOKINETICS

	Peak	Half-life	Excretion
PO	1.5-4h	2-3h	75%-95% in urine, c̄ 50% as unchanged drug
IM	1.6-2h	2-3h	75%-95% in urine, c̄ 50% as unchanged drug

CONTRAINDICATIONS: Hypersensitivity; adhesions between iris, lens; advanced hepatic/renal impairment, asthma, hiatal hernia associated c̄ reflux esophagitis, intestinal atony, myasthenia gravis, narrow-angle glaucoma, obstructive GI/GU conditions, severe ulcerative colitis.

DOSAGE

Pediatric *PO*	0.01mg/kg q4-6h
Anticholinergic *IM/IV/SC*	0.01mg/kg q4-6h
Antidote	0.5-1mg followed by 0.5mg q10-15m until signs of atropine toxicity appear
Pre-op	3kg, 0.1mg; 7-9kg, 0.2mg; 12-16kg, 0.3mg; 20-27kg, 0.4mg; 32kg, 0.5mg; 41kg, 0.6mg
Adult *PO*	0.1-1.2mg q4-6h
Anticholinergic *IM/IV/SC*	0.4-0.6mg q4-6h
Antidote	1-4mg followed by 1-2mg q5-10m until signs of atropine toxicity appear
Pre-op	0.4-1mg

SIDE/ADVERSE EFFECTS: CNS: mental confusion ▪ CV: tachycardia ▪ EENT: blurred vision, cycloplegia, mydriasis, ↑ IOP, photophobia ▪ GI: N/V, constipation, loss of taste, dysphagia ▪ GU: urinary retention ▪ INT: urticaria, skin rash ▪ Other: suppression of lactation/body secretions.

DRUG INTERACTIONS: Use c̄ antihistamines, phenothiazines, tricyclic antidepressants ↑ anticholinergic effects ▪ MAO-I ↑ activity by ↓ anticholinergic biotransformation.

NURSING MANAGEMENT

ADMINISTRATION: Assess for hx of hypersensitivity ▪ Administer tablets ac/hs ▪ Have physostigmine available for OD ▪ Parenteral antidotal therapy: first dose IV injection; repeated doses IM ▪ Elderly may require ↓ dosage (paradoxic rxs).

EVALUATION: Monitor VS, esp heart rate; I&O ▪ Observe for anticholinergic effects.

EDUCATION: Advise pt of expected anticholinergic side effects (dry mouth, photophobia, constipation) ▪ Notify physician *immediately* of skin rash, flushing of skin, eye pain; D/C drug ▪ Avoid concurrent antacid administration ▪ Avoid strenuous work/exercise during hot, humid weather ▪ Use sugarless gum/hard candy to diminish dry mouth ▪ Avoid OTC cough/hay fever preparations ▪ Avoid potentially hazardous activities ▪ ↑ Fluid intake (10-12 glasses/d).

NOTES:

auranofin • (au-rane-oh-fin)

CATEGORY: *Antiinflammatory*: gold compound

Rx; Preg Cat C

BRAND NAME	DOSAGE FORM
Ridaura (SKB)	Capsule: 3mg

ACTION: Antiinflammatory mechanism not determined.
USE: Treatment of rheumatoid arthritis.

PHARMACOKINETICS: Approximately 25% of gold absorbed, c̄ mean body half-life 80d; excretion of absorbed gold via urine (60%).

CONTRAINDICATIONS: Hx of gold-induced necrotizing enterocolitis, pulmonary fibrosis, exfoliative dermatitis, bone marrow aplasia, other severe blood dyscrasias.

DOSAGE

Adult *PO*	Initial dose 6mg/d given once or 3mg bid. May ↑ to 9mg/d after 6mo if response is inadequate

SIDE/ADVERSE EFFECTS: GI: *loose stools or diarrhea, abdominal pain, nausea,* vomiting, constipation, anorexia, flatulence, *stomatitis* ▪ GU: proteinuria, hematuria ▪ HEM: anemia, ***leukopenia, thrombocytopenia***, eosinophilia ▪ HEP: jaundice, ↑ enzyme levels ▪ INT: *rash, pruritus.*

DRUG INTERACTIONS: No significant rxs reported.

NURSING MANAGEMENT

ADMINISTRATION: Assess for hx of gold/heavy metal hypersensitivity ▪ Assess for hx of blood dyscrasia; do *not* administer ▪ Have emergency support equipment available.

EVALUATION: Monitor hepatic, renal status ▪ Monitor CBC, UA ▪ Assess joint function; comply c̄ physical therapy ▪ False(+): Tuberculin skin test.

EDUCATION: Take exactly as directed by physician even if symptom free ▪ Notify physician of diarrhea, itching ▪ D/C, notify physician of signs of bleeding (bruising, red pinpoint rash, black tarry stools) ▪ Keep scheduled appointments $\bar{c}$ physician/laboratory tests ▪ May produce changes in taste ▪ Maintain good oral hygiene; use soft toothbrush; avoid smoking, alcohol, acidic foods ▪ Check $\bar{c}$ physician before taking OTC/Rx preparations ▪ Full drug effect may require several months of therapy.

NOTES:

azithromycin • (a-zi-thro-my-sin)

CATEGORY: *Antibiotic*: macrolide antibiotic (semi-synthetic) Rx; Preg Cat B

BRAND NAME
Zithromax (Pfizer)

DOSAGE FORM
Capsule: 250mg

ACTION: Bacteriostatic activity due to inhibition of ribosomal protein synthesis in microorganisms. **USE:** Treatment of lower and upper respiratory, skin and sexually transmitted infections caused by susceptible strains of *Chlamydia trachomatis, Haemophilus influenzae, Moraxella catarrhalis, Staphylococcus aureus, Streptococcus agalactiae, Streptococcus pneumoniae, Streptococcus pyogenes.*

PHARMACOKINETICS

PO absorption	Peak	Half-life	Protein binding	Excretion
40%	2.5h	68h	Up to 51%	Via feces (biliary) and urine as unchanged drug

CONTRAINDICATIONS: Hypersensitivity to drug, erythromycin, or any macrolide.

DOSAGE
Adults/Children
16 or over *PO* — 500mg or single dose on day 1, then 250mg once/d 1h ac or 2h pc on days 2-5 (total dose of 1.5g). For chlamydia infection, 1g as single dose.

SIDE/ADVERSE EFFECTS: CNS: dizziness, headache, somnolence ▪ CV: chest pain, palpitations ▪ GI: N/V/D (highest dose: 1g), dyspepsia, flatulence, cholestatic jaundice, melena ▪ GU: monilia, nephritis, vaginitis ▪ INT: rash, photosensitivity ▪ Other: angioedema, fatigue.

DRUG INTERACTIONS: Bacteriostatic antibiotics can antagonize effects of bactericidal antibiotics ▪ Use c̄ carbamazepine, cyclosporine, digoxin, ergot alkaloids, phenytoin, theophylline, triazolam can ↑ their toxicity.

NURSING MANAGEMENT
ADMINISTRATION: Assess for hx of erythromycin/macrolide hypersensitivity ▪ Obtain C&S before therapy ▪

Assess hepatic status; ↓ dosage if impaired ▪ Administer 1h ac/2h pc $\bar{c}$ full glass H_2O (avoid citrus juice) ▪ Delay antacid administration for 2h after dose.

EVALUATION: Monitor VS, esp temperature; hepatic status ▪ Observe for signs of superinfection (diarrhea, perineal itching, oral ulcers).

EDUCATION: Complete full course of therapy ▪ Take on empty stomach, do *not* take $\bar{c}$ citrus juice ▪ Take at equal intervals around clock to maintain blood levels ▪ Diarrhea may occur.

NOTES:

aztreonam • (az-tree-oh-nam)

CATEGORY: *Antibiotic*: monobactam, synthetic β-lactam Rx; Preg Cat B

BRAND NAME
Azactam (Squibb)

DOSAGE FORMS
Powder for injection (IM/IV): 500mg; 1, 2g

ACTION: Bactericidal activity due to inhibition of mucopeptide cell wall synthesis in susceptible organisms. **USE:** Treatment of gynecologic, intraabdominal, lower respiratory, UTIs, and septicemia caused by susceptible strains of *Citrobacter* spp, *Enterobacter cloacae, Escherichia coli, Haemophilus influenzae, Klebsiella oxytoca, Klebsiella pneumoniae, Proteus mirabilis, Pseudomonas aeruginosa, Serratia* spp.

PHARMACOKINETICS

IM peak	Half-life	Protein binding	Excretion
1h	1.5-2h	56%	Complete w/in 12h primarily via urine

CONTRAINDICATIONS: Hypersensitivity.

DOSAGE
Adult *IM/IV* 500mg-1g q8-12h. For moderate infection 1-2g q8-12h. For life-threatening infection 2g q6-8h IV. Dosage must be ↓ c̄ renal impairment.

SIDE/ADVERSE EFFECTS: CNS: dizziness, confusion, headache, paresthesia ▪ CV: transient ventricular bigeminy, PVC, hypotension ▪ EENT: diplopia, tinnitus, nasal congestion ▪ GI: cramps, oral ulcers, taste change ▪ HEM: anemia, pancytopenia, neutropenia ▪ HEP: ↑ AST, ALT, alkaline phosphatase ▪ INT: pruritus, purpura, ***erythema multiforme, exfoliative dermatitis,*** urticaria ▪ Other: breast tenderness, muscular aches, vaginal monilia.

DRUG INTERACTIONS: Use c̄ furosemide/probenecid can cause slight ↑ in serum aztreonam levels ▪ In *Enterobacter* & *Pseudomonas* infections, avoid concurrent use c̄ β-lactamase-inducing antibiotics such as cefoxitin.

NURSING MANAGEMENT

ADMINISTRATION: Assess for hx of penicillin/cephalosporin hypersensitivity ▪ Obtain C&S before therapy ▪ IM/IV: reconstitute according to manufacturer's directions; shake well; discard unused solution.

EVALUATION: Monitor VS, esp temperature ▪ Monitor hepatic status ▪ Observe for signs of superinfection (diarrhea, perineal itching, oral ulcers) ▪ Check IV site carefully; monitor for phlebitis (red streak, heat, pain) ▪ Assess for ↑ serum creatinine; ↓ dose.

EDUCATION: Diarrhea may occur ▪ Maintain good personal hygiene (esp perineal, oral) ▪ Maintain fluid intake (6-8 glasses/d) ▪ Notify physician of symptoms of allergic rx (difficult breathing, rash) ▪ IM injection may be painful.

NOTES:

bacitracin/bacitracin sterile ▲• (bass-i-tray-sin) 26

CATEGORY: *Antibiotic:* polypeptide antibiotic Rx; Preg Cat NA

AVAILABLE PREPARATIONS

Bacitracin oint, ophthalmic oint (various)
Bacitracin powder for injection (various)

ACTION: Bactericidal activity due to inhibition of mucopeptide cell wall synthesis in susceptible organisms. **USE:** Treatment of topical infections caused by susceptible organisms ▪ Treatment of pneumonia, empyema in infants caused by susceptible strains of staphylococci.

PHARMACOKINETICS

IM absorption	Peak	Excretion
Complete	1-2h	Via urine

CONTRAINDICATIONS: Hypersensitivity.

DOSAGE

Infant *IM*	<2.5kg: 900U/kg/d in 2-3 divided doses >2.5g: 1000U/kg/d in 2-3 divided doses

SIDE/ADVERSE EFFECTS: CV: ↑ blood levels w/out ↑ in dosage ▪ GI: N/V ▪ GU: ***nephrotoxicity*** c̄ albuminuria, cylinduria, azotemia ▪ INT: skin rash ▪ Other: local pain at IM injection site.

DRUG INTERACTIONS: Use c̄ nephrotoxic drugs such as aminoglycosides, colistimethate sodium, polymyxin B, viomycin can result in significant toxicity ▪ Surgical neuromuscular blocking agent activity enhanced; can result in respiratory depression, paralysis.

NURSING MANAGEMENT

ADMINISTRATION: Assess for hx of hypersensitivity (incl neomycin) ▪ Obtain C&S before therapy ▪ IM: dilute; administer *deep, slowly* into gluteal UOQ; refrigerate ▪ Do *not* administer IV ▪ Avoid application to severely burned areas ▪ Maintain alkaline urine ▪ Maintain hydration.

EVALUATION: Monitor renal status ▪ Assess for skin rash; notify physician, D/C use ▪ Monitor I&O (IM) ▪ Monitor serum for ↑ BUN, creatinine.

Note: Side/adverse effects: common in *italic;* serious in ***boldface italic.*** *Available in Canada only.

EDUCATION: Notify physician of changes in urination ▪ ↑ Fluid intake (8-10 glasses/d) ▪ IM injection may be painful ▪ Ophthalmic application: wash hands; sterile technique, do *not* contaminate tip of tube; do *not* share $\bar{c}$ others; blurring of vision may occur ▪ D/C use, notify physician of burning, itching, difficult breathing.

NOTES:

benzquinamide hcl • (benz-kwin-a-mide)

CATEGORY: *Antiemetic* Rx; Preg Cat NA

BRAND NAME	**DOSAGE FORM**
Emete-con (Roerig)	Powder for injection (IM/IV): 50mg/vial

ACTION: Antiemetic activity probably due to inhibition of chemoreceptor trigger zone in medulla. **USE:** Treatment of N/V associated c̄ anesthesia/surgery.

PHARMACOKINETICS

Onset	IM peak	Duration	Half-life	Protein binding	Excretion
15m	30m	3-4h	40m	58%	95% via urine w/in 72h

CONTRAINDICATIONS: Hypersensitivity.

DOSAGE

Adult *IM* 0.5-1mg/kg IM; may be repeated in 1h. Subsequent doses q3-4h prn

IV 0.2-0.4mg/kg IV as single dose *slowly*. Subsequent doses IM

SIDE/ADVERSE EFFECTS: CNS: *Drowsiness*, headache, excitation, nervousness ▪ CV: hypertension, hypotension, atrial fibrillation, premature auricular/ventricular contractions ▪ EENT: blurred vision ▪ GI: anorexia, nausea, dry mouth, hiccoughs ▪ INT: hives, rash ▪ Other: shivering, sweating, shaking.

DRUG INTERACTIONS: Use c̄ epinephrine or other pressor agents may require dose adjustments ▪ Toxicity of concurrent drugs may be masked.

NURSING MANAGEMENT

ADMINISTRATION: Assess for hx of hypersensitivity ▪ Assess for cardiac hx; do *not* administer IV (hypotension, arrhythmias) ▪ Do *not* reconstitute c̄ NaCl (precipitation) ▪ IM: inject *deep, slowly* into gluteal UOQ ▪ Avoid exposure to cold, light during storage ▪ Administer *before* antineoplastic drugs.

EVALUATION: Monitor BP, heart rhythm ▪ Assess activity status (safety precautions) ▪ Monitor fluid/electrolyte balance if pt vomiting.

EDUCATION: Drowsiness may occur ▪ Notify nurse/physician *immediately* of dizziness, skipped heartbeats ▪ Use sugarless gum/hard candy to diminish dry mouth.

NOTES:

benzthiazide •(benz-thye-a-zide)

CATEGORY: *Thiazide diuretic*: antihypertensive Rx; Preg Cat C

BRAND NAME	DOSAGE FORM
Exna (Robins)	Tablet: 50mg

ACTION: Diuretic activity due to inhibition of Na^+ reabsorption primarily in ascending limb of loop of Henle, early distal tubule of nephron; K^+, bicarbonate, other ions, H_2O excreted w/out significant altering of urine pH; antihypertensive effect related to reduction in peripheral vascular resistance. **USE:** Treatment of hypertension as sole agent or c̄ other antihypertensives ▪ Treatment of edema related to renal dysfunction ▪ Adjunct in treating edema from CHF, hepatic cirrhosis, corticosteroid/estrogen therapy.

PHARMACOKINETICS

PO absorption	Onset	Peak	Duration	Excretion
Good	2h	4-6h	6-12h	Via urine as unchanged drug

CONTRAINDICATIONS: Hypersensitivity due to any thiazide or other sulfonamide-derivative drugs, anuria.

DOSAGE

Pediatric *PO*	1-4mg tid
Adult *PO*	50-200mg/d

SIDE/ADVERSE EFFECTS: CNS: *dizziness*, vertigo, paresthesia, headache ▪ EENT: blurred vision, xanthopsia ▪ GI: anorexia, gastric irritation, N/V/D, jaundice, ***pancreatitis*** ▪ HEM: ***agranulocytosis, aplastic anemia***, leukopenia, ***thrombocytopenia*** ▪ INT: purpura, urticaria, photosensitivity ▪ MET: ***hypokalemia***, glycosuria, hyperglycemia ▪ MS: *fatigue, leg cramps* ▪ RESP: respiratory distress ▪ Other: necrotizing angiitis.

DRUG INTERACTIONS: ↑ Dig toxicity due to hypokalemia ▪ Use c̄ corticosteroids produces ↑ hypokalemia ▪ Antidiabetic agents may require dose

Note: Side/adverse effects: common in *italic;* serious in ***boldface italic.***

*Available in Canada only.

adjustment ▪ Use c̄ diazoxide can produce significant diabetogenic effects.

NURSING MANAGEMENT

ADMINISTRATION: Assess for hx of hypersensitivity (incl sulfonamides) ▪ Assess renal function; do *not* administer if impaired ▪ Administer c̄ food or milk on arising ▪ Assess serum K^+ (normal: 3.5-5mEq/L) ▪ Elderly may require ↓ dosage.

EVALUATION: Monitor F/E, hepatic, renal status ▪ Monitor VS, esp BP, pulse ▪ Monitor serum for ↑ BUN, creatinine, uric acid; ↓ K^+ ▪ Diabetics: monitor blood glucose ▪ Monitor fluid retention (I&O, daily weight) ▪ Monitor digitalized pts closely (↓ K^+: ↑ dig toxicity).

EDUCATION: Expect ↑ urine output; have bathroom facilities easily accessible ▪ May cause weakness, lethargy ▪ Take c̄ food ▪ Take on waking up, at same time each day ▪ Take even if symptom free ▪ Used to control, *not* cure, hypertension ▪ Notify physician of signs of hypokalemia (muscle cramps, lethargy, nausea) ▪ Avoid changing positions (lying/sitting/standing) rapidly ▪ Take as directed by physician; do *not* skip doses ▪ Eat foods high in K^+ (bananas, citrus juices, raisins); avoid black licorice ▪ Avoid high Na^+ foods (canned soups, lunch meats, cheese) ▪ Maintain optimum weight ▪ Avoid exposure to direct sunlight/UV light ▪ Diabetics: check blood/urine glucose carefully ▪ Avoid smoking ▪ Use sugarless gum/hard candy to diminish dry mouth.

NOTES:

benztropine mesylate • (benz-troe-peen)

CATEGORY: *Anti-Parkinson agent:* anticholinergic — Rx; Preg Cat C

BRAND NAME
Cogentin (MSD)

DOSAGE FORMS
Injection (IM/IV): 1mg/ml
Tablet: 0.5, 1, 2mg

ACTION: Anti-Parkinson effect due to central anticholinergic inhibition of hyperactive cholinergic activity in striated fibers. **USE:** Adjunct to treatment of all forms of Parkinson disease ▪ Management of extrapyramidal symptoms (except tardive dyskinesia) induced by antipsychotic agents.

PHARMACOKINETICS: Not available.

CONTRAINDICATIONS: Hypersensitivity, glaucoma.

DOSAGE

Adults *PO/IM/IV*	Parkinson disease: 1-2mg/d c̄ range 0.5-6mg Drug-induced extrapyramidal symptoms: 1-4mg/d or bid

SIDE/ADVERSE EFFECTS: EENT: blurred vision ▪ GI: dry mouth, dysphagia, constipation, N/V ▪ Other: allergic rxs (rare).

DRUG INTERACTIONS: Use c̄ antihistamines, phenothiazines, tricyclic antidepressants will produce ↑ anticholinergic effects ▪ Amantadine can significantly ↑ anticholinergic effects of benztropine.

NURSING MANAGEMENT

ADMINISTRATION: Assess for hx of hypersensitivity ▪ Administer in divided doses c̄ meals, as single AM dose, or as single hs dose ▪ Avoid exposure to moisture during storage ▪ Avoid abrupt withdrawal ▪ Parenteral: avoid freezing ▪ Elderly may require ↓ dosage.

EVALUATION: Monitor GI, GU, CV status ▪ Assess for muscle weakness ▪ Observe for exaggerated anticholinergic effects ▪ Monitor VS ▪ Monitor I&O ▪ Assess IOP ▪ Assess for tolerance to therapeutic dose.

EDUCATION: Drowsiness may occur; use caution when engaging in potentially hazardous activities ▪ Avoid use c̄ alcohol, other CNS depressants ▪ Take c̄ meals ▪ Avoid extremes in exercise, hot climate ▪ Take as ordered by physician; do *not* ↑ dose ▪ Store in tightly closed container ▪ Schedule periodic eye exams ▪ Use sugarless gum/hard candy to diminish dry mouth ▪ Take antacid/antidiarrheal preparations at least 1h before or after taking drug ▪ Wear sunglasses to ↓ discomfort from bright light ▪ Avoid changing positions (lying/sitting/standing) rapidly ▪ Safety precautions $\bar{c}$ ↑ activity ▪ Women: avoid breastfeeding ▪ Full drug effects may require several days of therapy.

NOTES:

biperiden hcl/biperiden lactate▲ • (bye-per-i-den)

CATEGORY: *Anti-Parkinson agent*: anticholinergic Rx; Preg Cat C

BRAND NAME
Akineton (Knoll)

DOSAGE FORMS
Injection (IM/IV)▲: 5mg/ml
Tablet: 2mg

ACTION: Anti-Parkinson effect due to central anticholinergic inhibition of hyperactive cholinergic activity in striated fibers. **USE:** Adjunct in treatment of all forms of Parkinson disease ▪ Management of extrapyramidal symptoms (except tardive dyskinesia) induced by antipsychotic agents.

PHARMACOKINETICS: Good PO absorption; appears to peak after 1-1½ h; metabolic path not fully determined.

CONTRAINDICATIONS: Hypersensitivity.

DOSAGE

Adult	*PO*	Parkinson disease 2mg 3-4 times/d
		Extrapyramidal 2mg 1-3 times/d
	IM/IV	Extrapyramidal 2mg q1/2h until control is achieved; do *not* exceed 8mg/24h

SIDE/ADVERSE EFFECTS: EENT: blurred vision ▪ GI: dry mouth, dysphagia, constipation, N/V ▪ GU: urinary retention ▪ Other: allergic rxs.

DRUG INTERACTIONS: Use c̄ antihistamines, phenothiazines, tricyclic antidepressants will ↑ anticholinergic effects ▪ Amantadine can significantly ↑ anticholinergic effects.

NURSING MANAGEMENT

ADMINISTRATION: Assess for hx of hypersensitivity ▪ Administer in divided doses c̄ meals/pc ▪ Avoid exposure to moisture during storage ▪ Avoid abrupt withdrawal; D/C gradually ▪ Parenteral: avoid freezing ▪ Elderly may require ↓ dosage.

EVALUATION: Monitor CV, GI, GU status ▪ Assess for muscle weakness ▪ Observe for exaggerated anticholinergic effects ▪ Monitor VS ▪ Monitor I&O ▪ Assess IOP ▪ Assess for tolerance to therapeutic dose.

EDUCATION: Drowsiness may occur; use caution when engaging in potentially hazardous activities ▪ Avoid changing positions (lying/sitting/standing) rapidly ▪ Avoid use c̄ alcohol, other CNS depressants ▪ Take as ordered by physician ▪ Take c̄ /after meals ▪ Avoid extremes in exercise, temperature ▪ Store in tightly closed container ▪ Schedule periodic eye exams ▪ Use sugarless gum/hard candy to diminish dry mouth ▪ Take antacid preparations at least 1h before/after taking drug ▪ Wear sunglasses to ↓ discomfort from bright lights ▪ Safety precautions c̄ ↑ activity ▪ Full drug effects may require several days of therapy.

NOTES:

bisacodyl • (bis-a-koe-dill)

CATEGORY: *Laxative* OTC

BRAND NAMES / **DOSAGE FORMS**

Brand Names	Dosage Forms
**Bisacolax (ICN)*	
Dulcolax (Ciba)	Suppository: 10mg Tablet: 5mg
Fleet Laxative	Suppository: 10mg Tablet: 5mg

ACTION: Laxative activity due to direct stimulation to produce normal colon peristalsis. **USE:** Treatment of acute constipation ▪ Bowel evacuant for radiography, antepartum care, predelivery care, sigmoidoscopy, proctoscopy, colostomy.

PHARMACOKINETICS: Not applicable.

CONTRAINDICATIONS: Acute abdominal problem requiring surgery.

DOSAGE

Pediatric *PO*	5-10mg
Rectal	1/2 suppository for children <2y/o, whole suppository for older children
Adult *PO*	10-15mg for normal BM; up to 30mg as bowel evacuant for special procedures
Rectal	1 suppository (10mg)

SIDE/ADVERSE EFFECTS: GI: occasional abdominal cramps, possible rectal irritation.

NURSING MANAGEMENT

ADMINISTRATION: PO: administer hs or on arising; do *not* crush tablets; administer whole $\bar{c}$ full glass of liquid ▪ Suppository: administer just before desired effect ▪ Do *not* administer to tartrazine-sensitive pts ▪ Avoid exposure to heat during storage.

EVALUATION: Monitor bowel function ▪ Assess for rectal bleeding; notify physician ▪ Prolonged use: monitor blood glucose levels (↑), serum K^+ (↓).

Note: Side/adverse effects: common in *italic;* serious in ***boldface italic.***

*Available in Canada only.

EDUCATION: Avoid straining during BM ▪ Ingest high-fiber diet (cereal, fruit, vegetables) ▪ Maintain fluid intake (6-8 glasses/d) ▪ Encourage ventilation of feelings ▪ ↑ Daily exercise ▪ Do *not* take other medication w/in 2h of drug, milk or antacids w/in 1h ▪ Establish regular BM (pc) ▪ High laxative abuse potential ▪ Should have BM w/in 6h of administration.

NOTES:

bleomycin sulfate • (blee-oh-mye-sin)

CATEGORY: *Antineoplastic*: antibiotic

Rx; Preg Cat NA

BRAND NAME
Blenoxane (BM-ONC)
(*Bristol [Canada]*)

DOSAGE FORMS
Powder for injection (IM/IV/SC): 15U/vial

ACTION: Antineoplastic activity appears to be related to inhibition of DNA, RNA, protein synthesis. **USE:** Palliative treatment of squamous cell carcinoma of head-mouth area, neck; response is poor in pts who have undergone radiation therapy ▪ Palliative treatment of lymphomas incl Hodgkin's disease, lymphosarcoma, reticulum cell sarcoma ▪ Palliative treatment of testicular carcinoma.

PHARMACOKINETICS: Short half-life; excreted via urine as unchanged drug (70%).

CONTRAINDICATIONS: Hypersensitivity.

DOSAGE

IM/IV/SC Hodgkin's disease: 0.25-0.5U/kg 1-2 times/wk; after 50% response, maintenance dose 1U qd or 5U/wk IV or IM
Other cancers: 0.25-0.5U/kg 1-2 times/wk

SIDE/ADVERSE EFFECTS: GI: N/V, anorexia, fever, chills ▪ INT: *Most frequent (50%): alopecia, erythema,* hyperkeratosis, hyperpigmentation, nail changes, *pruritus, rash, stomatitis, striae, vesiculation* ▪ RESP: pulmonary toxicity (10%), dose or age related, esp c̄ high doses (>400U) or old age (70); pneumonitis, which can lead to fatal ***pulmonary fibrosis***.

DRUG INTERACTIONS: Use c̄ vinblastine has produced isolated Raynaud's disease in pts c̄ testicular carcinoma ▪ Use c̄ pulmotoxic/hepatotoxic drugs results in ↑ toxicity.

NURSING MANAGEMENT
ADMINISTRATION: Assess for hx of hypersensitivity ▪ Assess pulmonary function (chest x-ray, auscultation of lungs) ▪ Wear disposable surgical gloves, mask when

preparing solutions ▪ IM or SC: dissolve in 1-5ml sterile or bacteriostatic H_2O, CaCl, or 5% dextrose solution for injection ▪ IM: inject *deep, slowly* into gluteal UOQ; rotate sites ▪ IV: dissolve in 5ml NaCl or 5% dextrose solution for injection; administer *slowly*, over 10m ▪ Reconstituted solutions are stable for 24h (room temperature) or 7d (refrigerated) ▪ Have support equipment available for anaphylaxis ▪ Administer antiemetic before therapy ▪ Provide emotional support.

EVALUATION: Monitor hepatic, renal, hemopoietic status ▪ Monitor breath sounds, respiratory function (chest x-ray) ▪ Assess for hyperthermia (fever, chills); administer antipyretic as ordered ▪ Assess for skin rash; D/C drug ▪ Assess for infection, bleeding, anemia ▪ Assess hydration status (I&O, daily weight).

EDUCATION: Notify physician *immediately* of cough, shortness of breath ▪ Check all OTC preparations c̄ physician/pharmacist before use ▪ Darkened skin may occur ▪ Avoid smoking (↑ pulmonary toxicity) ▪ ↑ Fluid intake (10-12 glasses/d) ▪ Avoid exposure to infection ▪ Diet as tolerated; avoid spicy foods ▪ Maintain good oral hygiene; use soft-bristled toothbrush ▪ Loss of hair may occur (reversible after therapy) ▪ Notify physician of symptoms of bone marrow depression (fever, sore throat, bruising, bleeding, lethargy) ▪ Encourage ventilation of feelings ▪ Women: avoid breastfeeding ▪ Use contraception if sexually active.

NOTES:

bromocriptine mesylate • (broe-moe-krip-teen)

CATEGORY: *Dopaminergic*: dopamimetic, prolactin inhibitor — Rx; Preg Cat NA

BRAND NAME
Parlodel (Sandoz)

DOSAGE FORMS
Capsule 5mg, tablet 2.5mg
Snap Tabs: 2.5mg

ACTION: Dopaminergic receptor activity, esp c̄ D-2 dopamine receptors in CNS, produces significant amelioration of hyperprolactinemia, Parkinson disease; bromocriptine may cause symptoms of acromegaly to subside. **USE:** Treatment of idiopathic Parkinson disease ▪ Short-term treatment of amenorrhea/galactorrhea associated c̄ hyperprolactinemia ▪ Prevention of lactation; some pts may experience mild/moderate rebound lactation ▪ Treatment of acromegaly.

PHARMACOKINETICS

PO absorption	Peak	Protein binding	Excretion
28%	1-1.5h	90%-96%	Via bile (feces) as metabolites

CONTRAINDICATIONS: Hypersensitivity to drug/ergot alkaloids, uncontrolled hypertension, toxemia of pregnancy.

DOSAGE

Adult *PO*

Parkinson disease	Initial dose 1.25mg bid. Dosage may ↑ every 14-28d by 2.5mg/d. Do *not* exceed 100mg/d
Lactation	Therapy should start no sooner than 4h after delivery in pts c̄ stable VS. Usual dose 2.5mg bid for 14-21d
Acromegaly prevention	Initial dose 1.25-2.5mg hs c̄ food for 3d; c̄ 1.25-2.5mg increments q3-7d until satisfactory response obtained. Usual range 20-30mg/d. Do *not* exceed 100mg/d
Hyperprolactinemic indications	Initial dose 1.25-2.5mg/d. 2.5mg as tolerated may be added q3-7d. Usual dose 5-7.5mg/d c̄ a daily range of 2.5-15 mg

Note: Side/adverse effects: common in *italic;* serious in ***boldface italic.***

*Available in Canada only.

SIDE/ADVERSE EFFECTS: CNS: *dizziness, headache,* fatigue, lethargy, ***epileptiform seizures,*** nightmares, confusion ▪ CV: hypotension, edema, palpitations ▪ EENT: nasal congestion, visual disturbances ▪ GI: *N/V/D,* cramps, anorexia, constipation, dyspepsia, dry mouth, metallic taste ▪ GU: urinary frequency ▪ Other: symptoms of ergotism.

DRUG INTERACTIONS: Use c̄ hypotensive agents can produce significant hypotension ▪ Use c̄ levodopa can ↑ frequency of visual/auditory hallucinations ▪ Phenothiazines can ↑ prolactin levels, are best avoided.

NURSING MANAGEMENT

ADMINISTRATION: Assess for hx of ergot alkaloid hypersensitivity ▪ Avoid exposure to heat, moisture, light in storage ▪ Administer c̄ meals/milk ▪ Assess BP for stability before administration.

EVALUATION: Monitor hepatic/neuropsychiatric status ▪ Monitor VS, esp BP ▪ Pregnancy test at periodic intervals ▪ Assess serum FSH, LH, prolactin, urinary retention, pregnanediol prn ▪ Assess visual fields.

EDUCATION: Take c̄ meals ▪ Avoid alcohol ▪ May cause dizziness; use caution in potentially hazardous activities ▪ Avoid changing positions (lying/sitting/standing) rapidly ▪ Women: use birth control during therapy (unless for fertility), do *not* use oral contraceptives; avoid if breastfeeding ▪ Keep scheduled appointments c̄ physician ▪ May take >6wks for menses to recur ▪ Missed dose; if remembered >4h, do *not* take; do *not* double dose; resume regular dose schedule ▪ Store in tightly closed container.

NOTES:

bumetanide •(byoo-met-a-nide)

CATEGORY: *Loop diuretic* Rx; Preg Cat C

BRAND NAME
Bumex (Roche)

DOSAGE FORMS
Injection (IM/IV): 0.25 mg/ml
Tablet: 0.5, 1mg

ACTION: Diuretic activity due to excretion of H_2O, Na^+, Cl^-, other electrolytes by inhibiting tubular reabsorption, esp in medullary, cortical portions of ascending limb of loop of Henle. **USE:** Treatment of edema due to CHF, renal/hepatic dysfunction.

DOSAGE

Adult *PO*	0.5-2mg/d, to maximum 10mg
IM/IV	0.5-1mg given at 2-3h intervals. Do *not* exceed 10mg/d

SIDE/ADVERSE EFFECTS: CNS: dizziness, encephalopathy, headache ▪ CV: *hypotension*, ECG changes ▪ EENT: impaired hearing ▪ GI: *nausea*, vomiting, abdominal pain ▪ INT: pruritus, hives ▪ MET: hypoglycemia, hyperuricemia, metabolic alkalosis ▪ MS: *muscle cramps*, pain, arthritic pain.

PHARMACOKINETICS

PO absorption	Onset	Peak	Duration	Half-life	Protein binding	Excretion
85%-95%	30-60m	1-2h	4-6h	1-1.5h	95%-96%	Via urine, feces as metabolites, unchanged drug (45%)

CONTRAINDICATIONS: Hypersensitivity, hepatic coma, anuria, severe electrolyte depletion.

DRUG INTERACTIONS: Use c̄ neurotoxic drugs incl aminoglycosides, capreomycin, chloroquine, oxyphenbutazone, phenylbutazone, vancomycin, viomycin can result in significant toxicity ▪ Induced hypokalemia ↑ dig toxicity ▪ Avoid use c̄ nephrotoxic drugs, lithium, probenecid, indomethacin ▪ Antihypertensives may require dosage adjustment ▪ Use c̄ corticosteroids can produce severe hypokalemia.

NURSING MANAGEMENT

ADMINISTRATION: Assess for hx of hypersensitivity (incl sulfonamides) ▪ Assess renal function; do *not* administer if severely impaired ▪ PO: administer c̄ food/milk on arising ▪ IV: use infusion w/in 24h after preparation; administer *slowly* (2m) ▪ Do *not* use discolored/precipitated solutions ▪ Assess serum K^+ (normal: 3.5-5mEq/L) ▪ Elderly may require ↓ dosage ▪ Avoid exposure to light in storage ▪ IM: inject *deep, slowly* into gluteal UOQ.

EVALUATION: Monitor F/E, hepatic, renal status ▪ Monitor VS, esp BP, pulse ▪ Monitor serum for ↑ BUN, creatinine, uric acid; ↓ K^+ ▪ Diabetics: monitor blood glucose ▪ Monitor fluid retention (I&O, daily weight) ▪ Monitor digitalized pts closely (↓ K^+, ↑ dig toxicity) ▪ Assess for ↓ hearing (ototoxicity).

EDUCATION: Expect ↑ urine output; have bathroom facilities easily accessible ▪ May cause weakness, lethargy ▪ Take PO forms c̄ food ▪ Take on waking, at same time each day ▪ Take even if symptom free ▪ Notify physician of signs of hypokalemia (muscle cramps, lethargy, nausea), hyponatremia (thirst, dry mouth, drowsiness) ▪ Avoid changing positions (lying/sitting/standing) rapidly ▪ Take as directed by physician; do *not* skip doses ▪ Eat foods high in K^+ (bananas, citrus juices, raisins); avoid black licorice ▪ Avoid high-Na^+ foods (canned soup, lunch meats, cheese) ▪ Maintain optimum weight ▪ Check c̄ physician before taking OTC/Rx preparations ▪ Diabetics: check blood/urine glucose carefully.

NOTES:

bupropion hcl • (byoo-proe-pee-on)

CATEGORY: *Antidepressant*

Rx; Preg Cat B

BRAND NAME
Wellbutrin (B-W)

DOSAGE FORMS
Tablet: 75, 100mg

ACTION: Antidepressant mechanism not established.
USE: Treatment of depression. Avoid abrupt withdrawal of drug.

PHARMACOKINETICS

PO absorption	Peak	Half-life	Protein binding	Excretion
Good	2h	14h	80%	87% via urine and 10% via feces

CONTRAINDICATIONS: Hypersensitivity, seizure disorders, current or prior anorexia nervosa or bulimia, use of MAO-I.

DOSAGE

Adult *PO* Initial dose 200mg/d with a usual daily dose of 300mg after 3d. Do *not* exceed a single dose of 150mg, or a dose ↑ of 100mg/d in a 3d period. Maximum dose 450mg/d

SIDE/ADVERSE EFFECTS: CNS: *headache, migraine, insomnia,* dizziness, seizure disorders, neuropsychiatric disturbances, *agitation, tremor,* anxiety ▪ CV: edema, ECG abnormalities, rare phlebitis, tachycardia, cardiac arrhythmias ▪ ENT: visual & auditory disturbances ▪ GI: *dry mouth, N/V, constipation,* anorexia, rare colitis and bleeding ▪ GU: nocturia, menstrual complaints, male sexual dysfunction ▪ INT: rash, pruritus, dry skin, alopecia, hair color change ▪ Other: weight loss, dyspnea, gynecomastia, fatigue, arthritis.

DRUG INTERACTIONS: Use with phenelzine ↑ toxicity ▪ Use c̄ L-dopa may produce ↑ in adverse effects ▪ Use with drugs that reduce seizure threshold is best avoided ▪ Use c̄ carbamazepine, cimetidine, phenobarbital, phenytoin requires caution.

NURSING MANAGEMENT

ADMINISTRATION: Assess for hx of hypersensitivity ▪ Assess neurologic status; may potentiate if impaired ▪ Assess for hx of bulimia, anorexia nervosa (↑ seizures) ▪ Administer first dose >14d after MAO-I therapy ▪ Assess hepatic, renal status; ↓ dosage if impaired ▪ Administer in 3 equally divided doses/d ▪ Institute safety, seizure precautions ▪ Institute suicide precautions ▪ Avoid abrupt withdrawal; D/C gradually ▪ Heavy smokers may require ↑ dosage ▪ Elderly may require ↓ dosage.

EVALUATION: Monitor CV, hepatic, renal status ▪ Monitor fluid retention (I&O, daily weight), constipation ▪ Assess for symptoms of abrupt withdrawal (nausea, headache, malaise) ▪ Assess for actual swallowing of PO forms ▪ May ↑ serum prolactin ▪ Assess for restlessness, agitation, insomnia after starting therapy; notify physician.

EDUCATION: Dizziness/drowsiness may occur; use caution in potentially hazardous activities ▪ Avoid use of alcohol, other CNS depressants for up to 1wk after end of therapy ▪ Take as directed by physician ▪ Use sugarless gum/hard candy to diminish dry mouth ▪ Constipation may occur; ↑ fluids, bulk-containing foods ▪ Check c̄ physician/pharmacist before taking OTC/Rx preparations ▪ Notify physician/dentist of use before treatment ▪ Store in tightly closed container ▪ Encourage recreational/ diversional interests ▪ Notify physician of fever, sore throat, malaise ▪ Keep scheduled appointments c̄ physician ▪ Women: notify physician of pregnancy possibility; avoid breastfeeding ▪ Full drug effects may require several wks of therapy.

NOTES:

busulfan • (byoo-sul-fan)

CATEGORY: *Alkylating agent*: antineoplastic

Rx; Preg Cat D

BRAND NAME	**DOSAGE FORM**
Myleran (B-W)	Tablet: 2mg

ACTION: Antineoplastic activity due to alkylating effect on DNA replication; irreversible crosslinking of DNA strands results in disruption of DNA activity, inhibition of DNA replication, transcription of RNA; cytotoxic effect is produced, esp on myeloid elements. **USE:** Drug of choice for chronic myelocytic leukemia ▪ Treatment of polycythemia vera.

PHARMACOKINETICS: Rapid PO absorption, c̄ blood levels appearing in 0.5-2h; extensively metabolized; up to 50% of single dose excreted in urine w/in 24h.

CONTRAINDICATIONS: Prior drug resistance; use only in adequately diagnosed chronic myelogenous leukemia.

DOSAGE

Pediatric *PO*	60-120μg/kg/d or 1.8mg/m^2
Adult *PO*	4-8mg/d; maintenance dose 1-3mg when remission period is <3 mo

SIDE/ADVERSE EFFECTS: GI: *diarrhea,* N/V, glossitis ▪ GU: amenorrhea, gynecomastia ▪ HEM: dose-related myelosuppression resulting in ***thrombocytopenia,*** pancytopenia ▪ INT: *hyperpigmentation,* anhidrosis, alopecia ▪ MET: hyperuricemia ▪ Other: ***interstitial pulmonary fibrosis.***

DRUG INTERACTIONS: Live vaccines contraindicated during therapy.▪ Radiation or other myelosuppressive drugs produce additive bone marrow depression.

NURSING MANAGEMENT

ADMINISTRATION: Check hx for recent course of radiation or antineoplastic agents; report to physician ▪ Administer on empty stomach ▪ Avoid exposure to moisture during storage ▪ Administer antiemetic before therapy ▪ Provide emotional support.

EVALUATION: Monitor CBC throughout therapy ▪ Assess for infection, bleeding, anemia ▪ May produce ↑ serum uric acid level ▪ Monitor hepatic function ▪ Assess hydration status (I&O, daily weight).

EDUCATION: Store in dry, well-closed container ▪ ↑ Fluid intake (10-12 glasses/d) ▪ Avoid exposure to infection ▪ Check c̄ physician before immunization (pt, family) ▪ Diet as tolerated; avoid spicy foods ▪ Maintain good oral hygiene; use soft-bristled toothbrush ▪ Notify physician of symptoms of bone marrow depression (fever, sore throat, bruising, bleeding, lethargy) ▪ Loss of hair may occur (reversible after therapy) ▪ Compliance c̄ prescribed dosage regimen ▪ Women: avoid breastfeeding ▪ Encourage ventilation of feelings ▪ Use contraception if sexually active.

NOTES:

butorphanol tartrate • (byoo-tor-fa-nole)

CATEGORY: *Analgesic*: opioid agonist/antagonist   Rx; Preg Cat C

BRAND NAME
Stadol (MJP)

DOSAGE FORMS
Injection (IM/IV): 1, 2mg/ml
Nasal spray: 10mg/ml

ACTION: Analgesic mechanism not determined; possible site of activity may be subcortical areas of brain; narcotic agonist activity of 2mg approximately equivalent to 10-15mg morphine; narcotic antagonist activity equivalent to 1/40 that of naloxone. **USE:** relief of moderate/severe pain ▪ Preop medication and as a supplement to balanced anesthesia.

DOSAGE

Adult *IV/IM*

Pain	2mg IM q3-4h or 1mg IV q3-4h. For severe pain 4mg IM or 2mg IV may be required
Pre-op	2mg IM 60-90m before surgery
Balanced anesthesia	Usual incremental dose 0.5-1mg IV
Nasal spray	1mg (1 spray) in one nostril. Repeat in 60-90m prn

PHARMACOKINETICS

PO absorption	Onset	Peak	Duration	Protein binding	Excretion
Complete	10-30m	30-60m	3-4h	80%	85% via urine, 15% via feces

CONTRAINDICATIONS: Hypersensitivity.

SIDE/ADVERSE EFFECTS: CNS: *sedation*, euphoria, hallucinations, dizziness, vertigo, headache ▪ CV: palpitations, BP changes ▪ EENT: blurred vision ▪ GI: vomiting, dry mouth ▪ INT: rash, hives ▪ RESP: respiratory depression ▪ Other: *autonomic responses* (clammy sweating, flushing/warmth, sensitivity to cold).

DRUG INTERACTIONS: Use c̄ CNS depressant produces additive effects ▪ Use in narcotic-dependent pts can produce withdrawal symptoms.

NURSING MANAGEMENT

ADMINISTRATION: Assess for hx of opioid hypersensitivity ▪ Check compatibility chart for mixing preop IM preparations ▪ Do *not* administer if respirations are <12/m ▪ IM: inject *deep* into muscle; rotate sites ▪ IV: dilute; administer *slowly* ▪ Do *not* administer SC ▪ Have narcotic antagonist/support measures available ▪ Avoid administration in pts with suspected head injury ▪ Administer *before* pt has intense pain ▪ Avoid light, freezing in storage ▪ Utilize + power of suggestion ▪ Avoid abrupt withdrawal ▪ Elderly may require ↓ dosage.

EVALUATION: Monitor respirations, circulatory function ▪ Assess bowel function, abdominal distention ▪ Assess renal function, urinary retention ▪ Check for signs of dependence c̄ prolonged use (↑ drug request) ▪ Assess for potentiation of CNS depressant effect ▪ Assess for signs of overdose (coma, pinpoint pupils, respiratory depression).

EDUCATION: Avoid changing positions (lying/sitting/standing) rapidly ▪ Avoid excessive sensory stimulation ▪ Keep bedrails up when nonambulatory ▪ Obtain assistance prn when ambulatory ▪ Turn, cough, deep breathe after surgery ▪ Constipation may occur; ↑ fluid, bulk-containing foods ▪ Avoid potentially hazardous activities ▪ Avoid smoking while taking drug ▪ Indiscriminate use may lead to dependence ▪ Avoid alcohol, other CNS depressants.

OVERDOSE MANAGEMENT: naloxone hcl is specific antidote, in conjunction c̄ supportive therapy using oxygen, IV fluids, vasopressors.

NOTES:

calcium salts • (kal-see-um)

CATEGORY: *Antacid*: mineral supplement OTC

Calcium Carbonate
CATEGORY: *Antacid*: mineral supplement OTC

DOSAGE FORMS: Tablet: various strengths: 1g 1-3 times/d PO

Calcium Chloride
CATEGORY: *Electrolyte*: mineral Rx; Preg Cat C

DOSAGE FORMS: Injection (IV): 10%
1g calcium chloride = 13.6mEq calcium

USE: Treatment of acute hypocalcemic tetany secondary to array of causes ▪ Cardiac resuscitation.

DOSAGE

IV 500mg/1g; subsequent dose schedule dependent on response
Cardiac resuscitation: ≥200mg injected into ventricular cavity

Calcium Gluconate
CATEGORY: *Electrolyte*: mineral

DOSAGE FORMS: Injection (IV): 10%
Tablet: various strengths (OTC)
1g of calcium = 4.5mEq calcium

ACTION: Calcium is required for tissue growth/maintenance, regulation of physiologic activities; nerve transmission, muscular contraction, blood coagulation, renal function; involved c̄ activating enzymes, cell membrane & capillary permeability, neurotransmitter & hormone activity, maintenance of teeth & skeletal system. **USE:** Calcium supplement esp in pregnancy, lactation ▪ Treatment of hypocalcemic conditions ▪ Antidote for magnesium, oxalic acid, carbon tetrachloride fluoride, strontium.

DOSAGE

Pediatric	*PO*	125mg/kg 1-4 times/d
	IV	500mg/kg
Adult	*PO*	1-15g qd
	IV	500mg-2g

CONTRAINDICATIONS: Hypercalcemia, ventricular fibrillation, lithiasis.

SIDE/ADVERSE EFFECTS: CNS: tingling sensations c̄ parenteral administration, depression of nerve functions ▪ CV: ***cardiac arrhythmias*** ▪ GI: anorexia, abdominal pain, N/V, constipation c̄ PO administration ▪ Other: hypercalcemia, azotemia, renal calculi, depression of muscle function.

DRUG INTERACTIONS: Use c̄ dig can produce cardiac arrhythmias ▪ Use c̄ tetracycline is contraindicated.

NURSING MANAGEMENT

ADMINISTRATION: PO forms: take 2h ac/3h pc (antacid), 1h pc (electrolyte replacement), c̄ meals (antihyperphosphatemic); do *not* administer w/in 1-2h of other PO medication; do *not* administer c̄ milk ▪ PO suspension: shake well before pouring; high Na^+ content ▪ Assess for Chvostek, Trousseau signs (hypocalcemia) ▪ IV: warm to body temperature; administer *slowly* (1ml/m) into large vein; use infusion control device, cardiac monitoring; maintain supine position for 1h after administration ▪ Do *not* administer calcium chloride IM/SC, calcium gluconate IM ▪ ↓ Sensory stimulation if hypocalcemic ▪ Consult dietician re dietary restrictions.

EVALUATION: Monitor VS, esp BP ▪ Monitor bowel function (constipation) ▪ Observe for signs of hypercalcemia (↓ muscle tone, confusion, fatigue); D/C drug, notify physician ▪ Check IV insertion site carefully; avoid extravasation ▪ Monitor activity (safety precautions); pad bedrails if hypocalcemic ▪ Monitor serum calcium level (normal: 8.5-10.5mg/dl) ▪ Monitor serum phosphate level (normal: 3-4.5mg/dl).

EDUCATION: Chew tablets thoroughly before swallowing ▪ Do *not* take c̄ milk ▪ PO suspension: shake well before pouring ▪ Follow dietician's suggestions of foods to avoid ▪ Notify physician *immediately* of nausea, muscle weakness, confusion; D/C drug ▪ Keep scheduled appointments c̄ physician/blood work ▪ Constipation may occur; ↑ fluids, use prescribed stool softener.

NOTES:

captopril • (kap-toe-pril)

CATEGORY: *Antihypertensive*: angiotensin inhibitor — Rx; Preg Cat C/D†

BRAND NAME
Capoten (Squibb)

DOSAGE FORMS
Tablet: 12.5, 25, 50, 100mg

COMBINATION PRODUCTS Rx

Capozide (Squibb) captopril/HCT per tablet: 25mg/15mg, 25mg/25mg, 50mg/15mg, 50mg/25mg. Dosage must be individualized starting c̄ 25mg/15mg tablet

PHARMACOKINETICS

PO absorption no food	Peak	Half-life	Protein binding	Excretion
75%	1h	2h	25%-30%	95% via urine in 24h as metabolites (60%), unchanged drug (40%)

ACTION: Antihypertensive activity appears related to suppression of renin-angiotensin-aldosterone system by competitive inhibition of ACE, which produces angiotensin II from angiotensin I, resulting in ↓ of peripheral arterial resistance, ↓ in aldosterone secretion. **USE:** Treatment of hypertension as sole agent or c̄ other antihypertensives ▪ Treatment of heart failure not responsive to conventional dig, diuretic therapy.

CONTRAINDICATIONS: Hypersensitivity. D/C during pregnancy as soon as possible.

DOSAGE

Adult *PO* — Start c̄ 25mg bid or tid. ↑ slowly to 50 or 100mg bid or tid. Usual dose range 25-150mg bid or tid. Do *not* exceed 450mg/d

SIDE/ADVERSE EFFECTS: CV: hypotension, tachycardia, chest pain, palpitations, ***MI*** (rare), CHF, Raynaud syndrome ▪ HEM: ***agranulocytosis, neutropenia***, anemia, ***thrombocytopenia*** ▪ GU: proteinuria ▪ INT: rash, pruritus, angioedema ▪ Other: reversible loss of taste.

Note: Side/adverse effects: common in *italic;* serious in ***boldface italic.***

*Available in Canada only.
† 1st trimester, C; 2nd & 3rd trimesters, D.

DRUG INTERACTIONS: Aspirin, indomethacin, other NSAIA may antagonize therapeutic response ▪ Use potassium-sparing diuretics c̄ caution due to hyperkalemia.

NURSING MANAGEMENT

ADMINISTRATION: Assess for hx of hypersensitivity ▪ Assess BP; notify physician of extremes ▪ Assess renal function; may require ↓ dosage if impaired ▪ May crush, administer c̄ liquid; *best* on empty stomach (1h ac) ▪ Assess serum Na^+ (normal: 135-145Eq/L); notify physician of abnormalities ▪ Assess for rapid ↓ in BP w/in 3h after administration of 1st dose (occurs c̄ hyponatremia) ▪ SLE, elderly may require ↓ dosage ▪ Avoid abrupt withdrawal; D/C gradually.

EVALUATION: Monitor VS, esp BP ▪ Monitor CBC (esp WBC, differential) throughout therapy ▪ Monitor electrolyte status (↑ K^+; ↓ Na^+) ▪ Monitor I&O, daily weight ▪ Monitor renal function (proteinuria); notify physician ▪ Assess for loss of taste ▪ Assess for edema in extremities.

EDUCATION: Dizziness may occur; use caution when engaging in potentially hazardous activities ▪ Avoid changing positions (lying/sitting/standing) rapidly ▪ Notify physician of fever, sore throat, bruising/bleeding, swelling of feet/legs ▪ Take as ordered by physician even if symptom free; do *not* skip doses ▪ Take 1h ac ▪ Do *not* D/C w/out notifying physician ▪ Check c̄ physician/pharmacist before taking OTC/Rx preparations ▪ Avoid high-Na^+ foods (canned soups, lunch meats, cheese) ▪ Avoid high-K^+ foods (bananas, citrus juices, raisins) ▪ Check c̄ physician before using salt substitutes ▪ Avoid ↑ exercise, temperature extremes, smoking ▪ Loss of taste may occur ▪ Tablets may smell like sulfur ▪ Used to control, *not* cure, hypertension ▪ Maintain optimum weight ▪ Keep scheduled appointments c̄ physician; have BP checked at regular intervals ▪ Women: avoid breastfeeding ▪ Full drug effects may require several wks of therapy.

NOTES:

carbamazepine •(kar-ba-maz-e-peen)

CATEGORY: *Anticonvulsant:* analgesic

Rx; Preg Cat C

BRAND NAMES

Tegretol (Geigy)

**Azo-carbamazepine (Apotex)*

**Mazepine (ICN)*

DOSAGE FORMS

Tablet: 100, 200mg

Suspension: 200mg/5ml

DOSAGE

Epilepsy

Children/Adult *PO* — >12y/o: 200mg bid on d1. ↑ weekly by adding up to 200mg/d. Usual maintenance dose 800-1200mg/d. Do *not* exceed 1200mg/d in children, 1600mg in adults. 6-12y/o: 100mg bid on d1. ↑ weekly by adding up to 100mg/d. Usual maintenance dose 400-800mg/d. Do *not* exceed 1000mg/d

Neuralgia

Adult *PO* — 100mg bid on d1. ↑ slowly by adding up to 200mg/d. Do *not* exceed 1200mg/d

ACTION: Anticonvulsant activity not determined; analgesic activity in trigeminal neuralgia due to ↓ of synaptic activity in trigeminal nucleus. **USE:** Treatment of partial seizures c̄ complex symptoms, grand mal, mixed seizure patterns in pts who have not responded to treatment c̄ other agents ▪ Pain associated c̄ trigeminal, glossopharyngeal neuralgia.

PHARMACOKINETICS

PO absorption	Peak	Half-life	Protein binding	Excretion
Adequate	4-5h	25-65h 5-20h in multiple doses	76%	Via urine (72%), feces (28%) as metabolites

CONTRAINDICATIONS: Hypersensitivity to drug, tricyclic antidepressants, previous bone marrow depression.

SIDE/ADVERSE EFFECTS: CNS: *dizziness, drowsiness,* headache, abnormal involuntary movements, peripheral

Note: Side/adverse effects: common in *italic;* serious in ***boldface italic.***

*Available in Canada only.

neuritis, paresthesias ■ CV: edema, arrhythmias, hypotension, CHF, A-V block, thrombophlebitis ■ EENT: blurred vision, transient diplopia, nystagmus, tinnitus, lens opacities ■ GI: N/V/D, gastric distress, abdominal pain, anorexia, constipation, dry mouth ■ GU: acute urinary retention, oliguria, azotemia, impotence ■ HEM: ***aplastic anemia, agranulocytosis, thrombocytopenia,*** eosinophilia ■ HEP: cholestatic/***hepatocellular jaundice***, hepatitis ■ INT: pruritic/erythematous rashes, urticaria, ***Stevens-Johnson syndrome***, photosensitivity, ***exfoliative dermatitis*** LE, alopecia, ***erythema multiforme***/nodosum, purpura ■ MS: leg cramps, arching muscle/joints ■ RESP: dyspnea, pneumonitis, pneumonia.

DRUG INTERACTIONS: Use c̄ doxycycline, phenytoin, warfarin, theophylline significantly ↓ their half-lives ■ Avoid use c̄ MAO-I ■ Use c̄ other bone marrow depressants can produce significant bone marrow toxicity.

NURSING MANAGEMENT

ADMINISTRATION: Assess for hx of hypersensitivity (incl tricyclic antidepressants) ■ Assess hepatic, hematologic status ■ Administer c̄ meals ■ PO suspension: shake well before using ■ Avoid abrupt withdrawal ■ Institute strict seizure precautions if drug is abruptly withdrawn ■ Elderly may require ↓ dosage.

EVALUATION: Monitor occurrence/characteristics of seizures ■ Monitor hepatic, hematologic status ■ Monitor for ↑ IOP ■ Monitor elderly for CNS, cardiac effects ■ Monitor PT if taking oral anticoagulants; may ↓ effects ■ May ↑ urine glucose, albumin; ↓ thyroid function tests ■ Assess for skin rash; notify physician, D/C drug ■ Monitor activity status (safety precautions) ■ Assess for symptoms of abrupt withdrawal (tremors, abdominal/muscle cramps, convulsions) ■ Therapeutic blood level: 4-12μg/ml.

EDUCATION: Do *not* omit daily dose ■ Do *not* use for general pain relief ■ Take c̄ meals ■ Keep scheduled appointments for periodic eye exams ■ Women: avoid breastfeeding ■ Diabetics: may ↑ urine sugar; monitor blood sugar ■ Dizziness/drowsiness may occur; use caution in potentially hazardous activities ■ Avoid use c̄ alcohol, other CNS depressants ■ Avoid changing positions (lying/sitting/standing) rapidly ■ Use sugarless gum/hard candy to diminish dry mouth ■ Avoid exposure to direct sunlight, UV light ■ Notify physician of fever, sore throat, bruising/bleeding ■ Safety precautions may be instituted (bedrails) ■ Do *not* smoke after taking drug ■ Carry medical identification (MedicAlert) ■ Notify physician/dentist of use before treatment.

NOTES:

carteolol hcl/penbutolol sulfate • (car-tee-oh-lole/pen-byoo-toe-lole)

CATEGORY: *Beta-adrenergic blocker*: antihypertensive — Rx; Preg Cat C

BRAND NAMES	DOSAGE FORMS
carteolol	
Cartrol (Abbott)	Tablet: 2.5, 5mg
penbutolol	
Levatol (R-C)	Tablet: 20mg

ACTION: Blocks access of catecholamine neurotransmitters to $beta_1$, $beta_2$ receptors, resulting in bronchial constriction, decreased heart rate, myocardial contractility ▪ Antihypertensive effect not determined. **USE:** Treatment of hypertension as a sole agent or with other antihypertensive agents (esp thiazide diuretics).

PHARMACOKINETICS

PO absorption	Peak	Half-life	Protein binding	Excretion
carteolol				
Complete	1-3h	6h	23%-30%	50%-70% as unchanged drug via urine
penbutolol				
Complete	1.5-3h	5h	—	Via urine as unchanged drug and metabolites

CONTRAINDICATIONS: Hypersensitivity, asthma, cardiogenic shock, sinus bradycardia, greater than 1° heart block; CHF, severe bradycardia (carteold).

DOSAGE

Normal renal function

Adult *PO*

carteolol	Initial single dose of 2.5mg/d c̄ gradual ↑ to single dose of 5mg or 10mg/d. Usual maintenance range 2.5-5mg once/d
penbutolol	10-40mg once/d. Usual dose 20mg/d

SIDE/ADVERSE EFFECTS: CNS: somnolence, paresthesia, anxiety, dizziness, headache, abnormal dreams, bradycardia, cold extremities, chest pain, tiredness ▪ CV: angina, arrhythmia, palpitations, 2° heart block ▪ GI: D/N/V, constipation, dyspepsia, flatulence ▪ GU: impotence, urinary frequency, UTI ▪ HEM: agranulocytosis, thrombocytopenic purpura ▪ INT: pruritus, rash, sweating ▪ MS: *muscle cramps*, arthritis, gout ▪ RESP: nasal congestion, pharyngitis, bronchospasm, respiratory distress ▪ Other: *asthenia*, blurred vision, conjunctivitis, tinnitus.

DRUG INTERACTIONS: Use c̄ reserpine, other catecholamine-depleting drugs can result in serious adrenergic blockage ▪ Nonselective beta-adrenergics may antagonize therapeutic response ▪ Use of general anesthetics, MAO-I best avoided ▪ Use with IV Ca blockers may prolong AV conduction time (carteolol) ▪ Diabetics may require dosage adjustments of antidiabetic agent ▪ NSAIA may ↓ antihypertensive action of beta blockers.

NURSING MANAGEMENT

ADMINISTRATION: Assess for hx of hypersensitivity ▪ Assess apical pulse; if <60/m hold drug, notify physician ▪ Assess respiratory function; do *not* administer if impaired ▪ Administer consistently c̄ or w/out food ▪ Elderly may require ↓ dosage ▪ Avoid abrupt withdrawal; D/C gradually.

EVALUATION: Monitor VS, esp BP (lying/standing), heart rate ▪ Monitor I&O, daily weight ▪ Assess peripheral circulation ▪ Diabetics: closely monitor blood glucose (hypoglycemia) ▪ Assess for edema in extremities ▪ Monitor hepatic, CV, renal, hemopoietic status c̄ long-term use.

EDUCATION: Dizziness may occur; use caution in potentially hazardous activities ▪ Avoid changing positions (lying/sitting/standing) rapidly ▪ Procedure for checking radial pulse ▪ Check pulse before taking; if <60/m do *not* take drug, notify physician ▪ Take as ordered by physician, even if symptom free; do *not* change dose ▪ Take consistently c̄ or w/out food ▪ Used to control, *not* cure, hypertension ▪ Avoid use c̄ alcohol ▪ Avoid ↑ exercise, temperature extremes, smoking ▪ Notify physician of muscle cramps, difficult breathing, cold extremities, leg edema ▪ Keep scheduled appointments c̄ physician; have BP checked regularly ▪ Maintain optimum weight ▪ Avoid high-Na^+ foods (canned soups, lunch meats, cheese) ▪ Check c̄ physician/pharmacist before taking OTC preparations ▪ Notify physician/dentist of use before treatment ▪ Do *not* D/C drug w/out checking c̄ physician ▪ Carry medical identification (MedicAlert) if hypertensive ▪ Do *not* abstain from food >12h (low blood sugar).

NOTES:

cefaclor • (sef-a-klor)

CATEGORY: *Cephalosporin* (2nd generation): Antibiotic

Rx; Preg Cat B

BRAND NAME

Ceclor (Lilly)

DOSAGE FORMS

PO suspension: 125, 187, 250, 375mg/ml

Capsule: 250, 500mg

ACTION: Bactericidal activity due to inhibition of mucopeptide cell wall synthesis in susceptible organisms. **USE:** Treatment of infections caused by susceptible strains of *Escherichia coli*, group A β-hemolytic streptococci, *Haemophilus influenzae, Klebsiella* spp, staphylococci.

PHARMACOKINETICS

PO absorption	Peak	Half-life	Excretion
Good	30-60m	0.6-0.9h	Via urine as unchanged drug

CONTRAINDICATIONS: Hypersensitivity to any cephalosporin.

DOSAGE

Pediatric *PO*	20mg/kg/d in divided doses q8h. For severe infections, 40mg/kg/d in divided doses q8h (otitis media)
Adult *PO*	250mg q8h, range 1-4g/d

SIDE/ADVERSE EFFECTS: GI: *diarrhea*, N/V, symptoms of ***pseudomembranous colitis*** ▪ GU: vaginitis ▪ HEM: eosinophilia ▪ HEP: transitory ↑ in AST, ALT, BUN ▪ INT: pruritus, urticaria, morbilliform eruptions, ***erythema multiforme***.

DRUG INTERACTIONS: Bacteriostatic antibiotics can antagonize bactericidal activity ▪ Use c̄ PO anticoagulants may ↑ their activity ▪ Use c̄ aminoglycosides may produce additive nephrotoxicity ▪ Use c̄ probenecid will ↓ renal excretion.

NURSING MANAGEMENT

ADMINISTRATION: Assess for hx of cephalosporin/penicillin hypersensitivity ▪ Obtain C&S before therapy ▪

Assess renal function; ↓ dosage if impaired ▪ Administer 1h ac/2h pc ▪ PO suspension: reconstitute powder according to manufacturer's directions; shake well before using; store reconstituted for 14d in refrigerator ▪ Avoid exposure to moisture/light during storage.

EVALUATION: Monitor VS, esp temperature ▪ Monitor hepatic, renal status ▪ Monitor CBC ▪ Urine glucose: false (+) c̄ Clinitest; use Clinistix/Tes-Tape.

EDUCATION: Complete full course of therapy (usually 10d) even if symptoms subside ▪ Can be taken c̄ meals, but *best* on empty stomach ▪ Take at equal intervals around clock to maintain blood levels ▪ Diarrhea may occur ▪ PO suspension: refrigerate; shake well before use ▪ Store in dry, tightly closed container ▪ Discard outdated preparations ▪ Maintain good personal hygiene, esp perineal, oral ▪ ↑ Fluid intake (8-10 glasses/d) ▪ Use Clinistix/Tes-Tape for urine testing ▪ Notify physician of symptoms of allergic rx (fever, difficult breathing, rash) ▪ Carry identification (MedicAlert) if cephalosporin allergic.

NOTES:

cefadroxil • (sef-a-drox-ill)

CATEGORY: *Cephalosporin* (1st generation): antibiotic

BRAND NAMES

Duricef (Princeton)
(Bristol [Canada])

Ultracef (Bristol)

DOSAGE FORMS

Duricef: Capsule: 500mg; PO suspension: 125, 250, 500mg/5ml; Tablet: 1g

Ultracef: Capsule: 500mg; PO suspension: 125, 250mg/5ml; Tablet: 1g

ACTION: Bactericidal activity due to inhibition of mucopeptide cell wall synthesis in susceptible organisms. **USE:** Treatment of infections caused by susceptible strains of *Escherichia coli*, group A β-hemolytic streptococci, *Klebsiella* spp, *Proteus mirabilis*, staphylococci.

PHARMACOKINETICS

PO absorption	Peak	Half-life	Excretion
Complete	1.5h	1-2h	90% via urine in 24h as unchanged drug

CONTRAINDICATIONS: Hypersensitivity to any cephalosporin.

DOSAGE

Pediatric *PO*	30mg/kg/d in divided doses q12h
Adult *PO*	1-2g/d as single dose or divided bid

SIDE/ADVERSE EFFECTS: GI: *diarrhea*, N/V, symptoms of ***pseudomembranous colitis*** ▪ GU: vaginitis ▪ HEM: eosinophilia ▪ HEP: transitory ↑ in AST, ALT, BUN ▪ INT: pruritus, urticaria, morbilliform eruptions, ***erythema multiforme***.

DRUG INTERACTIONS: Bacteriostatic antibiotics can antagonize bactericidal activity ▪ Use c̄ PO anticoagulants may ↑ their activity ▪ Use c̄ aminoglycosides may produce additive nephrotoxicity ▪ Use c̄ probenecid will ↓ renal excretion

NURSING MANAGEMENT

ADMINISTRATION: Assess for hx of cephalosporin/penicillin hypersensitivity ▪ Obtain C&S before therapy ▪ Assess renal function; ↓ dosage if impaired ▪ Administer

1h ac/2h pc ▪ PO suspension: reconstitute powder according to manufacturer's directions; shake well before using; store reconstituted for 14d refrigerated ▪ Avoid exposure to moisture/light during storage.

EVALUATION: Monitor VS, esp temperature ▪ Monitor hepatic, renal status ▪ Monitor CBC ▪ Urine glucose: false (+) $\bar{c}$ Clinitest; use Clinistix/Tes-Tape.

EDUCATION: Complete full course of therapy (usually 10d) even if symptoms subside ▪ Can be taken $\bar{c}$ meals, but *best* on empty stomach ▪ Take at equal intervals around clock to maintain blood levels ▪ Diarrhea may occur ▪ PO suspension: refrigerate; shake well before use ▪ Store in dry, tightly closed container ▪ Discard outdated preparations ▪ Maintain good personal hygiene, esp perineal, oral ▪ ↑ Fluid intake (8-10 glasses/d) ▪ Use Clinistix/Tes-Tape for urine testing ▪ Notify physician of symptoms of allergic rx (fever, difficult breathing, rash) ▪ Carry identification (MedicAlert) if cephalosporin allergic.

NOTES:

cefamandole • (sef-a-man-dole)

CATEGORY: *Cephalosporin* (2nd generation): antibiotic — Rx; Preg Cat B

BRAND NAME
Mandol (Lilly)

DOSAGE FORMS
Powder for injection (IM/IV): 0.5, 1, 2, 10g vials

ACTION: Bactericidal activity due to inhibition of mucopeptide cell wall synthesis in susceptible organisms. **USE:** Treatment of infections caused by susceptible strains of *Enterobacter* spp, *Escherichia coli,* group A β-hemolytic streptococci, *Haemophilus influenzae, Klebsiella* spp, *Proteus mirabilis, Proteus* spp, *Staphylococcus aureus* (incl penicillinase-producing strains), *Staphylococcus epidermidis, Streptococcus pneumoniae.*

PHARMACOKINETICS

IM peak	Half-life	Protein binding	Excretion
30-120m	1h	55%-75%	85% via urine in 8h as unchanged drug

CONTRAINDICATIONS: Hypersensitivity to any cephalosporin.

DOSAGE

Pediatric *IM/IV*	50-100mg/kg/d in equal doses q4-8h. Severe infections, up to 150mg/kg/d
Adult *IM/IV*	500mg-1g q4-8h. Severe infections, 1g q4-8h. Life-threatening, 2g q4h

SIDE/ADVERSE EFFECTS: GI: symptoms of ***pseudomembranous colitis,*** N/V ▪ HEM: neutropenia, ***thrombocytopenia, hemolytic anemia*** ▪ INT: maculopapular rash, urticaria ▪ MS: pain, induration c̄ repeated IM injection ▪ Other: ***thrombophlebitis at IV site.***

DRUG INTERACTIONS: Bacteriostatic antibiotics can antagonize bactericidal activity ▪ Use c̄ PO anticoagulants may ↑ their activity ▪ Use c̄ aminoglycosides may produce additive nephrotoxicity ▪ Use c̄ probenecid will ↓ renal excretion ▪ Use c̄ alcohol may produce disulfiram rx.

NURSING MANAGEMENT

ADMINISTRATION: Assess for hx of cephalosporin/penicillin hypersensitivity ▪ Obtain C&S before therapy ▪ Assess for hx of bleeding disorder; avoid use ▪ Assess renal function; ↓ dosage if impaired ▪ IM: reconstitute according to manufacturer's directions; administer by *deep, slow* injection into gluteal UOQ ▪ IV: dilute according to manufacturer's directions, inject *slowly* (3-5m); avoid aminoglycoside administration at same site; may administer IVPB ▪ Assess IV compatibility; avoid Mg^{++}, Ca^{++} ion solutions ▪ Do *not* administer discolored/precipitated solutions; yellow-amber color does *not* indicate ↓ potency ▪ Use reconstituted preparations w/in 24h at room temperature, 96h refrigerated ▪ Do *not* store in syringe; fill immediately before use ▪ Have support equipment available for anaphylaxis ▪ Surgical prophylaxis: D/C w/in 24h after surgery ▪ Na^+ content: 3.3mEq (77mg)/g; calculate in Na^+-restricted diets ▪ Maintain hydration ▪ Avoid concurrent use of alcohol-containing products.

EVALUATION: Monitor VS, esp temperature ▪ Monitor renal, hepatic, hemopoietic status ▪ Urine glucose: false (+) $\bar{c}$ Clinitest; use Clinistix/Tes-Tape ▪ False (+): urine protein testing ▪ Monitor coagulation studies (PT); may potentiate bleeding ▪ Observe for signs of superinfection (diarrhea, itching, oral ulcers).

EDUCATION: Use Clinistix/Tes-Tape for urine testing ▪ Women: avoid breastfeeding ▪ Diarrhea may occur ▪ Maintain good personal hygiene (esp perineal, oral) ▪ ↑ Fluid intake (8-10 glasses/d) ▪ Notify nurse/physician of symptoms of allergic rx (difficult breathing, rash) ▪ Carry identification (MedicAlert) if cephalosporin allergic ▪ IM injection may be painful ▪ Avoid alcohol intake ▪ Report any signs of bleeding immediately.

NOTES:

cefmetazole • (sef-met-a-zol)

CATEGORY: *Cephalosporin* (2nd generation): antibiotic — Rx; Preg Cat B

BRAND NAME
Zefazone (Upjohn)

DOSAGE FORMS
IV powder for injection: 1, 2 vials

ACTION: Bactericidal activity due to inhibition of mucopeptide cell well synthesis in susceptible organisms. **USE:** Treatment of infections caused by susceptible strains of *Bacteroides* spp, *Clostridium perfringens, Escherichia coli, Haemophilus influenzae* (non-penicillinase producing), *Klebsiella* spp, *Morganella morganii, Proteus* spp, *Providencia stuartii*, staphylococci (incl penicillinase producing), *Streptococcus* spp ▪ Pre-op prophylaxis to ↓ incidence of abdominal/vaginal hysterectomy, caesarean section, cholecystectomy, colorectal surgery infections.

CONTRAINDICATIONS: Hypersensitivity (cross-hypersensitivity can occur in up to 10% of pts c̄ penicillin allergies).

DOSAGE: Adult *IV* (Must be ↓ in renal impairment)

Infection	Usual dose 2g q6-12h for 5-14 d. Mild to moderate: 2g q8h (6g/d). Severe to life-threatening: 2g q6h (8g/d) Urinary 2g q12h (4g/d)
Surgical Prophylaxis	
Hysterectomy	
Abdominal	1g 30-90m before surgery and repeated 8 and 16h later
Vaginal	2g as single dose 30-90m before surgery or 1g 30-90m before surgery and repeated 8 and 16h later

PHARMACOKINETICS

IV (2g q6h) Max	Trough	Plasma half-life	Protein binding	Excretion
138mg/ml	6mg/ml	1.2h	65%	85% via urine in 12h as unchanged drug

C-section	2g as single dose after clamping cord or 1g after clamping cord and repeated 8 and 16h later
Cholecystectomy (high risk)	1g 30-90m before surgery and repeated 8 and 16h later
Colorectal	2g as single dose 30-90m before surgery and repeated 8 and 16h later

SIDE/ADVERSE EFFECTS: CNS: headache, hot flashes ▪ CV: ***shock,*** hypotension ▪ EENT: color perception alteration ▪ GI: diarrhea (3.6%), nausea (1%), vomiting, pain bleeding, candidiasis, ***pseudomembranous colitis*** (mild to life-threatening) ▪ INT: rash (1.1.%), pruritus, generalized erythema ▪ Local: pain, swelling at site of administration, phlebitis, ***thrombophlebitis*** ▪ RESP: pleural effusion, dyspnea, epistaxis ▪ Other: joint pain/inflammation, fever, vaginitis, superinfection.

DRUG INTERACTIONS: Alcohol can cause a disulfiram-like reaction ▪ Bacteriostasis antibiotics can antagonize bactericidal activity ▪ Use c̄ PO anticoagulants may ↑ activity ▪ Use c̄ aminoglycosides may produce additive nephrotoxicity ▪ Use c̄ probenecid ↓ renal excretion

NURSING MANAGEMENT

ADMINISTRATION: Assess for hx of cephalosporin/penicillin hypersensitivity ▪ Obtain C&S before therapy ▪ Assess renal function; ↓ dosage if impaired ▪ Reconstitute & dilute according to manufacturer's directions; administer IVPB over 30-60m ▪ Do *not* administer discolored/precipitated solutions; yellow-amber color does *not* indicate ↓ potency ▪ Use reconstituted IV preparations w/in 24h at room temperature, 7d refrigerated ▪ Have support equipment available for anaphylaxis ▪ Avoid exposure to light during storage ▪ Maintain hydration.

EVALUATION: Monitor VS, esp temperature ▪ Monitor renal, hepatic, hemopoietic status ▪ Urine glucose: false (+) c̄ Clinitest; use Clinistix/Tes-Tape ▪ Observe for signs of superinfection (diarrhea, itching, oral ulcer) ▪ Check IV site closely (phlebitis) ▪ Monitor prothrombin levels; assess for bleeding.

EDUCATION: Use Clinistix/Tes-Tape for urine testing ▪ Women: avoid breastfeeding ▪ Diarrhea may occur ▪ Avoid use c̄ alcohol ▪ Maintain good personal hygiene (esp perineal, oral) ▪ ↑ Fluid intake (8-10 glasses/d) ▪ Notify nurse/physician of symptoms of allergic rx (difficult breathing, rash, fever, bleeding, diarrhea) ▪ Carry identification (MedicAlert) if cephalosporin allergic.

cefazolin sodium •(sef-a-zoe-lin)

CATEGORY: *Cephalosporin* (1st generation): antibiotic   Rx; Preg Cat B

BRAND NAMES	DOSAGE FORMS
Ancef (SKB)	Powder for injection (IM/IV): 0.25, 0.5, 1, 5, 10g vials
Kefzol (Lilly)	Powder for injection (IM/IV): 0.25, 0.5, 1, 10g vials
Zolicef (Squibb)	Powder for injection (IM/IV): 0.5, 1g vials

ACTION: Bactericidal activity due to inhibition of mucopeptide cell wall synthesis in susceptible organisms. **USE:** Treatment of infections caused by susceptible strains of *Enterobacter aerogenes, Escherichia coli,* group A β-hemolytic streptococci, *Haemophilus influenzae, Klebsiella* spp, *Proteus mirabilis,* staphylococci (incl penicillinase strains), *Streptococcus pneumoniae.*

PHARMACOKINETICS

IM peak	Half-life	Excretion
0.5-1h	1-2.2h	100% via urine in 24h as unchanged drug

CONTRAINDICATIONS: Hypersensitivity to any cephalosporin.

DOSAGE

Pediatric *IM/IV*	25-50mg/kg/d in 3-4 doses. Severe infections, 100mg/kg/d
Adult *IM/IV*	Usual range 250mg-1g q8-12h. Severe infections, dosage given q6-8h. Life threatening infections, 1-1.5g q6h

SIDE/ADVERSE EFFECTS: GI: Symptoms of ***pseudomembranous colitis,*** N/V ▪ HEM: neutropenia, ***thrombocytopenia, hemolytic anemia*** ▪ INT: maculopapular rash, urticaria ▪ MS: pain, induration c̄ repeated IM injection ▪ Other: ***thrombophlebitis at IV site.***

DRUG INTERACTIONS: Bacteriostatic antibiotics can antagonize bactericidal activity ▪ Use c̄ PO anticoagulants may ↑ their activity ▪ Use c̄ aminoglycosides may produce additive nephrotoxicity ▪ Use c̄ probenecid will ↓ renal excretion.

Note: Side/adverse effects: common in *italic;* serious in ***boldface italic.***   *Available in Canada only.

NURSING MANAGEMENT

ADMINISTRATION: Assess for hx of cephalosporin/penicillin hypersensitivity ▪ Obtain C&S before therapy ▪ Assess renal function; ↓ dosage if impaired ▪ IM: reconstitute according to manufacturer's directions; administer by *deep, slow* injection into gluteal UOQ ▪ IV: dilute according to manufacturer's directions; inject *slowly* (3-5m); avoid aminoglycoside administration in same site ▪ Do *not* administer discolored/precipitated solution; yellow-amber color does *not* indicate ↓ potency ▪ Thaw frozen preparations completely at room temperature; do *not* refreeze; stable 24h at room temperature, 10d refrigerated; do *not* use if cloudy/precipitated ▪ Use reconstituted preparations w/in 24h at room temperature, 96h refrigerated ▪ Have support equipment available for anaphylaxis ▪ Surgical prophylaxis: D/C w/in 24h after surgery ▪ Na^+ content: 2.2mEq (48mg)/g; calculate in Na^+-restricted diets ▪ Maintain hydration.

EVALUATION: Monitor VS, esp temperature ▪ Monitor renal, hepatic, hemopoietic status ▪ Observe for signs of superinfection (diarrhea, itching, oral ulcers).

EDUCATION: Use Clinistix/Tes-Tape for urine testing ▪ Women: avoid breastfeeding ▪ Diarrhea may occur ▪ Maintain good personal hygiene (esp perineal, oral) ▪ ↑ Fluid intake (8-10 glasses/d) ▪ Notify nurse/physician of symptoms of allergic rx (difficult breathing, rash) ▪ Carry identification (MedicAlert) if cephalosporin allergic ▪ IM injection may be painful.

NOTES:

cefixime • (se-fix-eem)

CATEGORY: *Cephalosporin* (3rd generation): antibiotic Rx; Preg Cat B

BRAND NAME
Suprax (Lederle)

DOSAGE FORMS
PO suspension: 100mg/5ml
Tablet: 200, 400mg

ACTION: Bactericidal activity due to inhibition of mucopeptide cell wall synthesis in susceptible organisms. **USE:** Treatment of otitis media, respiratory and urinary tract infections caused by susceptible strains of *Escherichia coli*, group A β-hemolytic streptococci, *Haemophilus influenzae, Moraxella catarrhalis, Proteus mirabilis* ▪ Treatment of otitis media requires use of PO suspension (peak is 25%-50% higher).

PHARMACOKINETICS

PO absorption	Peak	Half-life	Protein binding	Excretion
40%-50%	2-6h	3-4h	65%	Via urine in 24h

CONTRAINDICATIONS: Hypersensitivity to any cephalosporin.

DOSAGE

Pediatric *PO* — 8mg/kg/day as a single dose or 4mg/kg q12h

Adult *PO* — 400mg daily as a single dose or as 200mg q12h

SIDE/ADVERSE EFFECTS: CNS: headache, dizziness ▪ GI: *N/V/D,* symptoms of *pseudomembranous colitis* ▪ GU: vaginitis, candidiasis, ***toxic nephropathy*** ▪ HEM: transitory eosinophilia, leukopenia, thrombocytopenia, ***aplastic anemia*** ▪ HEP: transitory ↑ in AST, ALT, BUN ▪ INT: rash, urticaria, pruritus, ***erythema multiforme, Stevens-Johnson syndrome, toxic epidermal necrolysis*** ▪ Other: fever, positive direct Coombs test.

DRUG INTERACTIONS: Bacteriostatic antibiotics can antagonize bactericidal activity ▪ Use $\bar{c}$ PO anticoagulants may ↑ their activity ▪ Use $\bar{c}$ aminoglycosides may produce additive nephrotoxicity ▪ Use $\bar{c}$ probenecid will ↓ renal excretion.

NURSING MANAGEMENT

ADMINISTRATION: Assess for hx of cephalosporin/penicillin hypersensitivity ▪ Obtain C&S before therapy ▪ Assess renal function; ↓ dosage if impaired ▪ Administer 1h ac/2h pc; may administer c̄ food to ↓ GI irritation ▪ PO suspension: reconstitute powder according to manufacturer's directions; shake well before using; refrigerate reconstituted drug ▪ Avoid exposure to moisture, light in storage ▪ Maintain hydration.

EVALUATION: Monitor VS, esp temperature ▪ Monitor hepatic, renal status ▪ Monitor CBC ▪ Urine glucose: false (+) c̄ Clinitest; use Clinistix/Tes-Tape.

EDUCATION: Complete full course of therapy (usually 10d) even if symptoms subside ▪ Can be taken c̄ meals; *best* on empty stomach ▪ Take at equal intervals around clock to maintain blood levels ▪ Diarrhea may occur ▪ PO suspension: refrigerate; shake well before use; stable 14d after reconstitution ▪ Store in dry, tightly closed light-resistant container ▪ Discard outdated preparations ▪ Maintain good personal hygiene (esp perineal, oral) ▪ ↑ Fluid intake (8-10 glasses/d) ▪ Use Clinistix/Tes-Tape for urine testing ▪ Notify physician of symptoms of allergic rx (fever, difficult breathing, rash) ▪ Carry identification (MedicAlert) if cephalosporin allergic ▪ Women: avoid breastfeeding.

NOTES:

cefonicid sodium • (sef-fon-i-sid)

CATEGORY: *Cephalosporin* (2nd generation): antibiotic Rx; Preg Cat B

BRAND NAME
Monocid (SKB)

DOSAGE FORMS
Powder for injection (IM/IV): 0.5, 1, 10g vials

ACTION: Bactericidal activity due to inhibition of mucopeptide cell wall synthesis in susceptible organisms; exhibits good resistance to β-lactamases (penicillinase, cephalosporinase). **USE:** Treatment of infections caused by susceptible strains of *Escherichia coli*, group A β-hemolytic *Streptococcus, Haemophilus influenzae, Klebsiella pneumoniae, Proteus mirabilis, Staphylococcus aureus* (incl penicillinase-producing strains), *Staphylococcus epidermidis, Streptococcus agalactiae, Streptococcus pneumoniae.*

PHARMACOKINETICS

IM peak	Half-life	Protein binding	Excretion
1.3h	4.5h	>90%	99% via urine in 24h as unchanged drug

CONTRAINDICATIONS: Hypersensitivity to any cephalosporin.

DOSAGE
Adult *IM/IV* 1g q24h. For severe infections, 2g q24h

SIDE/ADVERSE EFFECTS: GI: diarrhea, symptoms of ***pseudomembranous colitis*** ▪ GU: moniliasis, vaginitis ▪ HEM: neutropenia, leukopenia ▪ HEP: ↑ AST, ALT, LDH, alkaline phosphatase ▪ Other: pain, induration at IM site; ***phlebitis at IV site***.

DRUG INTERACTIONS: Bacteriostatic antibiotics can antagonize bactericidal activity ▪ Use c̄ PO anticoagulants may ↑ their activity ▪ Use c̄ aminoglycosides may produce additive nephrotoxicity ▪ Use c̄ probenecid will ↓ renal excretion.

NURSING MANAGEMENT
ADMINISTRATION: Assess for hx of cephalosporin/penicillin hypersensitivity ▪ Obtain C&S before therapy ▪ Assess renal function; ↓ dosage if impaired ▪ Reconstitute c̄ sterile H_2O for injection: 2ml/500mg, 2.5ml/1g ▪ IM:

administer by *deep, slow* injection into gluteal UOQ ▪ IV: inject *slowly* (3-5m); avoid aminoglycoside administration at same site; may administer IVPB ▪ Do *not* administer discolored/precipitated solutions; yellow-amber color does *not* indicate ↓ potency ▪ Use reconstituted preparations w/in 24h at room temperature or 72h refrigerated ▪ Have supportive equipment available for anaphylaxis ▪ Surgical prophylaxis: D/C w/in 24h after surgery ▪ Na^+ content: 3.7mEq (85mg)/g; calculate in Na^+-restricted diets ▪ Avoid exposure to heat/light during storage ▪ Maintain hydration.

EVALUATION: Monitor VS, esp temperature ▪ Monitor renal, hepatic, hemopoietic status ▪ Observe for signs of superinfection (diarrhea, itching, oral ulcers). ▪ Urine glucose: false (+) $\bar{c}$ Clinitest; use Clinistix/Tes-Tape.

EDUCATION: Use Clinistix/Tes-Tape for urine testing ▪ Women: avoid breastfeeding ▪ Diarrhea may occur ▪ Maintain good personal hygiene (esp perineal, oral) ▪ ↑ Fluid intake (8-10 glasses/d) ▪ Notify nurse/physician of symptoms of allergic rx (difficult breathing, rash) ▪ Carry identification (MedicAlert) if cephalosporin allergic ▪ IM injection may be painful.

NOTES:

cefoperazone sodium • (sef-oh-per-a-zone)

CATEGORY: *Cephalosporin* (3rd generation): antibiotic Rx; Preg Cat B

BRAND NAME
Cefobid (Roerig)
(Pfizer [Canada])

DOSAGE FORMS
Powder for injection IM/IV): 1,2, 10g vials

ACTION: Bactericidal activity due to inhibition of mucopeptide cell wall synthesis in susceptible organisms; good resistance to beta lactamases (penicillinase, cephalosporinase). **USE:** Treatment of infections caused by susceptible strains of *Bacteroides* (incl *B. fragilis), Clostridium* spp, *Enterobacter* spp, *Enterococcus* spp, *Escherichia coli*, group A β-hemolytic streptococci, *Haemophilus influenzae, Klebsiella pneumoniae, Neisseria gonorrhoeae, Proteus* spp (indole[+]/[-]), *Pseudomonas aeruginosa*, staphylococci (incl penicillinase-producing strains), *Streptococcus agalactiae, Streptococcus pneumoniae.*

PHARMACOKINETICS

IM peak	Half-life	Protein binding	Excretion
1-2h	1.6-2.6h	82%-93%	Mainly via feces, 30% via urine

CONTRAINDICATIONS: Hypersensitivity to any cephalosporin.

DOSAGE

Adult *IM/IV* 2-4g/d in divided doses q12h. Severe infections, 6-12g/d in 2, 3, 4 doses

SIDE/ADVERSE EFFECTS: GI: N/V/D, symptoms of ***pseudomembranous colitis*** ▪ GU: moniliasis, vaginitis ▪ HEM: neutropenia, eosinophilia ▪ INT: rash, pruritus ▪ Other: pain at IM site, ***phlebitis at IV site***.

DRUG INTERACTIONS: Use c̄ alcohol may produce disulfiram rx ▪ Bacteriostatic antibiotics can antagonize bactericidal activity ▪ Use c̄ PO anticoagulants may ↑ their activity ▪ Use c̄ aminoglycosides may produce additive nephrotoxicity ▪ Use c̄ probenecid will ↓ renal excretion.

NURSING MANAGEMENT

ADMINISTRATION: Assess for hx of cephalosporin/penicillin hypersensitivity ▪ Obtain C&S before therapy ▪ Assess for hx of bleeding disorder; avoid use ▪ Assess hepatic function; ↓ dosage if impaired ▪ IM: reconstitu-

Note: Side/adverse effects: common in *italic;* serious in ***boldface italic.*** *Available in Canada only.

ture according to manufacturer's directions ▪ IV: dilute c̄ 2.8-5ml suitable diluent recommended by manufacturer; do *not* administer bolus ▪ Allow solution to stand after reconstitution; vigorous shaking may be required ▪ Do *not* administer discolored/precipitated solution; yellow-amber color does *not* indicate ↓ potency ▪ Use reconstituted preparations w/in 24h at room temperature, 5d refrigerated ▪ Na^+ content: 1.5mEq (34mg)/g; calculate in Na^+-restricted diets ▪ Maintain hydration.

EVALUATION: Monitor VS, esp temperature ▪ Monitor renal, hepatic, hemopoietic status ▪ Urine glucose: false (+) c̄ Clinitest; use Clinistix/Tes-Tape ▪ False (+): urine protein testing ▪ Monitor coagulation studies (PT); drug may potentiate bleeding ▪ Observe for signs of superinfection (diarrhea, itching, oral ulcers).

EDUCATION: Use Clinistix/Tes-Tape for urine testing ▪ Women: avoid breastfeeding ▪ Diarrhea may occur ▪ Maintain good personal hygiene (esp perineal, oral) ▪ ↑ Fluid intake (8-10 glasses/d) ▪ Notify nurse/physician of symptoms of allergic rx (difficult breathing, rash) ▪ Carry identification (MedicAlert) if cephalosporin allergic ▪ IM injection may be painful ▪ Avoid alcohol intake ▪ Report any signs of bleeding immediately.

NOTES:

ceforanide • (se-for-a-nide)

CATEGORY: *Cephalosporin* (2nd generation): antibiotic Rx; Preg Cat B

BRAND NAME
Precef (ICN)

DOSAGE FORMS
Powder for injection (IM/IV): 0.5, 1g vials

ACTION: Bactericidal activity due to inhibition of mucopeptide cell wall synthesis in susceptible organisms; good resistance to some beta lactamases. **USE:** Treatment of infections caused by susceptible strains of *Escherichia coli*, group A β-hemolytic streptococci, *Haemophilus influenzae, Klebsiella pneumoniae, Proteus mirabilis, Staphylococcus aureus* (incl penicillinase-producing strains), *Staphylococcus epidermidis, Streptococcus pneumoniae.*

PHARMACOKINETICS

IM peak	Half-life	Protein binding	Excretion
1h	2.9h	80%	78%-95% via urine in 12h as unchanged drug

CONTRAINDICATIONS: Hypersensitivity to any cephalosporin.

DOSAGE

Pediatric *IM/IV*	20-40mg/kg/d in equal doses q12h
Adult *IM/IV*	0.5-1g bid

SIDE/ADVERSE EFFECTS: GI: diarrhea, symptoms of ***pseudomembranous colitis*** ▪ GU: moniliasis, vaginitis ▪ HEM: neutropenia, leukopenia, thrombocytosis ▪ HEP: ↑ AST, ALT, LDH, alkaline phosphatase ▪ Other: pain, induration at IM site, ***phlebitis at IV site***.

DRUG INTERACTIONS: Bacteriostatic antibiotics can antagonize bactericidal activity ▪ Use c̄ PO anticoagulants may ↑ their activity ▪ Use c̄ aminoglycosides may produce additive nephrotoxicity ▪ Use c̄ probenecid will ↓ renal excretion.

NURSING MANAGEMENT

ADMINISTRATION: Assess for hx of cephalosporin/penicillin hypersensitivity ▪ Obtain C&S before therapy ▪ Assess renal function; ↓ dosage if impaired ▪ IM: reconstitute according to manufacturer's directions; administer by *deep, slow* injection into gluteal UOQ ▪ IV: dilute

Note: Side/adverse effects: common in *italic;* serious in ***boldface italic.*** *Available in Canada only.

according to manufacturer's directions; inject *slowly* (3-5m); avoid aminoglycoside administration at same site; may administer IVPB ▪ Do *not* administer discolored/precipitated solution; yellow-amber color does *not* indicate ↓ potency ▪ Use reconstituted IM preparations w/in 48h at room temperature, 14d refrigerated; IV preparations w/in 24h at room temperature ▪ Have support equipment available for anaphylaxis ▪ Surgical prophylaxis: D/C w/in 24h after surgery ▪ Maintain hydration.

EVALUATION: Monitor VS, esp temperature ▪ Monitor renal, hepatic, hemopoietic status ▪ Urine glucose: false (+) $\bar{c}$ Clinitest; use Clinistix/Tes-Tape ▪ Observe for signs of superinfection (diarrhea, itching, oral ulcers).

EDUCATION: Use Clinistix/Tes-Tape for urine testing ▪ Women: avoid breastfeeding ▪ Diarrhea may occur ▪ Maintain good personal hygiene (esp perineal, oral) ▪ ↑ Fluid intake (8-10 glasses/d) ▪ Notify nurse/physician of symptoms of allergic rx (difficult breathing, rash) ▪ Carry identification (MedicAlert) if cephalosporin allergic ▪ IM injection may be painful.

NOTES:

cefotaxime sodium • (sef-oh-taks-eem)

CATEGORY: *Cephalosporin* (3rd generation): antibiotic

Rx; Preg Cat B

BRAND NAME

Claforan (H-R)
(Roussel in Canada)

DOSAGE FORMS

Powder for injection (IM/IV): 1, 2, 10g vials
Frozen: 1, 2g in 5% dextrose

ACTION: Bactericidal activity due to inhibition of mucopeptide cell wall synthesis in susceptible organisms; drug exhibits good resistance to penicillinases, cephalosporinases. **USE:** Treatment of infections caused by susceptible strains of *Bacteroides* (incl *B. fragilis*), *Citrobacter* spp, *Clostridium* spp, *Enterobacter* spp, *Enterococcus* spp, *Escherichia coli,* group A β-hemolytic streptococci, *Haemophilus influenzae, Klebsiella* spp, *Morganella morganii, Neisseria gonorrhoeae, Peptococcus* spp, *Peptostreptococcus* spp, *Proteus mirabilis, Proteus vulgaris, Providencia rettgeri, Serratia marcescens, Staphylococcus* (incl penicillinase-producing strains), *Staphylococcus epidermidis, Streptococcus pneumoniae.*

PHARMACOKINETICS

IM peak	Half-life	Protein binding	Excretion
30m	1h	30%-50%	60% via urine in 6h as metabolites, unchanged drug

CONTRAINDICATIONS: Hypersensitivity to any cephalosporin.

DOSAGE

Pediatric *IM/IV*	0-1wk: 50mg/kg IV q12h 1-4wks: 50mg/kg IV q8h 1mo-12y/o: 50-180mg/kg IM/IV in 4-6 equal doses. Do *not* exceed 12g/d
Adult *IM/IV*	1-2g q12h. Moderate infections, 1-2g IV q8h, 2g IV q6-8h. Serious infections, 2g IV q4h

SIDE/ADVERSE EFFECTS: CNS: headache ▪ GI: colitis, N/V/D, ***symptoms of pseudomembranous colitis*** ▪ GU: moniliasis, vaginitis ▪ HEM: granulocytosis, eosinophilia, neutropenia ▪ HEP: ↑ AST, ALT, LDH, alkaline phosphatase ▪ INT: rash, pruritus ▪ Other: fever, local IV/IM site pain, induration, tenderness.

DRUG INTERACTIONS: Bacteriostatic antibiotics can antagonize bactericidal activity ▪ Use c̄ oral anticoagulants may ↑ their activity ▪ Use c̄ aminoglycosides may produce additive nephrotoxicity ▪ Use c̄ probenecid ↓ renal excretion.

NURSING MANAGEMENT

ADMINISTRATION: Assess for hx of cephalosporin/penicillin hypersensitivity ▪ Obtain C&S before therapy ▪ Assess renal function; ↓ dosage if severely impaired ▪ IM: reconstitute according to manufacturer's directions; administer 2g in divided doses at different sites by *deep, slow* injection into gluteal UOQ ▪ IV: dilute according to manufacturer's directions, inject *slowly* (3-5m); avoid aminoglycoside administration at same site; may administer IVPB ▪ Do *not* administer discolored/precipitated solutions; yellow-amber color does *not* indicate ↓ potency ▪ Use reconstituted preparations w/in 24h at room temperature, 10d refrigerated, 13wks frozen ▪ Have support equipment available for anaphylaxis ▪ Surgical prophylaxis: D/C w/in 24h after surgery ▪ Na^+ content: 2.2mEq(51mg)/g; calculate in Na^+-restricted diets ▪ Maintain hydration.

EVALUATION: Monitor VS, esp temperature ▪ Monitor renal, hepatic, hemopoietic status ▪ Urine glucose: false (+) c̄ Clinitest; use Clinistix/Tes-Tape ▪ Observe for signs of superinfection (diarrhea, itching, oral ulcers).

EDUCATION: Use Clinistix/Tes-Tape for urine testing ▪ Women: avoid breastfeeding ▪ Diarrhea may occur ▪ Maintain good personal hygiene (esp perineal, oral) ▪ ↑ Fluid intake (8-10 glasses/d) ▪ Notify physician of symptoms of allergic rx (difficult breathing, rash) ▪ Carry identification (MedicAlert) if cephalosporin allergic ▪ IM injection may be painful.

NOTES:

cefotetan disodium • (se-fo-tih-tan)

CATEGORY: *Cephalosporin* (3rd generation): antibiotic Rx; Preg Cat B

BRAND NAME
Cefotan (Stuart)

DOSAGE FORMS
Powder for injection (IM/IV): 1, 2, 10g vials

ACTION: Bactericidal activity due to inhibition of mucopeptide cell wall synthesis in susceptible organisms. **USE:** Treatment of infections caused by susceptible strains of *Bacteroides* spp, *Escherichia coli, Fusobacterium* spp, *Haemophilus influenzae, Klebsiella* spp, *Morganella morganii, Neisseria gonorrhoeae, Peptococcus* spp, *Peptostreptococcus* spp, *Proteus mirabilis, Proteus vulgaris, Staphylococcus aureus* (incl penicillinase producing), *Staphylococcus epidermidis, Streptococcus pneumoniae, Streptococcus pyogenes* ▪ Surgical infection prophylaxis.

PHARMACOKINETICS

Peak IM	Peak IV	Half-life	Protein binding	Excretion
1-3h	5-30m	3-4.6h	88%	51%-81% via urine, unchanged in 24h

CONTRAINDICATIONS: Hypersensitivity to any cephalosporin.

DOSAGE

Adult *IM/IV* 500mg-1g q12h. Severe infections may require 2g q12h IV. For life-threatening infection 3g q12h IV. Do *not* exceed 6g/d. Dosage must be ↓ c̄ renal impairment

SIDE/ADVERSE EFFECTS: GI: N/V/D, symptoms of ***pseudomembranous colitis*** ▪ GU: vaginitis ▪ HEM: eosinophilia ▪ HEP: transitory ↑ in AST, ALT, BUN ▪ INT: pruritus, urticaria, morbilliform eruptions, ***erythema multiforme***.

DRUG INTERACTIONS: Bacteriostatic antibiotics can antagonize bactericidal activity ▪ Use c̄ PO anticoagulants may ↑ their activity ▪ Use c̄ aminoglycosides may produce additive nephrotoxicity ▪ Use c̄ probenecid ↓ renal excretion.

Note: Side/adverse effects: common in *italic;* serious in ***boldface italic.***

*Available in Canada only.

NURSING MANAGEMENT

ADMINISTRATION: Assess for hx of cephalosporin/penicillin hypersensitivity ▪ Obtain C&S before therapy ▪ Assess for hx of impaired renal function; ↓ dosage ▪ IM: reconstitute according to manufacturer's directions; administer by *deep, slow* injection into gluteal UOQ ▪ IV: dilute c̄ sterile H_2O for injection; administer *slowly* (3-5m); avoid aminoglycoside administration at same site; may administer IVPB ▪ Do *not* administer discolored/precipitated solutions; yellow-amber color does *not* affect potency ▪ Frozen preparations: thaw completely at room temperature: do *not* refreeze; stable 24h at room temperature, 7d refrigerated ▪ Use reconstituted preparations w/in 18h at room temperature, 7d refrigerated ▪ Have support equipment available for anaphylaxis ▪ Na^+ content: 2.3mEq (54mg)/g; calculate in Na^+-restricted diets ▪ Maintain hydration.

EVALUATION: Monitor VS, esp temperature ▪ Monitor renal, hepatic, hematologic status ▪ Urine glucose: false (+) c̄ Clinitest; use Clinistix/Tes-Tape ▪ Observe for signs of superinfection (diarrhea, perineal itching, oral ulcers) ▪ Check IV site carefully; monitor for phlebitis (red streak, heat, pain).

EDUCATION: Use Clinistix/Tes-Tape for urine testing ▪ Women: avoid breastfeeding ▪ Diarrhea may occur ▪ Maintain good personal hygiene (esp perineal, oral) ▪ Maintain fluid intake (6-8 glasses/d) ▪ Notify physician of symptoms of allergic rx (difficult breathing, rash) ▪ Carry identification (MedicAlert) if cephalosporin allergic ▪ IM injection may be painful.

NOTES:

cefoxitin sodium • (se-fox-i-tin)

CATEGORY: *Cephalosporin* (2nd generation): antibiotic — Rx; Preg Cat B

BRAND NAME
Mefoxin (MSD)
(Frosst [Canada])

DOSAGE FORMS
Powder for injection (IM/IV): 1, 2, 10g vials
Frozen: 1, 2g in 5% dextrose injection

ACTION: Bactericidal activity due to inhibition of mucopeptide cell wall synthesis in susceptible organisms. **USE:** Treatment of infections caused by susceptible strains of *Bacteroides* spp, *Clostridium* spp, *Escherichia coli*, group B streptococci, *Haemophilus influenzae, Neisseria gonorrhoeae, Peptococcus* spp, *Peptostreptococcus* spp, *Proteus mirabilis, Proteus* spp (indole [+]), *Providencia* spp, staphylococci (incl penicillinase strains), *Streptococcus pneumoniae.*

PHARMACOKINETICS

IM peak	Half-life	Protein binding	Excretion
20-30m	64.8m	55%-75%	85% via urine in 6h as unchanged drug

CONTRAINDICATIONS: Hypersensitivity to any cephalosporin.

DOSAGE

Pediatric *IM/IV*	80-160mg/kg/d in 4-6 equal doses
Adult *IM/IV*	1-2g q6-8h. Severe infection, 1g q4h or 2g q6-8h (IV). Life-threatening infection, 2g q4h or 3g q6h (IV)

SIDE/ADVERSE EFFECTS: GI: symptoms of ***pseudomembranous colitis,*** N/V ▪ HEM: neutropenia, thrombocytopenia, hemolytic anemia ▪ INT: maculopapular rash, urticaria ▪ Other: pain, induration c̄ repeated IM injection; ***thrombophlebitis at iv site*** c̄ 6g dose given over 3d.

DRUG INTERACTIONS: Bacteriostatic antibiotics can antagonize bactericidal activity ▪ Use c̄ PO anticoagulants may ↑ their activity ▪ Use c̄ aminoglycosides may produce additive nephrotoxicity ▪ Use c̄ probenecid will ↓ renal excretion.

NURSING MANAGEMENT

ADMINISTRATION: Assess for hx of cephalosporin/penicillin hypersensitivity ▪ Obtain C&S before therapy ▪ Assess renal function; ↓ dosage if impaired ▪ IM: reconstitute c̄ 2ml sterile H_2O for injection or 0.5% or 1% lidocaine HCl injection (w/out epinephrine) ▪ IV: dilute c̄ sterile H_2O for injection; inject *slowly* (3-5m); avoid aminoglycoside administration at same site ▪ Do *not* administer discolored/precipitated solutions; yellow-amber color does *not* indicate ↓ potency ▪ Thaw frozen preparations completely at room temperature; do *not* refreeze; stable 24h at room temperature, 48h refrigerated ▪ Use reconstituted preparations w/in 24h at room temperature, 7d refrigerated, 30wks frozen ▪ Have support equipment available for anaphylaxis ▪ Surgical prophylaxis: D/C w/in 24h after surgery ▪ Na^+ content: 2.3mEq (54mg)/g; calculate in Na^+-restricted diets ▪ Avoid alkaline or strong acid solutions ▪ Maintain hydration.

EVALUATION: Monitor VS, esp temperature ▪ Monitor renal, hepatic, hemopoietic status ▪ Observe for signs of superinfection (diarrhea, itching, oral ulcers).

EDUCATION: Use Clinistix/Tes-Tape for urine testing ▪ Women: avoid breastfeeding ▪ Diarrhea may occur ▪ Maintain good personal hygiene (esp perineal, oral) ▪ ↑ Fluid intake (8-10 glasses/d) ▪ Notify nurse/physician of symptoms of allergic rx (difficult breathing, rash) ▪ Carry identification (MedicAlert) if cephalosporin allergic ▪ IM injection may be painful.

NOTES:

ceftazidime • (sef-tay-zi-deem)

CATEGORY: *Cephalosporin* (3rd generation): antibiotic Rx: Preg Cat B

BRAND NAMES	DOSAGE FORMS
Fortaz (Glaxo)	Powder for injection (IM/IV): 500mg; 1, 2, 6g Frozen: 1, 2g in 5% dextrose injection
Tazidime (Lilly)	Powder for injection (IM/IV): 500mg; 1, 2, 6g
Tazicef (SKB)	Powder for injection: 1, 2, 6g

ACTION: Bactericidal activity due to inhibition of mucopeptide cell wall synthesis in susceptible organisms. **USE:** Treatment of infections caused by susceptible strains of *Bacteroides* spp, *Citrobacter* spp, *Enterobacter* spp, *Escherichia coli, Haemophilus influenzae, Klebsiella* spp, *Neisseria meningitidis, Proteus mirabilis, Pseudomonas* spp, *Serratia* spp, *Staphylococcus aureus, Streptococcus pneumoniae, Streptococcus pyogenes.*

PHARMACOKINETICS

Peak		Half-	Protein	
IM	IV	life	binding	Excretion
1h	0.5h	2h	10%	80%-90% via urine unchanged in 24h

CONTRAINDICATIONS: Hypersensitivity to any cephalosporin.

DOSAGE

Pediatric *IV*	
Neonate	30mg/kg q12h
Infants/children	30-50mg/kg q8h. 6g/d may be required c̄ cystic fibrosis, meningitis, immunodeficiency
Adult *IM/IV*	250mg-1g q8-12h. For bone/joint infections, usually 2g q12h IV. For serious and life-threatening infection, 2g q8h IV. Dosage must be ↓ in renal impairment

SIDE/ADVERSE EFFECTS: GI: N/V/D, symptoms of ***pseudomembranous colitis*** ▪ UG: vaginitis ▪ HEM: eosinophilia ▪ HEP: transitory ↑ in AST, ALT, BUN ▪ INT: pruritus, urticaria, morbilliform eruptions, ***erythema multiforme.***

Note: Side/adverse effects: common in *italic;* serious in ***boldface italic.*** *Available in Canada only.

DRUG INTERACTIONS: Bacteriostatic antibiotics can antagonize bactericidal activity ▪ Use c̄ PO anticoagulants may ↑ their activity ▪ Use c̄ aminoglycosides may produce additive nephrotoxicity ▪ Use c̄ probenecid ↓ renal excretion.

NURSING MANAGEMENT

ADMINISTRATION: Assess for hx of cephalosporin/penicillin hypersensitivity ▪ Obtain C&S before therapy ▪ Assess renal status; ↓ dosage if impaired ▪ IM: reconstitute according to manufacturer's directions; administer by *deep, slow* injection into gluteal UOQ ▪ IV: dilute c̄ sterile H_2O for injection; administer *slowly* (3-5m); avoid aminoglycoside administration at same site; may administer IVPB ▪ Do *not* administer discolored/precipitated solutions; yellow-amber color does *not* indicate ↓ potency ▪ Frozen preparations: thaw completely at room temperature; do *not* refreeze; stable 24h at room temperature, 7d refrigerated ▪ Use reconstituted preparations w/in 18h at room temperature, 7d refrigerated ▪ Have support equipment available for anaphylaxis ▪ Na^+ content: 2.3mEq (54mg)/g; calculate in Na^+-restricted diets ▪ Maintain hydration.

EVALUATION: Monitor VS, esp temperature ▪ Monitor renal, hepatic, hematologic status ▪ Urine glucose: false (+) c̄ Clinitest; use Clinistix/Tes-Tape ▪ Observe for signs of superinfection (diarrhea, perineal itching, oral ulcers) ▪ Check IV site carefully; monitor for phlebitis (red streak, heat, pain).

EDUCATION: Use Clinistix/Tes-Tape for urine testing ▪ Women: avoid breastfeeding ▪ Diarrhea may occur ▪ Maintain good personal hygiene (esp perineal, oral) ▪ Maintain fluid intake (6-8 glasses/d) ▪ Notify physician of symptoms of allergic rx (difficult breathing, rash) ▪ Carry identification (MedicAlert) if cephalosporin allergic ▪ IM injection may be painful.

NOTES:

ceftizoxime • (sef-ti-zox-eem)

CATEGORY: *Cephalosporin* (3rd generation): antibiotic — Rx; Preg Cat B

BRAND NAME
Cefizox (Fujisawa)

DOSAGE FORMS
Powder for injection (IM/IV): 1, 2, 10g vials
Frozen: 1, 2g in 5% dextrose solution

PHARMACOKINETICS

IM peak	Half-life	Protein binding	Excretion
0.5-1.5h	1.7h	30%	Via urine in 24h as unchanged drug

ACTION: Bactericidal activity due to inhibition of mucopeptide cell wall synthesis in susceptible organisms; good resistance to β-lactamases (penicillinase, cephalosporinase). **USE:** Treatment of infections caused by susceptible strains of *Bacteroides* (incl *B. fragilis*), *Enterobacter* spp, *Escherichia coli*, group A β-hemolytic streptococci, *Haemophilus influenzae, Klebsiella* spp, *Morganella morganii, Neisseria gonorrhoeae, Peptococcus* spp, *Peptostreptococcus* spp, *Proteus mirabilis, Proteus vulgaris, Providencia rettgeri, Pseudomonas* spp, *Serratia* spp, staphylococci (incl penicillinase-producing strains), *Staphylococcus epidermidis, Streptococcus pneumoniae.*

CONTRAINDICATIONS: Hypersensitivity to any cephalosporin.

DOSAGE

Pediatric *IM/IV*	>6mo: 50mg/kg q6-8h. May be ↑ 200mg/kg/d if needed
Adult *IM/IV*	500mg-2g q8-12h. Life-threatening infections, 3-4g q8h

SIDE/ADVERSE EFFECTS: GI: N/V/D, symptoms of ***pseudomembranous colitis*** ▪ GU: moniliasis, vaginitis ▪ HEM: anemia, leukopenia, neutropenia, ***thrombocytopenia*** ▪ INT: rash, pruritus ▪ Other: pain, induration at IM site, ***phlebitis at IV site***.

DRUG INTERACTIONS: Bacteriostatic antibiotics can antagonize bactericidal activity ▪ Use c̄ PO anticoagulants may ↑ their activity ▪ Use c̄ aminoglycosides may produce additive nephrotoxicity ▪ Use c̄ probenecid will ↓ renal excretion.

NURSING MANAGEMENT

ADMINISTRATION: Assess for hx of cephalosporin/penicillin hypersensitivity ▪ Obtain C&S before therapy ▪ Assess renal function; ↓ dosage if impaired ▪ IM: reconstitute according to manufacturer's directions; administer 2g as divided doses at different sites by *deep, slow* injection into gluteal UOQ ▪ IV: dilute c̄ sterile H_2O for injection; administer *slowly* (3-5m); avoid aminoglycoside administration at same site; may administer IVPB ▪ Do *not* administer discolored/precipitated solutions; yellow-amber color does *not* indicate potency ▪ Thaw frozen preparations completely at room temperature; do *not* refreeze; stable 24h at room temperature, 10d refrigerated ▪ Use reconstituted preparations w/in 8h at room temperature, 48h refrigerated ▪ Have support equipment available for anaphylaxis ▪ Na^+ content: 2.6mEq (60mg)/g; calculate in Na^+-restricted diets ▪ Avoid exposure to light during storage ▪ Maintain hydration.

EVALUATION: Monitor VS, esp temperature ▪ Monitor renal, hepatic, hemopoietic status ▪ Urine glucose: false (+) c̄ Clinitest; use Clinistix/Tes-Tape ▪ Observe for signs of superinfection (diarrhea, itching, oral ulcers).

EDUCATION: Use Clinistix/Tes-Tape for urine testing ▪ Women: avoid breastfeeding ▪ Diarrhea may occur ▪ Maintain good personal hygiene (esp perineal, oral) ▪ ↑ Fluid intake (8-10 glasses/d) ▪ Notify nurse/physician of symptoms of allergic rx (difficult breathing, rash) ▪ Carry identification (MedicAlert) if cephalosporin allergic ▪ IM injection may be painful.

NOTES:

ceftriaxone sodium• (sef-try-ax-one)

CATEGORY: *Cephalosporin* (3rd generation): antibiotic   Rx; Preg Cat B

BRAND NAME
Rocephin (Roche)

DOSAGE FORMS
IM/IV powder: 0.25, 0.5, 1, 2, 10g vial
Frozen: 1, 2g in dextrose injection

ACTION: Bactericidal activity due to inhibition of mucopeptide cell wall synthesis in susceptible organisms. **USE:** Treatment of infections caused by susceptible strains of *Enterobacter* spp, *Escherichia coli* group A β-hemolytic streptococci, *Haemophilus influenzae, Haemophilus parainfluenzae, Klebsiella* spp, *Morganella morganii, Neisseria gonorrhoeae, Neisseria meningitidis, Proteus mirabilis, Proteus vulgaris, Pseudomonas aeruginosa, Serratia marcescens, Staphylococcus aureus* (incl penicillinase-producing strains), *Staphylococcus epidermidis, Streptococcus pneumoniae.*

PHARMACOKINETICS

IM peak	Half-life	Protein binding	Excretion
2h	5.8-8.7h	95%	33%-67% via urine as unchanged drug, remainder in feces as metabolites

CONTRAINDICATIONS: Hypersensitivity to any cephalosporin.

DOSAGE

Pediatric *IM/IV*	50-75mg/kg divided q12h. For meningitis, 100mg/kg divided q12h
Adult *IM/IV*	1-2g/d as single dose or divided. Do *not* exceed 4g/d

SIDE/ADVERSE EFFECTS: CNS: headache ▪ GI: N/V/D, taste impairment ▪ GU: moniliasis, vaginitis ▪ HEM: eosinophilia, thrombocytosis, leukopenia, anemia, neutropenia, ***thrombocytopenia*** ▪ HEP: ↑ AST, ALT, alkaline phosphatase, bilirubin ▪ INT: pruritus ▪ Other: pain, induration at IM site, phlebitis at IV site.

DRUG INTERACTIONS: Use $\bar{c}$ alcohol may produce disulfiram rx ▪ Use $\bar{c}$ oral anticoagulants may ↑ their activity ▪ Bacteriostatic antibiotics can antagonize bactericidal activity ▪ Use $\bar{c}$ probenecid will ↓ renal excretion.

NURSING MANAGEMENT

ADMINISTRATION: Assess for hx of cephalosporin/penicillin hypersensitivity ▪ Obtain C&S before therapy ▪ Assess renal function; ↓ dosage if impaired ▪ IM: reconstitute according to manufacturer's directions; administer by *deep, slow* injection into gluteal UOQ ▪ IV: dilute according to manufacturer's directions; avoid aminoglycoside administration at same site; may administer IVPB ▪ Frozen preparations: thaw completely at room temperature; do *not* refreeze ▪ Do *not* administer discolored/precipitated solutions; yellow-amber color does *not* indicate ↓ potency ▪ Use reconstituted IM/IV preparations w/in 3d at room temperature, 10d refrigerated ▪ Have support equipment available for anaphylaxis ▪ Surgical prophylaxis: D/C w/in 24h after surgery ▪ Na^+ content: 3.6mEq (83mg)/g; calculate in Na^+-restricted diets ▪ Avoid exposure to heat, light in storage ▪ Maintain hydration.

EVALUATION: Monitor VS, esp temperature ▪ Monitor renal, hepatic, hemopoietic status ▪ Urine glucose: false (+) $\bar{c}$ Clinitest; use Clinistix/ Tes-Tape ▪ Observe for signs of superinfection (diarrhea, itching, oral ulcers) ▪ Monitor PT.

EDUCATION: Use Clinistix/Tes-Tape for urine testing ▪ Women: avoid breastfeeding ▪ Diarrhea may occur ▪ Maintain good personal hygiene (esp perineal, oral) ▪ ↑ Fluid intake (8-10 glasses/d) ▪ Notify physician of symptoms of allergic rx (difficult breathing, rash) ▪ Carry identification (MedicAlert) if cephalosporin allergic ▪ IM injection may be painful.

NOTES:

cefuroxime sodium/cefuroxime axetil ▲• (se-fyoor-ox-eem)

CATEGORY: *Cephalosporin* (2nd generation): antibiotic Rx; Preg Cat B

BRAND NAMES

Ceftin ▲ *(A-H)*

Kefurox (Lilly)

Zinacef (Glaxo)

DOSAGE FORMS

Tablet: 125, 250, 500mg

IM/IV powder: 0.75, 1.5, 7.5g vial

IM/IV powder: 0.75, 1.5g vial

Frozen: 0.75, 1.5g

ACTION: Bactericidal activity due to inhibition of mucopeptide cell wall synthesis in susceptible organisms; drug exhibits good resistance to some β-lactamases.

USE: Treatment of infections caused by susceptible strains of *Enterobacter aerogenes, Escherichia coli*, group A β-hemolytic streptococci, *Haemophilus influenzae, Klebsiella pneumoniae, Neisseria gonorrhoeae, Neisseria meningitidis, Staphylococcus aureus* (incl penicillinase-producing strains), *Streptococcus pneumoniae.*

PHARMACOKINETICS

IM peak	Half-life	Protein binding	Excretion
15-60m	1-2h	35%-50%	89%-100% via urine in 24h as unchanged drug

CONTRAINDICATIONS: Hypersensitivity to any cephalosporin.

DOSAGE

Pediatric *IM/IV*	50-100mg/kg/d divided q6-8h >3mo: For meningitis, 200-240mg/kg/d divided q6-8h. ↓ To 100mg/kg/d after clinical improvement
Adult *IM/IV*	0.75-1.5g q8h. For serious infections, 1.5g q6h

SIDE/ADVERSE EFFECTS: GI: N/V/D, symptoms of ***pseudomembranous colitis*** ▪ GU: moniliasis, vaginitis ▪ HEM: ↓ hematocrit/hemoglobin, neutropenia, leukopenia ▪ HEP: ↑ AST, ALT, LDH, alkaline phosphatase, bilirubin ▪ Other: pain, induration at IM site, ***phlebitis*** at IV site.

DRUG INTERACTIONS: Bacteriostatic antibiotics can antagonize bactericidal activity ▪ Use c̄ PO anticoagulants may ↑ their activity ▪ Use c̄ aminoglycosides may produce additive nephrotoxicity ▪ Use c̄ probenecid ↓ renal excretion.

NURSING MANAGEMENT

ADMINISTRATION: Assess for hx of cephalosporin/penicillin hypersensitivity ▪ Obtain C&S before therapy ▪ Assess renal function; ↓ dosage if impaired ▪ IM: reconstitute c̄ 3.6ml sterile H_2O for injection; shake suspension well; administer by *deep, slow* injection into gluteal UOQ ▪ IV: dilute according to manufacturer's directions; inject *slowly* (3-5m); avoid aminoglycoside administration at same site; may administer IVPB ▪ Frozen preparations: thaw completely at room temperature; do *not* refreeze ▪ Do *not* administer discolored/precipitated solutions; yellow-amber color does *not* indicate ↓ potency ▪ Use reconstituted preparations w/in 24h at room temperature, 48h refrigerated ▪ Have support equipment available for anaphylaxis ▪ Surgical prophylaxis: D/C w/in 24h after surgery ▪ Na^+ content: 2.4mEq (55mg)/g; calculate in Na^+-restricted diets ▪ Avoid exposure to light in storage ▪ Maintain hydration ▪ PO: administer c̄ food; do *not* crush tablet (bitter); swallow whole.

EVALUATION: Monitor VS, esp temperature ▪ Monitor renal, hepatic, hemopoietic status ▪ Urine glucose: false (+) c̄ Clinitest; use Clinistix/Tes-Tape ▪ Blood glucose: false (-) c̄ ferricyanide methods ▪ Observe for signs of superinfection (diarrhea, itching, oral ulcers).

EDUCATION: Use Clinistix/Tes-Tape for urine testing ▪ Women: avoid breastfeeding ▪ Diarrhea may occur ▪ Maintain good personal hygiene (esp perineal, oral).

NOTES:

cephalexin/cephalexin hcl ▲ • (sef-a-lex-in)

CATEGORY: *Cephalosporin* (1st generation): antibiotic   Rx; Preg Cat B

BRAND NAMES	DOSAGE FORMS
**Ceporex (Glaxo)*	
Keflet (Dista)	Tablet: 0.25, 0.5, 1g
Keflex (Dista)	Capsule: 250, 500mg Pediatric drops: 100mg/ml PO suspension: 125, 250mg/5m
Keftab ▲ (Dista)	Tablet: 250, 500mg
**Novolexin (Novopharm)*	Tablet: 1g

ACTION: Bactericidal activity due to inhibition of mucopeptide cell wall synthesis in susceptible organisms. **USE:** Treatment of infections caused by susceptible strains of *Escherichia coli*, group A β-hemolytic streptococci, *Haemophilus influenzae, Klebsiella* spp, *Neisseria catarrhalis, Proteus mirabilis,* staphylococci, *Streptococcus pneumoniae.*

PHARMACOKINETICS

PO absorption	Peak	Half-life	Protein binding	Excretion
Rapid	1h	0.5-1.2h	5%-15%	90% via urine in 8h as unchanged drug

CONTRAINDICATIONS: Hypersensitivity to any cephalosporin.

DOSAGE

Pediatric *PO*	25-50mg/kg divided. For severe infections, 75-100mg/kg/d divided
Adult *PO*	250mg q6h, $\bar{c}$ range 1-4g/d

SIDE/ADVERSE EFFECTS: CNS: dizziness, fatigue, headache ▪ GI: N/V, dyspepsia, abdominal pain, symptoms of pseudomembranous colitis ▪ GU: vaginitis, vaginal discharge, moniliasis ▪ HEM: eosinophilia, neutropenia ▪ HEP: ↑ AST, ALT ▪ INT: urticaria, rash, angioedema ▪ Other: ***anaphylaxis.***

Note: Side/adverse effects: common in *italic;* serious in ***boldface italic.***

*Available in Canada only.

DRUG INTERACTIONS: Bacteriostatic antibiotics can antagonize bactericidal activity ▪ use c̄ oral anticoagulants may ↑ their activity ▪ Use c̄ aminoglycosides may produce additive nephrotoxicity ▪ Use c̄ probenecid will ↓ renal excretion.

NURSING MANAGEMENT

ADMINISTRATION: Assess for hx of cephalosporin/penicillin hypersensitivity ▪ Obtain C&S before therapy ▪ Assess renal function; ↓ dosage if impaired ▪ Administer 1h ac/2h pc ▪ PO suspension: reconstitute powder according to manufacturer's directions; shake well before using; store (reconstituted) for 14d refrigerated ▪ Avoid exposure to moisture, light in storage.

EVALUATION: Monitor VS, esp temperature ▪ Monitor hepatic, renal status ▪ Monitor CBC ▪ Urine glucose: false (+) Clinitest; use Clinistix/Tes-Tape.

EDUCATION: Complete full course of therapy (usually 10d) even if symptoms subside ▪ Can be taken c̄ meals; *best* on empty stomach ▪ Take at equal intervals around clock to maintain blood levels ▪ Diarrhea may occur ▪ PO suspension: refrigerate; shake well before use ▪ Store in dry tightly closed light-resistant container ▪ Discard outdated preparations ▪ Maintain good personal hygiene (esp perineal, oral) ▪ ↑ Fluid intake (8-10 glasses/d) ▪ Use Clinistix/Tes-Tape for urine testing ▪ Notify physician of symptoms of allergic rx (fever, difficult breathing, rash) ▪ Carry identification (MedicAlert) if cephalosporin allergic ▪ Procedure for pediatric gtt administration.

NOTES:

cephapirin sodium • (sef-a-pye-rin)

CATEGORY: *Cephalosporin* (1st generation): antibiotic Rx; Preg Cat B

BRAND NAME
Cefadyl (Apothecon)

DOSAGE FORMS
Powder for injection (IM/IV): 0.5, 1, 2, 4, 20g vials

ACTION: Bactericidal activity due to inhibition of mucopeptide cell wall synthesis in susceptible organisms. **USE:** Treatment of infections caused by susceptible strains of α-*Streptococcus viridans, Escherichia coli,* group A β-hemolytic streptococci, *Haemophilus influenzae, Klebsiella* spp, *Proteus mirabilis,* staphylococci (incl penicillinase-producing strains), *Streptococcus pneumoniae.*

PHARMACOKINETICS

IM peak	Half-life	Protein binding	Excretion
30m	36m	44%-50%	70%-94% via urine in 6h

CONTRAINDICATIONS: Hypersensitivity to any cephalosporin.

DOSAGE

Pediatric *IM/IV*	40-80mg/kg in 4 equal doses
Adult *IM/IV*	500mg-1g q4-6h. Severe infection may require 12g/d

SIDE/ADVERSE EFFECTS: GI: symptoms of ***pseudomembranous colitis*** ▪ HEM: neutropenia, ***thrombocytopenia,*** anemia ▪ INT: maculopapular rash, urticaria ▪ MS: pain, induration c̄ repeated IM injection ▪ Other: ***thrombophlebitis at IV site.***

DRUG INTERACTIONS: Bacteriostatic antibiotics can antagonize bactericidal activity ▪ Use c̄ PO anticoagulants may ↑ their activity ▪ Use c̄ aminoglycosides may produce additive nephrotoxicity ▪ Use c̄ probenecid will ↓ renal excretion.

NURSING MANAGEMENT
ADMINISTRATION: Assess for hx of cephalosporin/penicillin hypersensitivity ▪ Obtain C&S before therapy ▪ Assess renal function; ↓ dosage if impaired ▪ IM: reconstitute according to manufacturer's directions; administer

by *deep, slow* injection into gluteal UOQ ▪ IV: dilute according to manufacturer's directions; inject *slowly* (3-5m); avoid aminoglycoside administration at same site; may administer IVPB ▪ Do *not* administer precipitated solutions; color change does *not* indicate ↓ potency ▪ Use reconstituted preparations (depending on diluent) w/in 12-48h at room temperature, 10d refrigerated ▪ Have support equipment available for anaphylaxis ▪ Surgical prophylaxis: D/C w/in 24h after surgery ▪ Na^+ content: 2.4mEq (54mg)/g: calculate in Na^+-restricted diets ▪ Maintain hydration.

EVALUATION: Monitor VS, esp temperature ▪ Monitor renal, hepatic, hemopoietic status ▪ Observe for signs of superinfection (diarrhea, itching, oral ulcers) ▪ Urine glucose: false (+) Clinitest; use Clinistix/Tes-Tape.

EDUCATION: Use Clinistix/Tes-Tape for urine testing ▪ Women: avoid breastfeeding ▪ Diarrhea may occur ▪ Maintain good personal hygiene (esp perineal, oral) ▪ ↑ Fluid intake (8-10 glasses/d) ▪ Notify nurse/physician of symptoms of allergic rx (difficult breathing, rash) ▪ Carry identification (MedicAlert) if cephalosporin allergic ▪ IM injection may be painful.

NOTES:

cephradine • (sef-ra-deen)

CATEGORY: *Cephalosporin* (1st generation): antibiotic   Rx; Preg Cat B

BRAND NAME
Velosef (Apothecon)

DOSAGE FORMS
Capsule: 250, 500 mg
PO suspension: 125, 250mg/5ml
Powder for injection (IM/IV): 0.25, 0.5, 1, 2g

ACTION: Bactericidal activity due to inhibition of mucopeptide cell wall synthesis in susceptible organisms. **USE:** Treatment of infections caused by susceptible strains of *Escherichia coli*, group A β-hemolytic streptococci, *Haemophilus influenzae, Klebsiella* spp, *Proteus mirabilis*, staphylococci (incl penicillinase-producing strains), *Streptococcus pneumoniae.*

PHARMACOKINETICS

PO absorption	Peak	Half-life	Protein binding	Excretion
Rapid	1h	1-2h	8%-17%	90% via urine in 6h as unchanged drug

CONTRAINDICATIONS: Hypersensitivity to any cephalosporin.

DOSAGE

Pediatric *PO*		25-50mg/kg divided q6-12h. For otitis media, 75-100mg/kg/d divided q6-12h. Do *not* exceed 4g/d
	IM/IV	50-100mg/kg divided qid
Adult *PO*		250-500mg q6h may be required
	IM/IV	2-4g/d divided qid. Do *not* exceed 4g/d

SIDE/ADVERSE EFFECTS: GI; N/V/D, symptoms of ***pseudomembranous colitis*** ▪ GU: vaginitis ▪ HEM: eosinophilia ▪ HEP: ↑ AST, ALT, BUN ▪ INT: pruritus, urticaria, morbilliform eruptions, ***erythema multiforme***.

DRUG INTERACTIONS: Bacteriostatic antibiotics can antagonize bactericidal activity ▪ Use c̄ PO anticoagulants may ↑ their activity ▪ Use c̄ aminoglycosides may produce additive nephrotoxicity ▪ Use c̄ probenecid ↓ renal excretion.

Note: Side/adverse effects: common in *italic;* serious in ***boldface italic.***   *Available in Canada only.

NURSING MANAGEMENT

ADMINISTRATION: Assess for hx of cephalosporin/penicillin hypersensitivity ▪ Obtain C&S before therapy ▪ Assess renal function; ↓ dosage if impaired ▪ PO: administer 1h ac/2h pc ▪ PO suspension: reconstitute powder according to manufacturer's directions; shake well before using; store reconstituted for 7d at room temperature, 14d refrigerated ▪ IM: reconstitute according to manufacturer's directions; administer by *deep, slow* injection into gluteal UOQ; stable 2h at room temperature, 24h refrigerated ▪ IV: dilute according to manufacturer's directions; inject *slowly* (3-5m); avoid aminoglycoside administration at same site; may administer IVPB, stable 10h at room temperature, 48h refrigerated ▪ Do *not* mix $\bar{c}$ other injectable antibiotics; avoid Ca^{++} solutions ▪ Do *not* administer precipitated solutions; color change does *not* indicate ↓ potency ▪ Have support equipment available for anaphylaxis ▪ Na^{+} content: 6mEq (136mg)/g; calculate in Na^{+}-restricted diets ▪ Maintain hydration.

EVALUATION: Monitor VS, esp temperature ▪ Monitor hepatic, renal status ▪ Monitor CBC ▪ Urine glucose: false (+) Clinitest; use Clinistix/Tes-Tape.

EDUCATION: Complete full course of therapy (usually 10d) even if symptoms subside ▪ Can be taken $\bar{c}$ meals; *best* on empty stomach ▪ Take at equal intervals around clock to maintain blood levels ▪ Diarrhea may occur ▪ PO suspension: refrigerate; shake well before using ▪ Store in dry, tightly closed container ▪ Discard outdated preparations ▪ Maintain good personal hygiene (esp perineal, oral) ▪ ↑ Fluid intake (8-10 glasses/d) ▪ Use Clinistix/Tes-Tape for urine testing ▪ Notify physician of symptoms of allergic rx (fever, difficult breathing, rash) ▪ Carry identification (MedicAlert) if cephalosporin allergic.

NOTES:

chloral hydrate • (klor-al hye-drate)

CATEGORY: *Hypnotic:* sedative

Rx C-IV; Preg Cat C

BRAND NAMES

Aquachloral (Webcon)
Noctec (Apothecon)

**Novochlorohydrate (Novopharm)*

DOSAGE FORMS

Suppository: 324, 648mg
Capsule: 250, 500mg
Syrup: 500mg/5ml

DOSAGE

Pediatric *PO/Rectal*	Sedative, 25mg/kg/d divided. Hypnotic, 50mg/kg to maximum 1g/dose 15-30m before hs
Adult *PO/Rectal*	Sedative, 250mg tid pc. Hypnotic, 500mg-1g 15-30m before hs. 1/2h before surgery

ACTION: Drug metabolized into trichloroethanol (sedative/hypnotic substance); exact pharmacologic mechanism for chloral hydrate & its active metabolite unknown; drug has weak misuse potential, mild/moderate addictive liability. **USE:** Hypnotic, pre/post-op sedative.

PHARMACOKINETICS

PO absorption	Onset	Duration	Half-life	Excretion
Rapid	30m-1h	4-8h	8-10h	Via urine, feces

CONTRAINDICATIONS: Hypersensitivity, severe cardiac disease, hepatic/renal impairment, gastritis (PO only).

SIDE/ADVERSE EFFECTS: CNS: dizziness, nightmares, ataxia, disorientation, hangover ▪ GI: N/V, flatulence, gastric irritation, unpleasant taste ▪ HEM: leukopenia, eosinophilia ▪ INT: eczemoid dermatitis, urticaria, scarlatiniform exanthema.

DRUG INTERACTIONS: Use c̄ alcohol, antihistamines, barbiturates, narcotics, other CNS depressants ↑ depression ▪ May displace oral anticoagulants from protein binding sites; dosage adjustment may be required.

NURSING MANAGEMENT

ADMINISTRATION: Assess for hx of hypersensitivity ▪ Administer c̄ food/liquids; do *not* crush capsules (bitter) ▪ Administer hypnotic dose 15-30m before hs ▪ Avoid

Note: Side/adverse effects: common in *italic;* serious in ***boldface italic.***

*Available in Canada only.

abrupt withdrawal ▪ Do *not* administer for pain; may produce CNS stimulation ▪ Avoid exposure to heat, light in storage ▪ ↓ Environmental stimuli.

EVALUATION: Monitor hepatic, renal status ▪ Monitor PT if taking PO anticoagulants; may potentiate bleeding ▪ Urine glucose: false (+) Clinitest; use Clinistix/Tes-Tape ▪ Assess for symptoms of abrupt withdrawal (tremors, abdominal/muscle cramps, convulsions) ▪ Assess for actual swallowing of PO forms ▪ Check for signs of dependence (↑ drug request) ▪ Monitor activity status (safety precautions) ▪ Assess for tolerance to therapeutic dose ▪ Observe pt sleep patterns ▪ Suppository: check for anal irritation.

EDUCATION: Drowsiness may occur; use caution in potentially hazardous activities ▪ Avoid use c̄ alcohol, other CNS depressants ▪ Indiscriminate use may lead to dependence ▪ Do *not* keep at bedside ▪ Take as ordered by physician; do *not* ↑ dose ▪ Do *not* crush capsules, swallow whole ▪ Take c̄ food/full glass liquid ▪ Use Clinistix/Tes-Tape for urine testing ▪ Women: avoid breastfeeding ▪ Proper technique for suppository administration ▪ Store in tightly closed light-resistant container ▪ Safety precautions may be instituted (bedrails) ▪ Do *not* smoke when taking drug ▪ Utilize sleep producers (reading, warm milk, soft music).

OVERDOSE MANAGEMENT: Principal symptoms: gastric irritation, circulation collapse ▪ Lethal dose in adults approximately 10g ▪ Emergency treatment: remove drug by lavage/emesis; maintain respiration; administer IV fluids, maintain adequate BP.

NOTES:

chlorambucil • (klor-am-byoo-sill)

CATEGORY: *Alkylating agent*: antineoplastic

Rx; Preg Cat D

BRAND NAME	**DOSAGE FORM**
Leukeran (B-W)	Tablet: 2mg

ACTION: Antineoplastic activity due to alkylating effect on DNA replication. **USE:** Treatment of chronic lymphocytic leukemia, malignant lymphomas incl lymphosarcoma, giant follicular lymphoma, Hodgkin's disease.

PHARMACOKINETICS

PO absorption	Peak	Half-life	Protein binding	Excretion
Complete	1h	1.5h	99%	Very slow via urine as parent drug, metabolites

CONTRAINDICATIONS: Hypersensitivity, prior drug resistance.

DOSAGE

Pediatric/Adult *PO*	0.1-0.2mg/kg as single daily dose for 3-6wks. Usual maintenance dose 0.03-0.1mg/kg/d

SIDE/ADVERSE EFFECTS: GI: *N/V/D,* oral ulcers ▪ GU: sterile cystitis ▪ HEM: ***bone marrow depression*** resulting in neutropenia, thrombocytopenia ▪ HEP: hepatotoxicity ▪ MET: hyperuricemia ▪ Other: ***pulmonary fibrosis,*** drug fever.

DRUG INTERACTIONS: Live vaccines contraindicated during therapy ▪ Radiation/other myelosuppressive drugs will produce additive bone marrow depression.

NURSING MANAGEMENT

ADMINISTRATION: Assess for hx of hypersensitivity (incl melphalan) ▪ Check hx for recent course of radiation or antineoplastic therapy; report to physician ▪ Avoid exposure to moisture/light during storage ▪ Administer antiemetic before therapy ▪ Force fluids (3000ml/d) ▪ Provide emotional support.

EVALUATION: Monitor CBC throughout therapy ▪ Assess for infection, bleeding, anemia ▪ Assess for ↑ serum uric acid levels ▪ Monitor hepatic function during therapy ▪ Assess hydration status (I&O, daily weight).

EDUCATION: Store in dry, tightly closed, light-resistant container ▪ ↑ Fluid intake (10-12 glasses/d) ▪ Avoid exposure to infection ▪ Check c̄ physician before immunization (pt, family) ▪ Diet as tolerated; avoid spicy foods ▪ Maintain good oral hygiene; use soft-bristled toothbrush ▪ Notify physician of symptoms of bone marrow depression (fever, sore throat, brushing, bleeding, lethargy) ▪ Loss of hair may occur (reversible after therapy) ▪ Compliance c̄ prescribed dosage regimen ▪ Women: avoid breastfeeding ▪ Encourage ventilation of feeling ▪ Use contraception if sexually active ▪ Reduces fertility in both sexes.

NOTES:

chloramphenicol/chloramphenicol palmitate▲/ chloramphenicol sodium succinate △ • (klor-am-fen-i-kole)

CATEGORY: *Antibiotic*

Rx; Preg Cat NA

BRAND NAMES

Chloromycetin (P-D)
**Chloroptic (Allergan)*
**Fenical (Alcon)*
**Isopto Fenicol (Alcon)*
**Minims (S&N)*
**Novochlorocap (Novopharm)*
**Pentamycetin (Pentagone)*

DOSAGE FORMS

Capsules, ophthalmic drops and ointments, otic drops, PO suspension▲, powder for injection (IV)△, topical cream

ACTION: Antimicrobial activity due to inhibition of protein synthesis in susceptible organisms, usually a bacteriostatic effect. **USE:** Drug of choice for typhoid fever ▪ Treatment of serious infections caused by susceptible strains of *Haemophilus influenzae* and *Rickettsia*, lymphogranuloma, psittacosis ▪ Cystic fibrosis regimens ▪ Other susceptible organisms resistant to all other appropriate antimicrobial drugs.

PHARMACOKINETICS

PO absorption	Peak	Half-life	Excretion
Rapid	1-3h	1.5-4.1h	Via urine, feces as metabolites, unchanged drug

CONTRAINDICATIONS: Hypersensitivity, previous chloramphenicol toxicity, any minor infections.

DOSAGE

Neonatal *IV*	25mg/kg/d in 4 doses
Pediatric *PO*	50mg/kg/d in 4 doses
IV	50mg/kg/d in 4 doses
Adult *PO*	50-100mg/kg/d in 4 doses
IV	50mg/kg/d in 4 doses. Severe infections may require 100mg/kg/d, ⬇ as soon as possible as directed

SIDE/ADVERSE EFFECTS: CNS: headache, mild depression, optic/peripheral neuritis ▪ GI: N/V/D, glossitis, stomatitis, enterocolitis ▪ HEM: ***aplastic anemia***, hypoplastic anemia, ***thrombocytopenia***, granulocytopenia, irreversible bone marrow depression ▪ Other: fatal gray baby syndrome in newborn; ↓ dosage will usually preclude this syndrome.

DRUG INTERACTIONS: Use c̄ PO anticoagulants ↑ their effects ▪ Avoid use c̄ other bone marrow depressants ▪ Use may ↓ effects of vitamin B_{12}, folic acid, iron preparations in anemic pts.

NURSING MANAGEMENT

ADMINISTRATION: Assess for hx of hypersensitivity ▪ Assess hematologic, hepatic, renal function ▪ Obtain C&S before therapy ▪ PO: administer on empty stomach (1h ac/2h pc) c̄ full glass H_2O ▪ IV: dilute; administer *slowly* (over 1m) ▪ Topical: wash, dry area thoroughly before application ▪ Otic: do *not* contaminate dropper ▪ Switch from parenteral to PO dosage form as soon as possible ▪ Na^+ content: 72mg/g; calculate in Na^+-restricted diets.

EVALUATION: Monitor VS, esp temperature; blood glucose in diabetics (hypoglycemia) ▪ Observe for signs of superinfection (diarrhea, perineal itching, oral ulcers) ▪ Assess for bleeding, eye pain, rash; D/C drug, notify physician ▪ Therapeutic blood level: 5-20μg/ml.

EDUCATION: Complete full course in therapy even if symptoms subside ▪ PO: take on empty stomach at equal intervals around clock to maintain blood levels ▪ Unpleasant taste may occur c̄ IV injection ▪ Use Clinistix/Tes-Tape for urine glucose ▪ Diarrhea may occur ▪ Maintain fluid intake (6-8 glasses/d) ▪ Notify physician of symptoms of allergic rx (fever, difficult breathing, rash), sore throat, bruising/bleeding ▪ Women: avoid breastfeeding.

NOTES:

chlordiazepoxide/chlordiazepoxide hcl ▲ • (klor-dye-az-e-pox-ide)

CATEGORY: *Benzodiazepine*: antianxiety agent, anxiolytic   Rx C-IV; Preg Cat NA

BRAND NAMES	**DOSAGE FORMS**
**Apo-Chlorax (Apotex)*	
Libritabs ▲ (Roche)	Tablet: 5, 10, 25mg
Librium (Roche)	Capsule: 5, 10, 25mg, powder for injection (IM/IV): 20mg/ml
**Medilium (Medic)*	
**Novopoxide (Novopharm)*	
**Solium (Horner)*	

COMBINATION PRODUCTS Rx

Librax (Roche)	chlordiazepoxide clindinium bromide per capsule: 5mg/2.5mg
Limbitrol (Roche)	chlordiazepoxide amitriptyline HCl per tablet: 5mg/12.5mg
Limbitrol DS (Roche)	chlordiazepoxide amitriptyline HCl per tablet: 10mg/25mg

DOSAGE: 1-2 tablets 3-4 times/d

ACTION: Anxiolytic activity due to depression of CNS at brainstem reticular formation, limbic, thalamic areas.
USE: Treatment of anxiety, alcoholism withdrawal symptoms.

PHARMACOKINETICS

PO absorption	Half-life	Excretion
Very good	24-48h	Via urine as unchanged drug, metabolites

CONTRAINDICATIONS: Hypersensitivity.

DOSAGE

Pediatric *PO*	>6y/o: 5mg 2-4 times/d. May ↑ to 10mg 2-3 times/d
Adult *PO*	Mild/moderate anxiety: 5-10mg 3-4 times/d.
	Severe anxiety: 20-25mg 3-4 times/d
IM/IV	Severe anxiety: 50-100mg followed by 25mg 3-4 times/d

Adult *IM/IV*	Pre-op: 50-100mg IM before surgery Alcoholism: 50-100mg. May be repeated 2-4h prn. Do *not* exceed 300mg/24h

SIDE/ADVERSE EFFECTS: CNS: drowsiness, ataxia, confusion (esp in geriatric, debilitated pts), extrapyramidal symptoms, EEG pattern changes ▪ HEM: ***agranulocytosis*** ▪ HEP: jaundice, liver dysfunction.

DRUG INTERACTIONS: Use c̄ other CNS depressants produces additive effects ▪ Use c̄ MAO-I can produce serious toxic effects.

NURSING MANAGEMENT

ADMINISTRATION: Assess for hx of benzodiazepine hypersensitivity ▪ Do *not* mix parenteral preparations due to incompatibility ▪ IM: add 2ml special diluent to contents of ampule, avoid excessive pressure in injecting diluent to prevent bubbles; agitate gently until all powder is dissolved; inject *deep, slowly* into UOQ of buttock ▪ IV: add 5ml sterile H_2O for injection/normal saline solution, agitate until all powder is dissolved; do *not* use this solution for IM administration ▪ Parenteral: keep pt recumbent for 3h ▪ Avoid exposure to moisture, light in storage (PO form) ▪ Prepare parenteral solutions immediately before administration; discard unused portion ▪ Avoid abrupt withdrawal ▪ Have emergency support measures available ▪ Elderly may require ↓ dosage ▪ Problem discussion, sympathetic listening contributes to relief of anxiety.

EVALUATION: Monitor renal, hepatic status ▪ Assess for symptoms of abrupt withdrawal (tremors, abdominal/muscle cramps, convulsions) c̄ prolonged use ▪ Check for signs of dependence (↑ drug request) ▪ Monitor activity status (safety precautions) ▪ Assess for tolerance to therapeutic dose ▪ Assess for paradoxic rxs (CNS stimulation), esp in elderly ▪ Check for depression; suicide precautions prn ▪ Monitor serum for ↑ alkaline phosphatase, AST, ALT ▪ False (+) pregnancy test (Gravindex).

EDUCATION: Drowsiness may occur; use caution in potentially hazardous activities ▪ Avoid use c̄ alcohol, other CNS depressants ▪ Indiscriminate use may lead to dependence ▪ Do *not* keep at bedside ▪ Take as ordered by physicians; do *not* ↑ dose ▪ Check c̄ physician/pharmacist before taking OTC drugs ▪ Women: avoid breastfeeding ▪ Practice relaxation exercises, ventilation of feelings.

NOTES:

chlorothiazide/chlorothiazide sodium▲/hydrochlorothiazide •

(klor-oh-thye-a-zide/hye-droe-klor-oh-thye-a-zide)

CATEGORY: *Thiazide diuretic*: antihypertensive Rx; Preg Cat NA

BRAND NAMES	**DOSAGE FORMS**
chlorothiazide	
Diachlor (Major)	Tablet: 250, 500mg
Diuril (MSD) (Frosst in Canada)	PO suspension: 250mg/5ml Injection (IV)▲: 0.5g/vial Tablet: 250, 500mg
hydrochlorothiazide	
Esidrix (Ciba)	Tablet: 25, 50, 100mg
HydroDIURIL (MSD)	Tablet: 25, 50, 100mg
Oretic (Abbott)	Tablet: 25, 50mg

ACTION: Diuretic activity due to inhibition of Na^+ reabsorption, primarily in ascending limb of loop of Henle & early distal tubule of nephron; K^+, bicarbonate, other ions excreted w/out significant alteration of urine pH; antihypertensive activity due to reduction of peripheral vascular resistance. **USE:** Treatment of hypertension as sole agent/in combination c̄ other antihypertensives ▪ Treatment of edema due to renal dysfunction ▪ Adjunct in treating edema due to CHF, hepatic cirrhosis, corticosterids/estrogen therapy.

CONTRAINDICATIONS: Hypersensitivity due to any thiazide, other sulfonamide-derivative drugs, anuria.

DOSAGE

chlorothiazide

Pediatric *PO*	<6mo: 15mg/lb/d in 2 doses <2y/o: 125-375mg/d in 2 doses 2-12y/o: 375mg-1g/d in 2 doses
Adult *PO*	0.5-2g, usually divided
IV	0.5-1g/d divided

PHARMACOKINETICS

	PO absorption	Onset	Peak	Duration	Excretion
Chlorothiazide	Incomplete	2h	4h	6-12h	Via urine as unchanged drug
Hydrochlorothiazide	Good	2h	4h	6-12h	Via urine as unchanged drug

hydrochlorothiazide

Pediatric *PO*	< 6 mo: 1.5 mg/lb/d in 2 doses
	< 2 y/o: 12.5-37.5 mg/d in 2 doses
Adult *PO*	2-12y/o: 37.5-100 mg/d in 2 doses
	25-200 mg/d, usually divided

SIDE/ADVERSE EFFECTS: CNS: *dizziness,* vertigo, paresthesia, headache ▪ EENT: blurred vision, xanthopsia ▪ GI: anorexia, gastric irritation, N/V/D, jaundice ▪ HEM: ***agranulocytosis, aplastic anemia,*** leukopenia, ***thrombocytopenia*** ▪ INT: purpura, urticaria, photosensitivity ▪ MET: hypokalemia, glycosuria, hyperglycemia ▪ MS: *fatigue, leg cramps* ▪ Other: necrotizing angiitis ▪ RESP: respiratory distress.

DRUG INTERACTIONS: ↑ Dig toxicity due to hypokalemia ▪ Use c̄ corticosteroids ↑ hypokalemia ▪ Antidiabetic agents may require dose adjustment ▪ Use c̄ diazoxide can produce significant diabetogenic effects.

NURSING MANAGEMENT

ADMINISTRATION: Assess for hx of thiazide/sulfonamide hypersensitivity ▪ Administer c̄ food/milk, on arising ▪ Do *not* administer SC/IM ▪ IV: reconstitute c̄ 18ml sterile H_2O for injection, shake to dissolve; compatible c̄ dextrose, NaCl solutions; administer *slowly* (2m); stable for 24h at room temperature; *not* compatible c̄ whole blood/derivatives ▪ Assess serum K^+ (normal: 3.5-5mEq/L) ▪ Elderly may require ↓ dosage.

EVALUATION: Monitor VS, esp BP, pulse; serum for ↑ BUN, creatinine, uric acid; ↓ K^+; fluid retention (I&O, daily weight) ▪ Diabetics: closely monitor blood glucose.

EDUCATION: Expect ↑ urine output; have bathroom facilities easily accessible ▪ May cause lethargy ▪ Take PO forms c̄ food ▪ Take on waking, at same time each day ▪ Take even if symptom free ▪ Notify physician of signs of hypokalemia (muscle cramps, lethargy, nausea) ▪ Avoid changing positions rapidly ▪ Take as directed by physician; do *not* skip doses ▪ Eat foods high in K^+ (bananas, fruit juices); avoid black licorice ▪ Avoid high-Na^+ foods ▪ Avoid exposure to direct sunlight, UV light ▪ Diabetics: check blood/urine glucose ▪ Avoid smoking ▪ Use sugarless gum/hard candy to diminish dry mouth.

NOTES:

chlorotrianisene • (klor-oh-trye-an-i-seen)

CATEGORY: *Estrogenic agent* Rx; Preg Cat X

BRAND NAME
TACE (MMD)
(Merrell [Canada])

DOSAGE FORMS
Capsule: 12, 25mg

ACTION: Estrogens are required for development & maintenance of female reproductive system, secondary sex characteristics. **USE:** Prevention of postpartum breast enlargement ▪ Treatment of moderate/severe symptoms associated c̄ menopause ▪ Treatment of atrophic vaginitis, kraurosis, female hypogonadism, prostatic cancer.

PHARMACOKINETICS: Not available.

CONTRAINDICATIONS: Known/suspected pregnancy, estrogen-dependent neoplasia, breast cancer except in appropriately selected pts; abnormal genital bleeding, active thrombophlebitis, thromboembolic disorders or c̄ past hx that was estrogen associated (except for breast/prostatic cancer treatment).

DOSAGE

Adult *PO* Postpartum breast enlargement: 12mg qid for 7d or 50mg q6h for 6 doses or 72mg bid for 2d. First dose w/in 8h after delivery
Menopause: 12-25mg/d administered cyclically (3wks on, 1wk off). Attempts to D/C/taper dosage should be made at 3-6mo intervals
Atrophic vaginitis, kraurosis vulvae: 12-25mg/d administered cyclically for 30-60d
Hypogonadism: 12-25mg/d for 21d
Prostatic cancer: 12-25mg/d

SIDE/ADVERSE EFFECTS: CNS: headache, migraine, dizziness, mental depression ▪ EENT: intolerance to contact lens, steepening of corneal curvature ▪ GI: N/V, abdominal cramps, bloating ▪ GU: amenorrhea, breakthrough bleeding, dysmenorrhea, candidiasis, change in menstrual flow, spotting, ↑ uterine fibromyoma size ▪ INT: melasma, ***erythema multiforme***, erythema nodosum, alopecia, hirsutism, urticaria ▪ Other: weight changes, edema, ↓ carbohydrate tolerance, porphyria exacerbation.

Note: Side/adverse effects: common in *italic;* serious in ***boldface italic.*** *Available in Canada only.

DRUG INTERACTIONS: Use c̄ tricyclic antidepressants may result in toxic rxs.

NOTES:

NURSING MANAGEMENT

ADMINISTRATION: Assess for hx of estrogen hypersensitivity ▪ Administer c̄ food ▪ Do *not* crush capsule; administer whole ▪ Avoid abrupt withdrawal ▪ Avoid exposure to heat/moisture during storage.

EVALUATION: Monitor hepatic, renal status ▪ Monitor BP ▪ Assess for endometrial cancer (Pap test, physical exam) ▪ Monitor PT; may ↓ anticoagulant effect ▪ Diabetics: careful urine testing; may ↓ antidiabetic drug effect ▪ Assess for behavior changes, depression ▪ Monitor pt weight; observe for edema.

EDUCATION: Review package insert c̄ pt ▪ Nausea may occur during first 2wks of therapy ▪ Women: avoid pregnancy, breastfeeding ▪ Breast self-examination (incl male pts) ▪ Avoid smoking (↑ CV complications) ▪ Take c̄ food ▪ Notify physician/dentist of use before treatment ▪ Keep scheduled appointments c̄ physician ▪ Avoid direct sunlight/UV light ▪ D/C drug, notify physician if pregnancy suspected ▪ Notify physician *immediately* of chest/leg pain, unusual vaginal bleeding, difficult breathing, slurred speech ▪ Men: enlarged breasts, impotence are reversible after therapy ▪ Check weight, swelling in feet/legs daily.

chlorpromazine▲/chlorpromazine hcl • (klor-proe-ma-zeen)

CATEGORY: *Phenothiazine*: antipsychotic, neuroleptic — Rx; Preg Cat NA

BRAND NAMES

**Largactil (Rhone-Poulenc), Thorazine (SKB)*
**Chlor-Promanyl*

DOSAGE FORMS

Injection, concentrate, suppository ▲, capsule, syrup, tablet

ACTION: Antipsychotic activity appears associated c̄ ↓ neural transmission in central dopamine-dependent pathways, resulting in tranquilizing effect in psychotic pts; drug also exhibits anti-alpha adrenergic, anticholinergic, antiemetic, antiserotonin, ganglionic blocking activity.
USE: Treatment of psychotic states, pediatric behavioral problems ▪ Treatment of intractable hiccups, acute intermittent porphyria, nausea.

PHARMACOKINETICS: PO onset of 30-40m, peak in 4-6h.

CONTRAINDICATIONS: Hypersensitivity, comatose states, bone marrow depression, presence of large amounts of CNS depressants.

DOSAGE

Indication	Population	Route	Dose
Psychiatric			
	Pediatric	*PO*	50-200mg/d
		IM	≤5y/o: 40mg/d; 5-12y/o: 75mg/d
	Adult	*PO*	30-1000mg or more/d
		IM	25mg, then 25-50mg in 1h
Nausea/vomiting			
	Pediatric	*PO*	0.25mg/lb q4-6h
		IM/Rectal	0.25mg/lb q6-8h
	Adult	*PO*	10-25mg q4-6h
		IM	25mg, then 25-50mg q3-4h
		Rectal	100mg q6-8h
Hiccups	Adult	*PO*	25-50mg 3-4 times/d
		IM	25-50mg 3-4 times/d
Porphyria	Adult	*PO*	25-50mg 3-4 times/d
		IM	25mg 3-4 times/d
Pre-op	Pediatric	*PO*	0.25mg/lb 2-3h before surgery
		IM	0.25mg/lb 1-2h before surgery
	Adult	*PO*	25-50mg 2-3h before surgery
		IM	12.5-25mg 1-2h before surgery

*Available in Canada only.

SIDE/ADVERSE EFFECTS: CNS: drowsiness, extrapyramidal rxs, tardive dyskinesia ▪ CV: postural hypotension, tachycardia, ECG changes in Q, T waves ▪ EENT: blurred vision, corneal/lenticular changes, epithelial keratopathy, nasal congestion ▪ END: lactation, moderate breast enlargement in female pts ▪ HEM: ***agranulocytosis***, eosinophilia, leukopenia, ***hemolytic anemia***, thrombocytopenic purpura ▪ HEP: cholestatic jaundice ▪ INT: urticaria, photosensitivity ▪ PSYCH: adverse behavioral changes ▪ Other: fever, hyperpyrexia, neuroleptic malignant syndrome, hypothermia.

DRUG INTERACTIONS: Aluminum-magnesium antacid preparations ↓ absorption ▪ Use c̄ narcotics, barbiturates, other CNS depressants ↑ CNS depression ▪ Guanethidine, related antihypertensives antagonized.

NURSING MANAGEMENT

ADMINISTRATION: Assess for hx of phenothiazine hypersensitivity ▪ Assess VS, esp BP ▪ PO: administer c̄ food; do *not* crush/break SR capsules ▪ PO concentrate: dilute before administration c̄ >60ml fluid ▪ Syrup: shake well before using ▪ IM: inject *slowly, deep* into UOQ of buttock; keep pt lying down for 30m after injection ▪ Avoid SC injection ▪ IV: dilute according to manufacturer's directions; inject 1mg/m; maintain pt in supine position for 30m ▪ Discard discolored/precipitated solution ▪ Avoid exposure to moisture, light in storage ▪ Store suppositories at room temperature ▪ Avoid skin contact c̄ liquid forms (contact dermatitis) ▪ Avoid abrupt withdrawal ▪ Maintain hydration ▪ Elderly/debilitated may require ↓ dosage.

EVALUATION: Monitor hepatic, ophthalmic, renal status ▪ Monitor BP, CBC, fluid retention (I&O, daily weight), constipation ▪ Assess for extrapyramidal rx ▪ Seizure precautions in pts c̄ hx of convulsive disorders ▪ Long-term therapy: assess for jaundice, agranulocytosis.

EDUCATION: Dizziness/drowsiness may occur; use caution in potentially hazardous activities ▪ Avoid changing positions rapidly ▪ Avoid use of alcohol, other CNS depressants ▪ Store in tightly closed, light-resistant container ▪ Use sugarless gum/hard candy to diminish dry mouth ▪ Constipation may occur; ↑ fluids, bulk-containing foods ▪ May turn urine pink/red/brown ▪ Avoid contact c̄ liquid forms ▪ Women: avoid breastfeeding ▪ Take PO forms c̄ food; swallow SR capsules whole ▪ Avoid exposure to direct sunlight, UV light ▪ Notify physician of fever, sore throat, bruising/bleeding, tics/spasms, trembling, shuffling gait ▪ Avoid ↑ exercise, temperature extremes ▪ Check c̄ physician before taking OTC preparations ▪ Do *not* take antacids/antidiarrheals w/in 2h of drug ▪ Full drug effects may require several wks.

chlorthalidone • (klor-thal-i-done)

CATEGORY: *Diuretic:* antihypertensive

Rx; Preg Cat B

BRAND NAMES

**Apo-Chlorothalidone (Apotex)*
Hygroton (RPR) (Geigy [Canada])
**Novothalidone (Novopharm)*
**Uridon (ICN)*

DOSAGE FORMS

Tablet: 25, 50, 100mg

PHARMACOKINETICS

PO absorption	Onset	Duration	Half-life	Protein binding	Excretion
Good	2.6h	Up to 72h	40h	75%	Via urine primarily as unchanged drug

ACTION: Diuretic activity due to excretion of H_2O, Na^+, Cl^-, other electrolytes by inhibiting tubular reabsorption. **USE:** Treatment of hypertension as sole agent or in combination c̄ other antihypertensives ▪ Treatment of edema due to renal dysfunction ▪ Adjunct in treating edema due to CHF, hepatic cirrhosis, corticosteroid or estrogen therapy ▪ Investigational treatment of systolic hypertension.

CONTRAINDICATIONS: Hypersensitivity due to any thiazide or other sulfonamide-derivative drugs, anuria.

DOSAGE

Pediatric *PO*	2mg/kg 3 times/wk
Adult *PO*	50-100mg qd or 100mg on alternate d. 200mg qd may be needed

SIDE/ADVERSE EFFECTS: CNS: drowsiness, vertigo, paresthesia, headache ▪ EENT: blurred vision, xanthopsia ▪ GI: anorexia, gastric irritation, N/V/D, jaundice, ***pan-***

Note: Side/adverse effects: common in *italic;* serious in ***boldface italic.***

*Available in Canada only.

creatitis ▪ HEM: ***agranulocytosis, aplastic anemia***, leukopenia, ***thrombocytopenia*** ▪ INT: purpura, urticaria, photosensitivity ▪ MET: ***hypokalemia***, glycosuria, hyperglycemia ▪ MS: *fatigue, leg cramps* ▪ Other: necrotizing angiitis, respiratory distress.

DRUG INTERACTIONS: ↑ Dig toxicity due to hypokalemia ▪ Use c̄ corticosteroids produces ↑ hypokalemia ▪ Antidiabetic agents may require dose adjustments ▪ Use c̄ diazoxide can produce significant diabetogenic effects.

NURSING MANAGEMENT

ADMINISTRATION: Assess for hx of hypersensitivity (incl sulfonamides) ▪ Assess renal function; do *not* administer if impaired ▪ Administer c̄ food or milk on arising ▪ Assess serum K^+ (normal: 3.5-5mEq/L) ▪ Elderly may require ↓ dosage.

EVALUATION: Monitor F/E, hepatic, renal status ▪ Monitor VS, esp BP, pulse ▪ Monitor serum for ↑ BUN, creatinine, uric acid, ↓ K^+ ▪ Diabetics: closely monitor blood glucose ▪ Monitor fluid retention (I&O, daily weight) ▪ Monitor digitalized pts close (↓ K^+: ↑ dig toxicity).

EDUCATION: Expect ↑ urine output; have bathroom facilities easily accessible ▪ May cause weakness, lethargy ▪ Take c̄ food ▪ Take on waking, at same time each day ▪ Take even if symptom free ▪ Used to control, *not* cure, hypertension ▪ Notify physician of signs of hypokalemia (muscle cramps, lethargy, nausea) ▪ Avoid changing positions (lying/sitting/standing) rapidly ▪ Take as directed by physician; do *not* skip doses ▪ Eat foods high in K^+ (bananas, fruit juices, raisins); avoid black licorice ▪ Avoid high-Na^+ foods (canned soups, lunch meats, cheese) ▪ Maintain optimum weight ▪ Avoid exposure to direct sunlight/UV light ▪ Diabetics: check blood/urine glucose carefully ▪ Avoid smoking ▪ Use sugarless gum/hard candy to diminish dry mouth.

NOTES:

chlorzoxazone • (klor-zox-a-zone)

CATEGORY: *Skeletal muscle relaxant*

Rx; Preg Cat NA

BRAND NAMES
Paraflex (McNeil)
Parafon Forte DSC (McNeil)

DOSAGE FORMS
Tablet: 250mg
Tablet: 500mg

ACTION: Relaxant activity appears related to inhibition of multisynaptic reflex arcs in subcortical areas of brain, spinal cord; no direct relaxation, drug has CNS sedative properties. **USE:** Adjunct to relief of discomfort associated c̄ acute painful MS conditions.

PHARMACOKINETICS

PO absorption	Onset	Peak	Duration	Excretion
Complete	1h	3-4h	3-4h	Via urine as metabolites

CONTRAINDICATIONS: Hypersensitivity.

DOSAGE

Pediatric *PO* 125-500mg 3-4 times/d according to age, weight

Adult *PO* 250-500mg 3-4 times/d or 750mg 3-4 times/d. Maintenance dose after improvement, 250mg 3-4 times/d

Parafon Forte

Adult *PO* 1 tablet (caplet) 3-4 times/d

SIDE/ADVERSE EFFECTS: CNS: drowsiness, dizziness ▪ GI: some disturbances, rare bleeding ▪ INT: rash, petechiae, ecchymoses; angioneurotic edema ▪ Other: urine discoloration, malaise, hepatotoxicity.

DRUG INTERACTIONS: Use c̄ CNS depressants will result in additive depression.

NURSING MANAGEMENT

ADMINISTRATION: Assess for hx of hypersensitivity ▪ Administer c̄ meals; tablets can be crushed/mixed c̄ food/liquid ▪ Avoid exposure to moisture during storage ▪ Elderly may require ↓ dosage.

EVALUATION: Monitor hepatic status ▪ Monitor activity status (safety precautions) ▪ Assess for sensitivity rx (urticaria, skin redness, itching), liver dysfunction (jaundice, dark urine); D/C if present.

EDUCATION: Drowsiness may occur; use caution when engaging in potentially hazardous activities ▪ Avoid use $\bar{c}$ alcohol, other CNS depressants ▪ Take $\bar{c}$ food to ↓ GI distress ▪ Rest, physical therapy will promote comfort ▪ May turn urine orange or red-purple.

OVERDOSE MANAGEMENT: Principal symptoms: N/V, loss of muscle movement/deep tendon reflexes, respiratory depression ▪ Emergency treatment: remove drug by lavage or emesis, followed by activated charcoal; maintain respiration; administer IV fluids; maintain adequate BP; analeptic drugs are of no value.

NOTES:

cholestyramine resin • (koe-less-<u>tear</u>-a-meen)

CATEGORY: *Antilipemic*: ion-exchange resin Rx

BRAND NAMES	**DOSAGE FORMS**
Questran (Bristol) *(Bristol [Canada])*	Powder: 378g cans, 9g single-dose packets (9g powder contains 4g resin)
Questran Light (Bristol)	5g single-dose packets

ACTION: Resin binds bile acids in intestine to form insoluble complex, preventing reabsorption; loss of bile acids leads to ↑ oxidation of cholesterol, ↓ serum levels of cholesterol, beta lipoproteins. **USE:** Adjunct management of type II hyperlipoproteinemia (LDL) ▪ Relief of pruritus associated c̄ partial biliary obstruction.

PHARMACOKINETICS: Drug not absorbed.

CONTRAINDICATIONS: Hypersensitivity, complete biliary obstruction or where bile is not secreted into the intestine.

DOSAGE

Adult *PO* 9g 1-6 times/d as required

SIDE/ADVERSE EFFECTS: CNS: headache ▪ EENT: tinnitus, night blindness ▪ GI: *constipation*, N/V, anorexia, flatulence, bleeding, bloating, steatorrhea ▪ MS: osteoporosis ▪ Other: burnt odor to urine, urticaria.

DRUG INTERACTIONS: All drugs should be administered 1h before/4-6h after cholestyramine administration ▪ ↓ Fat-soluble vitamin absorption c̄ extremely high doses.

NURSING MANAGEMENT

ADMINISTRATION: Assess for hx of hypersensitivity ▪ Assess serum cholesterol, triglyceride levels ▪ Administer ac ▪ Place dose on surface of 4-6oz liquid, allow to stand for several minutes while swirling glass; stir, administer to pt; rinse glass c̄ more liquid, administer ▪ Avoid exposure to heat/light during storage ▪ Administer other medication 1h before/4-6h after.

EVALUATION: Monitor GI status ▪ Monitor elderly for GI irritation ▪ Monitor PT if taking PO anticoagulants; may potentiate bleeding ▪ Digitalized pts: maintain dig levels during therapy, after D/C (↓ absorption) ▪ Monitor serum triglyceride levels.

EDUCATION: Constipation/bad taste may occur ▪ Take ac ▪ Mix c̄ liquid, take drug; rinse glass c̄ liquid, drink; *never* take dry ▪ Follow prescribed diet (antihyperlipidemic) ▪ Check c̄ physician before taking any medication/OTC preparations ▪ Notify physician of changes in bowel function, bruising, bleeding ▪ ↑ Fluid intake (8-10 glasses/d), ↑ fiber in diet ▪ Do *not* skip doses ▪ Store in original container ▪ Take 1h after/4-6h before other medication.

NOTES:

cimetidine/cimetidine hcl▲ • (sye-met-i-deen)

CATEGORY: *H2 blocker:* antihistamine — Rx; Preg Cat B

BRAND NAMES
**Peptol*
Tagamet (SKB)

DOSAGE FORMS
Injection▲: 300mg/2ml
Liquid▲: 300mg/5ml, 300mg/50ml
Tablet: 200, 300, 400, 800mg

ACTION: H_2 antihistamine activity due to competitive inhibition of histamine at H_2 histamine receptors on parietal cells, resulting in ↓ gastric acid secretions; liquid, injection forms contain HCl salt. **USE:** Short-term treatment of gastric/duodenal ulcers ▪ Duodenal ulcer prophylaxis ▪ Treatment of pathologic hypersecretory conditions, eg, Zollinger-Ellison syndrome, systemic mastocytosis, multiple endocrine adenomas.

PHARMACOKINETICS

PO absorption	Peak	Half-life	Protein binding	Excretion
High	45-90m	2h	15%-20%	48% PO dose in 24h, 75% IM/IV dose in 24h, via urine

CONTRAINDICATIONS: No current contraindications.

DOSAGE

Adult *PO*	
Ulcers	800mg hs is the preferred dose, or 300mg qid c̄ meals & hs, or 400mg bid. Usual maintenance dose 400mg hs.
Pathologic hypersecretion	300mg qid c̄ meals & hs or higher if required. Do *not* exceed 2400mg/d
Adult Parenteral	
IM/IV	300mg q6-8h or higher if required. Do *not* exceed 2400mg/d
Intermittent *IV* infusion	300mg q6-8h infused over 15-20m. Do *not* exceed 2400mg/d
Continuous *IV* infusion	Usual dose 37.5mg/h. If required, a 150mg IV loading dose may precede the start of the infusion

Note: Side/adverse effects: common in *italic;* serious in ***boldface italic.***

*Available in Canada only.

SIDE/ADVERSE EFFECTS: CNS: dizziness, somnolence, mental confusion, anxiety ▪ END: gynecomastia ▪ GI: diarrhea, hepatitis, ***pancreatitis*** ▪ GU: ***interstitial nephritis***, urinary retention ▪ HEM: neutropenia, ***thrombocytopenia*** ▪ INT: rash, reversible alopecia ▪ MS: muscular pain ▪ Other: fever, local pain at IM site.

DRUG INTERACTIONS: Cimetidine can ↑ activity of coumarin anticoagulants, theophylline, propranolol, phenytoin, lidocaine.

NURSING MANAGEMENT

ADMINISTRATION: Assess for hx of hypersensitivity (incl rantidine) ▪ PO: Administer $\bar{c}$ meals, hs ▪ IM: dilution *not* required; may be painful ▪ IV injection: dilute to total vol 20ml (30mg); inject over 2m ▪ IV intermittent infusion: dilute to total vol 100ml (300mg); infuse over 15-20m ▪ May be mixed $\bar{c}$ 0.9% NaCl injection, 5% to 10% dextrose, lactated Ringer solution, 5% Na bicarbonate injection for direct IV injection/intermittent IV infusion ▪ Diluted injections stable for 48h at room temperature ▪ Avoid exposure to moisture, light in storage ▪ Avoid use in children <16 y/o ▪ Administer antacids prn 1h before/1h after ▪ Stable in hyperalimentation solutions.

EVALUATION: Monitor GI, neurologic, renal status ▪ Assess for reversible confusion in elderly/debilitated pts ▪ False (+): GI Hemoccult.

EDUCATION: Dizziness may occur; use caution in potentially hazardous activities ▪ Take $\bar{c}$ meals ▪ Women: avoid breastfeeding ▪ Men: breast enlargement may occur ▪ Avoid smoking ▪ Avoid GI irritating foods ▪ Check $\bar{c}$ physician before taking OTC preparations ▪ Avoid anxiety-producing situations ▪ Take as directed by physician ▪ Do *not* take w/in 1h of antacids ▪ Store in tightly closed, light-resistant container.

NOTES:

ciprofloxacin hcl • (sip-roe-flox-a-sin)

CATEGORY: *Synthetic antibacterial*: fluoroquinolone antiinfective Rx; Preg Cat C

BRAND NAME	DOSAGE FORMS
Cipro (Miles)	Tablet: 250, 500, 750mg

ACTION: Bactericidal activity due to interference with DNA gyrase enzyme (which is required for DNA synthesis) in susceptible organisms, especially gram-negative bacteria. **USE:** Treatment of bone, joint infection, infectious diarrhea, lower respiratory, skin, and urinary tract infection caused by susceptible strains of *Campylobacter jejuni, Morganella morganii, Citrobacter* spp, *Enterobacter cloacae, Escherichia coli, Haemophilus influenzae, Klebsiella pneumoniae, Proteus* spp, *Providencia* spp, *Pseudomonas aeruginosa, Serratia marcescens, Shigella* spp, *Staphylococcus* spp, *Streptococcus* spp.

PHARMACOKINETICS

PO absorption	Peak	Half-life	Protein binding	Excretion
Good	1-2h	4h	20%-40%	50% via urine as unchanged drug

CONTRAINDICATIONS: Hypersensitivity to drug or other quinolones.

DOSAGE

For normal renal function

Adult *PO* 250-500mg q12h for renal infections
500-750mg q12h for infectious diarrhea and bone, joint, lower respiratory, skin, & more complicated renal infections

SIDE/ADVERSE EFFECTS: CNS: headache, restlessness, dizziness, drowsiness, ***convulsive seizures***, hallucinations, nightmares, manic reactions ▪ CV: atrial flutter, palpitations, angina, hypertension, ***MI, cardiopulmonary arrest, cerebral thrombosis, ventricular ectopy*** ▪ EENT: blurred vision, color perception disorders, tinnitus, hearing loss ▪ GI: *N/V/D,* pain, ***intestinal perforation*** ▪ GU: vaginitis, ***interstitial nephritis, nephritis, renal failure***, urethral bleeding, voiding irregularities ▪ HEM: eosinophilia, leukopenia ▪ HEP: ↑ in ALT, AST, alkaline phosphatase, BUN ▪ INT: pruritus; urticaria; photosensitivity; erythema nodosum; edema of face, lips, neck;

Note: Side/adverse effects: common in *italic;* serious in ***boldface italic.***

*Available in Canada only.

hyperpigmentation; ***Stevens-Johnson syndrome; toxic epidermal necrolysis*** ▪ RESP: bronchospasm, edema, *embolism* ▪ Other: pain in joints, back, chest, gout exacerbation.

DRUG INTERACTIONS: Al and Mg antacids may ↓ PO absorption ▪ Nitrofurantoin can antagonize antibacterial activity ▪ Probenecid will ↓ renal excretion ▪ Use c̄ theophylline may ↑ theophylline toxicity.

NURSING MANAGEMENT

ADMINISTRATION: Assess for hx of quinolone derivative hypersensitivity ▪ Administer c̄ full glass H_2O 1h ac/2h pc at evenly spaced intervals ▪ Assess for CNS disorders; ↓ dosage if impaired ▪ Delay antacid administration for 2h after dose ▪ Avoid exposure to moisture, heat, light in storage ▪ Maintain hydration.

EVALUATION: Monitor VS, esp temperature ▪ Monitor I&O, hepatic, renal status ▪ Assess for CNS toxicity, crystalluria, nephrotoxicity, visual disturbances; D/C drug, notify physician ▪ May ↑ serum ALT, AST, alkaline phosphatase, creatinine, bilirubin, BUN.

EDUCATION: Drowsiness/dizziness may occur; use caution in potentially hazardous situations ▪ Take on empty stomach c̄ full glass of H_2O ▪ Take at equal intervals around clock to maintain blood levels ▪ Take antacids at least 2h after taking drug ▪ Complete full course of therapy even if symptoms subside ▪ ↑ Fluid intake (8-10 glasses/d) ▪ Avoid exposure to direct sunlight, UV light (sunlamp); use sunscreen, protective clothing ▪ Notify physician *immediately* of visual disturbances; D/C drug ▪ Store in dry, tightly closed, light-resistant container ▪ Discard outdated preparations ▪ May cause mouth discomfort, unpleasant taste ▪ Do *not* administer to infants, children ▪ Women: avoid breastfeeding.

NOTES:

cisplatin • (sis-pla-tin)

CATEGORY: *Alkylating agent*: antineoplastic   Rx; Preg Cat NA

BRAND NAME

Platinol (BM-ONC)
(Bristol in Canada)

DOSAGE FORMS

Powder for injection (IV)
10, 50mg/vial

ACTION: Antineoplastic activity due to alkylating effect on DNA replication; bifunctional activity causes inter-strand cross-linking of DNA. **USE:** Treatment of metastatic tumors of testes/ovaries, advanced bladder cancer.

PHARMACOKINETICS: Initial half-life 25-49m; post-distribution half-life 58-73h; approximately 27%-40% of drug excreted via urine in 5d.

CONTRAINDICATIONS: Hypersensitivity to drug/platinum, myelosuppression, renal/hearing impairment.

DOSAGE

Pediatric/Adult *IV*

Testicular cancer	20mg/m²/d for 5d q3wks for 3 courses, c̄ bleomycin sulfate 30U IV weekly on day 2 of each wk for 12 consecutive doses, vinblastine sulfate 0.15-0.2mg/kg IV on days 1, 2 q3wks for 4 courses
Ovarian cancer	Single agent: 100mg/m² once q4wks Therapy: 50mg/m² once q3wks, c̄ doxorubicin 50mg/m² IV once q3wks on day 1
Bladder cancer	50-70mg/m² IV once q3-4wks

SIDE/ADVERSE EFFECTS: CNS: peripheral neuropathy ▪ EENT: *ototoxicity* (up to 31% of patients c̄ single dose) ▪ GI: N/V, anorexia ▪ GU: dose-related ***nephrotoxicity*** (most limiting), more pronounced c̄ repeated treatment ▪ HEM: *leukopenia,* ***thrombocytopenia***.

Note: Side/adverse effects: common in *italic;* serious in ***boldface italic.***

*Available in Canada only.

DRUG INTERACTIONS: Live vaccines contraindicated during therapy ▪ Radiation, other myelosuppressive drugs produce additive bone marrow depression ▪ Ototoxic/nephrotoxic drugs produce additive toxicity.

NURSING MANAGEMENT

ADMINISTRATION: Reconstitute powder for injection c̄ 10ml sterile H_2O (10mg vial) or 50ml (50mg vial); produces 1mg/ml dilution ▪ Reconstituted solution stable for 20h at room temperature; do *not* refrigerate (precipitation) ▪ Administer antiemetic before therapy ▪ Administer IV fluids, mannitol 4h before, 24h after therapy to ensure urine output 100ml/h ▪ Administer by infusion over 6-8h ▪ Avoid using needles/IV sets c̄ aluminum-containing parts; precipitate will form c̄ drug contact ▪ Provide emotional support.

EVALUATION: Assess for hearing dysfunction ▪ Check IV site closely; avoid extravasation ▪ Assess serum for ↑ BUN, AST, ALT, creatinine ▪ Monitor neurologic, hepatic, renal function ▪ Assess for anaphylactic rxs; have support equipment available ▪ Monitor CBC throughout therapy, esp platelets ▪ Assess for ↑ serum uric acid levels ▪ Assess for infection, bleeding, anemia ▪ Assess hydration status (I&O, daily weight).

EDUCATION: ↑ Fluid intake (10-12 glasses/d) ▪ Avoid exposure to infection ▪ Check c̄ physician before immunization (pt, family) ▪ Diet as tolerated; avoid spicy foods ▪ Maintain good oral hygiene; use soft-bristled toothbrush ▪ Notify physician of symptoms of bone marrow depression (fever, sore throat, bruising, bleeding, lethargy) ▪ Report hearing difficulties to physician at once ▪ Women: avoid breastfeeding ▪ Encourage ventilation of feelings ▪ Use contraception if sexually active.

NOTES:

clarithromycin • (klah-rith-roe-mye-sin)

CATEGORY: *Antibiotic:* macrolide antibiotic (semi-synthetic) Rx; Preg Cat C

BRAND NAME
Biaxin (Abbott)

DOSAGE FORMS
Tablet: 250, 550mg

ACTION: Bacteriostatic activity due to inhibition of ribosomal protein synthesis in microorganisms. **USE:** Treatment of infections caused by susceptible strains of *Haemophilus influenzae, Moraxella catarrhalis, Mycoplasma pneumoniae, Staphylococcus aureus, Streptococcus pneumoniae, Streptococcus pyogenes.*

PHARMACOKINETICS

PO absorption	Peak	Half-life	Excretion
50%	2h	3-7h	Via urine, feces as unchanged drug, metabolites

CONTRAINDICATIONS: Hypersensitivity to drug or erythromycin.

DOSAGE

Adults/Children ≥12 *PO*	250mg q12h. Lower respiratory tract infections and acute sinusitis usually require 500mg q12h

SIDE/ADVERSE EFFECTS: CNS: headache ▪ GI: N/D, abnormal taste, dyspepsia, abdominal discomfort/pain, ***pseudomembranous colitis***.

DRUG INTERACTIONS: Bacteriostatic antibiotics can antagonize effects of bactericidal antibiotics ▪ Use c̄ carbamazepine, dig, PO anticoagulants, theophylline can ↑ their toxicity.

NURSING MANAGEMENT
ADMINISTRATION: Assess for hx of macrolide hypersensitivity, incl erythromycin ▪ Obtain C&S before therapy ▪ May administer w/out regard to meals ▪ Elderly, pts c̄ severe renal impairment may require ↓ dosage.

EVALUATION: Monitor VS, esp temperature ▪ Monitor renal status; may require ↓ dosage if severely impaired ▪ Observe for signs of superinfection (diarrhea, perineal itching, oral ulcers).

EDUCATION: Complete full course of therapy ▪ May be taken w/out regard to meals ▪ Take at equal intervals around clock to maintain blood levels ▪ Diarrhea may occur ▪ Women: avoid breastfeeding.

NOTES:

clofibrate • (kloe-fye-brate)

CATEGORY: *Antilipemic:* antilipidemic agent — Rx; Preg Cat NA

BRAND NAMES
Atromid S (W-A)
**Claripex (ICN);*
**Novofibrate (Novopharm)*

DOSAGE FORM
Capsule: 500mg

ACTION: Antilipemic mechanism not determined. **USE:** Drug of choice for type III hyperlipoproteinemia ▪ Treatment of types IV/V hyperlipoproteinemia.

PHARMACOKINETICS

PO absorption	Protein binding	Excretion
Good	>95%	Via urine primarily as metabolites

CONTRAINDICATIONS: Hypersensitivity, pregnant/nursing mothers, significant hepatic/renal dysfunction, primary biliary cirrhosis.

DOSAGE
Adult *PO* — Usual dose 2g/d divided

SIDE/ADVERSE EFFECTS: CNS: drowsiness, dizziness, headache ▪ CV: ***cardiac arrhythmias*** ▪ GI: *nausea,* V/D, upset, gallstones, stomatitis, polyphagia ▪ GU: impotence, dysuria, hematuria, proteinuria, ↓ urine output ▪ HEM: leukopenia ▪ INT: rash, pruritus, urticaria, alopecia ▪ MS: myalgia, arthralgia.

DRUG INTERACTIONS: Use c̄ PO anticoagulants ↑ their activity, requires dosage adjustment ▪ Furosemide may displace clofibrate from inactive storage sites.

NURSING MANAGEMENT
ADMINISTRATION: Assess for hx of hypersensitivity ▪ Assess serum cholesterol, triglyceride levels ▪ Administer c̄ meals to ↓ GI distress ▪ Assess hepatic, renal function; use c̄ caution if impaired ▪ Avoid exposure to light during storage.

EVALUATION: Monitor hepatic, renal status ▪ Monitor serum triglyceride levels ▪ Diabetics: closely monitor blood glucose (hypoglycemia) ▪ Monitor pt taking PO anticoagulants; may potentiate bleeding.

Note: Side/adverse effects: common in *italic;* serious in ***boldface italic.***

*Available in Canada only.

EDUCATION: Take c̄ meals to ↓ GI irritation ▪ Take as ordered by physician; do *not* change dose ▪ Check c̄ physician/pharmacist before taking OTC preparations ▪ Follow diet low in animal fats, triglycerides ▪ Women: use contraception for up to 2 mo after therapy is ended if sexually active ▪ Diabetics: hypoglycemia (anxiety, headache, fatigue, nausea, sweating) may occur; take sugar, notify physician ▪ Notify physician *immediately* of "flu-like" symptoms (fever, sore throat, weakness) ▪ Avoid use c̄ alcohol, barbiturates, narcotics ▪ Keep scheduled appointments c̄ physician/for blood work.

NOTES:

clomipramine hcl • (kloe-mip-ra-meen)

CATEGORY: *Tricyclic antidepressant*: antiobsessional Rx; Preg Cat C

BRAND NAME
Anafranil (Basel)

DOSAGE FORMS
Capsule: 25, 50, 75mg

ACTION: Exact mechanism of anticompulsive activity not determined but appears related to serotonergic neural transmission. Drug inhibits serotonin reuptake. **USE:** Treatment of obsession and/or compulsions in obsessive-compulsive disorder (OCD) syndrome. Long-term effectiveness (>10 wks) not currently evaluated, but treatment has lasted for at least 1 yr in selected pts.

PHARMACOKINETICS

PO absorption	Peak	Half-life	Protein binding	Excretion
Good	2-6	19-37h	97%	Via urine, glucuronic metabolites & other metabolites

CONTRAINDICATIONS: Hypersensitivity, MAO-I therapy, MI (acute recovery period).

DOSAGE

Children/ Adolescent *PO*	Initial dose 25mg/d c̄ gradual ↑ during the first 2 wks. Do *not* exceed 3mg/kg and/or 100mg/d. Follow by gradual ↑ *not* to exceed 3 mg/kg or 200mg/d (whichever is smaller). Maintenance dose lowest effective dose that can be given once/d hs
Adult *PO*	Initial dose 25mg/d c̄ gradual ↑ (2 wks) to 100mg/d. Follow by gradual ↑ to 250mg/d. Maintenance dose lowest effective dose that can be given once/d hs

SIDE/ADVERSE EFFECTS: CNS: somnolence, dizziness, tremor, nervousness, myoclonus, seizures ▪ CV: postural hypotension, tachycardia, palpitation ▪ GI: anorexia, constipation, nausea, dyspepsia, ↑ appetite, dry mouth ▪ INT: rash, pruritus, ↑ sweating ▪ Other: abnormal vision, tinnitus, weight gain, myalgia, micturition disorder, male sexual dysfunction.

DRUG INTERACTIONS: Significant depressant effects c̄ alcohol, other CNS depressants ▪ Use c̄ warfarin, digoxin can ↑ their effects by displacement from protein storage sites ▪ Use c̄ anticholinergics may produce ↑ atropine-like effects.

NURSING MANAGEMENT

ADMINISTRATION: Assess for hx of tricyclic antidepressant hypersensitivity, hepatitic dysfunction, glaucoma ▪ Assess VS, esp BP ▪ Administer c̄ food to ↓ GI irritation ▪ Avoid exposure to moisture, light in storage ▪ Avoid abrupt withdrawal; D/C *gradually* ▪ Maintain hydration ▪ Elderly/debilitated may require ↓ dosage ▪ ↑ Dosage *slowly* ▪ Heavy smokers may require ↑ dosage.

EVALUATION: Monitor CV, hepatic, ophthalmic, renal status ▪ Monitor BP, CBC, fluid retention (I&O, daily weight), constipation ▪ Assess mental status ▪ Assess for extrapyramidal symptoms (tics/spasms, trembling, shuffling gait) ▪ Institute seizure precautions in pts c̄ hx of convulsive disorders ▪ Assess for symptoms of abrupt withdrawal (nausea, headache, malaise) ▪ Assess IOP.

EDUCATION: Dizziness/drowsiness may occur; use caution in potentially hazardous activities ▪ Avoid changing positions (lying/sitting/standing) rapidly ▪ Avoid use c̄ alcohol, other CNS depressants for up to 1wk after therapy ▪ Take c̄ food ▪ Take as ordered by physician ▪ Constipation may occur; ↑ fluids, bulk-containing foods ▪ Store in tightly closed, light-resistant container ▪ Use sugarless gum/hard candy to diminish dry mouth ▪ Maintain fluid intake (6-8 glasses/d) ▪ Avoid exposure to direct sunlight, UV light (sunlamps); use sunscreen, protective clothing ▪ Notify physician of fever, sore throat, malaise ▪ Notify physician of extrapyramidal symptoms (tics/spasms, trembling, shuffling gait) ▪ Avoid ↑ exercise, temperature extremes ▪ Avoid smoking ▪ Check c̄ physician/pharmacist before taking OTC preparations ▪ Schedule periodic eye exams ▪ Full drug effects may require several wks of therapy ▪ Men: breast enlargement may occur ▪ May interfere c̄ sexual functioning.

NOTES:

clonazepam • (kloe-na-ze-pam)

CATEGORY: *Benzodiazepine*: anticonvulsant

Rx C-IV; Preg Cat NA

BRAND NAMES
Klonopin (Roche)
**Rivotril (Roche)*

DOSAGE FORMS
Tablet: 0.5, 1, 2mg
Tablet: 0.5, 2mg

ACTION: Anticonvulsant activity appears to be on subcortical level & in limbic system; about 30% of pts show loss of anticonvulsant activity. **USE:** Treatment of Lennox-Gastaut syndrome, akinesia, myoclonic seizures; may be useful in petit mal.

DOSAGE

Pediatric *PO* Up to 10y/o or 30kg: initial dose 0.01-0.03mg/kg/d in 2-3 divided doses. ↑ by no more than 0.25-0.5mg every 3d to maintenance dose 0.1-0.2mg/kg/d

Adult *PO* Initial dose *not* to exceed 1.5mg/d in 3 divided doses. ↑ by 0.5-1mg every 3d until seizures are controlled or adverse effects preclude further use. Do *not* exceed 20mg/d

PHARMACOKINETICS

PO absorption	Onset	Peak	Duration	Half-life	Excretion
Very good	20-60m	1-2h	6-12h	18-50h	Via urine as metabolites

CONTRAINDICATIONS: Hypersensitivity, narrow-angle/significant glaucoma.

SIDE/ADVERSE EFFECTS: CNS: drowsiness (50%), ataxia (30%), behavior problems (25%), choreiform movements, ***coma***, respiratory depression, hallucinations, psychosis, suicide attempts, dysarthria ▪ CV: palpitations,

Note: Side/adverse effects: common in *italic;* serious in ***boldface italic.***

*Available in Canada only.

ankle/facial edema ▪ EENT: abnormal eye movement, diplopia ▪ GI: anorexia, coated tongue, dry mouth, gastritis, nausea ▪ HEM: anemia, leukopenia, ***thrombocytopenia***, eosinophilia ▪ HEP: hepatomegaly ▪ MS: muscle weakness.

DRUG INTERACTIONS: Use c̄ other CNS depressants produces additive effects ▪ Use c̄ MAO-I, tricyclic antidepressants produces sedation.

NURSING MANAGEMENT

ADMINISTRATION: Assess for hx of benzodiazepine hypersensitivity ▪ Divide daily dose into 3 equal doses; if not possible, administer largest dose before hs ▪ Avoid use in pts with glaucoma ▪ Avoid exposure to heat, moisture, light in storage ▪ Avoid abrupt withdrawal; institute strict seizure precautions if drug is abruptly withdrawn ▪ Have emergency support measures available ▪ Elderly may require ↓ dosage.

EVALUATION: Assess for status epilepticus, hypoxia when therapy is D/C ▪ Assess serum for ↑ alkaline phosphatases, transaminases ▪ Monitor occurrence/characteristics of seizures ▪ Monitor hemopoietic, renal, hepatic status ▪ Assess for symptoms of abrupt withdrawal (tremors, abdominal/muscle cramps, convulsions) c̄ prolonged use ▪ Check for signs of dependence (↑ drug request) ▪ Monitor activity status (safety precautions) ▪ Assess for tolerance to therapeutic dose ▪ Assess for paradoxic rxs (CNS stimulation), esp in elderly ▪ Check for depression; suicide precautions prn.

EDUCATION: May cause ↑ salivation ▪ Carry medical identification (MedicAlert) ▪ Women: avoid breastfeeding ▪ Drowsiness may occur; use caution in potentially hazardous activities ▪ Avoid use c̄ alcohol, other CNS depressants ▪ Indiscriminate use may lead to dependence ▪ Do *not* keep at bedside ▪ Take as ordered by physician; do *not* omit daily dose ▪ Check c̄ physician/pharmacist before taking OTC drugs ▪ Store in tightly closed, light-resistant container.

NOTES:

clonidine hcl • (kloe-ni-deen)

CATEGORY: *Antihypertensive:* α_2 agonist

Rx; Preg Cat C

BRAND NAMES

Brand	DOSAGE FORMS
Catapres (B-I)	Tablet: 0.1, 0.2, 0.3mg Transdermal system (TTS): 1, 2, 3
**Dixarit (B-I)*	Tablet: 0.025mg

COMBINATION PRODUCTS

Combipres (B-I) 0.1	Clonidine 0.1mg/chlorthalidone 15mg per tablet
Combipres (B-I) 0.2	Clonidine 0.2mg/chlorthalidone 15mg per tablet
Combipres (B-I) 0.3	Clonidine 0.3mg/chlorthalidone 15mg per tablet

ACTION: Antihypertensive effect appears related to central α_2-adrenergic activity, which results in inhibition of bulbar sympathetic cardioaccelerator, sympathetic vasoconstriction centers. **USE:** Treatment of hypertension as sole agent or in combination c̄ other antihypertensive drugs.

PHARMACOKINETICS

PO absorption	Peak	Half-life	Excretion
Good	3-5h	6-20h	Via kidney, feces primarily as metabolites

CONTRAINDICATIONS: Hypersensitivity.

DOSAGE

Adult *PO*	Initial dose 0.1mg bid. Usual maintenance dose range 0.2-0.8mg/d. Maximum effect dose 2.4mg/d
Combripres	0.1mg tablet formulation bid, c̄ range 0.2-0.8mg/d in divided doses
Transdermal	Apply patch 1, 2, or 3 q7d

Note: Side/adverse effects: common in *italic;* serious in ***boldface italic.***

*Available in Canada only.

SIDE/ADVERSE EFFECTS: CNS: *drowsiness, sedation,* headache, vivid dreams, anxiety, mental depression ▪ CV: CHF, Raynaud's phenomenon, ECG changes (usually ventricular trigeminy), ***AV block*** ▪ EENT: nasal dryness, ocular irritation ▪ GI: *dry mouth*, constipation, anorexia, vomiting, parotid pain ▪ GU: urinary retention, impotence ▪ INT: rash, hives, alopecia, pruritus ▪ Other: ***angioneurotic edema.***

DRUG INTERACTIONS: Use c̄ alcohol, other CNS depressants produces additive depression.

NURSING MANAGEMENT

ADMINISTRATION: Assess for hx of hypersensitivity ▪ Assess renal function; may require ↓ dose if impaired ▪ Assess BP; if *hypotensive*, hold drug, notify physician ▪ Avoid abrupt withdrawal; D/C gradually ▪ Use c̄ diuretics will ↑ antihypertensive effect ▪ Elderly may require ↓ dosage.

EVALUATION: Monitor VS, esp BP ▪ Monitor I&O, daily weight ▪ Observe for mental depression; D/C drug, notify physician ▪ Assess for edema in extremities ▪ Schedule ophthalmic exams (retinopathy) ▪ Observe for signs of tolerance; notify physician.

EDUCATION: Drowsiness/dizziness may occur; use caution in potentially hazardous activities ▪ Avoid changing positions (lying/sitting/standing) rapidly ▪ Notify physician of fever, sore throat, bruising/bleeding ▪ Take as ordered by physician even if symptom free; do *not* skip doses ▪ Take last dose just before bedtime ▪ Do *not* stop taking w/out notifying physician ▪ Check c̄ physician/pharmacist before taking OTC/Rx preparations ▪ Avoid use c̄ alcohol, CNS depressants ▪ Avoid high-Na^+ foods (canned soups, lunch meats, cheese) ▪ Avoid ↑ exercise, temperature extremes, smoking ▪ Used to control, *not* cure, hypertension ▪ Maintain optimum weight ▪ Keep scheduled appointments c̄ physician/eye exams ▪ Use sugarless gum/hard candy to diminish dry mouth ▪ Carry identification (MedicAlert) if talking antihypertensives ▪ Procedure for transdermal patch application: Apply to hairless body area every 7 days; wash site c̄ soap, H_2O; dry thoroughly before applying; use firm pressure to ensure adherence to skin; rotate sites; do *not* apply to scarred or irritated area.

NOTES:

clorazepate dipotassium • (klor-az-e-pate)

CATEGORY: *Benzodiazepine:* antianxiety, anxiolytic — Rx C-IV; Preg Cat NA

BRAND NAMES	DOSAGE FORMS
Tranxene (Abbott)	Tablet: 3.75, 7.5, 15mg
Tranxene-SD (Abbott)	Tablet: 22.5mg
Tranxene-SD Half Strength (Abbott)	Tablet: 11.25mg

ACTION: Anxiolytic activity due to depression of CNS at brainstem reticular formation, limbic, thalamic areas. **USE:** Treatment of anxiety, acute alcohol withdrawal ▪ Adjunct in management of partial seizures.

PHARMACOKINETICS: Drug converted to nordiazepam (active metabolite) after PO absorption; excretion via urine, feces.

CONTRAINDICATIONS: Hypersensitivity, narrow-angle glaucoma.

DOSAGE

Anxiety	
Adult *PO*	Start c̄ 30mg/d divided, adjust gradually to 15-60mg/d
Geriatric *PO*	Start c̄ 7.5-15mg/d divided
Alcoholism	
Day 1	30mg followed by 30-60mg divided
Day 2	45-90mg divided
Day 3	22.5-45mg divided
Day 4	15-30mg divided Gradually ⬇ dose to 7.5-15mg/d. D/C when pt is stable
Seizures	
Pediatric *PO*	9-12y/o: Up to 7.5mg bid, adjust by 7.5mg increments weekly to maximum 60mg/d
Adult *PO*	Start c̄ 7.5mg tid, adjust by 7.5mg increments weekly to maximum 90mg/d

SIDE/ADVERSE EFFECTS: CNS: *drowsiness, fatigue, ataxia* ▪ CV: hypotension ▪ HEM: neutropenia (rare) ▪ PSYCH: paradoxical anxiety, hallucinations, hyperexcited states.

DRUG INTERACTIONS: Use c̄ other CNS depressants produces additive effects ▪ Use c̄ MAO-I can produce serious toxic effects.

NURSING MANAGEMENT

ADMINISTRATION: Assess for hx of benzodiazepine hypersensitivity ▪ Avoid exposure to heat, moisture, light in storage ▪ Avoid abrupt withdrawal ▪ Have emergency support measures available ▪ Elderly may require ↓ dosage ▪ Problem discussion, sympathetic listening contribute to relief of anxiety.

EVALUATION: Monitor renal, hepatic status ▪ Assess for symptoms of abrupt withdrawal (tremors, abdominal/muscle cramps, convulsions) c̄ prolonged use ▪ Check for signs of dependence (↑ drug request) ▪ Monitor activity status (safety precautions) ▪ Assess for tolerance to therapeutic dose ▪ Assess for paradoxic rxs (CNS stimulation), esp in elderly ▪ Check for depression; suicide precautions prn.

EDUCATION: Drowsiness may occur; use caution in potentially hazardous activities ▪ Avoid use c̄ alcohol, other CNS depressants ▪ Seizures: do *not* omit daily dose ▪ Indiscriminate use may lead to dependence ▪ Do *not* keep at bedside ▪ Take as ordered by physician; do *not* ↑ dose ▪ Women: avoid breastfeeding ▪ Check c̄ physician/pharmacist before taking OTC drugs ▪ Practice relaxation exercises; ventilation of feelings.

NOTES:

cloxacillin sodium/dicloxacillin sodium • (klox-a-sill-in)

CATEGORY: *Penicillinase-resistant penicillin:* antibiotic — Rx; Preg Cat B

BRAND NAMES

cloxacillin
- **Apo-Cloxi (Apotex)*
- **Bactopen (SKB)*
- *Cloxapen (SKB)*
- **Orbenin (Ayerst)*
- *Tegopen (Apothecon)*

dicloxacillin
- *Dycill (SKB)*
- *Dynapen (Apothecon)*
- *Pathocil (W-A)*

DOSAGE FORMS

cloxacillin:	Capsule, 250, 550mg
	PO suspension 125mg/5ml
dicloxacillin:	Capsule, 125, 250, 500mg
	PO suspension 62.5mg/5ml

ACTION: Bactericidal activity due to inhibition of mucopeptide cell wall synthesis in susceptible organisms. **USE:** Treatment of infections due to susceptible penicillinase-producing staphylococci.

CONTRAINDICATIONS: Hypersensitivity to any penicillin.

DOSAGE

cloxacillin

Pediatric *PO*	<20kg: 50-≥100mg/kg/dose divided, q6h >20kg: 250-≥500mg q6h
Adult *PO*	250-≥500mg q6h

dicloxacillin

Pediatric *PO*	<20kg: 12.5-≥25mg/kg/d divided
Adult *PO*	125-≥250mg q6h

SIDE/ADVERSE EFFECTS: CNS: neuropathy usually associated c̄ high parenteral doses ▪ GI: *N/V/D, epigastric distress,* black hairy tongue, flatulence, smell/taste disturbances ▪ GU: ***interstitial nephritis*** (rare) usually associated c̄ methicillin ▪ HEM: anemia, eosinophilia, leukope-

PHARMACOKINETICS

	PO absorption	Peak	Half-life	Protein binding	Excretion
cloxacillin	37%-68%	0.5-2h	0.4-0.8h	90%-96%	Via urine as unchanged
dicloxacillin	35%-76%	0.5-2h	0.7h	93%-96%	drug, metabolites

Note: Side/adverse effects: common in *italic;* serious in ***boldface italic.***

*Available in Canada only.

nia, neutropenia, ***thrombocytopenia*** ▪ HEP: ↑ serum AST, ALT, LDH ▪ INT: rash, pruritus, urticaria ▪ MS: arthralgia ▪ Other: fever, ***anaphylaxis***.

DRUG INTERACTIONS: Bacteriostatic antibiotics c̄ any penicillin can lead to antibiotic antagonism ▪ PO anticoagulant therapy may require dose adjustment.

NURSING MANAGEMENT

ADMINISTRATION: Assess for hx of penicillin/cephalosporin hypersensitivity ▪ Obtain C&S before therapy ▪ Use reconstituted solution w/in 14d refrigerated; shake well before administering ▪ Administer 1h ac/2h pc ▪ Do *not* administer bacteriostatic agents w/in 1h ▪ Avoid exposure to moisture in storage ▪ Have support equipment available for anaphylaxis.

EVALUATION: Monitor pts c̄ allergies/asthma (high risk for hypersensitivity) ▪ Monitor renal, hepatic, hemopoietic status ▪ Monitor VS, esp temperature ▪ Observe for signs of superinfection (diarrhea, perineal itching, oral ulcers).

EDUCATION: Complete full course of therapy (usually 10d) even if symptom free ▪ Take on empty stomach (1h ac/2h pc) at equal intervals around clock to maintain blood levels ▪ Do *not* take c̄ acid beverages (orange juice, carbonated beverage); take c̄ H_2O ▪ Diarrhea may occur ▪ Store in dry, tightly closed container ▪ Discard outdated preparations ▪ Maintain good personal hygiene (esp perineal, oral) ▪ Maintain fluid intake (6-8 glasses/d) ▪ Notify physician of symptoms of allergic rx (fever, difficult breathing, rash) ▪ Carry identification (MedicAlert) if penicillin allergic.

NOTES:

clozapine • (kloz-a-peen)

CATEGORY: *Antipsychotic:* neuroleptic

Rx; Preg Cat B

BRAND NAME
Clozaril (Sandoz)

DOSAGE FORMS
Tablet 25, 100mg

ACTION: Antipsychotic activity appears associated c̄ ↓ dopaminergic pathways, esp in limbic area, resulting in tranquilizing effect is psychotic pts. Drug is relatively free of extrapyramidal symptoms and exhibits antiadrenergic, anticholinergic, antihistaminic, and antiserotonin activity. **USE:** Treatment of severe schizophrenia that is unresponsive to standard antipsychotic regimens.

PHARMACOKINETICS

PO absorption	Peak	Half-life	Protein binding	Excretion
Good	2.5h	4-12h	95%	50% via urine, 30% via feces as metabolites

CONTRAINDICATIONS: Hypersensitivity, comatose states or severe CNS depression, bone marrow depression, severe granulocytopenia, hx of clozapine-induced agranulocytosis.

DOSAGE

Adults *PO* — Initial dose 25mg once or twice/d c̄ increments of 25-50mg/d until 300-450mg is reached by the end of 2 wks. Usual range 330-900mg/d with a usual dose of 600mg/d. Do *not* exceed 900mg/d

SIDE/ADVERSE EFFECTS: CNS: drowsiness, sedation, seizures, headache, tremor, syncope, sleep disorders, agitation, restlessness ▪ CV: tachycardia, hypotension, hypertension, chest pain, ECG changes ▪ GI: salivation, constipation, N/V, abdominal discomfort, dry mouth ▪ HEM: agranulocytosis, leukopenia, neutropenia ▪ Other: fever, rash, visual disturbances, weight gain.

DRUG INTERACTIONS: Use c̄ other CNS depressants will ↑ CNS depression ▪ Use c̄ warfarin, digoxin can ↑ their effects by displacement from protein storage sites ▪ Use c̄ anticholinergic drugs may ↑ atropine-like effects ▪ Use c̄ antihypertensives may ↑ hypotensive effect ▪ Avoid use c̄ other bone marrow depressants.

NURSING MANAGEMENT

ADMINISTRATION: Assess VS, esp BP ▪ Administer c̄ food/full glass of H_2O or milk ▪ Avoid exposure to moisture, light in storage ▪ Avoid abrupt withdrawal; D/C gradually ▪ Maintain hydration ▪ Elderly/debilitated may require ↓ dosage.

EVALUATION: Monitor hepatic, ophthalmic, renal status ▪ Monitor BP, CBC; fluid retention (I&O, daily weight), constipation ▪ Assess mental status ▪ Assess for extrapyramidal symptoms (tics/spasms, trembling, shuffling gait) ▪ Institute seizure precautions in pts c̄ hx of convulsive disorders ▪ Long-term therapy: assess for jaundice, agranulocytosis ▪ Assess for symptoms of abrupt withdrawal (nausea, dyskinesia, trembling, dizziness) ▪ Assess IOP.

EDUCATION: Dizziness/drowsiness may occur; use caution in potentially hazardous activities ▪ Avoid changing positions (lying/sitting/standing) rapidly ▪ Avoid use c̄ alcohol, other CNS depressants ▪ Take as ordered by physician ▪ Take c̄ food ▪ Constipation may occur; ↑ fluids, bulk-containing foods ▪ Store in tightly closed, light-resistant container ▪ Use sugarless gum/hard candy to diminish dry mouth ▪ Maintain fluid intake (6-8 glasses/d) ▪ Avoid exposure to direct sunlight, UV light (sunlamps); use sunscreen, protective clothing ▪ Notify physician of fever, sore throat, bruising/bleeding ▪ Notify physician of extrapyramidal symptoms (tics/spasms, trembling, shuffling gait) ▪ Avoid ↑ exercise, temperature extremes ▪ Avoid smoking ▪ Check c̄ physician/pharmacist before taking OTC preparations ▪ Schedule periodic eye exams ▪ Full drug effects may require several wks of therapy.

NOTES:

codeine phosphate/codeine sulfate • (koe-deen)

CATEGORY: *Narcotic:* opium alkaloid Rx C-II; Preg Cat C

AVAILABLE PREPARATIONS
Codeine phosphate (various)
Codeine sulfate (various)

DOSAGE FORMS: Hypodermic tablet: 15, 30, 60mg; injection: 15, 30, 60mg/ml; tablet: 15, 30, 60mg

Codeine phosphate has greater water solubility than does codeine sulfate.

ACTION: Narcotics produce analgesia, euphoria, sedation; codeine is a most popular antitussive & is included in many cough formulations; equianalgesic doses of codeine, morphine produce similar depression of respiration; 60mg codeine is approximately equal to 10mg morphine in analgesic activity. **USE:** Relief of moderate pain as sole agent or in combination c̄ nonnarcotic analgesics ▪ Antitussive (usually present in cough formulation).

PHARMACOKINETICS

PO absorption	Onset	Duration	Excretion
Good	15-30m	4-6h	Via urine primarily as metabolites

CONTRAINDICATIONS: Hypersensitivity; use c̄ extreme caution in head injuries.

DOSAGE

Pediatric *PO/SC/IM/IV* (IV not recommended)

Analgesic	6-11y/o: 5-10mg q4-6h. Do *not* exceed 60mg/d
Antitussive	2-5y/o: 2.5-5mg q4-6h. Do *not* exceed 30mg/d
Adult/Children	≥12y/o
Analgesic	15-60mg 3-4 times/d
Antitussive	10-20mg q4-6h. Do *not* exceed 120mg/d

SIDE/ADVERSE EFFECTS: CNS: *sedation, lightheadedness,* euphoria, dysphoria, tremors, disorientation, ↓ con-

Note: Side/adverse effects: common in *italic;* serious in ***boldface italic.*** *Available in Canada only.

vulsive threshold ▪ CV: hypotension, palpitations flushing of face ▪ EENT: miosis ▪ GI: *N/V*, dry mouth, constipation, biliary tract spasm ▪ GU: urine retention ▪ INT: pruritus, urticaria ▪ RESP: ***respiratory depression***.

DRUG INTERACTIONS: Use c̄ alcohol, antihistamines, barbiturates, benzodiazepines, methotrimeprazine, phenothiazines, other CNS depressants produces additive CNS depression; dosage reduction may be required ▪ Use c̄ tricyclic antidepressants may produce additive respiratory depression.

NURSING MANAGEMENT

ADMINISTRATION: Assess for hx of opioid hypersensitivity ▪ Assess quality, intensity, location of pain ▪ Store under double lock/key; document use accurately ▪ Check compatibility for mixing c̄ other drugs in solution ▪ Do *not* administer if respirations are <12/m ▪ IM: inject *deep* into muscle; rotate sites ▪ IV: dilute; administer *slowly*; keep supine for 2h ▪ Have narcotic antagonist (naloxone), support measures available ▪ Avoid administration in suspected head injury ▪ Administer *before* pt experiences intense pain ▪ Use + power of suggestion ▪ Avoid abrupt withdrawal; D/C gradually ▪ Elderly may require ↓ dosage.

EVALUATION: Monitor respirations, circulatory function ▪ Assess bowel function, abdominal distention ▪ Assess renal function, urinary retention ▪ Check for signs of dependence (↑ drug request) ▪ Assess for potentiation of CNS depressant effect ▪ Assess for N/V; administer antiemetic ▪ Assess for signs of overdosage (coma, pinpoint pupils, respiratory depression) ▪ SC: check for tissue irritation ▪ May produce ↑ CSF pressure.

EDUCATION: Avoid changing positions (lying/sitting/standing) rapidly ▪ Avoid excessive sensory stimulation ▪ Keep bedrails up when nonambulatory ▪ Turn, cough, deep breathe after surgery ▪ Constipation may occur; ↑ fluids, bulk-containing foods ▪ Avoid potentially hazardous activities ▪ Avoid smoking ▪ Take as ordered by physician; do *not* ↑ dose ▪ Indiscriminate use may lead to severe dependence ▪ Avoid use c̄ alcohol, other CNS depressants ▪ Women: avoid breastfeeding ▪ Notify physician/dentist of use before treatment.

OVERDOSE MANAGEMENT: *See* Narcotics.

NOTES:

colchicine • (kol-chi-seen)

CATEGORY: *Antigout agent* Rx; Preg Cat D

BRAND NAME
Colchicine (various)

DOSAGE FORMS
Injection (IV): 1mg/2ml
Tablet: 0.5, 0.6mg

ACTION: Complete mechanism not determined; antigout activity related to inhibition of leukocyte metabolism; reduction in lactic acid production in polymorphonuclear leukocytes results in retarding urate acid crystal deposition in joints; powerful inhibitor of cell mitosis, extremely toxic, no effect on uric acid excretion. **USE:** Drug of choice for treating acute attacks of gout ▪ Prevention of gout attacks.

PHARMACOKINETICS: Well absorbed PO, short plasma half-life, leukocyte half-life is about 60h; considerable enterohepatic recycling; excretion via feces as unchanged drug, metabolites.

CONTRAINDICATIONS: Hypersensitivity.

DOSAGE

Adult *PO*	Initial dose 0.6-1.2mg, then 0.6mg q1-2h until pain is relieved or until N/V/D develop. Prophylactic dose 0.6mg 1-4 times/wk or 0.6-1.2mg/d in more severe cases
IV	Initial dose 2mg, then 0.5mg q6h until condition improves. Do *not* exceed total of 4mg/d

SIDE/ADVERSE EFFECTS: GI: *N/V/D,* abdominal pain ▪ HEM: ***agranulocytosis, thrombocytopenia, aplastic anemia*** ▪ INT: alopecia, purpura ▪ Other: peripheral neuritis, chromosomal aberrations.

DRUG INTERACTIONS: Use $\bar{c}$ adrenergics, CNS depressants enhances effects ▪ Possible malabsorption syndrome for vitamin B_{12}.

NURSING MANAGEMENT
ADMINISTRATION: Assess for hx of hypersensitivity ▪ PO: administer $\bar{c}$ food/milk to ↓ GI distress ▪ Assess serum uric acid (normal: 3-7mg/dl) ▪ Assess hepatic, car-

diac, hematologic, renal function; use c̄ caution if impaired ▪ IV: administer *slowly* (2-5m); do *not* dilute/inject c̄ 5% dextrose, bacteriostatic solutions (precipitation) ▪ Do *not* use discolored/precipitated solutions ▪ Do *not* administer IM/SC ▪ ↑ Fluid intake (3000m/d) ▪ Avoid exposure to light during storage ▪ Elderly may require ↓ dosage.

EVALUATION: Monitor I&O, CBC ▪ Observe for signs of toxicity (N/D, abdominal pain): D/C drug, notify physician ▪ Check IV site carefully; avoid extravasation.

EDUCATION: Take c̄ food or milk ▪ Used to stop acute gout attack; always carry ▪ D/C drug if experiencing signs of toxicity (N/D, abdominal cramps); notify physician ▪ Limit purine dietary intake (organ meats, gravy, legumes) ▪ ↑ Fluid intake (10-12 glasses/d) ▪ Notify physician of fever, sore throat, bruising/bleeding, black/tarry stools ▪ Maintain optimum weight; *gradual* reduction ▪ Avoid use c̄ alcohol ▪ Notify physician/dentist of use before therapy.

NOTES:

cortisone • (kor-ti-sone)

CATEGORY: *Glucosteroid:* corticosteroid — Rx; Preg Cat NA

BRAND NAMES
Cortone Acetate
(MSD)
(Upjohn [Canada])

DOSAGE FORMS
IM suspension: 50mg/ml
Tablet: 25mg (also 5mg in Canada)

ACTION: Glucosteroids cause wide variety of pharmacologic activity; two major effects are potent antiinflammatory effect, inhibition of immune response. **USE:** Treatment of adrenocorticoid deficiency, adrenogenital syndrome, other endocrine disorders; allergic states, collagen diseases, dermatologic diseases, GI diseases, hematologic disorders, ophthalmologic disorders, respiratory diseases, rheumatic disorders ▪ Treatment of tubercular meningitis, neurologic or myocardial involvement associated c̄ trichinosis ▪ Remission of proteinuria in nephrotic syndrome, acute exacerbation of multiple sclerosis ▪ Palliative management of leukemia, lymphomas.

PHARMACOKINETICS: PO administration usually produces peak effect in 2h, duration about 1.5d.

CONTRAINDICATIONS: Systemic fungal infections, hypersensitivity.

DOSAGE

Pediatric *PO*	0.7-10mg/kg/d
Adult *PO/IM*	25-300mg/d

SIDE/ADVERSE EFFECTS: CNS: ***convulsions,*** headache, psychic impairment, mood swings, vertigo; pseudotumor cerebri may develop after treatment ▪ CV: edema due to Na^+ retention, CHF, hypertension ▪ EENT: ↑ IOP, glaucoma, posterior subcapsular cataracts, exophthalmos ▪ END: cushingoid states, growth suppression in children, menstrual irregularities, 2° adrenocortical/pituitary unresponsiveness, hyperglycemia, carbohydrate intolerance ▪ GI: peptic ulcer c̄ ***possible perforation, pancreatitis,*** abdominal distention, ulcerative esophagitis ▪ INT: poor wound healing, fragile skin, petechiae/ecchymoses facial erythema, ↑ sweating, urticaria, hirsutism ▪ MET: negative nitrogen balance, hypokalemic alkalosis ▪ MS: muscle weakness c̄ loss of mass, pathologic fracture of long bones, osteoporosis.

DRUG INTERACTIONS: Severe hypokalemia can occur c̄ diuretics (nonpotassium sparing) ▪ Use c̄ ulcerogenic drugs (aspirin, indomethacin) can produce additive effects ▪ Use c̄ antidiabetic agents may require higher doses of antidiabetic drugs.

NURSING MANAGEMENT

ADMINISTRATION: Assess for hx of hypersensitivity ▪ Administer single daily/alternate-day dose *before* 9AM; multiple doses at equal intervals ▪ PO: administer c̄ food, milk, antacid ▪ Do *not* administer IV ▪ IM: shake well; do *not* mix, dilute, freeze; inject *deep* into gluteal UOQ (avoid deltoid); rotate sites ▪ Avoid abrupt withdrawal ▪ Avoid exposure to heat, light in storage ▪ Elderly may require ↓ dosage; monitor BP.

EVALUATION: Monitor VS, esp BP ▪ Diabetics: closely monitor blood/urine glucose ▪ Assess mental/emotional status; avoid tricyclic antidepressants if depression induced ▪ Monitor serum electrolytes (esp K^+, Na^+), vision/IOP, stool for occult blood c̄ prolonged use ▪ Monitor hydration status (I&O, daily weight).

EDUCATION: Take c̄ food/milk (single dose *before* 9AM; multiple doses at equal intervals) ▪ Take as ordered by physician; do *not* ↑ dose ▪ Eat foods high in K^+, protein; avoid black licorice ▪ Follow low-Na^+ diet ▪ Check c̄ physician before immunization (pt, family) ▪ Avoid exposure to infection ▪ Report following symptoms *immediately* to physician: anorexia, difficult breathing, weakness, dizziness; may appear during periods of ↑ stress, trauma ▪ Notify physician of black/tarry stools, slow wound healing, blurred vision, bruising/bleeding, weight gain, emotional changes ▪ Diabetics: closely monitor blood/urine glucose ▪ Store in tightly closed, light-resistant container ▪ Do *not* D/C drug w/out checking c̄ physician ▪ Keep scheduled appointments c̄ physician/blood work/eye exams ▪ Women: avoid breastfeeding ▪ Body image changes (full face, ↑ facial hair, ↑ fat deposit) may occur c̄ prolonged use (reversible after therapy).

NOTES:

co-trimoxazole • (koe-trye-mox-a-zole)

CATEGORY: *Fixed-combination sulfonamide*: antiinfective Rx; Preg Cat C

COMBINATION PRODUCTS

**Apo-Sulfatrim (Apotex)*
Bactrim (Roche)
**Novotrimel (Novopharm)*
**Protrin (Pro-Dec)*
**Roubac (Rougier)*
Septra (B-W)

CONTRAINDICATIONS: Hypersensitivity, pregnancy at term, nursing mothers, infants <2mo of age (except in treatment of congenital toxoplasmosis), folate deficient megaloblastic anemia, urinary acidifier use.

DOSAGE FORMS

	IV	PO suspension	Pediatric suspension	Tablet	DS tablet
Sulfamethoxazole	80mg/ml	200mg/5ml	200mg/5ml	400mg	800mg
Trimethoprim	16mg/ml	40mg/5ml	40mg/5ml	80mg	160mg

ACTION: Bactericidal activity due to inhibition of two successive steps of folic acid synthesis. **USE:** Treatment of urinary tract infections caused by susceptible strains of *Enterobacter* spp, *Escherichia coli, Klebsiella* spp, *Morganella morganii, Proteus mirabilis, Proteus vulgaris* ▪ Treatment of pediatric otitis media, acute exacerbation of adult chronic bronchitis caused by susceptible strains of *Haemophilus influenzae, Streptococcus pneumoniae* ▪ Treatment of shigellosis caused by susceptible strains of *Shigella flexneri, S. sonnei* ▪ Treatment of *Pneumocystis carinii* pneumonitis.

DOSAGE

Pediatric *PO*

Ear, urinary infection	8mg/kg TMP, 40mg/kg SMZ in 24h in 2 doses/d for 10d
Shigellosis	8mg/kg TMP, 40mg/kg SMZ in 24h in 2 doses/d for 5d
Pneumonitis	20mg/kg TMP, 100mg/kg SMZ in 24h in 4 doses/d for 14d

Adult *PO*

Urinary infection, bronchitis	2 tablets, 1 DS tablet, 20ml suspension q12h for 10-14d

Note: Side/adverse effects: common in *italic;* serious in ***boldface italic.*** *Available in Canada only.

Shigellosis	2 tablets, 1 DS tablet, 20ml suspension, q12h for 5d
Pneumonitis	20mg/kg TMP, 100mg/kg SMZ in 24h in 4 doses/d for 14d
Pediatric/Adult *IV*	
Urinary infection	Based on TMP content 8-10mg/kg/d in 2-4 equal doses for 14d
Shigellosis	8-10mg/kg/d in 2-4 equal doses for 5d
Pneumocystis	15-20mg/kg/d in 2-4 equal doses

SIDE/ADVERSE EFFECTS: CNS: headache, peripheral neuritis, ataxia, ***convulsions*** ▪ GI: N/V/D, anorexia, abdominal pain, stomatitis ▪ GU: crystalluria, toxic nephrosis ▪ HEM: ***agranulocytosis, aplastic anemia, hemolytic anemia***, thrombocytopenic purpura, methemoglobinemia, hypoprothrombinemia, leukopenia ▪ INT: rash, pruritus, ***Stevens-Johnson syndrome, epidermal necrolysis, exfoliative dermatitis***, photosensitivity ▪ MET: ↑ Serum transaminase, creatinine, BUN ▪ MS: arthralgia ▪ Other: serum sickness, allergic myocarditis, periorbital edema.

DRUG INTERACTIONS: Avoid *p*-aminobenzoic preparations during therapy ▪ Increases activity of PO hypoglycemics, methotrexate, PO anticoagulants.

NURSING MANAGEMENT

ADMINISTRATION: Assess for hx of sulfonamide hypersensitivity; furosemide, thiazide diuretics ▪ Obtain C&S before therapy ▪ Maintain hydration ▪ Administer 1h ac/2h pc $\bar{c}$ full glass H_2O ▪ Avoid use in group A β-hemolytic streptococcal infections ▪ IV: dilute (5ml amp/125ml) 5% dextrose; administer w/in 2h after diluting; administer over 60-90m; flush lines at end of infusion to remove residual; store infusion at room temperature, do *not* refrigerate ▪ Do *not* administer IM rapidly, or by bolus injection ▪ Do *not* mix $\bar{c}$ other drugs/solutions.

EVALUATION: Monitor hepatic status, temperature, CBC, UA, I&O.

EDUCATION: Complete full course of therapy ▪ Take on empty stomach $\bar{c}$ full glass H_2O; if upset stomach occurs, take $\bar{c}$ food ▪ Take at equal intervals around clock ▪ ↑ Fluid intake (8-10 glasses/d) ▪ Women: avoid breastfeeding ▪ Notify physician/dentist of sulfonamide use before general anesthesia ▪ Notify physician of fever, sore throat, difficult breathing, rash, bruising/bleeding.

NOTES:

cyclobenzaprine hcl • (sye-kloe-ben-za-preen)

CATEGORY: *Skeletal muscle relaxant* Rx; Preg Cat B

BRAND NAME
Flexeril (MSD)

DOSAGE FORM
Tablet: 10mg

ACTION: Skeletal muscle relaxation mechanism not determined; primary site of activity appears to be w/in CNS at brain stem; no direct action on contractile mechanism of striated muscle, motor end plate, nerve fiber; anticholinergic activity; structurally related to tricyclic antidepressants. **USE:** Adjunct for relief of discomfort associated c̄ acute painful musculoskeletal conditions.

PHARMACOKINETICS

PO absorption	Peak	Half-life	Protein binding	Excretion
Complete	3-8h	1-3d	93%	Via urine, feces

CONTRAINDICATIONS: Hypersensitivity, arrhythmias, heart block/conduction disturbances, hyperthyroidism, recovery phase of MI, concurrent use c̄ MAO-I or w/in 14d of their discontinuance.

DOSAGE
Adult *PO* 10mg tid c̄ range 20-40mg/d for 2-3 wks

SIDE/ADVERSE EFFECTS: CNS: *drowsiness, dizziness,* paresthesia ▪ CV: ↑ heart rate ▪ EENT: blurred vision ▪ GI: *dry mouth,* nausea, dyspepsia.

DRUG INTERACTIONS: Use/sequential use (w/in 14d) c̄ MAO-I may cause significant hyperpyretic crisis ▪ Use c̄ anticholinergics, CNS depressants produces additive effects ▪ Use c̄ guanethidine-like drugs produces ↓ antihypertensive effects.

NURSING MANAGEMENT

ADMINISTRATION: Assess for hx of hypersensitivity ▪ Assess hepatic, ocular, renal function; use c̄ caution if impaired; do *not* use c̄ cardiac problems ▪ Administer c̄ food to ↓ GI distress ▪ Have physostigmine available for OD ▪ Avoid exposure to moisture during storage ▪ Elderly may require ↓ dosage.

EVALUATION: Monitor VS, esp BP ▪ Monitor hepatic, renal status (I&O) ▪ Monitor activity status (safety precautions) ▪ Observe for tachycardia; D/C drug, notify physician ▪ Glaucoma: monitor IOP (↑).

EDUCATION: Drowsiness may occur; use caution when engaging in potentially hazardous activities ▪ Take as ordered by physician; do *not* ↑ dose ▪ Take c̄ meals ▪ Avoid use c̄ alcohol, other CNS depressants ▪ Rest, physical therapy promote comfort ▪ Use sugarless gum/hard candy to diminish dry mouth ▪ Constipation may occur; ↑ fluids, bulk-containing foods ▪ Keep scheduled appointments for eye exams ▪ Women: avoid breastfeeding ▪ Notify physician *immediately* of eye pain; D/C drug.

NOTES:

cyclophosphamide • (sye-klow-foss-fa-mide)

CATEGORY: *Alkylating agent*: antineoplastic — Rx; Preg Cat NA

BRAND NAMES	DOSAGE FORMS
Cytoxan (BM-ONC) (Bristol in Canada)	Powder for injection (IV), tablet 25, 50mg
Neosar (Adria)	Powder for injection (IV)
**Procytox (Horner)*	Powder for injection, tablet

ACTION: Antineoplastic activity due to polyfunctional alkylating effects on DNA replication, RNA transcription; drug exhibits phosphorylating properties, immunosuppressive activity. **USE:** Treatment of malignant lymphomas incl Burkitt's lymphoma (drug of choice), follicular lymphoma, Hodgkin's disease, lymphoblastic lymphosarcoma, lymphocytic lymphosarcoma, reticulum cell sarcoma ▪ Treatment of leukemias incl acute pediatric lymphoblastic leukemias, acute myelogenous/monocytic leukemia, chronic granulocytic/lymphocytic leukemia ▪ Treatment of multiple myeloma, mycosis fungoides, solid malignancies, breast cancer.

PHARMACOKINETICS: IV half-life about 4h; excretion via kidneys as metabolites, unchanged drug w/in 48h.

CONTRAINDICATIONS: Hypersensitivity, severe depression of bone marrow function.

DOSAGE

Pediatric *PO/IV*	Induction: loading dose 2-8mg/kg/d divided for ≥6d
PO	Maintenance: 2-5mg/kg twice/wk
Adult *PO/IV*	Induction: 1-5mg/kg/d or 40-50mg/kg divided for 2-5d. Loading dose may require 1/3-1/2 reduction in presence of bone marrow dysfunction
PO	Maintenance: 1-5mg/kg/d
IV	10-15mg/kg q7-10d or 3-5mg/kg twice/wk

SIDE/ADVERSE EFFECTS: GI: *N/V/D,* oral ulcerations, ***hemorrhagic colitis*** ▪ GU: *hemorrhagic cystitis,* cystitis, fibrosis, amenorrhea, azoospermia ▪ HEM: *leukopenia,* ***thrombocytopenia***, anemia ▪ INT: *alopecia*, skin/fingernail darkening, nonspecific dermatitis ▪ MET: hyperuricemia ▪ Other: ***secondary malignancies*** (incl bladder, myeloproliferative/lymphoproliferative), interstitial pulmonary fibrosis.

Note: Side/adverse effects: common in *italic;* serious in ***boldface italic.***

*Available in Canada only.

DRUG INTERACTIONS: Live vaccines contraindicated during therapy ▪ Radiation, other myelosuppressive drugs produce additive bone marrow depression ▪ Steroids produce additive immunosuppressant activity ▪ Barbiturates may ↑ cyclophosphamide metabolism ▪ Doxorubicin may ↑ cardiac toxicity ▪ Allopurinol may ↑ bone marrow suppression.

NURSING MANAGEMENT

ADMINISTRATION: Check pt hx for recent course of radiation/antineoplastic therapy; report to physician ▪ Avoid exposure to moisture, light in storage ▪ Store between 36°-90° F ▪ PO: administer 1h ac/2h pc ▪ Reconstitute powder for injection c̄ 5ml sterile/bacteriostatic H_2O (100mg/vial), 120ml (200mg/vial), 25ml (250mg/vial); may be administered IV, IM, intraperitoneally, intrapleurally, by infusion (added to 5% dextrose/normal saline solution) ▪ Force fluids (3000ml/d) ▪ Use reconstituted injection w/in 24h at room temperature or 6d refrigerated ▪ Administer antiemetic before therapy ▪ Provide emotional support.

EVALUATION: Monitor CBC throughout therapy ▪ Assess for infection, bleeding, anemia ▪ Assess for ↑ serum uric acid levels ▪ Monitor hepatic, renal function during therapy ▪ Assess hydration status (I&O, daily weight) ▪ False (+): Pap test ▪ False (-): skin tests (*Candida*, mumps, PPD, trichophyton) ▪ Monitor wound healing (delay) ▪ Check IV site closely; avoid extravasation.

EDUCATION: ↑ Fluid intake (10-12 glasses/d) ▪ PO: take on empty stomach ▪ Avoid exposure to infection ▪ Check c̄ physician before immunization (pt, family) ▪ Diet as tolerated; avoid spicy foods ▪ Maintain good oral hygiene; use soft-bristled toothbrush ▪ Notify physician of symptoms of bone marrow depression (fever, sore throat, bruising, bleeding, lethargy) ▪ Loss of hair may occur (reversible) ▪ Women: avoid breastfeeding ▪ Encourage ventilation of feelings ▪ Use contraception if sexually active.

NOTES:

cyproheptadine hcl • (si-proe-<u>hep</u>-ta-deen)

CATEGORY: *Antihistamine:* H_1 blocker, antipruritic — Rx; Preg Cat B

BRAND NAMES

Periactin (MSD)
**Vimicon (Frosst)*

DOSAGE FORMS

Syrup: 2mg/5ml
Tablet: 4mg

ACTION: H_1 antihistamine activity due to competitive inhibition of histamine at H_1 histamine receptors on effector cells; drug exhibits antiserotonin activity, is structurally related to azatadine maleate. **USE:** Symptomatic treatment of allergic disorders mediated by histamine.

PHARMACOKINETICS: 40% of single dose excreted in urine, 2%-20% in feces.

CONTRAINDICATIONS: Hypersensitivity, neonates, nursing mothers, lower respiratory tract symptoms.

DOSAGE

Pediatric *PO*	2-6y/o: 2mg 2-3 times/d. Do *not* exceed 12mg/d 7-14y/o: 4mg 2-3 times/d. Do *not* exceed 16mg/d
Adult *PO*	4-20mg/d divided. Doses of 32mg/d may be required. Do *not* exceed 0.5mg/kg/d

SIDE/ADVERSE EFFECTS: CNS: *drowsiness,* dizziness, fatigue, euphoria, paresthesias ▪ CV: hypotension, palpitations, tachycardia, extrasystole ▪ EENT: blurred vision, nasal stuffiness ▪ GI: N/V, anorexia ▪ GU: early menses ▪ HEM: ***agranulocytosis, hemolytic anemia, thrombocytopenia*** ▪ INT: drug rash, photosensitivity ▪ RESP: thickening of bronchial secretions, wheezing ▪ Other: anticholinergic effects.

DRUG INTERACTIONS: Use c̄ anticholinergics, CNS depressants, tricyclic antidepressants produces additive effects ▪ MAO-I can intensity anticholinergic effects of antihistamines.

Note: Side/adverse effects: common in *italic;* serious in ***boldface italic.***

*Available in Canada only.

NURSING MANAGEMENT

ADMINISTRATION: Assess for hx of antihistamine hypersensitivity ▪ Administer c̄ food ▪ Have support equipment available for anaphylaxis ▪ Avoid exposure to moisture, light in storage ▪ Maintain hydration.

EVALUATION: Monitor VS, esp BP ▪ Assess for excessive drowsiness, dizziness, weakness ▪ Monitor CBC c̄ prolonged therapy ▪ Monitor children for paradoxic rxs (CNS stimulation) ▪ Assess for tolerance to therapeutic dose; notify physician, another antihistamine may be substituted.

EDUCATION: Drowsiness, dizziness, lightheadedness may occur; use caution in potentially hazardous activities ▪ Avoid use c̄ alcohol, other CNS depressants ▪ Take c̄ meals ▪ Store in tightly closed, light-resistant container ▪ Use sugarless gum/hard candy to diminish dry mouth ▪ ↑ Fluid intake (8-10 glasses/d) ▪ Notify physician of symptoms of allergic rx (fever, difficult breathing, rash) ▪ Women: avoid breastfeeding ▪ Carry identification (MedicAlert) if antihistamine allergic ▪ Notify physician of antihistamine use before allergy testing.

NOTES:

cytarabine • (sye-tare-a-been)

CATEGORY: *Antineoplastic*: antimetabolite — Rx; Preg Cat D

BRAND NAME
Cytosar-U (Upjohn)

DOSAGE FORMS
Powder for injection (IV/SC): 100, 500mg, 1, 2g vials

ACTION: Antimetabolic activity due to inhibition of DNA polymerase, resulting in cytotoxic effect in cells c̄ high rates of proliferation; exhibits immunosuppressive activity. **USE:** Treatment of acute myelocytic, lymphocytic leukemia, non-Hodgkin lymphoma in children, intrathecal use in meningeal leukemia. Drug is not active PO.

PHARMACOKINETICS: Route of administration determines peak, duration, half-life; protein binding about 13%; metabolized in liver, excreted via urine.

CONTRAINDICATIONS: Hypersensitivity/severe preexisting drug-induced bone marrow suppression.

DOSAGE: *IV/SC* or *intrathecally*

Children/Adult

Nonlymphocytic leukemia	$100mg/m^2/d$ by continuous IV infusion days 1-7 or $100mg/m^2$ IV q12h
Acute lymphocytic leukemia	Consult latest recommendations
Meningeal leukemia	Most frequent intrathecal dose $30mg/m^2$ q4d until cerebrospinal fluid is normal. Usual dose range $5\text{-}75mg/m^2$

SIDE/ADVERSE EFFECTS: CNS: dizziness, neuritis, neural toxicity ▪ CV: chest pain ▪ EENT: conjunctivitis ▪ GI: *anorexia, V/D, oral/anal ulceration*, sore throat, esophageal ulcers, abdominal pain, bowel neurosis ▪ HEM: ***bone marrow suppression*** resulting in anemia, leukopenia, ***thrombocytopenia,*** megaloblastosis ▪ HEP: dysfunction, jaundice ▪ INT: rash, skin ulceration, freckling, alopecia, pruritus, urticaria ▪ Other: ***bleeding, thrombophlebitis.***

DRUG INTERACTIONS: Use of live vaccines contraindicated during therapy.

NURSING MANAGEMENT

ADMINISTRATION: Check hx for recent course of radiation or antineoplastic agents; report to physician ▪ IV: reconstitute, dilute according to manufacturer's directions; stable for 48h at room temperature ▪ Do *not* administer discolored/precipitated solutions ▪ Avoid direct administration c̄ other antineoplastic agents (physical incompatibility) ▪ Administer antiemetic before therapy ▪ Provide emotional support.

EVALUATION: Monitor CBC throughout therapy ▪ Assess for infection, bleeding, anemia ▪ May produce ↑ serum uric acid level ▪ Monitor hepatic function ▪ Assess hydration status (I&O, daily weight) ▪ Check IV insertion site carefully (cellulitis).

EDUCATION: ↑ Fluid intake (8-10 glasses/d) ▪ Avoid exposure to infection ▪ Check c̄ physician before immunization (pt, family) ▪ Diet as tolerated; avoid spicy foods ▪ Avoid alcoholic beverages ▪ Maintain oral hygiene; use soft-bristled toothbrush ▪ Notify physician of symptoms of bone marrow depression (fever, sore throat, bruising, bleeding, lethargy) ▪ Loss of hair may occur (reversible after therapy is ended) ▪ Women: avoid breastfeeding ▪ Encourage ventilation of feelings ▪ Use contraception if sexually active.

NOTES:

dexamethasone/dexamethasone acetate/ dexamethasone sodium phosphate • (dex-a-meth-a-sone)

CATEGORY: *Glucosteroid:* corticosteroid Rx; Preg Cat NA

BRAND NAMES	DOSAGE FORMS
dexamethasone	Elixir, tablet
Decadron (MSD)	Elixir, tablet
**Dexasone (ICN)*	Elixir, tablet
Hexadrol (Organon)	
dexamethasone acetate	
Decadron-LA (MSD)	Injection suspension
dexamethasone sodium phosphate	
Decadron Phosphate (MSD)	Aerosol, injection
Hexadrol (Organon)	Injection

ACTION: Glucosteroids produce potent antiinflammatory effect, inhibit immune response. **USE:** Treatment of adrenocortical deficiency, allergic states, inflammatory/ autoimmune disorders, cerebral edema, septic shock, TB meningitis ▪ Palliation of leukemia, lymphomas ▪ Remission of proteinuria in nephrotic states and acute multiple sclerosis.

PHARMACOKINETICS: PO administration usually produces peak effect in 1-2h, c̄ duration about 3d.

CONTRAINDICATIONS: Systemic fungal infections.

DOSAGE

Pediatric *Aerosol*	2 inhalations (0.3mg) 3-4 times/d. Do *not* exceed 8/d
Adult *PO*	0.75-9mg/d
IM/IV	0.5-9mg/d; intraarticular, intralesional, soft tissue, 0.2-6mg once q3-5d to once q2-3wks
IM suspension	8-16mg q1-3wks prn. Intraarticular, 4-16mg q1-3wks prn. Intralesional, 0.8-1.6mg/injection site
Aerosol	3 inhalations (0.3mg) 3-4 times/d. Do *not* exceed 12/d

SIDE/ADVERSE EFFECTS: CNS: ***convulsions***, headache, psychic impairment, mood swings, vertigo; ↑ intracranial pressure c̄ papilledema may develop ▪ CV: CHF, hypertension ▪ EENT: ↑ IOP, cataracts, exophthalmos ▪ END: cushingoid states, growth suppression in children, menstrual irregularities, 2° adrenocortical/pituitary unrespon-

Note: Side/adverse effects: common in *italic;* serious in ***boldface italic.***

*Available in Canada only.

siveness, hyperglycemia, carbohydrate intolerance ▪ GI: peptic ulcer, ulcerative esophagitis ▪ INT: poor wound healing, fragile skin, petechiae/ecchymoses, facial erythema, ↑ sweating, urticaria, hirsutism ▪ MET: (-) nitrogen balance, hypokalemic alkalosis, edema ▪ MS: muscle weakness/loss of mass, pathologic fracture of long bones, osteoporosis, necrosis of femoral/humeral heads ▪ Other: ↑ susceptibility to infection.

DRUG INTERACTIONS: Severe hypokalemia can occur c̄ diuretics (nonpotassium sparing) ▪ Use c̄ ulcerogenic drugs (eg, aspirin, indomethacin) can produce additive effects ▪ Use c̄ antidiabetic agents may require higher doses of antidiabetic drugs

NURSING MANAGEMENT

ADMINISTRATION: Assess for hx of hypersensitivity ▪ PO: administer c̄ food, milk, antacids ▪ Do *not* administer acetate suspension IV ▪ IM: shake suspension well; do *not* freeze; inject *deep* into gluteal UOQ (avoid deltoid); rotate sites ▪ Avoid abrupt withdrawal ▪ Elderly may require ↓ dosage.

EVALUATION: Monitor VS, esp BP; mental status, blood glucose in diabetics (hyperglycemia), I&O, weight, serum K^+, Na^+; vision/IOP; stools for occult blood.

EDUCATION: Take c̄ food/milk (single daily dose *before* 9AM; multiple doses at equal intervals) ▪ Take as ordered by physician; do *not* ↑ dose, D/C ▪ Eat foods high in K^+, protein, calcium, vitamin D; avoid black licorice ▪ Follow low-Na^+ diet ▪ Check c̄ physician before immunization ▪ Avoid infection ▪ Report anorexia, difficult breathing, weakness, dizziness to physician *immediately* ▪ Notify physician of black/tarry stools, slow wound healing, blurred vision, bruising/bleeding, weight gain, emotional changes ▪ Avoid alcohol, caffeine ▪ Diabetics: closely monitor blood/urine glucose ▪ Safety precautions c̄ ↑ activity/exercise ▪ Notify physician/dentist of use before treatment ▪ Carry medical identification (MedicAlert) ▪ Keep appointment c̄ physician ▪ Women: avoid breastfeeding ▪ Body image changes may occur c̄ prolonged use.

NOTES:

dextroamphetamine hcl • (dex-troe-am-fet-a-meen)

CATEGORY: *Anorexiant, CNS stimulant*: sympathomimetic Rx C-II; Preg Cat C

BRAND NAME
Dexedrine (SKB)

DOSAGE FORMS
Elixir: 5mg/5ml
Sustained-release capsule (Spansules): 5, 10, 15mg
Tablet: 5mg

ACTION: Weak, indirect acting sympathomimetic c̄ strong CNS stimulant activity; peripheral effects incl respiratory stimulant activity, ↑ in BP, weak bronchodilation; CNS effects incl alerting rxs. **USE:** Treatment of narcolepsy, behavioral syndrome (minimal brain dysfunction) in children ▪ Control of exogenous obesity.

PHARMACOKINETICS: Good PO absorption; hepatic metabolism c̄ 10-12h half-life in adults, 7h in children.

CONTRAINDICATIONS: Hypersensitivity, advanced arterial sclerosis, symptomatic CV disease, significant hypertension, hypothyroidism, glaucoma.

DOSAGE

Pediatric	Behavioral: 3-5y/o Initial dose 2.5mg/d, raised in 2.5mg increments wkly until desired effect is reached ≥6y/o Initial dose 5mg 1-2 times/d, raised in 5mg increments wkly until desired effect is reached. Some cases may require ≥40mg/d Narcolepsy: 6-12y/o 5mg/d, raised in 5mg increments wkly until desired effect is reached
Adult *PO*	Obesity: 10-15mg/d Narcolepsy: 5-60mg/d depending on response

SIDE/ADVERSE EFFECTS: CNS: dizziness, insomnia, euphoria, dyskinesia, headache, exacerbation of tics, rare psychotic episodes, *restlessness* ▪ CV: ↑ in BP, palpitations, tachycardia ▪ GI: anorexia, dry mouth, diarrhea, constipation, unpleasant taste ▪ GU: impotence ▪ INT: urticaria.

DRUG INTERACTIONS: Use c̄ MAO-I can produce hypertensive crisis ▪ Use can antagonize effects of guanethidine-like drugs ▪ Diabetic pts may require insulin adjustments ▪ Urinary alkalizers will ↓ urinary excretion, prolong activity.

NURSING MANAGEMENT

ADMINISTRATION: Assess for hx of catecholamine hypersensitivity ▪ Do *not* administer w/in 6h of hs or w/in 14d after MAO-I therapy ▪ Administer tablets ac for obesity ▪ Do *not* crush Spansule; administer whole ▪ Avoid abrupt withdrawal; D/C gradually.

EVALUATION: Monitor VS, esp BP/pulse ▪ Assess for tolerance to therapeutic effect ▪ Diabetics: closely monitor blood glucose ▪ Check for signs of dependence.

EDUCATION: Dizziness, restlessness may occur; use caution when engaging in potentially hazardous activities ▪ Take as directed by physician; do *not* ↑ dose ▪ Swallow Spansule whole ▪ Do *not* take w/in 6h of hs; may cause insomnia ▪ Avoid caffeine-containing products ▪ Weight-reduction diet ▪ Diabetics: monitor blood/urine glucose carefully ▪ Physical dependence may occur ▪ Use sugarless gum/hard candy to diminish dry mouth ▪ Notify physician of nervousness, dizziness, insomnia ▪ Women: avoid breast-feeding ▪ Check c̄ physician/pharmacist before taking OTC cough/cold preparations.

NOTES:

diazepam • (dye-az-e-pam)

CATEGORY: *Benzodiazepine:* antianxiety agent, anxiolytic, anticonvulsant Rx C-IV; Preg Cat NA

BRAND NAMES

**E-Pam (ICN)*
**Meval (Medic)*
**Rival (Riva)*
Valium (Roche)
Valrelease (Roche)
**Vivol (Horner)*

DOSAGE FORMS: Capsule, injection (IM/IV), tablet, timed-release tablet.

ACTION: Anxiolytic activity due to depression of CNS at brainstem reticular formation, limbic, thalamic areas. Drug exhibits muscle relaxant and moderate anticonvulsant properties. **USE:** Treatment of anxiety, tension, alcohol withdrawal symptoms ▪ Convulsive disorders ▪ Preop/instrumental examination anxiety ▪ Adjunct for relief of skeletal muscle spasm.

CONTRAINDICATIONS: Hypersensitivity, narrow-angle glaucoma.

DOSAGE

PO: anxiety, alcoholism, spasm, convulsive disorders

Pediatric >6mo	1.25mg 3-4 times/d
Adult	2-10mg 2-4 times/d
Geriatric	2-2.5mg 1-2 times/d

PHARMACOKINETICS

	Onset	Peak	Duration	Half-life	Protein binding	Excretion
PO	30-60m	1-2h	3h	20-50h	80%-98%	As conjugates in urine
IM	15-30m	Erratic	1-3h	20-50h	80%-98%	
IV	1-5m	—	15m-1h	20-50h	80%-98%	

Note: Side/adverse effects: common in *italic;* serious in ***boldface italic.***

*Available in Canada only.

Parenteral *(IM/IV)*
Pediatric

Tetanus	>30d: 1-2mg, repeat in 3-4h prn ≥5y/o: 5-10mg, repeat in 3-4h prn
S. epilepticus	>30d: 0.2-0.5mg q2-5m to a maximum of 5mg ≥5y/o: 1mg q2-5m to a maximum of 10mg

Adult

Anxiety	2-10mg, repeat in 3-4h prn
Alcoholism	10mg, then 5-10mg in 3-4h prn
Cardioversion	5-10mg IV w/in 5-10m before procedure
Endoscopy	10-20mg IV before procedure
Pre-op	10mg IM before surgery
Spasm	5-10mg, repeat in 3-4h prn
S. epilepticus	5-10mg, repeat at 10-15m interval to a maximum of 30mg. Repeat in 3-4h prn

SIDE/ADVERSE EFFECTS: CNS: *drowsiness, fatigue*, ataxia ▪ CV: hypotension ▪ HEM: neutropenia (rare) ▪ PSYCH: paradoxical anxiety, hallucinations, hyperexcited states.

DRUG INTERACTIONS: Use c̄ other CNS depressants produces additive effects ▪ Use c̄ MAO-I can produce toxic effects.

NURSING MANAGEMENT

ADMINISTRATION: Assess for hx of benzodiazepine hypersensitivity ▪ Do *not* mix/dilute parenteral preparations (incompatibility) ▪ IM: inject *deep, slowly* into large muscle mass ▪ IV: assess respirations before each dose; administer *slowly* (5mg/1m) as close to venipuncture site as possible; keep pt recumbent for 3h ▪ Avoid abrupt withdrawal.

EVALUATION: Assess for symptoms of abrupt withdrawal (tremors, abdominal/muscle cramps, convulsions) c̄ prolonged use ▪ Check for signs of dependence (↑ drug request)/tolerance ▪ Monitor activity status (safety precautions) ▪ Assess for paradoxic rxs (CNS stimulation), esp in elderly ▪ Check for depression; suicide precautions prn.

EDUCATION: Use caution in potentially hazardous activities ▪ Avoid use c̄ alcohol, CNS depressants ▪ Indiscriminate use may lead to dependence ▪ Do *not* keep at bedside ▪ Take as ordered by physician; do *not* ↑ dose ▪ Women: avoid breastfeeding.

OVERDOSE MANAGEMENT: *See* Benzodiazepines.

diazoxide • (dye-az-ox-ide)

CATEGORY: *Antihypertensive:* antihypoglycemic

Rx; Preg Cat C

BRAND NAMES

Hyperstat IV (Schering)
Proglycem (Baker Norton)
(Schering [Canada])

DOSAGE FORMS

Injection (IV): 300mg/20m
Capsule: 50mg
PO Suspension: 50mg/ml

CONTRAINDICATIONS: Hypersensitivity (incl other sulfonamide-like drug allergies), compensatory hypertension associated c̄ coarctation/arteriovenous shunt; functional hypoglycemia.

ACTION: Antihypertensive effect (IV administration) due to direct relaxing of smooth muscle in peripheral vascular beds; PO use produces antihypoglycemic effect due to inhibition of insulin release from pancreas & by ↑ hepatic glucose release. **USE:** IV: management of hypertensive emergencies ▪ PO: management of hypoglycemia due to hyperinsulinism associated c̄ extrapancreatic malignancy, inoperable islet cell adenoma/carcinoma, leucine sensitivity/nesideroblastosis.

DOSAGE

Adult *IV* — Bolus dose 300mg or a mini bolus dose 1-3mg/kg repeated at 5-15m intervals. Mini bolus dosage has become the most recommended schedule because it produces a more controlled reduction of BP. Maintenance doses can be given at 4-24h intervals if needed. Pediatric dose: mini bolus schedule

PHARMACOKINETICS

	Onset	Duration	Half-life	Protein binding	Excretion
PO	1h	Up to 8h	20-36h	>90%	Slowly via urine as unchanged
IV	5m	Up to 12h	20-36h	>90%	drug, metabolites

Note: Side/adverse effects: common in *italic;* serious in ***boldface italic.***

*Available in Canada only.

Adult/ Pediatric *PO*	3-8mg/kg in 2-3 equal doses q8-12h
Neonates/ Infants *PO*	8-15mg/kg in 2-3 equal doses q8-12h

SIDE/ADVERSE EFFECTS: CNS: cerebral ischemia, *dizziness*, lightheadedness, drowsiness, anxiety, headache ▪ CV: sodium/H_2O retention, *orthostatic hypotension*, ***arrhythmias***, bradycardia ▪ GI: N/V, anorexia, abdominal discomfort, ***acute pancreatitis*** (rare) ▪ INT: hirsutism in women (PO) ▪ MET: hyperglycemia in diabetic pts (IV).

DRUG INTERACTIONS: Use c̄ PO anticoagulants may require dosage reduction due to displacement of anticoagulant from protein storage sites ▪ Use c̄ thiazides can produce additive hyperglycemic/antihypertensive activity ▪ Use c̄ hydralazine may cause severe hypotension ▪ Avoid IV use for 6h after administration of antihypertensives, papaverine-like drugs, nitrites.

NURSING MANAGEMENT

ADMINISTRATION: Assess for hx of hypersensitivity (incl sulfonamides) ▪ Assess BP, pulse; notify physician of extremes ▪ Assess renal function; may require ↓ dosage if impaired ▪ Assess serum electrolytes, blood glucose, CBC ▪ IV: place pt in supine position, maintain for 1h after injection; inject over 10-30s ▪ Do *not* administer IM or SC ▪ PO suspension: shake well before pouring ▪ Do *not* administer discolored/precipitated solutions ▪ Administer c̄ diuretic to ↓ Na^+ H_2O retention, esp with multiple doses.

EVALUATION: Monitor BP q5m, then qh when stable ▪ Monitor I&O, daily weight ▪ Assess for CHF (dyspnea, peripheral edema, ↑ weight); notify physician ▪ Diabetics: closely monitor blood glucose (hyperglycemia) ▪ Check IV insertion site carefully; avoid extravasation ▪ May produce ↑ serum uric acid.

EDUCATION: Dizziness may occur; use caution in potentially hazardous activities ▪ Avoid changing positions (lying/sitting/standing) rapidly ▪ Notify physician of abnormal rxs (difficulty breathing, chest pain, irregular heartbeat) ▪ Diabetics: monitor blood/urine glucose carefully ▪ Excessive hair growth may occur c̄ prolonged PO therapy (reversible after therapy).

NOTES:

diclofenac • (die-klo-fen-ack)

CATEGORY: *Antiinflammatory*: NSAIA

Rx; Preg Cat B

BRAND NAME	DOSAGE FORMS
Voltaren (Geigy)	Enteric-coated tablet: 25, 50, 75mg

ACTION: Antiinflammatory activity appears related to inhibition of prostaglandin synthesis. **USE:** Treatment of rheumatoid/osteoarthritis and ankylosing spondylitis.

PHARMACOKINETICS

PO absorption	Peak	Protein binding	Excretion
Complete	2-3h	99%	Via urine and bile as conjugates

CONTRAINDICATIONS: Hypersensitivity, aspirin/other antiinflammatory agent hypersensitivity.

DOSAGE

Adult *PO*

Osteoarthritis	100-150mg/d divided 2-3 times/d. A daily dose above 150mg not currently evaluated
Rheumatoid arthritis	150-200mg/d divided 3-4 times/d. A daily dose above 200mg not currently evaluated.
Ankylosing spondylitis	100-125mg/d given as 25mg qid and 25mg hs if needed. A daily dose above 125mg not currently evaluated.

SIDE/ADVERSE EFFECTS: CNS: *headache, dizziness,* depression, anxiety ▪ CV: palpitations, chest pain, tachycardia, PVC, possible and rare ***MI*** ▪ EENT: amblyopia, night blindness, vitreous floaters, blurred vision, tinnitus, reversible hearing loss ▪ GI: *pain, cramps, constipation, nausea,* stomatitis, ***GI bleeding,*** colitis, V/D, flatulence ▪ GU: oliguria, proteinuria, ***acute renal failure, interstitial nephritis, nephrotic syndrome, papillary necrosis*** ▪ HEM: leukopenia, ***thrombocytopenia, agranulocytosis, aplastic anemia*** ▪ INT: rash, urticaria, photosensitivity, ***Stevens-Johnson syndrome, erythema multiforme*** ▪ Other: asthma, excessive perspiration.

DRUG INTERACTIONS: use $\bar{c}$ ulcerogenic drugs produces additive effects ▪ Use $\bar{c}$ PO anticoagulants may ↑ their activity ▪ Use $\bar{c}$ aspirin will ↓ diclofenac plasma levels ▪ Use c̄ methotrexate, digoxin, cyclosporin may ↑ their toxicity ▪ Use c̄ lithium requires monitoring of lithium levels.

NURSING MANAGEMENT

ADMINISTRATION: Assess for hx of NSAIA, salicylate hypersensitivity ▪ Avoid administration to pts c̄ hx of asthma, bleeding disorders, salicylate hypersensitivity ▪ Assess GI, renal, hepatic function; use caution if impaired ▪ May be administered c̄ food, milk, antacid; *best* on empty stomach (1h ac/2h pc); do *not* crush tablets (enteric coated) ▪ Administer c̄ full glass of liquid; encourage upright position for 15-30m ▪ Avoid exposure to moisture during storage ▪ *Not* recommended for pts c̄ restricted Na^+ intake ▪ Elderly may require ↓ dosage.

EVALUATION: Monitor hepatic, renal status c̄ prolonged use ▪ Monitor pt receiving anticoagulant therapy; may potentiate bleeding ▪ Monitor I&O, daily weight ▪ Monitor AST, ALT ▪ Assess for edema in extremities ▪ Assess for visual/hearing disturbances; D/C drug, notify physician.

EDUCATION: Dizziness/drowsiness may occur; use caution in potentially hazardous activities ▪ Take on empty stomach (1h ac/2h pc), c̄ food/milk if GI distress occurs; swallow tablet whole; take c̄ a full glass of liquid; maintain upright position for 15-30m ▪ Take as ordered by physician; do *not* ↑ dose ▪ Notify physician *immediately* of bleeding, ↓ urine output, swelling of feet/legs, lethargy, GI distress, jaundice, visual/hearing disturbances ▪ Avoid taking c̄ aspirin, other NSAIAs ▪ Avoid use c̄ alcohol ▪ Check c̄ physician/pharmacist before taking OTC preparations ▪ Notify physician/dentist of use before treatment ▪ Store in tightly closed container ▪ Women: avoid breastfeeding ▪ Full drug effects may require several wks of therapy.

NOTES:

didanosine (ddI) • (dye-<u>dan</u>-o-seen)

CATEGORY: *Antiviral*

Rx; Preg Cat B

BRAND NAME

Videx (Bristol)

DOSAGE FORMS

Powder for PO solution: 100, 167, 250, 375mg foil packets
Ped powder for PO solution: 2g (4oz), 4g (8oz) bottles
Chewable tablet: 25, 50, 100, 150mg

ACTION: Antiviral activity due to inhibition of viral replication in HIV; drug is a nucleoside analogue of deoxyadenosine that is converted by cellular enzymes into the active antiviral metabolite dideoxyadenosine triphosphate (dd ATP), which when incorporated into viral DNA leads to chain termination and subsequent inhibition of viral replication. In addition, dd ATP inhibits HIV reverse transcriptase enzymes required for viral DNA synthesis. **USE:** Management of advanced HIV infection in adults and children over 6 mo of age who have significant immunologic deterioration or are intolerant to zidovidine therapy.

PHARMACOKINETICS

PO absorption (ac)	Half-life	Excretion
33%-37%	8-24h	Via urine as metabolites

CONTRAINDICATIONS: Hypersensitivity.

DOSAGE

Pediatric *PO*

Body Surface Area (m^2)	Tablets	Pediatric Solution
1.1-1.4	100mg bid	125mg/12.5ml bid
0.8-1.0	75mg bid	94mg/9.5ml bid
0.5-0.7	50mg bid	62mg/6ml bid
≤0.5	25mg bid	31mg/3ml bid

Adult *PO*

Weight	Tablets	Solution (packet)
≤75kg	300mg bid	375mg bid
50-74kg	200mg big	250mg bid
35-49kg	125mg bid	167mg bid

SIDE/ADVERSE EFFECTS: CNS: headache, peripheral neuropathy, insomnia, depression, dizziness ▪ CV: hypertension, vasodilation ▪ GI: anorexia, N/V/D, abdominal pain, constipation, stomatitis, taste changes, dry mouth, pancreatitis ▪ HEM: ***leukopenia***, granulocytopenia, ***thrombocytopenia*** ▪ INT: alopecia, rash, pruritus, eczema ▪ MS: arthritis, myalgia, asthenia ▪ RESP: asthma, cough, rhinitis, rhinorrhea ▪ Other: otic pain, malaise, photophobia.

DRUG INTERACTIONS: Use c̄ tetracycline best avoided ▪ Administer drugs such as dapsone, ketoconazole, whose absorption is affected by stomach acidity 2h before didanosine administration ▪ Use c̄ drugs that cause peripheral neuropathy, pancreatitis requires close monitoring.

NURSING MANAGEMENT

ADMINISTRATION: Assess for hx of hypersensitivity ▪ Administer on empty stomach (1h ac/2h pc) ▪ Chewable tablets: chew thoroughly or mix in 1oz H_2O to form dispersion; drink immediately ▪ PO solution: reconstitute & dilute c̄ antacid according to manufacturer's directions; shake admixture well before use; refrigerate, store in tightly closed container.

EVALUATION: Monitor VS, esp temperature ▪ Assess for development of neuropathy (numbness, tingling, pain in distal extremities) ▪ Monitor hepatic, renal status.

EDUCATION: Take as ordered by physician at equal intervals around clock to maintain blood levels; do *not* ↑ dose ▪ Do *not* share drug ▪ Women: avoid breastfeeding ▪ Used to control, *not* cure, HIV infections ▪ Notify physician of any change in health status ▪ Check c̄ physician/pharmacist before taking OTC preparations ▪ Avoid sexual contact, blood donation (risk of HIV transmission) ▪ Keep scheduled appointments c̄ physician/for blood work.

NOTES:

diethylstilbestrol/diethylstilbestrol diphosphate • (dye-eth-ul-stil-bess-trole)

CATEGORY: *Estrogenic agent* Rx; Preg Cat X

AVAILABLE PREPARATIONS	DOSAGE FORMS
Diethylstilbestrol (various)	Tablet: 0.1, 0.25, 0.5, 1, 5mg
Diethylstilbestrol Diphosphate *Stilphostroll (Miles)*	Injection (IV): 0.25g/ampule Tablet: 50mg

ACTION: Drug appears to have same mechanism as natural estrogens: development, maintenance of female reproductive system, secondary sex characteristics. **USE:** Palliation of breast/prostatic cancer. Diphosphate salt is currently limited to prostatic cancer palliation.

PHARMACOKINETICS: Drug exhibits good PO absorption, slow metabolism, and is excreted as metabolites via urine and feces.

CONTRAINDICATIONS: Known/suspected pregnancy, estrogen-dependent neoplasms, breast cancer except in appropriately selected pts; abnormal genital bleeding, active or in pts c̄ a past hx of thrombophlebitis/thrombophlebitic disorders (except breast/prostate cancer treatment).

DOSAGE FORMS

Adult *PO* Usual palliation dose for prostate cancer 1-3mg/d which can be ↓ to 1mg/d. Usual dose for breast cancer 15mg/d.
Dose of diphosphate salt 50mg tid and ↑ depending on pt tolerance. Do *not* exceed 1g/d. Usual IV dose 0.5g/d and ↑ to 1g on subsequent days for ≥5d followed by 0.25-0.5g maintenance dose 1-2 times/wk

SIDE/ADVERSE EFFECTS: CNS: headache, migraine, dizziness, mental depression ▪ EENT: intolerance to contact lenses, steepening of corneal curvature ▪ GI: N/V, abdominal cramps, bloating ▪ GU: amenorrhea, breakthrough bleeding, dysmenorrhea, candidiasis, change in menstrual flow, spotting, ↑ size of uterine fibromyomas ▪ INT: melasma, ***erythema multiforme***/nodosum, alopecia, hirsutism, urticaria ▪ MET: ↓ carbohydrate tolerance ▪ Other: weight changes, edema, porphyria exacerbation.

DRUG INTERACTIONS: Use c̄ tricyclic antidepressants may result in toxic rxs.

NURSING MANAGEMENT

ADMINISTRATION: Assess for hx of hypersensitivity ▪ Administer cyclically (3wks on, 1wk off) c̄ meals ▪ Do *not* crush enteric-coated tablets; administer whole ▪ Schedule pregnancy test for sexually active women before administration ▪ Avoid abrupt withdrawal; D/C gradually.

EVALUATION: Monitor hepatic, renal status ▪ Monitor BP ▪ Assess PT; may ↓ anticoagulant effect ▪ Diabetics: careful blood/urine testing; may ↓ antidiabetic drug effect ▪ Assess for behavioral changes, depression ▪ Monitor pt weight; observe for edema.

EDUCATION: Review package insert c̄ pt ▪ Nausea may occur during first 2wks of therapy ▪ Women: avoid pregnancy, breastfeeding ▪ Breast self-exam (incl men) ▪ Avoid smoking (↑ CV complications) ▪ Take c̄ food ▪ Notify physician/dentist of use before treatment ▪ Keep scheduled appointments c̄ physician ▪ Avoid exposure to direct sunlight, UV light (sunlamps); use sunscreen, protective clothing ▪ D/C drug, notify physician if pregnancy is suspected ▪ Vaginal: procedure for suppository insertion; use sanitary napkin (avoid tampons) to protect clothing ▪ Notify physician *immediately* of chest/leg pain, unusual vaginal bleeding, difficult breathing, slurred speech ▪ Men: enlarged breasts, impotence reversible ▪ Check weight, swelling in feet/legs daily.

NOTES:

diflunisal • (dye-floo-ni-sal)

CATEGORY: *Salicylate:* analgesic, antiinflammatory Rx; Preg Cat C

BRAND NAME
Dolobid (MSD) (Frosst in Canada)

DOSAGE FORMS
Tablet: 250, 500mg

DOSAGE
Adult *PO*

Pain	1g followed by 500mg q8-12h Geriatric: 500mg followed by 250mg q8-12h
Arthritis	500-1000mg/d divided. Do *not* exceed 1500mg/d

ACTION: Produces analgesia by ↑ in pain threshold, ↓ in synthesis of prostaglandins; antiinflammatory effect due to ↓ in prostaglandin synthesis, release. **USE:** Analgesic for mild/moderate pain ▪ Treatment of rheumatoid/osteoarthritis.

PHARMACOKINETICS

PO absorption	Onset	Peak	Duration	Half-life	Protein binding	Excretion
98%-100%	1h	2-3h	8-12h	8-12h	99%	90% in urine as glucuronide conjugates

CONTRAINDICATIONS: Hypersensitivity to diflunisal, aspirin, other NSAIAs.

Side/Adverse Effects: CNS: dizziness, tinnitus ▪ GI: *epigastric distress incl N/V,* flatulence, ulcers, ***bleeding*** ▪ HEM: ***thrombocytopenia*** ▪ HEP: ↑ serum AST, ALT, creatinine ▪ INT: rash, ***erythema multiforme, Stevens-Johnson syndrome.***

DRUG INTERACTIONS: ↓ absorption c̄ antacids ▪ ↑ PO anticoagulant activity ▪ ↓ Renal excretion of naproxen, sulindac ▪ ↑ Serum levels of acetaminophen, hydrochlorothiazide, indomethacin ▪ ↓ Hyperuricemic effect of furosemide, hydrochlorothiazide.

NURSING MANAGEMENT

ADMINISTRATION: Assess for hx of NSAIA hypersensitivity ▪ Avoid administration to individuals c̄ hx of asthma, bleeding disorders, salicylate hypersensitivity ▪ Avoid use in children c̄ chickenpox, flulike symptoms; may precipitate Reye's syndrome ▪ Administer c̄ food if GI irritation occurs ▪ Do *not* crush tablets; administer whole ▪ Avoid large amount of concurrent antacid suspensions.

EVALUATION: Assess for bleeding (GI, GU, skin, mucous membrane) ▪ Monitor pt receiving anticoagulant therapy; may potentiate bleeding ▪ Assess hepatic, renal status.

EDUCATION: Take c̄ food if GI irritation occurs ▪ Avoid large amounts of concurrent antacid suspension ▪ Avoid chewing/crushing tablets; swallow whole ▪ Avoid taking c̄ aspirin, acetaminophen, other NSAIAs.

OVERDOSE MANAGEMENT: Symptoms incl disorientation, stupor ▪ Remove drug by emesis/gastric lavage.

NOTES:

digitoxin • (di-ji-tox-in)

CATEGORY: *Cardiac glycoside*

Rx; Preg Cat C

BRAND NAME
Crystodigin (Lilly)

DOSAGE FORMS
Tablet: 0.05, 0.1mg

ACTION: Dig glycosides ↑ force of myocardial contractions; ↑ refractory period of AV, SA nodes; ↓ conductivity of AV node, bundle of His, heart rate. **USE:** Treatment of CHF, supraventricular arrhythmias.

DOSAGE: Dig doses usually administered w/in 24h divided.

Pediatric *PO*	Dig dose usually divided, ≥6h between doses Premature: 0.022mg/kg Newborn: 0.025mg/kg 2wks-1yr: 0.040-0.045mg/kg 1-2y/o: 0.040mg/kg 2-12y/o: 0.020-0.030mg/kg
Adult *PO*	Dig dose usually 0.6mg followed by 0.4mg & 0.2mg at 4-6 intervals. Usual maintenance dose 0.05-0.3mg/d

PHARMACOKINETICS

Route	Absorption	Onset	Peak	Half-life	Protein binding	Excretion
PO	Complete	30m-2h	4-12h	120-168h	97%	Up to 14-21d for complete renal excretion; also in feces
IM/IV	——	24m-2h	4-12h	120-168h	97%	

Note: Side/adverse effects: common in *italic;* serious in ***boldface italic.***

*Available in Canada only.

CONTRAINDICATIONS: Hypersensitivity, ventricular tachycardia, presence of toxic effects.

SIDE/ADVERSE EFFECTS: CNS: apathy, headache, psychosis (rare) ▪ CV: conduction disturbances, PVCs ▪ EENT: blurred, yellow/red/green vision ▪ GI: N/V/D, anorexia ▪ Other: diaphoresis, gynecomastia, fatigue.

DRUG INTERACTIONS: Acetazolamide, amphotericin B, chlorthalidone, ethacrynic acid, ethoxazolamide, furosemide, laxatives, thiazides, other K^+-reducing agents ↑ dig toxicity by inducing hypokalemia ▪ Parenteral Ca administration can produce serious arrhythmias ▪ Antacids, antidiarrhals, ion-exchange resins ↓ PO dig absorption ▪ Barbiturates, hydantoins, phenylbutazone ↓ dig activity by enzyme induction ▪ Use cautiously c̄ adrenergics, beta blockers, quinidine, procainamide.

NURSING MANAGEMENT

ADMINISTRATION: Loading dose must be administered to achieve therapeutic blood levels; assess for dig ingestion w/in past 2 wks ▪ Assess for toxicity before administering each dose (N/V, bradycardia, arrhythmias) ▪ Check apical pulse for 1m before administration; if <60/>120 hold dose, notify physician ▪ Administer single PO dose in AM c̄ food ▪ IV: preferred parenteral route; administer *slowly* ▪ Elderly may require ↓ dosage.

EVALUATION: Monitor serum electrolytes (hypokalemia, hypercalcemia, hypomagnesemia ↑ dig toxicity) ▪ Check cardiac monitor for arrhythmias ▪ Assess cardiopulmonary, renal status; monitor I&O ▪ Therapeutic serum dig level: 25-35ng/ml.

EDUCATION: Take as ordered by physician; do *not* skip dose w/out notifying physician ▪ Notify physician of symptoms of toxicity (loss of appetite, N/D, visual problems, irregular heartbeat) ▪ Eat foods high in K^+, esp if taking diuretics; avoid licorice ▪ Procedure for radial pulse determination ▪ Check radial pulse each AM for 1m; notify physician if slow (<60)/irregular ▪ Maintain optimum weight; avoid high-Na^+ substances ▪ Check c̄ physician before taking other medications ▪ Store in cool, dry, light-resistant container.

OVERDOSE MANAGEMENT: *See* Cardiac Glycosides.

NOTES:

digoxin • (di-jox-in)

CATEGORY: *Cardiac glycoside*

Rx; Preg Cat C

BRAND NAMES

Lanoxicaps (B-W)
Lanoxin (B-W)

DOSAGE FORMS

Capsule: 0.05, 0.1, 0.2mg
Pediatric elixir: 0.05mg/ml
Pediatric injection: 0.1mg/ml
Injection: 0.25mg/ml
Tablet: 0.125, 0.25, 0.5mg

ACTION: Dig glycosides ↑ force of myocardial contraction; ↑ refractory period of AV, SA nodes; ↓ conductivity of AV node, bundle of His, heart rate. **USE:** Treatment of CHF, supraventricular arrhythmias.

DOSAGE: Dig doses usually given w/in 24h; first dose 50% of total dose, followed by two 25% doses given at 48h intervals.

Pediatric *IV*
Premature: 0.015-0.025mg/kg
Newborn: 0.020-0.030mg/kg
1mo-2y/o: 0.030-0.050mg/kg
2-5y/o: 0.025-0.035mg/kg
5-10y/o: 0.015-0.030mg/kg
>10y/o: 0.080-0.012mg/kg

PO
Premature: 0.020-0.030mg/kg
Newborn: 0.025-0.035mg/kg
1mo-2y/o: 0.035-0.060mg/kg
2-5y/o: 0.030-0.040mg/kg

PHARMACOKINETICS

	PO absorption	Onset	Peak	Duration	Half-life	Protein binding	Excretion
PO	50%-90%	50m-2h	2-6h	2-4d	36h	20%-25%	Renal, Feces
IV	—	5-30m	1-4h	2-4d	36h	20%-25%	Renal, Feces

CONTRAINDICATIONS: Hypersensitivity, ventricular tachycardia, presence of toxic effects.

	5-10y/o: 0.020-0.035mg/kg
	>10y/o: 0.010-0.015mg/kg
	Usual ped maintenance dose is 20-35% of dig dose
Adult *PO/IV*	Usual dig dose 1-1.5mg/d, $\bar{c}$ usual maintenance dose 0.125-0.5mg/d

SIDE/ADVERSE EFFECTS: CNS: apathy, headache, psychosis (rare) ▪ CV: conduction disturbances, PVCs, bradycardia ▪ EENT: blurred, yellow/red/green vision ▪ GI: N/V/D, anorexia ▪ Other: diaphoresis, gynecomastia, fatigue.

DRUG INTERACTIONS: Acetazolamide, amphotericin B, chlorthalidone, ethacrynic acid, ethoxazolamide, furosemide, laxatives, thiazides, other K^+-reducing agents ↑ dig toxicity by inducing hypokalemia ▪ Parenteral Ca administration can produce serious arrhythmias ▪ Antacids, antidiarrheals, ion-exchange resins ↓ PO dig absorption ▪ Barbiturates, hydantoins, phenylbutazone ↓ dig activity by enzyme induction ▪ Use cautiously $\bar{c}$ adrenergics, beta blockers, quinidine, procainamide.

NURSING MANAGEMENT

ADMINISTRATION: Loading dose must be administered to achieve therapeutic blood levels; assess for dig ingestion w/in past 2 wks ▪ Assess renal function; may require ↓ dosage ▪ Assess for toxicity before administering each dose (N/V, bradycardia, arrhythmias) ▪ Check apical pulse for 1m before administration; if <60/>120 hold dose, notify physician ▪ Administer single PO dose in AM $\bar{c}$ food ▪ IV: preferred parenteral route; administer *slowly* ▪ Elderly may require ↓ dosage.

EVALUATION: Monitor serum electrolytes (K^+, Ca^{++}, Mg^{++}) ▪ Monitor I&O ▪ Therapeutic serum digoxin level: 0.5-2.5ng/ml.

EDUCATION: Take as ordered by physician; do *not* skip dose w/out notifying physician ▪ Notify physician of symptoms of toxicity (loss of appetite, N/D, visual problems, irregular heartbeat) ▪ Eat foods high in K^+, esp if taking diuretics; avoid licorice ▪ Check radial pulse each AM for 1m; notify physician if slow (<60)/irregular ▪ Maintain optimum weight; avoid high-Na^+ substances ▪ Check $\bar{c}$ physician before taking other medications ▪ Store in cool, dry, light-resistant container.

OVERDOSE MANAGEMENT: *See* Cardiac Glycosides.

diltiazem hcl • (dil-tye-a-zem)

CATEGORY: *Calcium blocker*: antianginal, slow channel blocker   Rx; Preg Cat C

BRAND NAMES

Cardizem (Marion)

(Nordic [Canada])

Dilacor xr (RPR)

DOSAGE FORMS

SR capsule: 60, 90, 120mg
Tablet: 30, 60, 90, 120mg
IV injection: 5mg/ml
Capsule: 180, 240mg

ACTION: Antianginal effect due to inhibition of extracellular calcium-ion transmembrane migration in cardiac, vascular smooth muscle via slow channel passageway, resulting in coronary vasodilation; ↑ myocardial oxygen supply, ↓ oxygen consumption. **USE:** Treatment of chronic stable/vasospastic angina pectoris ▪ Treatment of hypertension as a sole agent or in combination c̄ other antihypertensives (SR capsule) ▪ Treatment of atrial fibrillation/flutter, paroxysmal supraventricular tachycardia.

CONTRAINDICATIONS: Hypersensitivity, sick sinus syndrome or 2nd/3rd° AV block (except in presence of pacemaker), hypotension (<90 systolic), acute MI and pulmonary congestion (documented by x-ray).

DOSAGE

Adult *PO*	Initial dose 30mg qid (ac, hs). Usual daily range 180-240mg divided in 3-4 doses/d
IV	Bolus dose 0.25mg/kg over 2m. Second dose 0.35 mg/kg over 2m after 15m prn. Then 5-10mg/h or higher by continuous infusion.

PHARMACOKINETICS

PO absorption	Onset	Peak	Half-life	Protein binding	Excretion
80%	30m	2-3h	3.5-9h	70%-85%	Via urine, feces primarily as metabolites

Note: Side/adverse effects: common in *italic;* serious in ***boldface italic.***   *Available in Canada only.

SIDE/ADVERSE EFFECTS: CNS: *headache, dizziness,* nervousness, sleep disturbances ▪ CV: *peripheral edema,* ***arrhythmias***, palpitations, CHF, *bradycardia* ▪ GI: *nausea,* diarrhea, constipation ▪ INT: rash, pruritus, photosensitivity.

DRUG INTERACTIONS: Use c̄ dig may ↑ dig serum level ▪ Use c̄ beta blockers may prolong cardiac conduction time.

NURSING MANAGEMENT

ADMINISTRATION: Assess for hx of hypersensitivity ▪ Assess for hx of heart failure; use c̄ caution ▪ Assess BP, heart rate; if apical pulse <60, hold dose, notify physician ▪ Administer ac, hs; may crush tablets ▪ Elderly may require ↓ dosage.

EVALUATION: Monitor VS, esp BP, pulse ▪ Monitor I&O ▪ Monitor hepatic, renal status ▪ Assess for CHF (dyspnea, peripheral edema, ↑ weight); notify physician ▪ Monitor PR interval (may ↑) ▪ Digitalized pts: assess for dig toxicity (bradycardia, anorexia, palpitations).

EDUCATION: Dizziness may occur; use caution in potentially hazardous activities ▪ Avoid changing positions (lying/sitting/standing) rapidly ▪ Procedure for checking radial pulse ▪ If pulse slow (<60)/irregular, do *not* take dose; notify physician ▪ Avoid caffeine ▪ Check c̄ physician/pharmacist before taking OTC preparations ▪ Take as ordered by physician; do *not* change dosage ▪ Notify physician of difficult breathing, chest pain, swelling of hands/legs; D/C drug ▪ Keep scheduled appointments c̄ physician ▪ Continue SL nitroglycerin (if ordered) to relieve sudden chest pain or for prophylaxis before exertion ▪ Avoid use c̄ alcohol.

NOTES:

diphenhydramine hcl • (dye-fen-hye-dra-meen)

CATEGORY: *Antihistamine: H_1 blocker* — Rx/OTC; Preg Cat B

BRAND NAMES	DOSAGE FORMS
**Allerdryl (ICN)*	Capsule: 25.5mg
Benadryl (P-D)	Capsule: 25, 50mg
	Elixir: 12.5mg/ml
	Injection (Rx): 10, 50mg/ml
**Insomnal (Welcker-Lyster)*	Capsule: 25mg

ACTION: Antihistamine activity due to competitive inhibition of histamine at H_1 histamine receptors on effector cells; exhibits good anticholinergic, antitussive, antiemetic, sedative properties. **USE:** Symptomatic treatment of allergic disorders mediated by histamine ▪ Treatment of motion sickness, Parkinson disease; nighttime sleep aid ▪ Adjunct to epinephrine in anaphylactic rx.

PHARMACOKINETICS

PO absorption	Peak	Half-life	Protein binding	Excretion
Good	1-4h	2-7h	82%	Via urine primarily as metabolites

CONTRAINDICATIONS: Hypersensitivity, neonates, nursing mothers, lower respiratory tract symptoms.

DOSAGE

Pediatric	*PO*	>20lbs: 12.5-25mg 3-4 times/d. Do *not* exceed 300mg/d
	IM/IV	5mg/kg/d. Do *not* exceed 300mg/d
Adult	*PO*	24-50mg 3-4 times/d, 50mg hs as sleep aid
	IM/IV	10-50mg c̄ maximum 400mg/d. Do *not* exceed 300mg/d

SIDE/ADVERSE EFFECTS: CNS: *drowsiness,* dizziness, fatigue, euphoria, paresthesias ▪ CV: hypotension, palpitations, tachycardia, extrasystole ▪ EENT: blurred vision, nasal stuffiness ▪ GI: epigastric distress, nausea ▪ HEM: ***agranulocytosis, hemolytic anemia, thrombocytopenia*** ▪ INT: drug rash, photosensitivity ▪ RESP: thickening of bronchial secretions, wheezing ▪ Other: anticholinergic effects.

Note: Side/adverse effects: common in *italic;* serious in ***boldface italic.***

*Available in Canada only.

DRUG INTERACTIONS: Use c̄ anticholinergics, CNS depressants, tricyclic antidepressants produces additive effects ▪ MAO-I can ↑ anticholinegic effects of antihistamines.

NURSING MANAGEMENT

ADMINISTRATION: Assess for hx of antihistamine hypersensitivity ▪ PO: administer c̄ food ▪ IM: inject *deep* into large muscle mass ▪ IV: use only preparations w/out preservatives; administer *slowly* ▪ Avoid exposure to moisture, light in storage ▪ Maintain hydration ▪ Elderly may require ↓ dosage.

EVALUATION: Monitor VS, esp BP ▪ Assess for excessive drowsiness, dizziness, weakness ▪ Monitor CBC c̄ prolonged therapy ▪ Monitor children for paradoxic rxs (CNS stimulation) ▪ Assess for tolerance to therapeutic dose; notify physician, another antihistamine may be substituted.

EDUCATION: Drowsiness, dizziness, lightheadedness may occur; use caution in potentially hazardous activities ▪ Avoid use c̄ alcohol, other CNS depressants ▪ Take PO forms c̄ meals ▪ Store in tightly closed, light-resistant container ▪ Use sugarless gum/hard candy to diminish dry mouth ▪ ↑ Fluid intake (8-10 glasses/d) ▪ Motion sickness: take 30m before motion-producing event ▪ Notify physician of symptoms of allergic rx (fever, difficult breathing, rash) ▪ Women: avoid breastfeeding ▪ Carry identification (MedicAlert) if antihistamine allergic ▪ Notify physician of antihistamine use before allergy testing.

NOTES:

diphenoxylate hcl/atropine sulfate • (dye-fen-ox-i-late/a-troe-peen)

CATEGORY: *Antidiarrheal combination*

Rx C-V; Preg Cat C

BRAND NAME
Lomotil (Searle)

DOSAGE FORMS
Diphenoxylate/atropine per 5ml liquid/tablet: 2.5mg/0.025mg

ACTION: Antidiarrheal effect due to slowing of intestinal motility. **USE:** Adjunct in management of diarrhea.

PHARMACOKINETICS: Combination has good PO absorption, rapid metabolism, and is excreted primarily as metabolites via urine and feces.

CONTRAINDICATIONS: Hypersensitivity, diarrhea associated c̄ pseudomembranous enterocolitis, obstructive jaundice.

DOSAGE

Pediatric *PO*
- 2y/o: 1.5-3ml qid
- 3y/o: 2-3ml qid
- 4y/o: 2-4ml qid
- 5y/o: 2.5-4.5ml qid
- 6-8y/o: 2.5-5ml qid
- 9-12y/o: 3.5-5ml qid

Adult *PO* — 2 tablets/10ml liquid qid. Control usually maintained c̄ 2 tablets/10ml/d

SIDE/ADVERSE EFFECTS: CNS: sedation, dizziness, depression, numbness of extremities, euphoria, lethargy ▪ GI: N/V, abdominal discomfort, paralytic ileus, toxic megacolon, anorexia ▪ INT: pruritus ▪ Other: anticholinergic: normal effects due to atropine (eg, dry mouth, blurred vision), respiratory depression, angioneurotic edema, swollen gums.

DRUG INTERACTIONS: Use c̄ CNS depressants produces additive effects ▪ Use c̄ anticholinergics produces additive effects.

NURSING MANAGEMENT

ADMINISTRATION: Assess for hx of hypersensitivity to either compounds ▪ Assess F/E balance; do *not* administer if severely impaired ▪ Assess hepatic function; ↓ dosage if impaired ▪ Avoid exposure to moisture, light in storage; do *not* freeze liquid form ▪ May crush tablet, administer c̄ food.

EVALUATION: Monitor bowel function; ↓ dose as diarrhea is controlled ▪ Assess for atropinism (dry mouth, blurred vision, tachycardia) ▪ Assess hydration status (I&O, daily weight) ▪ Check for signs of dependence $\bar{c}$ prolonged use ▪ Assess for abdominal distention; D/C drug ▪ Monitor children, elderly closely (↑ susceptibility to adverse effects).

EDUCATION: Follow clear liquid/bland diet until diarrhea subsides ▪ Take as directed by physician; do *not* ↑ dose ▪ Avoid use of alcohol, caffeine ▪ Do *not* take $\bar{c}$ CNS depressants ▪ May cause drowsiness/dizziness; use caution in potentially hazardous activities ▪ Indiscriminate use may lead to dependence ▪ Use sugarless gum/hard candy to diminish dry mouth ▪ Maintain fluid intake (6-8 glasses/d) ▪ Store in tightly closed, light-resistant container ▪ Women: avoid breastfeeding ▪ Notify physician if diarrhea persists (>48h), fever occurs.

NOTES:

dipyridamole • (dye-peer-id-a-mole)

CATEGORY: *Platelet inhibitor:* anticoagulant Rx; Preg Cat B

BRAND NAMES	DOSAGE FORMS
**Apo-Dipyridamole (Apotex)*	Tablet: 25, 50, 75mg
Persantine (B-I)	Tablet: 25, 50, 75mg

ACTION: Anticoagulant activity due to a dose-dependent lengthening of abnormally shortened platelet survival time that occurs c̄ prosthetic heart valve replacement.
USE: Adjunct to coumarin anticoagulants in preventing postoperative thromboembolic rxs in prosthetic heart valve replacement.

PHARMACOKINETICS: Exhibits slow absorption c̄ a peak in about 75m; high protein binding; fecal (biliary) excretion as glucuronide conjugates.

CONTRAINDICATIONS: Hypersensitivity.

DOSAGE

Adult *PO* Usual adjunct dose 75-100mg qid

SIDE/ADVERSE EFFECTS: CNS: headache, dizziness, syncope ▪ GI: nausea, distress ▪ INT: skin rash ▪ Other: flushing, weakness.

DRUG INTERACTIONS: Use c̄ heparin requires caution ▪ Use c̄ aspirin produces additive antiplatelet activity.

NURSING MANAGEMENT

ADMINISTRATION: Assess for hx of hypersensitivity ▪ Administer 1h ac/2h pc c̄ full glass H_2O; may crush, mix c̄ food; may administer c̄ meals if GI distress occurs.

EVALUATION: Monitor VS, esp BP ▪ Assess for bleeding, esp c̄ anticoagulants, aspirin.

EDUCATION: Dizziness may occur; use caution in potentially hazardous activities ▪ Avoid changing positions (lying/sitting/standing) rapidly ▪ Take as ordered by physician; do *not* change frequency ▪ May take c̄ meals; *best* on empty stomach (1h before/2h after eating) ▪

Avoid changing brand-name preparations ▪ Avoid use $\bar{c}$ alcohol ▪ Avoid smoking ▪ Check $\bar{c}$ physician/pharmacist before taking OTC preparations ▪ Notify physician of unusual bleeding/bruising ▪ Full drug effects may require several wks of therapy.

NOTES:

disopyramide phosphate • (dye-soe-peer-a-mide)

CATEGORY: *Antiarrhythmic* Rx; Preg Cat C

BRAND NAMES	DOSAGE FORMS
Norpace (Searle)	Capsule: 100, 150 mg Controlled-release (CR) Capsule: 100, 150mg
**Rythmodan (Rouscel)*	Capsule: 100,150mg

ACTION: Antiarrhythmic effect similar to procainamide, quinidine (type 1 antiarrhythmics); ↓ rate of diastolic depolarization in cells c̄ augmented automaticity, upstroke velocity, while ↑ action potential duration of normal cardiac cells. **USE:** Treatment of cardiac arrhythmias incl unifocal, multifocal premature (ectopic) ventricular contractions, paired premature ventricular contractions, episodes of ventricular tachycardia.

PHARMACOKINETICS

PO absorption	Peak	Half-life	Protein binding	Excretion
Complete	2h	6.7h	50%-65%	Via urine as unchanged drug, metabolites

CONTRAINDICATIONS: Hypersensitivity, cardiogenic shock, preexisting 2nd, 3rd° AV block (if no pacemaker present), congenital Q-T prolongation.

DOSAGE

Adult *PO* — Usual dose 150mg q6h, 300mg (CR) q12h, c̄ daily range 400-800mg divided

SIDE/ADVERSE EFFECTS: CNS: dizziness, headache, nervousness, depression, insomnia ▪ CV: ***hypotension***, ↑ CHF, conduction disturbances, esp ***QRS widening*** ▪ EENT: blurred vision; dry nose, throat, eyes ▪ GI: *dry mouth, gas bloating* c̄ pain, constipation, anorexia, N/V/D ▪ GU: *urinary hesitancy*, impotence, dysuria ▪ INT: rash, dermatoses, pruritus ▪ MET: hypokalemia ▪ MS: muscle aches, pains.

DRUG INTERACTIONS: Use c̄ anticholinergics produces additive effects ▪ Use c̄ phenytoin (enzyme inducer) produces ↓ blood levels.

Note: Side/adverse effects: common in *italic;* serious in ***boldface italic.***

*Available in Canada only.

NURSING MANAGEMENT

ADMINISTRATION: Assess for hx of hypersensitivity ▪ Assess for hx of heart failure; use $\bar{c}$ caution ▪ Assess apical pulse; if <60/>120, hold dose, notify physician ▪ Monitor ECG; D/C if widened QRS/↑ arrhythmias ▪ Assess hepatic, renal function, IOP in glaucoma; notify physician if abnormal, hold drug ▪ Assess serum K^+ (normal: 3.5-5mEq/L) correct imbalances ▪ Administer 1h ac/2h pc ▪ Administer SR capsules whole; do *not* crush ▪ Avoid abrupt withdrawal; D/C gradually ▪ Elderly may require ↓ dosage.

EVALUATION: Monitor hepatic, renal status ▪ Monitor VS, esp BP, heart rate ▪ Monitor I&O, daily weight ▪ Assess for CHF (dyspnea, peripheral edema, ↑ weight); notify physician ▪ Monitor serum K^+, glucose levels (hypoglycemia) ▪ Therapeutic blood levels: 2-4μg/ml.

EDUCATION: Take on empty stomach (1h ac/2h pc); swallow SR capsules whole ▪ Take as ordered by physician; do *not* change dose or time intervals ▪ Check $\bar{c}$ physician/pharmacist before taking any OTC preparations ▪ Use sugarless gum/hard candy to diminish dry mouth ▪ Avoid exposure to direct sunlight/UV light (sunlamps); use sunscreen, protective clothing ▪ Dizziness, blurred vision may occur; use caution in potentially hazardous activities ▪ Avoid alcohol ▪ Constipation may occur; ↑ fluid, roughage in diet ▪ Notify physician of eye pain, swelling in hands/legs ▪ Avoid ↑ exercise, temperature extremes ▪ Diabetics: hypoglycemia may occur; take sugar, notify physician.

NOTES:

dobutamine hcl • (doe-byoo-ta-meen)

CATEGORY: *Sympathomimetic:* β_1-adrenergic Rx; Preg Cat NA

BRAND NAME
Dobutrex (Lilly)

DOSAGE FORMS
Powder for injection (IV): 250mg/vial

DOSAGE
Adult *IV infusion* Usual dose 2.5-10μg/kg/m. Doses up to 40μg/kg/m may be required

ACTION: β_1-Receptor activity produces cardiac stimulation, positive inotropic effect, ↑ cardiac output, ↑ stroke volume; ↓ peripheral resistance; does not cause release of norepinephrine. **USE:** Short-term treatment of cardiac decompensation due to depressed contractility associated c̄ organic heart disease or cardiac surgical procedures.

PHARMACOKINETICS

Onset	Peak	Half-life	Excretion
1-2m	Up to 10m	2m	Primarily via urine as metabolites

CONTRAINDICATIONS: Hypersensitivity, idiopathic hypertrophic subaortic stenosis.

SIDE/ADVERSE EFFECTS: CNS: headache ▪ CV: *dose-related* ↑ *heart rate*, BP, ***ventricular ectopic activity;*** palpitation, anginal pain ▪ GI: nausea ▪ RESP: shortness of breath.

DRUG INTERACTIONS: Use c̄ nitroprusside may result in ↑ cardiac output, ↓ pulmonary wedge pressure ▪ Use c̄ beta blockers antagonizes therapeutic effects ▪ Use c̄ halogenated general anesthetics may cause serious arrhythmias ▪ Use c̄ MAO-I will ↑ pressor effects; ↓ doses are needed.

NURSING MANAGEMENT
ADMINISTRATION: Assess for hx of catecholamine hypersensitivity ▪ Assess fluid balance; correct hypovolemia ▪ Do *not* mix c̄ sodium bicarbonate, other alka-

line solutions ▪ Reconstitute c̄ 10ml sterile H_2O for injection/5% dextrose injection; if not completely dissolved, add 10ml diluent; further dilute to 50ml, administer c̄ 5% dextrose/0.9% NaCl/sodium lactate injection, use w/in 24h; administer via infusion pump ▪ Reconstituted solution stable 6h at room temperature, 48h refrigerated ▪ Do *not* freeze (crystallizes) ▪ Pink discoloration does *not* affect potency ▪ Do *not* mix in same IV line with heparin, hydrocortisone, cefazolin, cefamandole, cephalothin, penicillin, sodium ethacrynate.

EVALUATION: Monitor VS, esp BP, heart rate q2-5m ▪ Monitor ECG, hemodynamic status q15m ▪ Monitor I&O q15-30m ▪ Check IV infusion site carefully; avoid extravasation.

EDUCATION: Notify nurse/physician of abnormal rxs (difficult breathing, chest pain, irregular heartbeat).

NOTES:

dopamine • (doe-pa-meen)

CATEGORY: *Sympathomimetic:* β_1 adrenergic   Rx; Preg Cat C

BRAND NAMES
Intropin (Du Pont)
(AHS [Canada])
**Revimine (USV)*

DOSAGE FORMS
Injection (IV): 40, 80, 160mg/ml
Injection (IV): 40mg/ml

ACTION: Direct stimulation of β_1-receptors, dopaminergic receptors; in high doses, affects alpha receptors; sum total of adrenergic, dopaminergic activity results in positive inotropic effect, ↑ renal & mesenteric blood flow; alpha adrenergic effects more pronounced c̄ higher doses, produces vasoconstriction, ↑ BP. **USE:** Treatment of shock syndrome due to chronic cardiac decompensation, endotoxic septicemia, myocardial infarction, open-heart surgery, renal failure, trauma.

PHARMACOKINETICS

Onset	Half-life	Excretion
3-5m	2m	Via urine as metabolites in 24h

CONTRAINDICATIONS: Pheochromocytoma.

DOSAGE

Adult *IV infusion*	Start c̄ 1-5μg/kg/m. May be ↑ if needed. In severe cases, start c̄ 5μg/kg/m, gradually ↑ in 5-10μg/m increments to 20-50μg/kg/m if needed

SIDE/ADVERSE EFFECTS: CNS: headache ▪ CV: anginal pain, ***ectopic beats,*** hypotension, tachycardia, vasoconstriction ▪ GI: N/V ▪ RESP: dyspnea ▪ Other: necrosis, tissue sloughing c̄ extravasation.

DRUG INTERACTIONS: Use c̄ cyclopropane/halogenated general anesthetics may cause serious arrhythmias ▪ Use with MAO-I will ↑ pressor effects, ↓ doses are needed.

NURSING MANAGEMENT

ADMINISTRATION: Assess for hx of catecholamine hypersensitivity ▪ Assess fluid balance; correct hypovolemia ▪ Monitor ABG; correct acidosis ▪ Dilute (stable for 24h); infuse into large vein, titrate rate according to

Note: Side/adverse effects: common in *italic;* serious in ***boldface italic.***   *Available in Canada only.

findings following physician guidelines; use infusion pump ▪ Do *not* mix c̄ sodium, bicarbonate, other alkaline solutions ▪ Do *not* mix alkaline drugs in same IV line ▪ Do *not* use discolored/precipitated solutions ▪ Have phentolamine available for extravasation ▪ Avoid exposure to light.

EVALUATION: Monitor VS, esp BP, heart rate (assess for ↓ BP when infusion is stopped) ▪ Monitor ECG, hemodynamic status q5-15m ▪ Monitor I&O q5-15m ▪ Check IV insertion site carefully; avoid extravasation ▪ Observe pts c̄ hx of peripheral vascular disease for change in color/temperature of extremities; assess peripheral pulses; notify physician of abnormalities.

EDUCATION: Notify nurse/physician of abnormal rxs (difficult breathing, chest pain, irregular heartbeat, pain at IV insertion site).

NOTES:

doxepin hcl • (dox-e-pin)

CATEGORY: *Tricyclic antidepressant*: mood elevator Rx; Preg Cat C

BRAND NAME
Sinequan (Roerig)
(Pfizer [Canada])

DOSAGE FORMS
Capsule: 10, 25, 50, 75, 100, 150mg
PO concentrate: 10mg/ml

ACTION: Antidepressant activity appears related to inhibition of norepinephrine reuptake in central adrenergic neurons. **USE:** Treatment of endogenous depression ▪ Treatment of depression/anxiety c̄ alcoholism or organic disease ▪ Treatment of psychotic depressive disorders c̄ anxiety and manic-depressive conditions.

PHARMACOKINETICS

PO absorption	Peak	Half-life	Excretion
Rapid	2h	6-8h	Via urine as metabolites

CONTRAINDICATIONS: Hypersensitivity, MAO-I therapy, myocardial infarction (acute recovery period), glaucoma, urinary retention.

DOSAGE
Adult *PO* 75-150mg/d. Do *not* exceed 300mg/d

SIDE/ADVERSE EFFECTS: CNS: *drowsiness,* dizziness, headache, incoordination, tremors, extrapyramidal symptoms, paresthesia (extremities), insomnia ▪ CV: ***arrhythmias, myocardial infarction (rare),*** stroke (rare), ***heart block*** (rare), orthostatic hypotension ▪ EENT: tinnitus ▪ GI: anorexia, N/V/D, stomatitis, cramps, black tongue, dry mouth, constipation ▪ GU: gynecomastia, testicular swelling, galactorrhea, breast enlargement, urinary hesitancy, urinary retention ▪ HEM: ***agranulocytosis,*** eosinophilia, ***thrombocytopenia*** ▪ HEP: cholestatic jaundice ▪ INT: skin rash, photosensitivity, alopecia ▪ PSYCH: disorientation, delusions, hallucinations, exacerbation of psychosis, confusion ▪ Other: parotid swelling.

DRUG INTERACTIONS: Significant depressant effects c̄ alcohol ▪ Anticholinergics, chlorpromazine produce ↑ atropinelike effects; paralytic ileus could occur ▪ Significant ↑ in activity c̄ epinephrine, levarterenol, other adrenergic agents ▪ Significant antagonism to effects of reserpine, clonidine, guanethidine-type antihypertensives ▪ Use c̄ MAO-I best avoided.

NURSING MANAGEMENT

ADMINISTRATION: Assess for hx of tricyclic antidepressant hypersensitivity ▪ Assess for impaired hepatic, renal function; hx of glaucoma, prostatic hypertrophy; may require ↓ dosage ▪ PO: administer as single dose/d at hs c̄ food ▪ PO concentrate: use calibrated dropper; dilute in 120ml H_2O, milk, fruit or tomato juice before administrating; do *not* mix c̄ carbonated beverages ▪ Institute safety precautions ▪ Institute suicide precaution ▪ ↑ Dosage *slowly*; maintenance dose lowest dose that will maintain remission of depression ▪ Avoid abrupt withdrawal; D/C gradually ▪ Heavy smokers may require ↑ dosage ▪ Elderly may require ↓ dosage.

EVALUATION: Monitor CV, hepatic, renal status ▪ Monitor VS, esp BP ▪ Monitor CBC, esp long-term ▪ Monitor fluid retention (I&O, daily weight), constipation ▪ Assess for symptoms of abrupt withdrawal (nausea, headache, malaise) ▪ Assess for actual swallowing of PO forms.

EDUCATION: Dizziness/drowsiness may occur; use caution in potentially hazardous activities ▪ Avoid changing positions (lying/sitting/standing) rapidly ▪ Avoid use of alcohol, other CNS depressants up to 1 wk after ending therapy ▪ Take PO forms c̄ food to ↓ GI irritation ▪ Take as directed by physician ▪ Use sugarless gum/hard candy to diminish dry mouth ▪ Constipation may occur; ↑ fluids, bulk-containing foods ▪ Check c̄ physician before taking OTC/Rx preparations ▪ May produce peculiar taste ▪ Notify physician/dentist of use before treatment ▪ Store in tightly closed container ▪ Avoid exposure to direct sunlight, UV light (sunlamps); use sunscreen, protective clothing ▪ Encourage recreational/diversional interests ▪ Notify physician of fever, sore throat, malaise ▪ Keep scheduled appointments c̄ physician ▪ Full drug effects may require several wks of therapy.

NOTES:

doxycycline hyclate/minocycline hcl •

(dox-i-sye-kleen/mi-noe-sye-kleen)

CATEGORY: *Tetracycline*: broad-spectrum antibiotic Rx; Preg Cat D

BRAND NAMES	DOSAGE FORMS
doxycycline	Capsule, injection (IV), PO suspension, syrup, tablet
Doryx (P-D)	
Doxychel (Rachelle)	
Vibramycin (Pfizer)	
Vibra-Tabs (Pfizer)	
minocycline	
Minocin (Lederle)	Capsule, injection (IV), syrup

ACTION: Bacteriostatic effect due to inhibition of ribosomal protein synthesis. **USE:** Drug(s) of choice for chlamydial, mycoplasmal, rickettsial infections; acne control, balantidiasis, brucellosis, chancroid, cholera, granuloma inguinale, shigellosis, spirochetal relapsing fever ▪ Alternative in penicillin allergy, infections where bacteriologic testing indicates good activity ▪ Infections due to susceptible strains of *Escherichia coli, Enterobacter aerogenes, Francisella tularensis,* gonococcal (male) urethritis, *Haemophilus influenzae, Klebsiella* spp, *Yersinia pestis.*

CONTRAINDICATIONS: Hypersensitivity, pregnancy, nursing mothers, children <8y/o.

DOSAGE

doxycycline *PO/IV*

Pediatric	>8y/o: 2mg/lb d 1, then 1-2mg/lb/d
Adult	200mg d 1, then 100-200mg/d

minocycline *PO/IV*

Pediatric	>8y/o: 4mg/kg followed by 2mg/kg q12h
Adult	200mg followed by 100mg q12h. Do *not* exceed 400mg/d IV

PHARMACOKINETICS

	PO absorption		PO	Half-	Protein	
	No food	Food	Peak	life	binding	Excretion
doxycycline	90%-100%	70%-80%	2-12h	14-24h	30%-90%	Via feces, urine
minocycline	90%-100%	70%-80%	2-12h	11-26h	55%-80%	Via feces, urine

Note: Side/adverse effects: common in *italic;* serious in ***boldface italic.*** *Available in Canada only.

SIDE/ADVERSE EFFECTS: GI: gastric upset, diarrhea, bleeding, enterocolitis ▪ GU: dose-related ↑ BUN ▪ HEM: ***hemolytic anemia, thrombocytopenia***, ▪ INT: monilial overgrowth, maculopapular rash, ***exacerbation of SLE***, photosensitivity ▪ MS: reversible bulging fontanel in neonates, fetal skeletal retardation, discoloration of teeth ▪ Other: phlebitis at infusion site.

DRUG INTERACTIONS: Do *not* use c̄ antacids, antidiarrheals, bactericidal antibiotics, dairy products, methoxyflurane ▪ PO anticoagulants may require ↓ doses, esp during extended antibiotic therapy.

NURSING MANAGEMENT

ADMINISTRATION: Assess for hx of tetracycline hypersensitivity ▪ Obtain C&S before therapy ▪ Avoid PO administration c̄ milk, dairy products, antacids/antidiarrheal suspensions, iron salts ▪ Shake PO suspensions well before pouring ▪ Administer PO dose c̄ full glass H_2O ▪ IV: dilute; administer *slowly* (over 1h) ▪ Use reconstituted IV solution immediately ▪ Avoid exposure to heat, moisture, light in storage ▪ Do *not* administer to pregnant women, neonates, children <8y/o (permanent discoloration of teeth, ↓ bone growth).

EVALUATION: Monitor pt receiving anticoagulant therapy; may potentiate bleeding ▪ Assess renal, hepatic status ▪ Monitor VS, esp temperature ▪ Observe for signs of superinfection (diarrhea, itching, coated tongue) ▪ Assess for ↑ BUN, AST, creatinine.

EDUCATION: Complete full course of therapy (usually 10d), even if symptoms subside ▪ Avoid prolonged exposure to direct sunlight, UV light ▪ Take c̄ full glass H_2O; do *not* take w/in 1h of hs ▪ Take at equal interval around clock to maintain blood levels ▪ Diarrhea may occur ▪ Store in dry, tightly closed, light-resistant container ▪ Avoid taking products containing Al^{+++}, Mg^{++}, Ca^{++}, Fe^{++}, Zn^{++} concurrently ▪ Discard outdated preparations ▪ Can be taken c̄ meals; avoid dairy products ▪ Women: avoid breastfeeding.

NOTES:

edrophonium chloride • (ed-roe-foe-nee-um)

CATEGORY: *Parasympathomimetic*: anticholinesterase Rx; Preg Cat NA

BRAND NAME	DOSAGE FORMS
Tensilon (ICN)	Injection (IM/IV): 10mg/ml

ACTION: Anticholinesterase activity results in higher levels of acetylcholine, which produces indirect parasympathomimetic activity; ↑ acetylcholine levels at somatic myoneural nicotinic receptors alleviate symptoms of myasthenia gravis. **USE:** Differential diagnosis of myasthenia gravis; adjunct in evaluating treatment ▪ To reverse neuromuscular blockage of curare-like drugs.

PHARMACOKINETICS

IV onset	Duration	Excretion
30-60s	10m	Route, metabolism not determined

CONTRAINDICATIONS: Hypersensitivity, mechanical urinary obstructions.

DOSAGE FORMS

Pediatric	*IV*	1mg for children ≤75 lbs, 2mg for children ≥75 lbs. If no response after 45s, dose may be titrated up to 5mg in children <75 lbs, up to 10mg in bigger children, given at increments of 1mg q30-45s 0.5mg for infants
	IM	2mg for children ≤75 lbs, 5mg for children ≥75 lbs. Rx time delayed 2-10m
Adult	*IV*	Start $\bar{c}$ 10mg dose, $\bar{c}$ 2mg administered in 15-30s. If no response after 45s, remaining 8mg injected. If muscarinic rx $\bar{c}$ 2mg dose, test stopped, atropine 0.4-0.5mg given. As antagonist to curare-like drugs, 10mg IV over 30-40s. Repeat if needed. Do *not* exceed maximum dose 40mg
	IM	10mg; repeat in 30m $\bar{c}$ 2mg to rule out false negative

SIDE/ADVERSE EFFECTS: CNS: ***convulsions***, dysarthria, dysphonia ▪ CV: bradycardia, hypotension ▪ EENT: miosis, ↑ lacrimation ▪ GI: ↑ secretions, N/V, abdominal cramps, dysphagia ▪ GU: urinary frequency.

DRUG INTERACTIONS: Use c̄ caution in pts already receiving anticholinesterase therapy.

NURSING MANAGEMENT

ADMINISTRATION: Assess for hx of hypersensitivity ▪ Assess for hx of cardiac problems; test dose administered ▪ Administered by physician; assist as necessary ▪ Do *not* administer c̄ other cholinergics ▪ Monitor BP, pulse, respirations throughout administration ▪ Have atropine injection available for OD ▪ Have emergency support equipment available ▪ Test for myasthenia gravis; assess muscle strength before, after administration ▪ Use protective measures (bedrails) to prevent injury from possible restlessness.

EVALUATION: Monitor VS, esp respirations ▪ Myasthenic crisis (↑ respiratory status); cholinergic crisis (↓ respiratory status).

EDUCATION: Notify nurse/physician *immediately* of sweating, abdominal cramps, salivation ▪ Effects of drug will last approximately 30m.

NOTES:

enalapril maleate/enalaprilat ▲ • (e-nal-a-pril)

CATEGORY: *Antihypertensive*: angiotensin inhibitor — Rx; Preg Cat C/D†

BRAND NAME
Vasotec (MSD)

DOSAGE FORMS
IV injection▲: 1.25mg/ml
Tablet: 2.5, 5, 10, 20mg

ACTION: Antihypertensive activity appears related to suppression of renin-angiotensin-aldosterone system by competitive inhibition of ACE, which produces angiotensin II from angiotensin I; this results in reduction of peripheral arterial resistance, aldosterone secretion.

USE: Treatment of hypertension as sole agent or in combination c̄ other antihypertensives ▪ Adjunct in heart failure management.

DOSAGE

Adult *PO*	Start c̄ 5mg/d. ↑ slowly to 10-40mg/d as single dose or in 2 equal doses. Usual dose range 5-20mg/d in 2 divided doses for heart failure control
IV	1.25 mg q6h over a 5m period

SIDE/ADVERSE EFFECTS: CNS: *headache, dizziness* ▪ CV: hypotension, tachycardia, chest pain, palpitations, ***MI*** (rare), CHF, Raynaud's syndrome ▪ GI: V/D, pain, dyspepsia ▪ HEM: ***agranulocytosis***, neutropenia, anemia, ***thrombocytopenia*** ▪ INT: rash, pruritus, ***angioedema*** ▪ Other: loss of taste (reversible), *fatigue*.

PHARMACOKINETICS

PO absorption	Onset	Peak	Half-life	Duration	Excretion
60%	1h	4-6h	1-1.5h	Up to 24h	95% via urine in 24h

CONTRAINDICATIONS: Hypersensitivity; hx of angioedema c̄ other ACE-1. D/C during pregnancy as soon as possible.

DRUG INTERACTIONS: Aspirin, indomethacin, other NSAIA may antagonize therapeutic response Use K^+-sparing diuretics c̄ caution (hyperkalemia). Use c̄ lithium requires caution.

Note: Side/adverse effects: common in *italic;* serious in ***boldface italic***

*Available in Canada only.
† 1st trimester, C; 2nd & 3rd trimesters, D.

NURSING MANAGEMENT

ADMINISTRATION: Assess for hx of hypersensitivity ▪ Assess BP; notify physician of extremes ▪ Assess renal function; may require ↓ dosage if impaired ▪ Diuretics may be D/C for 2-3d before beginning drug to avoid hypotension ▪ PO: may crush, administer c̄ liquid; *best* on empty stomach (1h ac) ▪ IV: administer slowly (over 5m); may be diluted c̄ up to 50ml compatible diluent ▪ Assess serum Na^+ (normal: 135-145mEq/L) ▪ Assess for rapid ↓ in BP w/in 3h after administration of 1st dose (c̄ hyponatremia) ▪ SLE, elderly may require ↓ dosage ▪ Avoid abrupt withdrawal; D/C gradually.

EVALUATION: Monitor VS, esp BP ▪ Monitor CBC (esp WBC, differential) throughout therapy ▪ Monitor electrolyte status (↑K^+, ↓Na^+) ▪ Monitor I&O, daily weight ▪ Monitor renal function (proteinuria); notify physician ▪ Assess for loss of taste ▪ Assess for edema in extremities.

EDUCATION: Dizziness may occur; use caution in potentially hazardous activities ▪ Avoid changing positions (lying/sitting/standing) rapidly ▪ Notify physician of fever, sore throat, bruising/bleeding, swelling of feet/legs ▪ Take as ordered by physician even if symptom free; do *not* skip doses ▪ Take 1h ac ▪ Do *not* D/C w/out notifying physician ▪ Check c̄ physician/pharmacist before taking OTC/Rx preparations ▪ Avoid high Na^+ foods (canned soups, lunch meats, cheese) ▪ Avoid high K^+ foods (bananas, citrus juices, raisins) ▪ Check c̄ physician/pharmacist before using salt substitutes ▪ Avoid ↑ exercise, temperature extremes, smoking ▪ Loss of taste may occur, which may result in loss of appetite ▪ Tablets may smell like sulfur ▪ Used to control, *not* cure, hypertension ▪ Maintain optimum weight ▪ Keep scheduled appointments c̄ physician; have BP checked regularly ▪ Women: avoid breastfeeding ▪ Full drug effects may require several wks of therapy.

NOTES:

ephedrine sulfate • (e-fed-rin)

CATEGORY: *Sympathomimetic*: adrenergic, bronchodilator, decongestant

Rx/OTC; Preg Cat C

AVAILABLE PREPARATIONS
Capsule (OTC): 15, 25, 30, 50mg
Injection (IM/IV/SC) (Rx): 5, 25, 50mg/ml
Nose drops (OTC): 0.5%, 1%, 3%
Syrup (OTC): 11, 20mg/5ml

ACTION: Sympathomimetic effect due to activity on alpha-, beta-adrenergic receptors, resulting in vasoconstriction, ↑ BP, stimulation of heart, dilation of bronchioles; drug exhibits strong CNS stimulation. **USE:** Symptomatic treatment of asthma ▪ Topical, systemic decongestant ▪ Pressor agent for hypotension, shock ▪ Treatment of enuresis.

PHARMACOKINETICS: Complete PO, parenteral absorption; bronchodilation onset 15-60m PO, c̄ duration 2-4h; cardiac, pressor duration IV about 1h; drug extensively metabolizes, excreted via urine.

CONTRAINDICATIONS: Hypersensitivity, narrow-angle glaucoma, psychoneurosis.

DOSAGE

Pediatric *PO*	2-3mg/kg/d in 4-6 divided doses
IM/IV/SC	3mg/kg/d divided in 4-6 doses
Topical	1-3gtt q3-4h for nasal decongestion
Adult *PO*	12.5-50mg 3-4 times/d
IM/IV/SC	25-50 mg. Do *not* exceed daily maximum dose of 150mg
Topical	1-3gtt q3-4h for nasal decongestion

SIDE/ADVERSE EFFECTS: CNS: *nervousness*, insomnia, ***restlessness***, headache ▪ CV: ***arrhythmias***, precordial pain, palpitations ▪ EENT: rebound nasal congestion c̄ long-term/excessive local application ▪ GU: vesicle sphincter spasm, possible urinary retention ▪ PSYCH: mood changes, hallucinations.

DRUG INTERACTIONS: Use c̄ MAO-I can produce hypertensive crisis ▪ Use c̄ dig, anesthetics may cause arrhythmias ▪ Use c̄ other sympathomimetics, tricyclic antidepressants best avoided ▪ Use c̄ guanethidine, reserpine, hydralazine can antagonize antihypertensive effects ▪ Use c̄ beta-adrenergic blocking agents can antagonize their effects.

NURSING MANAGEMENT

ADMINISTRATION: Assess for hx of catecholamine hypersensitivity ▪ Assess BP, hx of cardiac problems; do *not* administer ▪ Do *not* crush timed-release preparations ▪ Do *not* administer discolored/precipitated solutions; discard unused portions ▪ PO: do *not* administer just before hs ▪ IV: inject *slowly* ▪ Protect from light; do *not* freeze ▪ Elderly may require ↓ dosage.

EVALUATION: Monitor VS, esp BP, heart rate ▪ Monitor I&O ▪ Assess for tolerance to therapeutic effect; D/C for few days, then resume.

EDUCATION: Avoid taking before hs; insomnia may occur ▪ Notify physician of pressure sensation in eyes, heart/bladder problems; stop taking drug ▪ Take as ordered by physician; do *not* ↑ dosage ▪ Check c̄ physician/pharmacist before using OTC cough/cold preparations ▪ Procedure for intranasal administration.

NOTES:

epinephrine • (ep-i-nef-rin)

CATEGORY: *Sympathomimetic*: bronchodilator, vasopressor — Rx/OTC; Preg Cat C

BRAND NAMES

Adrenalin (P-D)
AsthmaHaler (Norcliff Thayer)
Bronitin Mist (Whitehall)
Bronkaid Mist (Winthrop)
**Dysne-Inhal (Rougier)*
**Epifrin (Allergan)*
**Glaucon (Alcon)*
Medihaler-Epi (3M)
Primatene Mist (Whitehall)

DOSAGE FORMS

Aerosol (OTC); injection (Rx); nasal solution (OTC), ophthalmic solution (Rx)

ACTION: Sympathomimetic effect due to direct activity on both alpha-, beta-adrenergic receptors, resulting in vasoconstriction, increased BP, stimulation of heart, dilation of bronchioles. **USE:** To relieve respiratory distress due to bronchospasm ▪ Treatment of mucosal congestion, hypersensitivity rxs, esp anaphylaxis ▪ To prolong activity of infiltration local anesthetics ▪ To restore cardiac rhythm in cardiac arrest ▪ Hemostatic agent ▪ Management of open-angle glaucoma, ophthalmic/nasal congestion.

PHARMACOKINETICS: Onset in asthma attacks instant via inhalation, about 5-10m SC; excretion via urine primarily as metabolites.

CONTRAINDICATIONS: Hypersensitivity, narrow-angle glaucoma, organic brain damage; shock due to trauma, cyclopropane, halogenated general anesthetics, c̄ local anesthetics for use in toes/fingers, labor, coronary insufficiency.

DOSAGE

Pediatric	*Parenteral*	10μg/kg/dose SC
Adult	*Parenteral*	100μg-1mg SC/IM, 25-400μg IV
Adult/Pediatric	*Inhalation*	Proper dose automatically dispensed by nebulizer/aerosol dosage unit
	Ophthalmic	1-2 drops in eye prn

*Available in Canada only.

SIDE/ADVERSE EFFECTS: CNS: headache, *restlessness*, tremor, insomnia ▪ CV: *palpitations*, chest pain ▪ EENT: dry mouth, sore throat c̄ aerosol ▪ PSYCH: transient anxiety ▪ Other: tissue necrosis from repeated injections.

DRUG INTERACTIONS: Use c̄ MAO-I produces significant hypertension ▪ Use c̄ adrenergic blockers antagonizes their effects ▪ Use c̄ other sympathomimetics may cause additive effects, ↑ toxicity.

NURSING MANAGEMENT

ADMINISTRATION: Assess for hx of catecholamine hypersensitivity ▪ Administer while awake (except in cardiac arrest) ▪ Auscultate breath sounds; notify physician if abnormal ▪ Check preparation, dosage calculations c̄ another RN for accuracy ▪ Do *not* expose to light ▪ SC: refrigerate suspension; shake well before administration, use TB syringe; massage injection site (↓ vasoconstriction); rotate sites ▪ IV: use cardiac monitoring; check compatibility chart for mixing; dilute 1mg (1:1000 solution) c̄ 10ml NaCl injection to produce 1:10,000 solution, inject *slowly* (1mg/m); may dilute further c̄ 5% dextrose solution; discard unused portion. ▪ IM: do *not* inject intragluteally; use deltoid ▪ Do *not* use discolored/precipitated solution ▪ Ophthalmic: put pressure on lacrimal sac for 1m after instillation.

EVALUATION: Monitor VS, esp BP, heart rate ▪ Monitor respiratory status ▪ Assess I&O, urinary retention ▪ Assess for signs of excessive CNS stimulation; hold drug, notify physician ▪ Diabetics: closely monitor blood glucose (hyperglycemia).

EDUCATION: Take as ordered by physician; do *not* ↑ dose ▪ Diabetics: check blood/urine glucose carefully ▪ Notify physician of irritability, difficult breathing, chest pain, insomnia ▪ Check c̄ physician/pharmacist before taking OTC preparations ▪ Women: avoid breastfeeding ▪ Procedure for ophthalmic, intranasal, inhalation, SC (Autoinjector) administration.

NOTES:

ergonovine maleate • (er-goe-noe-veen)

CATEGORY: *Oxytoxic*

Rx; Preg Cat NA

BRAND NAME
Ergotrate Maleate (Lilly)

DOSAGE FORMS
Injection (IM/IV): 0.2mg/ml
Tablet: 0.2mg

ACTION: Oxytoxic effect due to direct stimulation of uterine smooth muscle, resulting in intense contractions followed by periods of relaxation; accordingly, ↑ uterine tone, ↓ postpartum uterine bleeding; drug can occasionally produce severe hypertensive episodes, esp in toxemic pts. **USE:** Treatment/prevention of postpartum/postabortal hemorrhage due to uterine atony.

PHARMACOKINETICS

Onset			Duration	Excretion
PO	IM	IV		
10m	2-5m	Immediate	≥3h	Primarily via feces

CONTRAINDICATIONS: Hypersensitivity, threatened spontaneous abortion.

DOSAGE

Adult *PO*	Initial dose 0.2mg, usually IM, followed by 0.2-0.4mg PO q6-12h until danger of atony is over (approximately 48h)
IM	0.2mg; may be repeated for severe hemorrhage
IV	Route should be restricted to excessive hemorrhage because of higher rate of side effects, esp N/V

SIDE/ADVERSE EFFECTS: CNS: headache ▪ CV: hypertension, particularly when administered IV ▪ GI: N/V ▪ Other: possible symptoms of ergot poisoning.

DRUG INTERACTIONS: Concurrent/sequential use c̄ vasoconstrictors/regional anesthesia may affect BP.

NURSING MANAGEMENT
ADMINISTRATION: *Not* routinely used before delivery ▪ Assess BP ▪ Assess serum calcium; IV calcium gluconate if hypocalcemic ▪ PO: avoid excessive moisture in storage ▪ Injection: store in cold place (<46° F); do *not* exceed 60d at room termperature ▪ Do *not* administer discolored/precipitated solutions ▪ IV: use infusion con-

trol device; administer *slowly* ▪ Have emergency support equipment available ▪ Provide emotional support.

EVALUATION: Monitor BP, pulse ▪ Monitor serum calcium ▪ Observe for signs of ergotism (N/V, dizziness, cramps, headache, confusion) ▪ Postpartum: monitor fundal height/tone; assess amount/character of lochia.

EDUCATION: Explain procedure, rationale to pt, family ▪ Occurrence of contractions ▪ Relaxation techniques ▪ Comfort measures ▪ Store in tightly closed container ▪ Avoid smoking ▪ Notify physician of infection, signs of ergotism (cramps, vomiting, thirst, weakness, tingling in extremities).

NOTES:

ergotamine tartrate • (er-got-a-meen)

CATEGORY: *Alpha-adrenergic blocker:* antimigraine, sympatholytic Rx; Preg Cat X

BRAND NAMES	DOSAGE FORMS
Ergostat (P-D)	Sublingual tablets: 2mg
Medihaler Ergotamine (3M)	0.36 mg metered/dose

Combination Products

Caffergot (Sandoz)	Ergotamine/caffeine
Wigraine (Organon)	1mg/100mg per tablet
	2mg/100 mg per suppository

ACTION: Produces direct vasoconstriction on cranial blood vessels to relieve vascular pulsations probably responsible for vascular headache; exhibits oxytoxic activity. **USE:** Treatment of vascular headache.

PHARMACOKINETICS

Peak	Half-life	Excretion
0.5-3h	2.7h, then 27h	90% in bile as metabolites; unmetabolized in saliva

CONTRAINDICATIONS: Coronary heart disease, hypersensitivity, hypertension, impaired hepatic/renal function, peripheral vascular disease, pregnancy, sepsis.

DOSAGE

Adult *SL*	2mg, repeat at 1/2h intervals. Do *not* exceed 6mg/d, 10mg/wk
Aerosol	One inhalation (0.36mg), repeat at ≥5m intervals. Do *not* exceed 6 inhalations/d, 15/wk
Cafergot/Wigraine	
PO	2 tablets, then 1 q1/2h to a maximum of 6 tablets/attack, or 10/wk
Rectal	1 supp., then 1 in one h. (Maximum of 2/attack or 5/wk)

SIDE/ADVERSE EFFECTS: CNS: headache, tremors, convulsions ▪ CV: blood vessel contraction (↓ circulation esp limbs; ***gangrene*** possible) ▪ GI: N/V.

DRUG INTERACTIONS: Propranolol, other beta blockers may interfere c̄ activity of ergotamine.

NURSING MANAGEMENT

ADMINISTRATION: Used to abort *acute* vascular headache; administer at onset of pain/during prodromal stage ▪ Assess characteristics of pain ▪ Assess psychosocial factors associated c̄ pain ▪ Aerosol: shake well before use ▪ Provide pt comfort during headache attacks ▪ Provide ↓ environmental stimuli ▪ Avoid exposure to moisture, light in storage; use original container.

EVALUATION: Observe for signs of ergotism (N/V/D, drowsiness, dizziness, headache, mental confusion) ▪ Monitor hepatic status ▪ Monitor VS, esp heart rate ▪ Assess peripheral pulses c̄ prolonged therapy.

EDUCATION: Take drug when pain starts (used to stop *acute* attacks) ▪ Lie down in darkened, quiet room for several hrs after taking drug ▪ Compliance c̄ prescribed dosage regimen; do *not* exceed recommended dose/wk allowable ▪ Notify physician immediately of signs of ergotism (N/V/D, drowsiness, dizziness, headache, mental confusion) ▪ Store in tightly closed, light-resistant container ▪ Women: avoid breastfeeding ▪ Procedure for inhalation/SL administration.

NOTES:

erythromycin ophthalmic ointment • (eh-rith-roe-mye-sin)

CATEGORY: *Antibiotic:* macrolide antibiotic Rx

BRAND NAME	DOSAGE FORMS
Ak-Mycin (Akorn)	Ophthalmic ointment: 0.5% (5mg/g)
Ilotycin (Dista) (Lilly in Canada)	Ophthalmic ointment: 0.5% (5mg/g)

ACTION: Bacteriostatic activity due to inhibition of ribosomal protein synthesis in susceptible microorganisms; topical ophthalmic application has limited tissue penetration, may fail to protect against gonococcal penicillinase-producing strains of *Neisseria gonorrhoeae.* **USE:** Treatment of ophthalmic infections due to susceptible organisms ▪ Prophylaxis of gonococcal/chlamydial ophthalmia neonatorum.

CONTRAINDICATIONS: Hypersensitivity.

DOSAGE

Ophthalmic infection	Apply ribbon (approximately 1cm) of ointment to infected eye(s), usually in conjunctival sac, ≥1 time/d
Ophthalmia neonatorum	Use new tube for each infant. Apply ribbon (0.5-1cm) of ointment in each conjunctival sac *not* later than 1h after delivery

SIDE/ADVERSE EFFECTS: EENT: local ophthalmic irritation ▪ Other: possible overgrowth of nonsusceptible organisms.

NURSING MANAGEMENT

ADMINISTRATION: Assess for hx of hypersensitivity ▪ Avoid contamination of ointment tube tip ▪ Use new tube of ointment for each neonate ▪ Apply thin strip into lower conjunctival sac after delivery ▪ Do *not* flush from eye after administration ▪ Avoid excessive heat, light in storage; do *not* freeze.

EVALUATION: Observe for signs of local hypersensitivity; notify physician.

EDUCATION: Explain procedure, rationale to family ▪ Report signs of local hypersensitivity (redness, tearing, irrigation) immediately ▪ Avoid using common towels/wash cloths among family members ▪ Procedure for ophthalmic administration.

NOTES:

erythromycin salts • (eh-rith-roe-mye-sin)

CATEGORY: *Antibiotic*: macrolide antibiotic

Rx; Preg Cat NA

BRAND NAMES

Erythromycin base

E-Mycin (Boots), Ery-Tab (Abbott), ERYC (P-D)

Erythromycin estolate

Ilosone (Dista) (Lilly in Canada)

Erythromycin ethylsuccinate

*EES (various), *Erythrocin (Abbott) Ery Ped (Abbott)*

Erythromycin gluceptate

Ilotycin Gluceptate IV (Dista) (Lilly in Canada)

Erythromycin lactobionate

Erythrocin Lactobionate IV (Abbott)

Erythromycin stearate

Erypar (P-D), Erythrocin Stearate (Abbott), Wyamycin S (W-A)

DOSAGE FORMS

Capsules, chewable tablet, injection (IV), suspension, tablet

USE: Treatment of systemic infections caused by susceptible strains of α-hemolytic streptococci, *Bordetella pertussis, Chlamydia trachomatis, Chlamydia urethritis, Entamoeba histolytica* (intestinal amebiasis only), group A β-hemolytic streptococci, *Haemophilus influenzae, Legionella pneumophila, Listeria monocytogenes, Mycoplasma pneumoniae, Neisseria gonorrhoeae,* staphylococci, *Streptococcus pneumoniae, Treponema pallidum, Ureaplasma* urethritis ▪ Treatment of erythrasma (*Corynebacterium minutissimum)* ▪ Adjunct to antitoxin therapy in treating *Corynebacterium* diphtherial infections ▪ Treatment of diphtheria carriers.

PHARMACOKINETICS

PO absorption	Peak	Half-life	Protein binding	Excretion
Good	1-4h	1.5-2h	73%-96%	Primarily via feces as unchanged drug

ACTION: Bacteriostatic activity due to inhibition of ribosomal protein synthesis in susceptible organisms.

*Available in Canada only.

CONTRAINDICATIONS: Hypersensitivity.

DOSAGE

Base, estolate, stearate	
Pediatric *PO*	30-50mg/kg/d divided. Severe infection, up to 60-100mg/kg/d
Adult *PO*	250mg qid. Severe infection, ≤4g/d. Primary syphilis, 30-50g divided, for 10-15d. Urethritis, 500mg qid for 7d
Ethyl succinate	
Adult *PO*	400mg qid. Primary syphilis, 48-64g divided, for 10-15d. Urethritis, 800mg tid for 7d
Gluceptate, Glactobionate	
Pediatric/Adult *IV*	15-20mg/kg/d. Severe infection, higher doses

SIDE/ADVERSE EFFECTS: EENT: hearing loss (reversible) ▪ GI: *abdominal cramps,* N/V/D ▪ HEP: hepatotoxicity ▪ INT: urticaria, rash ▪ Other: ***anaphylaxis,*** thrombophlebitis (IV).

DRUG INTERACTIONS: Bacteriostatic antibiotics can antagonize effects of bacterial antibiotics ▪ Use c̄ carbamazepine, PO anticoagulants, theophylline can ↑ their toxicity.

NURSING MANAGEMENT

ADMINISTRATION: Assess for erythromycin sensitivity ▪ Obtain C&S before therapy ▪ PO: administer 1h ac/2h pc c̄ full glass H_2O (avoid citrus juice); do *not* crush delayed-release/enteric-coated preparations; estolate, ethylsuccinate, enteric-coated preparations can be taken w/out regard to meals ▪ IV: dilute c̄ 10ml (250, 500mg vial), 20ml (1g vial) sterile H_2O for infection; further dilute to 1g/L normal saline, lactated Ringer, 5% dextrose solution according to manufacturer's directions; administer via *slow,* continuous infusion (20-60m).

EVALUATION: Monitor VS, esp temperature; hepatic status ▪ Observe for signs of superinfection (diarrhea, perineal itching, oral ulcers).

EDUCATION: Complete full course of therapy ▪ Take on empty stomach; estolate, ethylsuccinate, enteric-coated preparations can be taken c̄ meals (avoid citrus juice); swallow delayed-release, enteric-coated preparations whole; shake suspension well before pouring, keep refrigerated; chewable tablet should *not* be swallowed whole, chew thoroughly ▪ Take at equal intervals around clock to maintain blood levels ▪ Diarrhea may occur.

estazolam/quazepam • (ess-taz-oh-lam/kway-ze-pam)

CATEGORY: *Benzodiazepine*: hypnotic

Rx C-IV; Preg Cat X

BRAND NAME
estazolam
ProSom (Abbott)
quazepam
Doral (Wallace)

DOSAGE FORMS
Tablet: 1, 2mg
Tablet: 7.5, 15mg

ACTION: Hypnotic activity improves total sleep time, ↓ number of nocturnal awakenings; REM sleep not affected. **USE:** Short-term use as hypnotic.

DOSAGE: *PO*

estazolam	
Adult	1-2mg hs
Geriatric	0.5mg or higher hs
quazepam	
Adult	7.5 or 15mg hs
Geriatric	Adult dosage ↓ after 1-2 d

PHARMACOKINETICS

	PO absorption	Peak	Half-life	Protein binding	Excretion
estazolam	Readily	2h	18.4h	93%	96% via urine, 4% via feces as metabolites
quazepam	Rapid	2h	39h	95%	23% via urine, 31% via feces as metabolites over 5d period

CONTRAINDICATIONS: Hypersensitivity.

SIDE/ADVERSE EFFECTS: CNS: *drowsiness*, headache, hypokinesia, nervousness, dizziness, hangover ▪ CV: infrequent flushing, palpitation ▪ GI: dry mouth, N/V ▪ HEM: leukopenia (rare) ▪ Other: asthenia, abnormal vision, malaise.

DRUG INTERACTIONS: Use c̄ other CNS depressants produces additive effects ▪ Use c̄ MAO-I can produce serious toxic effects.

NURSING MANAGEMENT

ADMINISTRATION: Assess for hx of benzodiazepine hypersensitivity ▪ Avoid exposure to heat, moisture, light in storage ▪ Avoid abrupt withdrawal ▪ Elderly may require ↓ dosage ▪ ↓ Environmental stimuli.

EVALUATION: Monitor renal, hepatic status ▪ Assess for symptoms of abrupt withdrawal (tremors, abdominal/muscle cramps, convulsions) c̄ prolonged use ▪ Check for signs of dependence (↑ drug request)/tolerance ▪ Monitor activity status (safety precautions) ▪ Assess for paradox rxs (CNS stimulation), esp in elderly ▪ Check for depression; suicide precautions prn ▪ Assess pt sleep patterns.

EDUCATION: Drowsiness may occur; use caution in potentially hazardous activities ▪ Avoid use c̄ alcohol, other CNS depressants ▪ Indiscriminate use may lead to dependence ▪ Do *not* smoke after taking drug ▪ Do *not* keep at bedside ▪ Take as ordered by physician; do *not* ↑ dose ▪ Women: avoid breastfeeding ▪ Check c̄ physician/pharmacist before taking OTC drugs ▪ Practice relaxation exercises, ventilation of feelings ▪ Utilize sleep producers (reading, warm milk, soft music).

NOTES:

estradiol • (ess-tra-dye-ole)

CATEGORY: *Estrogenic agent* Rx; Preg Cat X

BRAND NAMES	DOSAGE FORMS
Estrace (MJP) *(Bristol [Canada])*	Tablet: 1, 2mg Vaginal cream: 0.01% (NA in Canada)
Estraderm (Ciba)	Transdermal patch: 0.05, 0.1mg/d

ACTION: Estrogens required for development, maintenance of female reproductive system, 2° sex characteristics. **USE:** Treatment of moderate/severe symptoms associated c̄ menopause, atrophic vaginitis, kraurosis vulvae, female hypogonadism, female castration, breast/prostate cancer palliation, osteoporosis prevention, primary ovarian failure.

PHARMACOKINETICS: Rapid PO absorption, extensive protein binding and metabolism, excretion via urine.

CONTRAINDICATIONS: Known/suspected pregnancy, estrogen-dependent neoplasia, breast cancer except in appropriately selected pts; abnormal genital bleeding, active or past hx of estrogen associated thrombophlebitis/thromboembolic disorders (except for breast/prostate cancer treatment).

DOSAGE: Drug should be given cyclically for short-term use; lowest dose that will control symptoms should be chosen, D/C as soon as possible; administer for 3wks, then skip 1 wk; attempts to D/C or taper medication should be made at 3-6mo intervals.

PO	Usual initial dose 1-2mg/d administered cyclically For cancer palliation, usual starting dose 1-2mg tid
Vaginal	2-4g cream (marked on applicator)/d for 1-2wks. Gradually reduce to half initial dose for similar period. Usual maintenance dose 1g 1-3 times/wk
Transdermal	Initiate c̄ 0.5mg/d patch 2 times/wk, adjust for control of symptoms

SIDE/ADVERSE EFFECTS: CNS: headache, migraine, dizziness, mental depression ▪ CV: edema ▪ EENT: intolerance to contact lenses, steepening of corneal curvature ▪ GI: *nausea*, vomiting, abdominal cramps, bloating ▪ GU: amenorrhea, breakthrough bleeding, dysmenorrhea, candidiasis, change in menstrual flow, spotting, ↑ size of uterine fibromyomas ▪ INT: melasma, ***erythema multiforme***/nodosum, alopecia, hirsutism, urticaria ▪ MET: ↓ carbohydrate tolerance ▪ Other: weight changes, porphyria exacerbation.

DRUG INTERACTIONS: Use c̄ tricyclic antidepressants may result in toxic rxs.

NURSING MANAGEMENT

ADMINISTRATION: Assess for hx of hypersensitivity ▪ PO: administer cyclically (3wks on, 1wk off) c̄ meals ▪ Avoid abrupt withdrawal; D/C gradually ▪ Vaginal: apply c̄ plastic dose applicator; maintain in recumbent position 30m after application.

EVALUATION: Monitor BP ▪ Monitor hepatic, renal status ▪ Assess for endometrial cancer (Pap test, physical exam) ▪ Monitor PT; may ↓ anticoagulant effect ▪ Diabetics: careful blood/urine testing; may ↓ antidiabetic drug effect ▪ Assess for behavioral changes, depression ▪ Monitor weight; observe for edema.

EDUCATION: Review package insert c̄ pt ▪ Take PO dosage form c̄ food ▪ Nausea may occur during first 2wks of therapy ▪ Women: avoid pregnancy, breastfeeding ▪ Breast self-examination (incl men) ▪ Avoid smoking (↑ CV complications) ▪ Notify physician/dentist of use before treatment ▪ Avoid exposure to direct sunlight, UV light (sunlamps); use sunscreen, protective clothing ▪ D/C drug, notify physician if pregnancy is suspected ▪ Vaginal: apply at hs; use sanitary napkin (avoid tampons) to protect clothing; procedure for using plastic dose applicator ▪ Notify physician *immediately* of chest/leg pain, unusual vaginal bleeding, difficult breathing, slurred speech ▪ Men: enlarged breasts, drug-related impotence reversible after therapy ▪ Check weight, swelling in feet/legs daily ▪ Keep scheduled appointments c̄ physician (Pap test, physical exam).

NOTES:

estrogens, conjugated • (<u>ess</u>-troe-jenz)

CATEGORY: *Estrogenic agent* Rx; Preg Cat X

BRAND NAMES
**C.E.S. (ICN)*
Premarin (W-A)

DOSAGE FORMS
Powder for injection (IM/IV): 25mg/vial
Tablet: 0.3, 0.625, 0.9, 1.25, 2.5mg
Vaginal cream: 0.625mg/g

ACTION: Estrogens required for development, maintenance of female reproductive system, 2° sex characteristics. **USE:** Treatment of moderate/severe symptoms associated c̄ menopause ▪ Treatment of atrophic vaginitis, kraurosis vulvae, female hypogonadism, female castration, breast/prostatic cancer palliation, primary ovarian failure ▪ Prevention of postpartum breast enlargement ▪ Probably effective for estrogen deficiency-induced osteoporosis in conjunction c̄ diet.

PHARMACOKINETICS: Rapid PO absorption, wide tissue distribution, high protein binding, urinary excretion.

CONTRAINDICATIONS: Known/suspected pregnancy, estrogen-dependent neoplasms, breast cancer except in appropriately selected pts; abnormal genital bleeding, active past hx estrogen associated thrombophlebitis/thromboembolic disorders (except for breast/prostatic cancer treatment).

DOSAGE

Adult *PO*	
Menopause	1.25mg/d. If pt is menstruating, start on day 5 of bleeding for cyclic administration
Atrophic vaginitis, kraurosis valvae	≥0.3mg/d, depending on response. Administer cyclically
Hypogonadism	2.5-7.5mg/d divided, or 20d, followed by rest period of 10d
Castration, ovarian-failure	1.25mg/d, cyclically
Postpartum breast enlargement	3.75mg q4h for 5 doses. 1.25mg q4h for 5d
Prostatic cancer	1.25-2.5mg tid
Breast cancer	10mg tid for at least 3mo
IM/IV	
Abnormal uterine bleeding	25mg, repeat in 6-12h prn. Start PO doses as soon as possible

Cream

Atrophic vaginitis, kraurosis vulvae	1/2-1 applicator (2-4g) intravaginally/topical

SIDE/ADVERSE EFFECTS: CNS: headache, migraine, dizziness, mental depression ▪ EENT: intolerance to contact lenses ▪ GI: N/V, abdominal cramps, bloating ▪ GU: amenorrhea, breakthrough bleeding, dysmenorrhea, candidiasis, ↑ size of uterine fibromyomas ▪ INT: melasma, **erythema multiforme**/nodosum, alopecia, hirsutism, urticaria ▪ MET: ↓ carbohydrate tolerance ▪ Other: weight changes, porphyria exacerbation.

DRUG INTERACTIONS: Use c̄ tricyclic antidepressants may produce toxic rxs.

NURSING MANAGEMENT

ADMINISTRATION: PO: administer cyclically (3wks on, 1wk off) c̄ meals ▪ Avoid abrupt withdrawal ▪ Parenteral: reconstitute by withdrawing 5ml air from container, inject 5ml sterile diluent against container side, gently agitate, do *not* shake; compatible c̄ normal saline, dextrose, invert sugar solutions; *not* compatible c̄ acidic solutions; stable for 60d refrigerated, protect from light ▪ IM: administer *deep, slowly* into gluteal UOQ; use dry syringe, 21-gauge needle for oil preparations ▪ IV: preferred route; administer *slowly*; do *not* administer oil preparations IV ▪ Vaginal: apply c̄ plastic dose applicator.

EVALUATION: Monitor BP, PT ▪ Assess for endometrial cancer (Pap test, physical exam) ▪ Diabetics: careful blood/urine testing ▪ Assess for behavioral changes, depression ▪ Monitor pt weight; observe for edema.

EDUCATION: Nausea may occur during first 2wks of therapy ▪ Women: avoid pregnancy, breastfeeding ▪ Breast self-exam (incl men) ▪ Avoid smoking ▪ Take PO dosage form c̄ food ▪ Notify physician/dentist of use before treatment ▪ Keep appointments c̄ physician ▪ Avoid direct sunlight, UV light ▪ D/C drug, notify physician if pregnancy suspected ▪ Vaginal: apply hs; use sanitary napkin ▪ Notify physician *immediately* of chest/leg pain, unusual vaginal bleeding, difficult breathing, slurred speech ▪ Men: enlarged breasts, impotence (reversible).

NOTES:

ethambutol hcl • (e-tham-byoo-tole)

CATEGORY: *Antitubercular*

Rx; Preg Cat NA

BRAND NAMES
**Etibi (ICN)*
Myambutal (Lederle)

DOSAGE FORMS
Tablet: 100, 400mg

ACTION: Tuberculostatic activity due to interference of protein synthesis by inhibition of RNA synthesis in actively growing susceptible tubercular bacilli; use c̄ isoniazid ↓ mycobacterial resistance to isoniazid. **USE:** Combined treatment of pulmonary TB c̄ isoniazid, streptomycin, both, or other agents.

PHARMACOKINETICS

PO absorption	Peak	Half-life	Protein binding	Excretion
75%-80%	2-4h	3.3h	22%	50% via urine as unchanged drug in 24h, 8%-15% as metabolites

CONTRAINDICATIONS: Hypersensitivity, known optical neuritis (unless clinically required).

DOSAGE

Adult *PO*	Initial dose 15mg/kg as single daily dose. Retreatment dose 25mg/kg as single daily dose

SIDE/ADVERSE EFFECTS: CNS: optic/peripheral neuritis, headache, dizziness, mental confusion, possible hallucinations ▪ EENT: dose-related loss of visual acuity (optic neuritis) ▪ GI: gastric distress, anorexia N/V, abdominal pain ▪ INT: dermatitis, pruritus ▪ MS: joint pain, exacerbation of gout ▪ Other: fever.

DRUG INTERACTIONS: None currently reported.

NURSING MANAGEMENT

ADMINISTRATION: Assess for hx of hypersensitivity ▪ Obtain sputum C&S before therapy ▪ May administer c̄ food ▪ Avoid exposure to heat, moisture, light in storage ▪ Assess renal function; ↓ dose if impaired.

EVALUATION: Monitor hepatic, renal status ▪ Assess for visual disturbances (ocular toxicity) ▪ Monitor serum for ↑ uric acid, AST, ALT.

EDUCATION: Take as directed by physician; do *not* skip doses ▪ May take $\bar{c}$ food ▪ Keep scheduled appointments for eye exams ▪ Notify physician *immediately* of visual problems ▪ Women: avoid pregnancy, breastfeeding ▪ May produce gouty symptoms ▪ Emotional support during long-term therapy.

NOTES:

ethosuximide • (eth-oh-sux-i-mide)

CATEGORY: *Anticonvulsant*

Rx; Preg Cat NA

BRAND NAME
Zarontin (P-D)

DOSAGE FORMS
Capsule: 250mg
Syrup: 250mg/5ml

ACTION: Anticonvulsant activity due to motor cortex depression, ↑ in convulsive threshold; drug ↓ paroxysmal spike/wave patterns of petit mal seizure. **USE:** Drug of choice for petit mal.

PHARMACOKINETICS

PO absorption	Peak	Half-life	Excretion
Good	4h	30-60h	Primarily via urine as metabolites

CONTRAINDICATIONS: Hypersensitivity.

DOSAGE

Pediatric *PO*	3-6y/o: Start c̄ 250mg/d, adjust to achieve control ≥6y/o: Start c̄ 500mg/d, adjust to achieve control. 20mg/kg/d is optimal dose in most children
Adult *PO*	Start c̄ 500mg/d, ↑ by 250mg q4-7d to achieve control. Doses >1.5g require close supervision. Usual maintenance dose 5000mg-1.5g/d

SIDE/ADVERSE EFFECTS: CNS: *drowsiness*, headache, dizziness, euphoria, sleep disturbances, hiccoughs, ataxia, agitation, aggressiveness ▪ GI: N/V/D, anorexia, cramps, pain ▪ GU: vaginal bleeding ▪ HEM: ***agranulocytosis, aplastic anemia,*** leukopenia, pancytopenia, eosinophilia ▪ INT: urticaria, erythematous rash, ***Stevens-Johnson syndrome, SLE*** ▪ Other: gum hypertrophy, swollen tongue.

DRUG INTERACTIONS: Use c̄ chloramphenicol, other bone marrow depressants results in significant blood dyscrasia.

NURSING MANAGEMENT

ADMINISTRATION: Assess for hx of anticonvulsant hypersensitivity ▪ Assess hepatic, hematologic, renal function ▪ Administer c̄ food/milk ▪ Avoid abrupt withdrawal; institute strict seizure precautions if drug abruptly withdrawn ▪ Avoid exposure to light (syrup), moisture in storage; do *not* freeze syrup.

EVALUATION: Monitor occurrence/characteristics of seizures ▪ Monitor hepatic, hematologic, renal status ▪ Assess for behavioral changes ▪ Assess for skin rash; notify physician, D/C drug ▪ Monitor activity status (safety precautions) ▪ Assess for symptoms of abrupt withdrawal (tremors, abdominal/muscle cramps, convulsions) ▪ Therapeutic blood level: 40-100mg/ml.

EDUCATION: Do *not* omit doses ▪ Drowsiness/dizziness may occur; use caution in potentially hazardous activities ▪ Do *not* smoke after taking drug ▪ Take c̄ food/milk ▪ Carry medical identification (MedicAlert) ▪ Take at equal intervals ▪ Keep scheduled appointments c̄ physician ▪ Store in tightly closed container ▪ Syrup: do *not* freeze; protect from light, moisture ▪ Check c̄ physician/pharmacist before taking OTC/Rx preparations.

NOTES:

etodolac • (eh-toe-doe-lack)

CATEGORY: *Antiinflammatory:* analgesic, NSAIA

Rx; Preg Cat C

BRAND NAME
Lodine (W-A)

DOSAGE FORMS
Capsules: 200, 300mg

ACTION: Antiinflammatory, analgesic activity appears related to inhibition of prostaglandin synthesis. **USE:** Treatment of acute and long-term osteoarthritis ▪ Relief of mild/moderate pain.

PHARMACOKINETICS

PO absorption	Onset	Peak	Duration	Protein binding	Excretion
100%	1/2h	1-2h	4-6h	99%	70%-75% via urine and feces primarily as metabolites

CONTRAINDICATIONS: Hypersensitivity, pts c̄ aspirin or other NSAIA-induced allergies (asthma, rhinitis, etc.)

DOSAGE

Adult *PO*

Osteoarthritis	Initial dose of 800-1200mg/d divided. Then adjust between 600-1200mg/d. Do *not* exceed 1200mg/d, or 20mg/kg for pts ≤60kg
Pain	200-400mg q6-8h prn. Do *not* exceed 1200mg/d, or 20mg/kg for pts ≤60kg

SIDE/ADVERSE EFFECTS: CNS: confusion, paresthesia, dizziness, depression ▪ CV: fluid retention, edema, hypertension ▪ EENT: blurred vision, tinnitus, taste changes ▪ GI: dyspepsia, abdominal pain, bleeding, N/V/D, flatulence ▪ GU: dysuria, urinary frequency ▪ HEM: anemia ▪ INT: pruritus, rash ▪ Other: asthenia, asthma.

DRUG INTERACTIONS: Use c̄ ulcerogenic drugs produces additive effects ▪ Phenylbutazone will ↑ plasma levels due to protein displacement ▪ Use c̄ cyclosporine, digoxin, lithium methotrexate can ↑ their activity.

NURSING MANAGEMENT

ADMINISTRATION: Assess for hx of NSAIA hypersensitivity ▪ Avoid administration to pts c̄ hx of asthma, bleeding disorders, salicylate hypersensitivity ▪ Obtain C&S before therapy ▪ Assess for hx of peptic ulcer; use c̄ caution if impaired ▪ Administer c̄ food/milk to ↓ GI irritation; encourage upright position for 15-30m ▪ Avoid exposure to moisture in storage ▪ Elderly may require ↓ dosage.

EVALUATION: Monitor hepatic, renal status c̄ prolonged use ▪ Monitor pts receiving anticoagulant therapy; may potentiate bleeding ▪ Monitor I&O, daily weight ▪ Assess for edema in extremities ▪ Assess for visual/hearing disturbances; D/C drug, notify physician.

EDUCATION: Dizziness/drowsiness may occur; use caution in potentially hazardous activities ▪ Take c̄ food/milk to ↓ GI distress; maintain upright position for 15-30m ▪ Take as ordered by physician; do *not* ↑ dose ▪ Notify physician *immediately* of bleeding, ↓ urine output, swelling of feet/legs, lethargy, GI distress, jaundice, visual disturbance ▪ Avoid taking c̄ aspirin, other NSAIAs ▪ Avoid use c̄ alcohol ▪ Check c̄ physician/pharmacist before taking OTC preparations ▪ Notify physician/dentist of use before treatment ▪ Store in tightly closed container ▪ Schedule eye exams c̄ prolonged use ▪ Women: avoid breastfeeding ▪ Full drug effects may require several wks of therapy.

NOTES:

famotidine • (fa-moe-ti-deen)

CATEGORY: *H_2 blocker:* antihistamine   Rx; Preg Cat B

BRAND NAME
Pepcid (MSD)

DOSAGE FORMS
IV injection: 10mg/ml
PO suspension: 40mg/5ml
Tablet: 20, 40mg

ACTION: H_2 antihistaminic activity due to competitive inhibition of histamine at H_2 histamine receptors on parietal cells, resulting in ↓ gastric acid secretions. **USE:** Short-term treatment of gastric/duodenal ulcers ▪ Duodenal ulcer prophylaxis ▪ Treatment of pathologic hypersecretory conditions—eg, Zollinger-Ellison syndrome, multiple endocrine adenomas.

PHARMACOKINETICS

PO absorption	Peak	Half-life	Protein binding	Excretion
40%-45%	1-3h	2.5-3.5h	15%-20%	30% PO dose and 65%-70% IV dose as unchanged drug via urine

CONTRAINDICATIONS: Hypersensitivity.

DOSAGE

Adult *PO*	
Ulcers	40mg/d hs or 20mg bid. Usual maintenance dose 20mg/d hs
Pathologic hypersecretions	20-160mg q6h
Prophylaxis/maintenance	20mg/d hs
IV	20mg q12h

SIDE/ADVERSE EFFECTS: CNS: *headache, dizziness,* depression, anxiety, grand mal seizure ▪ CV: palpitations ▪ EENT: tinnitus ▪ GI: N/V, dry mouth ▪ HEM: ***thrombocytopenia*** ▪ HEP: cholestatic jaundice ▪ INT: acne, alopecia, urticaria, rash, pruritus ▪ Other: bronchospasm, arthralgia, angioedema, facial edema, rare gynecomastia.

DRUG INTERACTIONS: None currently reported.

NURSING MANAGEMENT

ADMINISTRATION: Assess for hx of H_2 blocker sensitivity ▪ Avoid exposure to moisture in storage ▪ PO: administer c̄ food; PO suspension: add 46ml distilled H_2O; shake well before pouring; discard unused portion after 30d ▪ IV injection: dilute to total vol 5-10ml 0.9% NaCl injection; inject over 2m ▪ IV intermittent infusion: dilute to total vol 100ml D_5W injection; infuse over 15-30m; do *not* use if discolored, precipitation present ▪ Diluted injection is stable for 48h at room temperature ▪ Elderly may require ↓ dosage.

EVALUATION: Monitor GI, hepatic, neurologic, renal status.

EDUCATION: Take c̄ food, hs ▪ May be taken w/out regard to antacids ▪ Dizziness may occur; use caution in potentially hazardous activities ▪ Avoid smoking ▪ Avoid GI irritating foods ▪ Check c̄ physician/pharmacist before taking OTC preparations ▪ Avoid anxiety-producing situations ▪ Notify physician of H_2 blocker use before allergy & gastric acid secretion testing ▪ Store in tightly closed container in cool, dry area ▪ Take as ordered by physician; do *not* change or skip dosage ▪ Women: avoid breastfeeding.

NOTES:

fenopropfen calcium • (fen-oh-proe-fen)

CATEGORY: *Antiinflammatory*: analgesic — Rx; Preg Cat NA

BRAND NAME
Nalfon (Distal)
(Lilly in Canada)

DOSAGE FORMS
Capsule (Pulvule): 200, 300mg
Tablet: 600mg

ACTION: Antiinflammatory, analgesic activity appears related to inhibition of prostaglandin synthesis. **USE:** Treatment of rheumatoid, osteoarthritis ▪ Relief of mild/moderate pain.

PHARMACOKINETICS

PO absorption	Peak	Half-life	Protein binding	Excretion
Rapid	2h	2-4h	99%	90% via urine primarily as metabolities in 24h

CONTRAINDICATIONS: Hypersensitivity, aspirin hypersensitivity, impaired renal function.

DOSAGE
Adult *PO*

Pain	200mg q4-6h prn
Arthritis	Starting dose 300-600mg qid. Do *not* exceed 3200mg/d

SIDE/ADVERSE EFFECTS: CNS: *headache, somnolence,* dizziness, tremor, confusion ▪ CV: palpitations, tachycardia ▪ EENT: tinnitus, hearing, blurred vision ▪ GI: *dyspepsia,* constipation, N/V, pain, anorexia, flatulence, dry mouth, ***hemorrhage*** ▪ INT: pruritus, rash, urticaria.

DRUG INTERACTIONS: Use c̄ ulcerogenic drugs produces additive effects ▪ Use c̄ PO anticoagulants, thrombolytic agents may ↑ their activity ▪ Use c̄ aspirin will ↓ fenoprofen plasma levels.

NURSING MANAGEMENT
ADMINISTRATION: Assess for hx of NSAIA, salicylate hypersensitivity ▪ Avoid administration to pts c̄ hx of asthma, bleeding disorders, salicylate hypersensitivity ▪ Assess GI, renal, hepatic function; use caution if

Note: Side/adverse effects: common in *italic;* serious in ***boldface italic.***

*Available in Canada only.

impaired ▪ May be administered c̄ food, milk, antacid; *best* on empty stomach (1h ac/2h pc); tablets may be crushed, capsules opened; encourage upright position for 15-30m ▪ Avoid exposure to moisture during storage ▪ Elderly may require ↓ dosage.

EVALUATION: Monitor hepatic, renal status c̄ prolonged use ▪ Monitor pt receiving anticoagulant therapy; may potentiate bleeding ▪ Monitor I&O, daily weight ▪ Assess for edema in extremities ▪ Assess for visual/hearing disturbances; D/C drug, notify physician

EDUCATION: Dizziness/drowsiness may occur; use caution in potentially hazardous activities ▪ Take on empty stomach (1h ac/2h pc), c̄ food/milk if GI distress occurs; maintain upright position for 15-30m ▪ Take as ordered by physician; do *not* ↑ dose ▪ Notify physician *immediately* of bleeding, urine output, swelling of feet/legs, lethargy, GI distress, jaundice, visual/hearing disturbances ▪ Avoid taking c̄ aspirin, other NSAIAs ▪ Avoid use c̄ alcohol ▪ Check c̄ physician/pharmacist before taking OTC preparations ▪ Notify physician/dentist of use before treatment ▪ Store in tightly closed container ▪ Full drug effects may require several wks of therapy.

NOTES:

fentanyl citrate • (fen-ta-nil)

CATEGORY: *Narcotic*: synthetic opiate

Rx C-II; Preg Cat C

BRAND NAMES
Sublimaze (Janssen)
Duragesic (Janssen)

DOSAGE FORMS
Injection (IM/IV): 0.5mg/ml
Transdermal 25, 50, 75, 100

ACTION: Narcotics produce analgesia, euphoria, sedation; 0.1mg dose approximately equivalent to 10mg morphine, 75mg meperidine. **USE:** Relief of moderate/severe pain ▪ Preop sedation; operative, preop analgesia ▪ Relief of chronic pain requiring opioids (transdermal).

PHARMACOKINETICS

	Onset	Peak	Half-life	Excretion
IM	7-15m	1-2h	1.5-6h	Via urine as unchanged drug, metabolites
IV	1-3m	30-60m	6-8m	

Transdermal provides a dose of 25, 50, 75, or 100 μg/hr for 72 hr

CONTRAINDICATIONS: Hypersensitivity; use c̄ extreme caution in head injuries.

DOSAGE

Pediatric *IM/IV* (2-12y/o)	Induction, maintenance: 0.02-0.03mg/kg
Adult *IM/IV*	
Pre-op	0.05-0.1mg IV before surgery
Adjunct to general anesthesia	Induction: low dose 0.002mg/kg; moderate dose 0.002-0.02mg/kg; high dose 0.02-0.05mg/kg Maintenance: low dose 0.002mg/kg; moderate dose 0.002-0.02mg/kg; high dose 0.02-0.5mg/kg
Adjunct to regional anesthesia	0.05-0.1mg. May be repeated
Post-op	0.05-0.1mg. May be repeated in 1-2h prn
Adult Transdermal	Start c̄ 25μg/hr and adjust

SIDE/ADVERSE EFFECTS: CNS: *sedation, lightheadedness*, euphoria, dysphoria, tremor, disorientation, ↓ convulsive threshold ▪ CV: hypotension, palpitations, flushing of face, phlebitis at IV site ▪ EENT: miosis ▪ GI: N/V, dry mouth, constipation, biliary tract spasm ▪ GU: urinary retention ▪ INT: pruritus, urticaria ▪ RESP: ***respiratory depression***.

DRUG INTERACTIONS: Use c̄ alcohol, antihistamines, barbiturates, benzodiazepines, methotrimeprazine, phenothiazines, other CNS depressants produces additive CNS depression; ↓ dosage may be required ▪ Use c̄ tricyclic antidepressants may product additive respiratory depression.

NURSING MANAGEMENT

ADMININISTRATION: Assess for hx of hypersensitivity ▪ Store under double lock/key; document use accurately ▪ Check compatibility for mixing c̄ other drugs in solution ▪ Do *not* administer if respirations are < 12/m ▪ IM: inject *deep* into muscle ▪ IV: dilute; administer *slowly* (1-2m) ▪ Have narcotic antagonist, support measures available ▪ Elderly may require ↓ dosage ▪ Administer subsequent initial narcotic analgesic at ↓ dosage (1/4 - 1/3 usual dose).

EVALUATION: Monitor VS, esp BP, respirations ▪ Assess renal function, urinary retention ▪ Assess for potentiation of CNS depressant effect ▪ Assess for signs of overdose (coma, pinpoint pupils, respiratory depression).

EDUCATION: Avoid excessive sensory stimulation ▪ Keep bedrails up ▪ Turn, cough, deep breathe after surgery ▪ Avoid changing positions (lying/sitting/standing) rapidly ▪ Avoid smoking.

NOTES:

flecaininde acetate • (flek-a-nide)

CATEGORY: *Antiarrhythmic*

Rx; Preg Cat C

BRAND NAME
Tambocor (3M)

DOSAGE FORMS
Tablet: 50, 100, 150mg

ACTION: Antiarrhythmic effect due to dose-related depression of cardiac conduction, esp in His-Purkinje system; drug has not appreciable effect on atrial arrhythmias, produces effects similar to group 1C antiarrhythmics, is reserved for documented serious ventricular arrhythmias. **USE:** Treatment of documented ventricular arrhythmias.

PHARMACOKINETICS

PO absorption	Peak	Half-life	Protein binding	Excretion
Almost complete	3h	20h	40%	Via urine as unchanged drug, metabolites

CONTRAINDICATIONS: Hypersensitivity, cardiogenic shock, second/third-degree AV block, right bundle branch block when associated c̄ left hemiblock w/out pacemaker.

DOSAGE

Adult *PO*

Sustained ventricular tachycardia	Initial dose 100mg q12h, c̄ 50mg increments if needed ↑ 50 mg bid q4d until satisfactory response. Usual dose 150mg q12h, c̄ daily maximum 400mg
Nonsustained tachycardia, ventricular complexes	Initial dose 100mg q12h, c̄ 50mg increments if needed bid q4d until satisfactory response. Usual range 200-400mg/d, c̄ maximum 600mg/d

SIDE/ADVERSE EFFECTS: CNS: *dizziness, headache, tremor,* convulsions, confusion, paresthesia, depression, drowsiness ▪ CV: CHF, ***proarrhythmic effect,*** palpitations, ***heart block,*** bradycardia, angina, hypotension, hypertension, chest pain ▪ EENT: *blurred vision,* visual spots, tinnitus, photophobia ▪ GI: N/V, anorexia, constipation, abdominal pain ▪ GU: impotence ▪ HEM: leukopenia, ***thrombocytopenia*** ▪ INT: rash, urticaria, pruritus, ***exfoliative dermatitis*** ▪ MS: arthralgia ▪ RESP: *dyspnea.*

Note: Side/adverse effects: common in *italic;* serious in ***boldface italic.***

*Available in Canada only.

DRUG INTERACTIONS: Use c̄ propranolol will ↑ plasma levels of both drugs, possible summation of negative inotropic effects ■ Use c̄ disopyramide or verapamil requires extreme caution.

NURSING MANAGEMENT

ADMINISTRATION: Assess for hx of hypersensitivity ■ Assess hepatic, renal function; may require ↓ dosage if impaired ■ May be administered w/out regard to meals ■ Assess serum K^+ levels (normal: 3.5-5mEq/L); correct imbalances before administration ■ Maintain blood levels; administer at equal intervals around clock ■ Avoid exposure to moisture during storage ■ Elderly may require ↓ dosage.

EVALUATION: Monitor VS, esp heart rate, BP ■ Assess for CHF (dyspnea, peripheral edema, ↑ weight); notify physician ■ Monitor serum for ↑ alkaline phosphatase c̄ prolonged use ■ Monitor ECG, CBC, blood levels throughout therapy ■ Assess for tremors (signifies maximum dose) ■ Therapeutic blood levels: 0.4-1.0μg/ml.

EDUCATION: Dizziness may occur; use caution in potentially hazardous activities ■ Avoid changing positions (lying/sitting/standing) rapidly, esp elderly ■ Take as ordered by physician even if symptom free; do *not* skip doses ■ Take at equal intervals around clock ■ Procedure for checking radial pulse ■ Notify physician *immediately* of irregular pulse, fever, sore throat, bruising/bleeding ■ Keep scheduled appointments c̄ physician ■ Notify physician/dentist of use before treatment ■ Full drug effect may require several days of therapy.

NOTES:

fluconazole • (floo-koe-na-zole)

CATEGORY: *Broad-spectrum antifungal*

Rx; Preg Cat C

BRAND NAME

Diflucan (Roerig)

DOSAGE FORMS

IV infusion: 2mg/ml in 100, 200ml units

Tablet: 50, 100, 200mg

ACTION: Antifungal activity may be related to selective inhibition of fungal sterol demethylation (cytochrome P-450 sterol C-14 alpha-demethylation) resulting in the accumulation of 14 alpha-methyl sterols, which are fungistatic. **USE:** Treatment of oropharyngeal, esophageal, and serious systemic UTI, pneumonia, and peritonitis caused by susceptible strains of *Candida* spp. ▪ Treatment of cryptococcal meningitis.

PHARMACOKINETICS

PO absorption	Peak	Half-life	Protein binding	Excretion
Almost complete	1-2h	30h	11%-20%	Primarily as unchanged drug via urine

CONTRAINDICATIONS: Hypersensitivity.

DOSAGE: For pts $\bar{c}$ normal renal function. The PO and IV dose are the same. The IV dose should be administered at a maximum rate of about 200mg/h as a continuous infusion.

Adult

Candidiasis

Oropharyngeal	Initial dose 200mg/d followed by 100mg once/d for at least 2 wks. Doses up to 400mg/d may be required
Esophageal	Initial dose 200mg/d followed by 100mg once/d. Doses up to 400mg/d may be used. Minimum treatment time is at least 3 wks and 2 or more wks following resolution of symptoms
Systemic	Initial dose 400mg/d followed by 200mg once/d for at least 4 wks and at least 2 wks following resolution of symptoms

Meningitis	Initial dose 400mg/d followed by 200mg once/d for 10-12 wks after negative CSF cultures. Prophylactic dose of 200mg/d required in AIDS pts

SIDE/ADVERSE EFFECTS: Substantially higher c̄ HIV-infected pts ▪ CNS: *headache* ▪ GI: N/V, abdominal pain, diarrhea ▪ HEP: ↑ in serum transaminase ▪ INT: ***Stevens-Johnson syndrome.***

DRUG INTERACTIONS: Use c̄ PO anticoagulants can ↑ PT & requires careful monitoring ▪ Use c̄ phenytoin and cyclosporine can ↑ their plasma concentrations ▪ Use c̄ PO hypoglycemic agents will ↓ their metabolism and ↑ their plasma concentrations, and dosage adjustments may be required.

NURSING MANAGEMENT

ADMINISTRATION: Assess for hx of hypersensitivity to azole antifungal agent ▪ Obtain C&S before therapy ▪ Assess hepatic, renal function; ↓ dosage if impaired ▪ IV: Administer via continuous infusion at a maximum rate of 200mg/h; do *not* use if solution is cloudy or precipitated; do *not* add other medication to the IV solution; do *not* administer IM or SC ▪ Avoid exposure to moisture in storage.

EVALUATION: Monitor VS, esp temperature ▪ Monitor hepatic function ▪ Assess for occurrence of rash; D/C drug, notify physician.

EDUCATION: Take as ordered by physician at same time qd; do *not* change dose ▪ Take c̄ food to avoid GI upset ▪ Report skin rash to physician *immediately*; D/C drug ▪ Check c̄ physician/pharmacist before taking OTC drugs ▪ Store in tightly closed container.

NOTES:

fluorouracil • (flure-oh-yoor-a-sill)

CATEGORY: *Antineoplastic*: antimetabolite

Rx; Preg Cat D

BRAND NAMES	**DOSAGE FORMS**
Adrucil (Adria)	Injection (IV): 50mg/ml
Efudex (Roche)	Topical cream: 5% Solution: 2%, 5%
Fluroplex (Herbert)	Topical cream: 1% (5% in Canada) Solution: 1%

ACTION: Antimetabolite activity due to competitive inhibition of enzyme thymidylate synthetase, resulting in deficiency of thymidine, which inhibits DNA synthesis. **USE:** Palliative treatment of colon, rectum, breast, stomach, pancreas cancer ▪ Topical treatment of superficial basal cell carcinomas when conventional treatment is impractical ▪ Topical treatment of actinic or solar keratosis.

PHARMACOKINETICS: After IV administration, drug is distributed into bone marrow, intestinal mucosa, liver, tumors; no intact drug can be detected in blood after 3h; excretion via urine primarily as metabolites.

CONTRAINDICATIONS: Depressed bone marrow function, poor nutritional state, serious infections; topical: local hypersensitivity.

DOSAGE

Adult *IV*	Start c̄ 12mg/kg/d for 4 successive d. Do *not* exceed total daily dose 800mg. If no toxicity, give 6mg/kg on days 6, 8, 10, 12, do not give on days 5, 7, 9, 11, D/C on day 12 For poor-risk pts, start c̄ 6mg/kg/d for 3 successive d. If no toxicity, give 3mg/kg on days 5, 7, 9, do not give on days 4, 6, 8. Do *not* exceed total daily dose 400mg. Usual maintenance dose 10-15mg/kg/wk, c̄ reduced doses for poor-risk pts. Do *not* exceed 1g/wk
Topical	
Actinic/solar keratosis	Apply cream/solution bid to lesions. Continue until inflammatory response reaches erosion, necrosis, ulceration stage. Usually requires 2-4 wks, complete healing may require up to 2mo

Superficial basal cell carcinoma	Apply 5% cream/solution bid to lesions for at least 3-6 wks. Therapy may require 10-12 wks

SIDE/ADVERSE EFFECTS: GI: esophagopharyngitis, stomatitis, anorexia, N/V/D ▪ HEM: ***myelosuppression, thrombocytopenia*** ▪ INT: alopecia, dermatitis, dry skin, loss of nails ▪ Other: photophobia, lacrimation, ***acute cerebellar syndrome*** ▪ Topical: local pain, burning, pruritus, hyperpigmentation, scarring, suppuration, scaling, swelling.

DRUG INTERACTIONS: Radiation therapy, other myelosuppressive drugs produce additive bone marrow depression.

NURSING MANAGEMENT

ADMINISTRATION: Check hx for radiation/antineoplastic therapy ▪ IV: dilute according to manufacturer's directions; administer antiemetic before therapy; administer via direct injection (1-2m) or slow IV infusion (2-24h); precipitate may form when exposed to cold temperatures; heat to 60°C to redissolve, shake vigorously; cool to body temperature before using ▪ Topical: cleanse area, apply c̄ applicator/fingers; wash hands before, after application ▪ Provide emotional support ▪ Assess oral cavity for ulceration; notify physician ▪ Avoid exposure to heat, moisture, light in storage ▪ Contact dermatitis may occur.

EVALUATION: Monitor hepatic, renal function; CBC, esp WBC, platelets throughout therapy; notify physician if ↓ ▪ Assess for infection, bleeding, anemia ▪ May produce ↑ serum uric acid level ▪ Assess hydration status (I&O, daily weight) ▪ Check IV insertion site carefully (cellulitis).

EDUCATION: ↑ Fluid intake (8-10 glasses/d) ▪ Avoid exposure to infection ▪ Check c̄ physician before immunization ▪ Diet as tolerated; avoid spicy foods ▪ Maintain oral hygiene; use soft-bristled toothbrush ▪ Notify physician of symptoms of bone marrow depression ▪ Loss of hair may occur (reversible) ▪ Women: avoid breastfeeding ▪ Use contraception if sexually active ▪ Topical: avoid exposure to direct sunlight, UV light (sunlamps); use sunscreen; avoid application near eyes, nose, mouth; local discomfort may occur; apply as ordered; store in tightly closed, light-resistant container; wash hands before, after application.

NOTES:

fluoxetine hcl • (floo-ox-uh-teen)

CATEGORY: *Antidepressant* Rx; Preg Cat B

BRAND NAME
Prozac (Dista)

DOSAGE FORM
Tablet: 20mg

ACTION: Antidepressant activity appears related to inhibition of serotonin reuptake in the CNS. **USE:** Treatment of depression that closely resembles DSM-III category of major depressive disorder. Long-term use (>5-6 wks) requires reevaluation of clinical effectiveness.

PHARMACOKINETICS

PO absorption	Peak	Half-life	Protein binding	Excretion
Good ac/pc	6-8h	7-9d	94.5%	Mainly as inactive metabolites via urine

CONTRAINDICATIONS: Hypersensitivity.

DOSAGE

Adult *PO* Usual dose 20mg/d in AM. If no clinical improvement is obtained after several wks, ↑ may be required. Doses >20mg/d require bid administration, in the AM and at noontime. Do *not* exceed 80mg/d.

SIDE/ADVERSE EFFECTS: CNS: *anxiety, nervousness, insomnia, drowsiness, tremor, headache,* dizziness, abnormal dreams ▪ CV: angina, hot flashes, palpitations, rare conduction disturbances, lymphadenopathy ▪ GI: *anorexia* c̄ significant weight loss, N/D, dry mouth, dyspepsia, constipation, abdominal pain ▪ GU: frequent urination, painful menstruation, sexual dysfunction ▪ INT: *rash, pruritus, excessive sweating, erythema multiforme* ▪ RESP: flulike symptoms, pharyngitis, bronchitis ▪ Other: *fatigue,* visual disturbances, tinnitus, anemia.

DRUG INTERACTIONS: Use c̄ MAO-I and tryptophan is best avoided ▪ Use c̄ diazepam may ↑ its half-life ▪ Use c̄ highly protein bound drugs (digitoxin, warfarin, etc.) can result in adverse effects of these drugs and/or fluoxetine because of protein displacement.

NURSING MANAGEMENT

ADMINISTRATION: Assess for hx of hypersensitivity ▪ Assess for hx of seizures; use caution ▪ Assess hepatic, renal status; ↓ dosage if impaired ▪ Administer consistently c̄ or w/out food; single dose in AM, divided dose in AM & noon ▪ Institute safety, seizure precautions ▪ Institute suicide precautions ▪ Avoid abrupt withdrawal;

D/C gradually ▪ Avoid moisture, heat, direct light in storage ▪ Elderly may require ↓ dosage.

EVALUATION: Monitor CV, hepatic, renal status ▪ Monitor fluid retention (I&O, daily weight), constipation ▪ Assess for weight loss (anorectic effect) ▪ Assess for symptoms of abrupt withdrawal (nausea, headache, malaise) ▪ Assess for actual swallowing of PO forms ▪ Assess for skin rash, hives; notify physician, D/C drug.

EDUCATION: Dizziness/drowsiness may occur; use caution in potentially hazardous activities ▪ Avoid changing positions (lying/sitting/standing) rapidly ▪ Avoid use of alcohol, other CNS depressants for up to 1 wk after end of therapy ▪ Take consistently c̄ or w/out food ▪ Take as directed by physician ▪ Use sugarless gum/hard candy to diminish dry mouth ▪ Constipation may occur; ↑ fluids, bulk-containing foods ▪ Notify physician of skin rash, hives; D/C drug ▪ Check c̄ physician/pharmacist before taking OTC/Rx preparations ▪ Notify physician/dentist of use before treatment ▪ Store in tightly closed, light-resistant container ▪ Encourage recreational/diversional interests ▪ Notify physician of weight loss, fever, sore throat, malaise ▪ Keep scheduled appointments c̄ physician ▪ Women: notify physician of pregnancy possibility; avoid breastfeeding ▪ Full drug effects may require several wks of therapy.

NOTES:

fluphenazine decanoate/enanthate/hcl • (floo-fen-a-zeen)

CATEGORY: *Phenothiazine*: antipsychotic, neuroleptic — Rx; Preg Cat NA

BRAND NAMES / **DOSAGE FORMS**

Brand Names	Dosage Forms
**Modecate (Squibb)*	Injection (SC/IM): 5mg/ml, 25mg/5ml
**Moditen (Squibb)*	Injection (SC/IM): 5mg/ml, 25mg/5ml
Permitil (Schering)	PO concentrate: 5mg/ml Tablet: 2.5, 5, 10mg
Proloxin Decanoate (Princeton)	Injection (SC/IM): 25mg/ml
Prolixin Enanthate (Princeton)	Injection (SC/IM): 25mg/ml
Prolixin (Princeton)	Elixir: 2.5mg/5ml Injection (IM): 2.5 mg/ml PO concentrate: 5mg/ml Tablet: 1, 2.5, 5, 10mg

ACTION: Antipsychotic activity appears associated c̄ ↓ in neural transmission in central dopamine-dependent pathways, resulting in tranquilizing effect; decanoate/enanthate injection effects have onset between 24-72h, psychotic symptoms controlled w/in 48-96h. **USE:** Treatment of psychoses.

PHARMACOKINETICS

PO absorption	Onset	Peak	Duration	Excretion
Rapid	1h	2h	6-8h	Via urine, feces

CONTRAINDICATIONS: Hypersensitivity, comatose states, bone marrow depression, presence of large amounts of CNS depressants, liver impairment, renal damage.

DOSAGE

decanoate/enanthate	
Adult *SC/IM*	12.5-25mg usually adequate. Do *not* exceed 100mg/dose
hcl	
Adult *PO*	0.5-20mg/d
IM	2.5-10mg/d
Geriatric *PO*	1-2.5mg/d

SIDE/ADVERSE EFFECTS: CNS: drowsiness, extrapyramidal rxs, tardive dyskinesia, seizures, depression, catatonia-like states ▪ CV: postural hypotension, tachycardia, ECG changes ▪ EENT: blurred vision; corneal, lenticular changes; nasal congestion ▪ END: menstrual irregularities, galactorrhea ▪ HEM: ***agranulocytosis***, eosinophilia, ***hemolytic anemia***, thrombocytopenic purpura ▪ HEP: cholestatic jaundice ▪ INT: urticaria, photosensitivity, ***exfoliative dermatitis*** ▪ Other: fever, hyperpyrexia, hypothermia.

DRUG INTERACTIONS: Al^{+++}/Mg^{++} antacid preparations ↓ absorption ▪ Use c̄ narcotics, barbiturates, other CNS depressants ↑ CNS depression ▪ Guanethidine, related antihypertensive effects antagonized.

NURSING MANAGEMENT

ADMINISTRATION: Assess for hx of phenothiazine hypersensitivity ▪ Assess VS, esp BP ▪ PO: administer c̄ food ▪ PO concentrate: dilute before administration c̄ >60ml fluid ▪ IM/SC: keep pt lying down for 30m after injection ▪ Discard markedly discolored/precipitated solution ▪ Avoid skin contact c̄ liquid forms (contact dermatitis) ▪ Avoid abrupt withdrawal; D/C gradually ▪ Heavy smokers may require ↑ dosage.

EVALUATION: Monitor hepatic, ophthalmic, renal status; BP, CBC; fluid retention; constipation; seizures ▪ Assess for extrapyramidal symptoms (tics/spasms, trembling, shuffling gait); jaundice, agranulocytosis ▪ Assess for symptoms of abrupt withdrawal (nausea, dyskinesia, trembling, dizziness).

EDUCATION: Dizziness/drowsiness may occur; use caution in potentially hazardous activities ▪ Avoid changing positions rapidly ▪ Avoid alcohol, other CNS depressants ▪ Take PO forms c̄ meals ▪ Store in tightly closed, light-resistant container ▪ Use sugarless gum/hard candy to diminish dry mouth ▪ Constipation may occur; ↑ fluids, bulk-containing foods ▪ May turn urine pink/red/brown ▪ Avoid contact c̄ liquid forms ▪ Women: avoid breastfeeding ▪ Avoid exposure to temperature extremes; direct sunlight, UV light (sunlamps); use sunscreen, protective clothing ▪ Notify physician of fever, sore throat, bruising/bleeding, extrapyramidal symptoms (tics/spasms, trembling, shuffling gait) ▪ Take as directed by physician ▪ Check c̄ physician before taking OTC preparations ▪ Extended-action injectable effects may last up to 6 wks ▪ Do *not* take antacids/antidiarrheals w/in 2h of drug ▪ Full drug effects may require several wks of therapy.

OVERDOSE MANAGEMENT: *See* Phenothiazines.

flurazepam hcl • (flure-az-e-pam)

CATEGORY: *Benzodiazepine*: hypnotic

Rx C-IV; Preg Cat X

BRAND NAMES	DOSAGE FORMS
**Apo-Flurazepam (Apotex)*	
Dalmane (Roche)	Capsule 15, 30mg
**Somnol (Horner)*	
**Som-Pam (ICN)*	

ACTION: Hypnotic activity extends to all stages (0-4) of sleep; improves total sleep time; ↓ number of nocturnal awakenings. **USE:** Short-term use as hypnotic.

PHARMACOKINETICS

PO absorption	Peak	Half-life	Excretion
Rapid	30-60m	2-3h	Via urine primarily as metabolites, which have long half-life

CONTRAINDICATIONS: Hypersensitivity, pregnancy.

DOSAGE

Adult *PO*	15-30mg hs
Geriatric/debilitated	15mg hs

SIDE/ADVERSE EFFECTS: CNS: *drowsiness, fatigue, ataxia* ▪ CV: hypotension ▪ EENT: dry mouth ▪ HEM: neutropenia (rare) ▪ INT: skin rash ▪ PSYCH: paradoxical anxiety, hallucinations, hyperexcited states.

DRUG INTERACTIONS: Use c̄ other CNS depressants produces additive effects ▪ Use c̄ MAO-I can produce serious toxic effects.

NURSING MANAGEMENT

ADMINISTRATION: Assess for hx of benzodiazepine hypersensitivity ▪ Avoid exposure to heat, moisture, light in storage ▪ Avoid abrupt withdrawal ▪ Elderly may require ↓ dosage ▪ ↓ Environmental stimuli.

EVALUATION: Monitor renal, hepatic status ▪ Assess for symptoms of abrupt withdrawal (tremors, abdominal/muscle cramps, convulsions) c̄ prolonged use ▪ Check for signs of dependence (↑ drug request) ▪ Monitor activity status (safety precautions) ▪ Assess for tolerance to therapeutic dose ▪ Assess for paradoxical rxs (CNS stimulation), esp in elderly ▪ Check for depression, suicide precautions prn ▪ Assess pt sleep patterns.

EDUCATION: Drowsiness may occur; use caution in potentially hazardous activities ▪ Avoid use $\bar{c}$ alcohol, other CNS depressants ▪ Indiscriminate use may lead to dependence ▪ Do *not* smoke after taking drug ▪ Do *not* keep at bedside ▪ Take as ordered by physician; do *not* ↑ dose ▪ Women: avoid breastfeeding ▪ Check $\bar{c}$ physician/ pharmacist before taking OTC drugs ▪ Practice relaxation exercises, ventilation of feelings ▪ Utilize sleep producers (reading, warm milk, soft music).

NOTES:

flurbiprofen • (flur-bi-proe-fen)

CATEGORY: *Antiinflammatory*: analgesic, NSAIA   Rx; Preg Cat B

BRAND NAME
Ansaid (Upjohn)

DOSAGE FORMS
Tablet: 50, 100mg

ACTION: Antiinflammatory, analgesic activity appears related to inhibition of prostaglandin synthesis. **USE:** Treatment of rheumatoid/osteoarthritis.

PHARMACOKINETICS

PO absorption	Peak	Half-life	Protein binding	Excretion
Good	1.5h	5.7h	99%	Via urine as conjugates (90%)

CONTRAINDICATIONS: Hypersensitivity, aspirin/other antiinflammatory agent hypersensitivity.

DOSAGE
Adult *PO*

Arthritis	200-300mg/d divided 2, 3, or 4 times/d. Do *not* exceed a single dose of 100mg. Total daily dose above 300mg not currently recommended

SIDE/ADVERSE EFFECTS: CNS: *headache*, nervousness, dizziness, drowsiness ▪ CV: hypertension, heart failure, edema ▪ EENT: tinnitus, conjunctivitis ▪ GI: *abdominal pain, N/D,* ***GI bleeding****,* vomiting, flatulence ▪ GU: symptoms of renal infection, ***interstitial nephritis****,* hematuria ▪ HEM: ***hemolytic anemia, thrombocytopenia,*** leukopenia ▪ INT: rash, urticaria, pruritus, photosensitivity, ***toxic epidermal necrolysis,*** exfoliative dermatitis ▪ Other: asthma, hyperuricemia.

DRUG INTERACTIONS: Use c̄ ulcerogenic drugs produces additive effects ▪ use c̄ PO anticoagulants may ↑ their activity ▪ Aspirin will ↓ flurbiprofen plasma levels ▪ Use with furosemide requires monitoring.

NURSING MANAGEMENT

ADMINISTRATION: Assess for hx of NSAIA, salicylate hypersensitivity ▪ Avoid administration to pts c̄ hx of asthma, bleeding disorders, salicylate hypersensitivity ▪ Assess GI, renal, hepatic function; use caution if impaired ▪ May be administered c̄ food, milk, antacid; *best* on empty stomach (1h ac/2h pc); tablets may be crushed; administer c̄ full glass of liquid; encourage upright position for 15-30m ▪ Avoid exposure to moisture during storage ▪ Elderly may require ↓ dosage.

EVALUATION: Monitor VS, esp BP ▪ Monitor hepatic, renal status c̄ prolonged use ▪ Monitor pt receiving anticoagulant therapy; may potentiate bleeding ▪ Monitor stool for occult blood ▪ Monitor I&O, daily weight ▪ Assess for edema in extremities ▪ Assess for visual disturbances; D/C drug, notify physician.

EDUCATION: Dizziness/drowsiness may occur; use caution in potentially hazardous activities ▪ Take on empty stomach (1h ac/2h pc) c̄ food/milk if GI distress occurs; take c̄ full glass liquid; maintain upright position for 15-30m ▪ Take as ordered by physician; do *not* ↑ dose ▪ Notify physician *immediately* of bleeding, ↓ urine output, swelling of feet/legs, lethargy, GI distress, jaundice, visual disturbances ▪ Avoid taking c̄ aspirin, other NSAIAs ▪ Avoid use c̄ alcohol ▪ Check c̄ physician/pharmacist before taking OTC preparations ▪ Notify physician/dentist of use before treatment ▪ Women: avoid breastfeeding ▪ Store in tightly closed container ▪ Full drug effects may require several wks of therapy.

NOTES:

foscarnet (phosphonoformic acid) • (foss-car-net)

CATEGORY: *Antiviral*

Rx; Preg Cat C

BRAND NAME	DOSAGE FORM
Foscavir (Astra)	IV injection 24mg/ml

ACTION: Antiviral activity due to inhibition of viral replication of herpes viruses including cytomegalovirus (CMV), herpes HS-1, herpes HS-2, human herpes HHV-6, Epstein-Barr, and varicella-zoster virus; drug is an organic analog of inorganic pyrophosphate that inhibits virus-specific DNA polymerase and reverse transcriptase enzymes required for DNA synthesis. USE: Treatment of cytomegalovirus retinitis in AIDS pts.

PHARMACOKINETICS

Protein binding	Half-life	Excretion
14%-17%	3h	80%-90% via urine as unchanged drug

CONTRAINDICATIONS: Hypersensitivity.

DOSAGE: For normal renal function

Adult *IV* Initial dose 60mg/kg (adjusted for renal function) given over a minimum of 1h q8h for 2-3 wks. Usual maintenance range 90-120mg/kg/d over 2h

SIDE/ADVERSE EFFECTS: CNS: seizures (10%), headache (26%), dizziness, neuropathy (both central and peripheral), cerebral edema, ***encephalopathy,*** tremor, paresthesia, extrapyramidal symptoms, neuralgia, ataxia, EEG abnormalities, aphasia, paraplegia, tetany, dementia, confusion, anxiety, hallucinations ▪ CV: ***ECG abnormalities, cardiomyopathy, cardiac failure and arrest,*** palpitations, arrhythmias ▪ EENT: vision abnormalities, eye pain, conjunctivitis, photophobia blindness, retinal detachment, tinnitus, otitis ▪ GI: diarrhea (30%), nausea (47%), vomiting, anorexia, rectal hemorrhage, ***pseudomembranous colitis,*** abdominal pain, flatulence, dry mouth, ulcers (duodenal and esophageal), ulcerative proctitis and stomatitis, constipation, pancreatitis ▪ HEM: anemia (33%), granulocytopenia, leukopenia, ***pulmonary embolism, thrombosis, thrombocytopenia*** ▪ INT:

Note: Side/adverse effects: common in *italic;* serious in ***boldface italic.***

*Available in Canada only.

pruritus, rash, ulceration, acne, alopecia, urticaria ▪ MET: hypocalcemia (15%), hypomagnesemia (15%), hypokalemia (16%), hypophosphatemia (8%), hyperphosphatemia (6%) ▪ Renal: albuminuria, dysuria, ***acute renal failure,*** hematuria, ***glomerulonephritis,*** UTIs, nocturia ▪ RESP: coughing, dyspnea, pneumonia, sinusitis, pulmonary infiltration ▪ Other: neoplasms, ↑ AST, ↑ ALT, fever (65%), arthralgia, myalgia, inflammation/pain at local injection site.

DRUG INTERACTIONS: Use c̄ nephrotic drugs produces additive effects ▪ Use c̄ pentamidine can ↑ hypocalcemia ▪ Use c̄ zidovudine can produce additive anemia.

NURSING MANAGEMENT

ADMINISTRATION: Assess for hx of hypersensitivity ▪ Assess for renal impairment; requires ↓ dosage ▪ Administer via infusion control device at rate <1mg/kg/m ▪ Administer c̄ NSS or 5% dextrose solution; do *not* add another drug/supplement to IV line ▪ Maintain hydration.

EVALUATION: Monitor VS, esp temperature ▪ Monitor hepatic, renal status ▪ Monitor electrolyte balance; notify physician of abnormalities ▪ Assess for paresthesias; notify physician ▪ May ↑ serum creatinine ▪ Seizure precautions, esp in pts c̄ hx of convulsive disorders ▪ Assess for visual disturbances.

EDUCATION: Used to control, *not* cure, HIV-related infections ▪ Notify physician of any change in health status ▪ Avoid sexual contact, blood donation (risk of HIV transmission) ▪ Keep scheduled appointments c̄ physician/ for blood work ▪ Notify physician of numbness, tingling in extremities ▪ ↑ Fluid intake (8-10 glasses/d) ▪ Women: avoid breastfeeding ▪ IV injection site may be painful ▪ Loss of taste may occur ▪ Keep appointments c̄ physician for eye exams.

NOTES:

furosemide • (fur-oh-se-mide)

CATEGORY: *Loop diuretic*: antihypertensive

Rx; Preg Cat C

BRAND NAMES
**Furoside (ICN)*
Lasix (H-R)
(Hoechst in Canada)
**Neo-Renal (Neolab)*
**Novosemide (Novopharm)*
**Uritol (Horner)*

DOSAGE FORMS
Injection (IM/IV): 10mg/ml; PO solution: 10mg/ml; tablet: 20, 40, 80mg

ACTION: Diuretic activity due to excretion of H_2O, Na^+, Cl^-, other electrolytes by inhibiting tubular reabsorption, esp in medullary, cortical portions of ascending limb of loop of Henle; antihypertensive effect due to reduction in peripheral vascular resistance. **USE:** Treatment of edema due to renal dysfunction ▪ Treatment of hypertension as sole agent/in combination c̄ other antihypertensives ▪ Adjunct in treating edema due to CHF, hepatic cirrhosis, acute pulmonary edema.

CONTRAINDICATIONS: Hypersensitivity, anuria, severe electrolyte imbalance.

DOSAGE

Pediatric *PO*	2mg/kg as single dose. Do *not* exceed 6mg/kg/d
IM/IV	1mg/kg
Adult *PO*	
Edema	20-80mg/d as single dose. Refractory pts may require 600mg/d as single dose or divided
Hypertension	40mg bid. Adjust dosage according to response
Adult *IM/IV*	
Edema	20-40mg. May be repeated in 2h
Acute pulmonary edema	40mg IV, repeat 1-1.5h later prn

PHARMACOKINETICS

PO absorption	Onset	Peak	Duration	Half-life	Protein binding	Excretion
60%	1h	1-2h	6-8h	30-50m	95%	50% via urine in 24h

Note: Side/adverse effects: common in *italic;* serious in ***boldface italic.***

*Available in Canada only.

SIDE/ADVERSE EFFECTS: CNS: dizziness, paresthesia, headache ▪ CV: orthostatic hypotension ▪ EENT: blurred vision, hearing loss, tinnitus ▪ GI: anorexia, N/V, cramping, jaundice, ***pancreatitis*** ▪ HEM: anemia, leukopenia, ***thrombocytopenia, aplastic anemia*** ▪ INT: purpura, rash, urticaria, ***exfoliative dermatitis, erythema multiforme***, photosensitivity.

DRUG INTERACTIONS: Use c̄ neurotoxic drugs incl aminoglycosides, capreomycin, chloroquine, oxyphenobutazone, phenylbutazone, vancomycin, viomycin can result in significant toxicity ▪ Induced hypokalemia ↑ dig toxicity ▪ Avoid use c̄ lithium, clofibrate ▪ Use c̄ corticosteroid can produce severe hypokalemia ▪ Use c̄ tubocurarine can ↑ its activity.

NURSING MANAGEMENT

ADMINISTRATION: Assess for hx of hypersensitivity (incl sulfonamides) ▪ PO: administer c̄ food/milk on arising ▪ IV: use infusion w/in 24h after preparation; administer *slowly* (2m), hearing loss may occur c̄ rapid bolus ▪ Slight discoloration of tablets does *not* affect potency ▪ Assess serum K^+ (normal level: 3.5-5mEq/L) ▪ Elderly may require ↓ dosage ▪ IM: inject *deep, slowly* into gluteal UOQ.

EVALUATION: Monitor VS, esp BP, pulse; fluid retention (I&O, daily weight) ▪ Monitor serum for ↑ BUN, creatinine, uric acid; ↓ K^+ ▪ Assess for ↓ hearing (ototoxicity).

EDUCATION: Expect ↑ urine output ▪ May cause weakness, lethargy ▪ Take PO forms c̄ food ▪ Take on waking up, at same time qd ▪ Take even if symptom free ▪ Notify physician of signs of hypokalemia (muscle cramps, lethargy, nausea)/hyponatremia (thirst, dry mouth, drowsiness) ▪ Avoid changing positions rapidly ▪ Take as directed; do *not* skip doses ▪ Eat foods high in K^+; avoid black licorice ▪ Avoid high-Na^+ foods ▪ Check c̄ physician/pharmacist before taking OTC/Rx preparations ▪ Diabetics: check blood/urine glucose carefully ▪ Women: avoid breastfeeding ▪ Avoid exposure to direct sunlight, UV light ▪ May produce sweet taste.

NOTES:

gentamicin sulfate • (jen-ta-mye-sin)

CATEGORY: *Aminoglycoside:* antibiotic

Rx; Preg Cat C

BRAND NAMES
**Alcomicin (Alcon)*
**Cidomycin (Roussel)*
Garamycin (Schering)

DOSAGE FORMS
Injection, ophthalmic gtt/ointment, pediatric injection, topical cream/ointment

ACTION: Bactericidal activity due to inhibition of ribosomal protein synthesis in susceptible organisms. **USE:** Treatment of infections caused by susceptible strains of *Enterobacter aerogenes, Escherichia coli, Klebsiella pneumoniae, Proteus* spp, *Pseudomonas aeruginosa, Salmonella* spp, *Serratia* (nonpigmented), *Shigella* spp ▪ Alternate for penicillin-resistant staphylococcal infections ▪ In combination $\bar{c}$ carbenicillin for treating stubborn *Pseudomonas* infection ▪ With penicillin for treating sepsis, staphylococcal pneumonia in neonates.

PHARMACOKINETICS

IM peak	Half-life	Protein binding	Excretion
0.5-1h	2-2.5h	0%-30% in 24h	70% unchanged in urine

CONTRAINDICATIONS: Hypersensitivity, previous hx of serious aminoglycoside toxicity.

DOSAGE: For pts $\bar{c}$ normal renal function; treatment usually 7-10d; dosage for pts $\bar{c}$ impaired renal function must be adjusted according to manufacturer's recommendation.

Pediatric *IM/IV*	Neonates (<1wk old): 5mg/kg/d or 2.5mg/kg q12h Neonates/infants: 7.5mg/kg/d or 2.5mg/kg q12h Children: 6-7mg/kg/d q8h in equal doses
Adult *IM/IV*	3mg/kg/d q8h in equal doses Serious infection: 5mg/kg/d in 3-4 doses. ⬇ to 3mg/kg/d when clinically indicated
Topical/Ophthalmic	Apply to affected area as directed by physician

SIDE/ADVERSE EFFECTS: CNS: headache, paresthesia ▪ EENT: ***ototoxicity*** (auditory/vestibular damage: dizziness, vertigo, tinnitus, roaring in ears, hearing loss) ▪ REN:

nephrotoxicity (casts, proteinuria, ↑ BUN, NPN, serum creatinine) ▪ INT: rash ▪ Other: fever.

DRUG INTERACTIONS: Avoid use c̄ neurotoxic/nephrotoxic drugs (eg, other aminoglycosides, colistin, ethacrynic acid, furosemide, polymyxin B, vancomycin, viomycin) ▪ Dimenhydrinate can mask aminoglycoside ototoxicity ▪ ↑ Activity of succinylcholine/tubocurarine; Ca salts can reverse blockade ▪ PO anticoagulant activity may ↑ due to ↓ intestinal vitamin K synthesis.

NURSING MANAGEMENT

ADMINISTRATION: Assess for hx of aminoglycoside hypersensitivity ▪ Obtain C&S before therapy ▪ Obtain pt weight for dose calculation ▪ Determine creatinine clearance before administration ▪ IV: single dose may be diluted in 50-250ml sterile normal saline/5% dextrose solution; infuse over 1/2-1h; use less diluent for pediatric IV; may mix c̄ dextrose, lactated Ringer, Ringer injection, normal saline solution ▪ Do *not* mix c̄ other drugs, incl carbenicillin, other extended-spectrum penicillins ▪ IM: administer by *deep, slow* injection; rotate sites; avoid inflamed areas ▪ Do *not* administer SC ▪ Maintain hydration ▪ Elderly may require ↓ dosage ▪ Therapeutic blood levels: 4-10μg/ml.

EVALUATION: Assess for hearing dysfunction ▪ Monitor VS, esp temperature ▪ Assess for edema in extremities ▪ Assess for neuromuscular blockade, respiratory paralysis, nephrotoxicity ▪ Observe for signs of superinfection (diarrhea, URI, coated tongue) ▪ Assess peak (<12μg/ml), trough (<2μg/ml) serum concentrations.

EDUCATION: Report hearing, balance difficulties to physician at once ▪ ↑ Fluid intake (10-12 glasses/d) ▪ Notify physician of symptoms of allergic rx (fever, difficult breathing, rash, burning/stinging in eyes).

NOTES:

glipizide/glyburide • (glip-i-zide/glye-byoo-ride)

CATEGORY: *Oral hypoglycemic*: sulfonylurea — Rx; Preg Cat C/B

BRAND NAMES	DOSAGE FORMS
glipizide	
Glucotrol (Roerig)	Tablet: 5, 10mg
glyburide	
DiaBeta (H-R)	Tablet: 1.25, 2.5, 5mg
**Euglucon (USV)*	Tablet: 5mg
Glynase Pres Tab (Upjohn)	Tablet: 1.5, 3mg
Micronase (Upjohn)	Tablet: 1.25, 2.5, 5mg

ACTION: Antidiabetic activity due to stimulation of insulin release from functioning beta cells of pancreas; drug appears to ↑ action of insulin at peripheral postreceptor sites. **USE:** Management of type II (non-insulin-dependent) diabetes that cannot be controlled by diet alone.

CONTRAINDICATIONS: Hypersensitivity, diabetic ketoacidosis $\overline{c}$, w/out coma.

DOSAGE: Adult *PO*

glipizide	Must be individualized. Usual maintenance range 2.5-40mg/d
glyburide	Must be individualized. usual maintenance range 1.25-20mg/d

SIDE/ADVERSE EFFECTS: GI: *nausea,* epigastric fullness, heartburn ▪ HEM: ***aplastic anemia, agranulocytosis,*** leukopenia, ***hemolytic anemia,*** pancytopenia, ***thrombocytopenia*** ▪ INT: erythema, morbilliform/maculopapular

PHARMACOKINETICS

	PO absorption	Onset	Peak	Duration	Half-life	Binding	Excretion
glipizide	Rapid	1h	1-3h	Up to 24h	2-4h	98%-99%	90% via urine as metabolites
glyburide	Rapid	1-2h	3-4h	Up to 24h	10h	NA	50% via bile, 50% via urine

Note: Side/adverse effects: common in *italic;* serious in ***boldface italic.***

*Available in Canada only.

eruptions, photosensitivity ▪ MET: ***hypoglycemia***.

DRUG INTERACTIONS: Use c̄ alcohol, MAO-I, phenylbutazones, beta blockers can significantly ↑ hypoglycemic effects ▪ Use c̄ anabolic steroids, chloramphenicol, guanethidine, PO anticoagulants, probenecid, salicylates, sulfinpyrazone, sulfonamides ↑ hypoglycemic effects ▪ Use c̄ adrenergics, corticosteroids, phenytoin, thiazides, thyroid preparations ↓ hypoglycemic effects.

NURSING MANAGEMENT

ADMINISTRATION: Assess for hx of hypersensitivity (incl sulfonamides) ▪ Administer 1/2h ac in single AM dose/divided doses ▪ Avoid exposure to moisture, light in storage ▪ Elderly may require ↓ dosage.

EVALUATION: Monitor hepatic, renal, hematologic status ▪ Monitor FBS ▪ Evaluate pt closely during first wk to assess effectiveness ▪ Monitor for signs of hypo/hyperglycemia.

EDUCATION: Compliance c̄ special diet therapy ▪ Blood/urine glucose/ketone testing procedure ▪ Symptoms of hypoglycemia (anxiety, headache, fatigue, nausea, sweating); notify physician *immediately* ▪ Always carry lump of sugar/candy for quick use in hypoglycemia ▪ Avoid alcohol ▪ Check c̄ physician before taking OTC preparations ▪ Symptoms of hyperglycemia (excessive hunger, thirst, urination, rapid pulse, sweet-smelling breath, weight loss); notify physician *immediately* ▪ Maintain good personal hygiene ▪ Carry medical identification (MedicAlert) ▪ Store in tightly closed container ▪ Keep scheduled appointments c̄ physician/for blood glucose determinations ▪ Schedule periodic eye exams ▪ Maintain optimum body weight ▪ Avoid prolonged exposure to sunlight; use sunscreen, protective clothing ▪ Women: avoid breastfeeding ▪ PO hypoglycemic needs may change c̄ ↑ stress, ↑ exercise, ↓ appetite; notify physician ▪ Report skin rash, itching to physician.

NOTES:

guanabenz acetate • (gwahn-a-benz)

CATEGORY: *Antihypertensive:* α_2-adrenergic Rx; Preg Cat C

BRAND NAME
Wytensin (W-A)

DOSAGE FORMS
Tablet: 4, 8mg

ACTION: Antihypertensive effect due to agonist activity c̄ central α_2-receptors, resulting in ↓ sympathetic outflows from bulbar level of brain to circulatory system. **USE:** Treatment of hypertension as sole agent or in combination c̄ thiazide diuretic.

PHARMACOKINETICS

PO absorption	Peak	Half-life	Protein binding	Excretion
75%	2-5h	4-14h	90%	Via urine primarily as metabolites

CONTRAINDICATIONS: Hypersensitivity.

DOSAGE

Adult *PO* Starting dose 4mg bid. May be ↑ in 4-8mg increments/d q1-2wks. Doses > 32mg bid may be required in rare cases

SIDE/ADVERSE EFFECTS: CNS: *drowsiness, dizziness, headache*, anxiety, depression, sleep disturbances ▪ CV: ***arrhythmias***, palpitations, edema, chest pain ▪ EENT: blurred vision, nasal congestion ▪ END: gynecomastia ▪ GI: dry mouth, N/V/D, pain, constipation, taste disorders ▪ GU: urinary frequency, sex function disturbances ▪ INT: rash, pruritus ▪ MS: muscle aches.

DRUG INTERACTIONS: Use c̄ CNS depressants produces additive sedation.

NURSING MANAGEMENT

ADMINISTRATION: Assess for hx of hypersensitivity ▪ Assess BP; notify physician of extremes ▪ Administer last dose at hs ▪ Elderly may require ↓ dosage ▪ Avoid abrupt withdrawal; D/C gradually.

EVALUATION: Monitor VS, esp BP ▪ Monitor electrolyte status ▪ Monitor I&O, daily weight ▪ Assess for edema in extremities.

EDUCATION: Dizziness/drowsiness may occur; use caution in potentially hazardous activities ▪ Avoid changing positions (lying/sitting/standing) rapidly ▪ Take last dose at hs ▪ Take as ordered by physician even if symptom free; do *not* skip doses ▪ Use sugarless gum/hard candy to diminish dry mouth ▪ Used to control, *not* cure, hypertension ▪ Do *not* D/C w/out notifying physician ▪ Check $\bar{c}$ physician/pharmacist before taking OTC/Rx preparations ▪ Do *not* use $\bar{c}$ alcohol, other CNS depressants ▪ Avoid high-Na^+ foods (canned soups, lunch meats, cheese) ▪ Avoid ↑ exercise, cold, smoking ▪ Maintain optimum weight ▪ Check for swelling in feet/legs daily; notify physician if present.

NOTES:

guanethidine monosulfate • (gwahn-eth-i-deen)

CATEGORY: *Antihypertensive*: norepinephrine depletor — Rx; Preg Cat C

BRAND NAMES	DOSAGE FORMS
**Apo-Guanethidine (Apotex); Ismelin (Ciba)*	Tablet: 10, 25mg

COMBINATION PRODUCT	
Esimil (Ciba)	Guanethidine 10mg/hydrochlorothiazide 25mg/tablet

ACTION: Antihypertensive effect due to slow depletion, inhibition of norepinephrine release at sympathetic fibers. **USE:** Treatment of hypertension as sole agent or in combination c̄ other antihypertensives ▪ Treatment of renal hypertension.

PHARMACOKINETICS: PO absorption is incomplete, up to 50% of single dose reaches circulatory system; at least 2wks required for full therapeutic effect; excretion via urine as unchanged drug, metabolites.

CONTRAINDICATIONS: Hypersensitivity, pheochromocytoma, use c̄ MAO-I, frank CHF not due to hypertension.

DOSAGE

Pediatric *PO*	Initial dose 0.2mg/kg/d, ↑ by same amount if needed q7-10d to maximum dose 3mg/kg/d
Adult *PO*	Initial dose 10mg/d, ↑ gradually if needed. For hospitalized pts, initial dose 25-50mg, ↑ by 25-50mg/d qod if needed
Esimil	Usual adult starting dose 2 tablets/d

SIDE/ADVERSE EFFECTS: CNS: dizziness, syncope, mental depression, weakness ▪ CV: bradycardia, edema, CHF, postural/exertional hypotension ▪ EENT: blurred vision, parotid tenderness, nasal congestion ▪ GI: ↑ bowel movement/diarrhea, dry mouth ▪ GU: inhibition of ejaculation, urinary incontinence ▪ HEM: anemia, leukopenia ▪ INT: alopecia ▪ MS: myalgia ▪ RESP: asthma ▪ Other: weight gain.

DRUG INTERACTIONS: Use c̄ amphetamines, MAO-I, tricyclic antidepressants, phenothiazines, oral contracep-

Note: Side/adverse effects: common in *italic;* serious in ***boldface italic.***

*Available in Canada only.

tives may antagonize effects of guanethidine ▪ Use c̄ epinephrine, other direct-acting adrenergics may ↑ their vasopressor effect ▪ Use c̄ *Rauwolfia* derivatives may cause significant hypotension, bradycardia, mental depression.

NURSING MANAGEMENT

ADMINISTRATION: Assess for hx of hypersensitivity ▪ Assess BP, apical pulse; if <60/m, hold drug, notify physician ▪ May crush tablet ▪ Avoid abrupt withdrawal; D/C gradually ▪ Elderly may require ↓ dosage.

EVALUATION: Monitor VS, esp BP ▪ Monitor electrolyte status ▪ Monitor I&O, daily weight ▪ Assess for edema in extremities.

EDUCATION: Dizziness/drowsiness may occur, use caution in potentially hazardous activities ▪ Avoid changing positions (lying/sitting/standing) rapidly ▪ Avoid ↑ exercise, temperature extremes, smoking ▪ Procedure for checking radial pulse ▪ Check pulse before taking; if <60/m, do *not* take drug, notify physician ▪ Take as ordered by physician even if symptom free; do *not* skip doses ▪ Used to control, *not* cure, hypertension ▪ Do *not* D/C w/out notifying physician ▪ Check c̄ physician/pharmacist before taking OTC/Rx preparations ▪ Do *not* use c̄ alcohol or other CNS depressants ▪ Avoid high-Na^+ foods (canned soups, lunch meats, cheese) ▪ Maintain optimum weight ▪ Check for swelling in feet/legs daily; notify physician if present ▪ Men: impotence may occur; inform physician ▪ Notify physician/dentist of use before treatment ▪ Notify physician of diarrhea, frequent dizziness/fainting.

NOTES:

guanfacine hcl • (gwahn-fa-seen)

CATEGORY: *Antihypertensive:* α_2-adrenergic

Rx; Preg Cat B

BRAND NAME
Tenex (Robins)

DOSAGE FORMS
Tablet: 1, 2mg

ACTION: Antihypertensive effect due to agonist activity at central α_2 receptors, resulting in ↓ sympathetic outflow from bulbar level of brain to circulatory system, which produces a ↓ in peripheral vascular resistance & heart rate. **USE:** Treatment of hypertension as a sole agent or in combination c̄ other antihypertensives.

PHARMACOKINETICS

PO absorption	Peak	Half-life	Protein binding	Excretion
Good	1-4h	10-30h	70%	Via urine as unchanged drug and metabolites

CONTRAINDICATIONS: Hypersensitivity.

DOSAGE

Adult *PO* — Usual dose is 1mg hs. May ↑ to 2 or 3mg/d hs after 3-4 wks

SIDE/ADVERSE EFFECTS: CNS: *somnolence, dizziness, headache, insomnia,* depression ▪ CV: bradycardia, palpitations ▪ EENT: tinnitus, vision irregularities, conjunctivitis, rhinitis, taste perversion ▪ GI: *dry mouth, constipation,* pain, D/N, dyspepsia ▪ INT: rash, pruritus, purpura ▪ Other: asthenia, dyspnea, leg cramps, hypokinesia, fatigue, impotence, paresthesia.

DRUG INTERACTIONS: Use c̄ CNS depressants produces additive sedation.

NURSING MANAGEMENT

ADMINISTRATION: Assess for hx of hypersensitivity ▪ Assess renal function; may require ↓ dosage if impaired ▪ Assess BP; if hypotensive, hold drug, notify physician ▪ Administer at hs ▪ Avoid abrupt withdrawal; D/C gradually ▪ Use c̄ diuretics will ↑ antihypertensive effects ▪ Elderly may require ↓ dosage ▪ Avoid moisture, heat, light in storage.

EVALUATION: Monitor VS, esp BP ▪ Monitor I&O, daily weight ▪ Observe for mental depression; D/C drug, notify physician ▪ Observe for signs of tolerance; notify physician.

EDUCATION: Drowsiness/dizziness may occur; use caution in potentially hazardous activities ▪ Avoid changing positions (lying/sitting/standing) rapidly ▪ Take as ordered by physician, even if symptom free; do *not* skip doses ▪ Take last dose just before hs ▪ Do *not* D/C w/out notifying physician ▪ Check c̄ physician/pharmacist before taking OTC/Rx preparations ▪ Avoid use c̄ alcohol, CNS depressants ▪ Avoid high-Na^+ foods (canned soups, lunch meats, cheese) ▪ Avoid ↑ exercise, temperature extremes, smoking ▪ Used to control, *not* cure, hypertension ▪ Maintain optimum weight ▪ Keep scheduled appointments c̄ physician; have BP regularly checked ▪ Use sugarless gum/hard candy to diminish dry mouth ▪ Carry identification (MedicAlert) if hypertensive.

NOTES:

haloperidol/haloperidol decanoate▲ • (ha-loe-per-i-dole)

CATEGORY: *Antipsychotic*: butyrophenone neuroleptic — Rx; Preg Cat C

BRAND NAMES	DOSAGE FORMS
Haldol (McNeil)	Injection (IM): 5mg/ml PO concentrate: 2mg/ml Tablet: 0.5, 1, 2, 5, 10, 20mg
Haldol Decanoate (McNeil)▲	Injection (IM): 50mg/ml, 100mg/ml

ACTION: Antipsychotic activity may be due to brainstem depression; drug inhibits ascending reticular activating system of brainstem; exhibits anti-alpha-adrenergic, anticholinergic, antiemetic, antidopaminergic, hypotensive, hypothermic, sedative properties. **USE:** Treatment of psychotic states (Decanoate salt is intended for chronic psychotic patients) ▪ Treatment of Gilles de la Tourette syndrome ▪ Treatment of severe behavior problems in children ▪ Short-term treatment in hyperactive children.

PHARMACOKINETICS

PO absorption	Peak	Protein binding	Excretion
Good (70%)	2-6h	92%	Via urine, feces

CONTRAINDICATIONS: Hypersensitivity, comatose states, presence of large amount of CNS depressants, Parkinson disease.

DOSAGE

Pediatric *PO*	
Psychosis	0.05-0.15 mg/kg/d
Tourette syndrome & nonpsychotic behavior	0.05-0.075mg/kg/d
Adult *PO*	
Moderate psychosis	0.5-2mg 2-3 times/d or more
Severe psychosis	3-5mg 2-5 times/d or up to 100mg/d
IM	2-5mg q4-8h. Initial dose of decanoate salt is calculated to be 10-15 times previous daily PO dose and should *not* exceed 100mg. Doses >300mg/mo not well studied. Dosing intervals usually 4wks
Geriatric/debilitated *PO*	0.5-2mg 2-3 times/d or more

SIDE/ADVERSE EFFECTS: CNS: *drowsiness*, extrapyramidal rxs, tardive dyskinesia ▪ CV: hypotension, tachycardia, ECG changes ▪ END: lactation, breast enlargement, menstrual irregularities, gynecomastia, impotence ▪ GI: anorexia, N/V, dry mouth ▪ GU: urinary retention ▪ HEM: anemia, lymphomonocytosis, ***agranulocytosis*** ▪ INT: acneiform maculopapular rash, photosensitivity, alopecia ▪ RESP: bronchospasm, laryngospasm ▪ Other: neuroleptic malignant syndrome.

DRUG INTERACTIONS: Use c̄ lithium can produce significant encephalopathic syndrome ▪ Use c̄ alcohol, narcotics, barbiturates, other CNS depressants will ↑ CNS depression.

NURSING MANAGEMENT

ADMINISTRATION: Assess VS, esp BP ▪ PO concentrate: dilute before administration c̄ >60ml H_2O; do *not* use coffee, tea, lithium citrate syrup ▪ PO: administer c̄ food/full glass of H_2O or milk ▪ IM: inject *slowly, deep* into UOQ of buttock; keep pt lying down for 1/2h after injection ▪ Avoid exposure to moisture, light in storage ▪ Avoid abrupt withdrawal; D/C gradually ▪ Maintain hydration ▪ Elderly/debilitated may require ↓ dosage ▪ Avoid administration c̄ lithium.

EVALUATION: Monitor, hepatic, ophthalmic, renal status ▪ Monitor BP, CBC ▪ Monitor fluid retention (I&O, daily weight) ▪ Assess for extrapyramidal symptoms (tics/spasms, trembling, shuffling gait) ▪ Seizure precautions in pts c̄ hx of convulsive disorders ▪ Long-term therapy: assess for jaundice, agranulocytosis ▪ Assess for symptoms of abrupt withdrawal (nausea, dyskinesia, trembling, dizziness) ▪ Assess IOP.

EDUCATION: Dizziness/drowsiness may occur; use caution in potentially hazardous activities ▪ Avoid changing positions (lying/sitting/standing) rapidly ▪ Avoid use c̄ alcohol, CNS depressants ▪ Take as ordered by physician ▪ Take PO forms c̄ meals ▪ Store in tightly closed, light-resistant container ▪ Use sugarless gum/hard candy to diminish dry mouth ▪ Maintain fluid intake (6-8 glasses/d) ▪ Avoid exposure to direct sunlight, UV light (sunlamps); use sunscreen, protective clothing ▪ Notify physician of fever, sore throat, bruising/bleeding ▪ Notify physician of extrapyramidal symptoms (tics/spasms, trembling, shuffling gait) ▪ Avoid ↑ exercise, temperature extremes ▪ Avoid smoking ▪ Check c̄ physician/pharmacist before taking OTC preparations ▪ Schedule periodic eye exams ▪ Full drug effects may require several wks of therapy ▪ Procedure for PO concentrate administration.

NOTES:

heparin sodium • (hep-a-rin)

CATEGORY: *Anticoagulant* Rx; Preg Cat C

BRAND NAMES
**Calilean (Harris)*
Hep-Lock (Elkins-Sinn)
**Hepalean (Harris)*
Liquaemin Sodium (Organon)

DOSAGE FORM
Injection (IV/SC)

ACTION: Anticoagulant activity due to inhibition of conversion of prothrombin to thrombin; heparin also appears to have antithrombin action, ↓ agglutination of platelets; has no effect on existing clots; does not cross placental barrier. **USE:** Prophylaxis, treatment of arterial embolism, pulmonary embolism, venous thrombosis & extensions ▪ Atrial fibrillation c̄ embolization ▪ Prevention of clotting during arterial/heart surgery ▪ Diagnosis, treatment of acute/chronic consumption coagulopathies (disseminated intravascular coagulation) ▪ Anticoagulant for use in blood transfusion, extracorporeal circulation, dialysis, laboratory blood samples ▪ Controversial adjunct in treating coronary occlusion c̄ acute myocardial infarction.

PHARMACOKINETICS

Onset		Half-life	Excretion
SC	IV		
20-60m	Immediate	1-2h	Reticular endothelial system; small amount excreted via urine

CONTRAINDICATIONS: Hypersensitivity, any uncontrolled bleeding.

DOSAGE

Pediatric *IV*	Usual dose 50U/kg followed by 100U/kg q4h
Adult *SC*	Usual dose 10,000-20,000U followed by 8,000-10,000U tid
IV	Usual dose 10,000U followed by 5,000-10,000U 4-6 times/d Usual infusion dose 20,000-40,000U/d

SIDE/ADVERSE EFFECTS: CV: hemorrhage (10%), vasospastic rx may develop ▪ HEM: acute reversible thrombocytopenia, rebound hyperlipemia ▪ Other: ↓

Note: Side/adverse effects: common in *italic;* serious in ***boldface italic.*** *Available in Canada only.

renal function, osteoporosis c̄ long-term therapy; local irritation at SC site.

DRUG INTERACTIONS: Aspirin, other drugs that affect platelet function (esp cefamandole, cefoperazone, moxalactam) ↑ anticoagulant effect ▪ PO anticoagulants ↑ anticoagulant effect ▪ Use c̄ streptokinase, urokinase is best avoided.

NURSING MANAGEMENT

ADMINISTRATION: Assess for hx of hypersensitivity ▪ Administer by deep SC injection, intermittent IV injection, continuous IV infusion ▪ Avoid IM (danger of hematoma formation) ▪ Can be mixed c̄ dextrose, dextrose/NaCl, normal saline, invert sugar, protein hydrolysate, Ringer solution; lactated Ringer injection ▪ Prepare fresh solutions; avoid storage for > 24 h ▪ Do *not* use discolored/precipitated solutions ▪ SC: use lower abdomen; change needle after preparation; do *not* aspirate; rotate sites; check for hemorrhage; avoid massaging ▪ IV: use infusion pump ▪ Regulate dosage according to APTT, coagulation studies ▪ Avoid mixing c̄ other drugs in solution ▪ Have protamine sulfate available for OD ▪ Elderly may require ↓ dosage.

EVALUATION: Monitor hepatic, CV, renal status ▪ Monitor APTT; maintain at 1.5-2.5 times control value ▪ Observe for signs of hemorrhage, incl abdominal/lumbar pain; treat c̄ protamine sulfate (w/in 30m of heparin administration).

EDUCATION: Report any bleeding/bruising *immediately* ▪ Avoid smoking, alcohol ▪ Use electric razor/depilatory for hair removal ▪ Avoid aspirin-containing products ▪ Check c̄ physician/pharmacist before taking OTC products ▪ Women: avoid breastfeeding.

OVERDOSE MANAGEMENT: *See* Protamine Sulfate.

NOTES:

hydralazine hcl • (hye-dral-a-zeen)

CATEGORY: *Antihypertensive*

Rx; Preg Cat C

BRAND NAMES

Alazine (Major)
Apresoline HCl (Ciba)

DOSAGE FORMS

Tablet: 10, 25, 50mg
Injection (IM/IV): 20mg/ml
Tablet: 10, 25, 50, 100mg

COMBINATION PRODUCTS

Apresazide 25/25 (Ciba), Aprozide 25/25 (Major)	hydralazine hcl/hydrochlorothiazide per capsule: 25mg/25mg
Apresazide 50/50 (Ciba), Aprozide 50/50 (Major)	hydralazine hcl/hydrochlorothiazide per capsule: 50mg/50mg
Apresazide 100/50 (Ciba), Aprozide 100/50 (Major)	hydralazine hcl/hydrochlorothiazide per capsule: 100mg/50mg
Ser-Ap-Es (Ciba)	Reserpine/hydralazine hcl/hydrochlorothiazide per tablet: 0.1mg/25mg/15mg

ACTION: Antihypertensive effect due to direct relaxing, vasodilation of arteriolar smooth muscle. **USE:** Treatment of hypertension as sole agent/in combination c̄ other antihypertensives.

PHARMACOKINETICS

PO absorption	Peak	Half-life	Protein binding	Excretion
Rapid	1-2h	3-7h	87%	Via urine primarily as metabolites

CONTRAINDICATIONS: Hypersensitivity, coronary artery disease, mitral valvular/rheumatic heart disease.

DOSAGE

Pediatric *PO*	0.75mg/kg divided, ↑ slowly for 2-3wks to daily maximum 7.5mg/kg prn
Adult *PO*	Initial dose 10mg qid for 2-4d, ↑ to 25mg qid for balance of wk, 50mg qid wk 2. Adjust to lowest effective dose for maintenance
IM/IV	20-40mg, repeat prn. Switch to PO as soon as possible.

Combination products	Dosage must be adjusted for each pt, in general 1-2U (capsules/tablets) 1-3 times/d

SIDE/ADVERSE EFFECTS: CNS: *headache,* peripheral neuritis, dizziness, tremors, anxiety, psychotic rxs ▪ CV: *palpitations, tachycardia, angina pectoris,* edema, paradoxical hypertension ▪ EENT: nasal congestion, conjunctivitis ▪ GI: *anorexia, N/V/D,* constipation, paralytic ileus ▪ GU: difficult urination ▪ HEM: anemia, leukopenia, ***agranulocytosis,*** lymphadenopathy ▪ HEP: hepatitis ▪ INT: rash, urticaria, pruritus ▪ RESP: dyspnea.

DRUG INTERACTIONS: Use c̄ adrenergic drugs may antagonize hypotensive effect ▪ Use c̄ other antihypertensives, MAO-I produces additive hypotensive effects.

NURSING MANAGEMENT

ADMINISTRATION: Assess for hx of hypersensitivity ▪ Assess renal function; ↓ dosage if impaired ▪ PO: administer c̄ meals; switch from parenteral form w/in 48h ▪ IV: administer *slowly* (10mg/m); monitor BP, heart rate ▪ Elderly may require ↓ dosage ▪ Avoid abrupt withdrawal ▪ Have pyridoxine (vitamin B_6) available for neurotoxicity.

EVALUATION: Monitor VS, esp BP, electrolyte status, I&O, daily weight ▪ Assess for edema in extremities; mental status (depression, disorientation, anxiety).

EDUCATION: Dizziness/drowsiness may occur; use caution in potentially hazardous activities ▪ Avoid changing positions rapidly ▪ Take as ordered by physician, even if symptom free; do *not* skip doses ▪ Take c̄ meals ▪ Do *not* D/C w/out notifying physician ▪ Check c̄ physician/pharmacist before taking OTC/Rx preparations ▪ Notify physician *immediately* of tingling/numbness of hands/feet; D/C drug ▪ Physician may order vitamin B_6 supplements to alleviate neurotoxic effects ▪ Avoid high-Na^+ foods ▪ Avoid ↑ exercise, temperature extremes, smoking ▪ Used to control, *not* cure, hypertension ▪ Maintain optimum weight ▪ Avoid use c̄ alcohol, CNS depressants ▪ Keep scheduled appointments c̄ physician; have BP checked regularly ▪ Check for swelling in feet/legs daily ▪ Men: impotence may occur.

NOTES:

hydroxyzine hcl/hydroxyzine pamoate▲ • (hye-drox-i-zeen)

CATEGORY: *Antianxiety*: antihistamine

Rx; Preg Cat NA

BRAND NAMES

Atarax (Roerig) (Pfizer in Canada)
**Multipax (U.S.U.)*
Vistaril (Pfizer)

DOSAGE FORMS

Capsule▲, injection, PO suspension▲, syrup, tablet

ACTION: Anxiolytic activity appears related to depression of CNS at brainstem reticular formation, hypothalamus; drug also exhibits antiemetic, antihistamine properties. **USE:** Treatment of anxiety, tension ▪ Pre/postop sedative ▪ Management of N/V, allergic pruritus.

PHARMACOKINETICS: Rapid PO absorption c̄ 4-6h sedation; excretion via feces primarily as metabolites.

CONTRAINDICATIONS: Hypersensitivity.

DOSAGE

Pediatric	
Anxiety/pruritus *PO*	<6y/o: 50mg/d divided ≥6y/o: 50-100mg/d divided
Sedation *PO*	Pre-/Post-op: 0.6mg/kg
Nausea/vomiting *IM*	0.5mg/lb
Adult	
Anxiety *PO*	50-100mg qid
IM	50-100mg q4-6h prn
Pruritus *PO*	25mg 3-4 times/d
Sedation *PO*	Pre/postop: 50-100mg
IM	Pre/postop, pre/postpartum: 25-100mg
Nausea/vomiting *IM*	25-100mg

SIDE/ADVERSE EFFECTS: Drowsiness, dry mouth, involuntary motor activity (rare).

DRUG INTERACTIONS: use c̄ CNS depressant ↑ depression, may require dosage adjustments ▪ Use c̄ anticholinergics, tricyclic antidepressants may produce ↑ anticholinergic effects.

Note: Side/adverse effects: common in *italic;* serious in ***boldface italic.***

*Available in Canada only.

NURSING MANAGEMENT

ADMINISTRATION: Assess for hx of hypersensitivity ▪ PO: may crush tablets/open capsules ▪ PO suspension: shake well before administering ▪ IM: inject *deep, slowly* into large muscle mass; rotate sites; do *not* administer IV/SC ▪ Avoid abrupt withdrawal; D/C gradually ▪ Avoid exposure to heat, moisture, light in storage ▪ Elderly may require ↓ dosage ▪ Problem discussion, sympathetic listening contribute to relief of anxiety.

EVALUATION: Monitor renal, hepatic status ▪ Assess for symptoms of abrupt withdrawal (tremors, abdominal/muscle cramps, convulsions) $\bar{c}$ prolonged use ▪ Check for signs of dependence (↑ drug request) ▪ Monitor activity status (safety precautions) ▪ Assess for tolerance to therapeutic dose ▪ Check for depression; suicide precautions prn.

EDUCATION: Dizziness/drowsiness may occur; use caution in potentially hazardous activities ▪ Avoid use $\bar{c}$ alcohol, CNS depressants ▪ Indiscriminate use may lead to dependence ▪ Do *not* keep at bedside ▪ Take as ordered by physician; do *not* ↑ dose ▪ Use sugarless gum/hard candy to diminish dry mouth ▪ Maintain good oral hygiene; use soft-bristled toothbrush ▪ Check $\bar{c}$ physician/pharmacist before taking OTC/Rx preparations ▪ Women: avoid breast-feeding ▪ Store in tightly closed, light-resistant container ▪ Practice relaxation exercises, ventilation of feelings, stress management techniques.

NOTES:

ibuprofen • (eye-byoo-proe-fen)

CATEGORY: Antiinflammatory: analgesic, antipyretic

Rx/OTC▲; Preg Cat NA

BRAND NAMES	DOSAGE FORMS
Advil▲ *(Whitehall)*	Caplet: 200mg Tablet: 200mg
**Amersol (Horner)*	Capsule: 200, 300, 400mg
Medipren▲ *(McNeil)*	Caplet: 200mg Tablet: 200mg
Motrin (Upjohn)	Tablet: 300, 400, 600, 800mg
Motrin IB▲ *(Upjohn)*	Caplet: 200mg Tablet: 200mg
**Novoprofen (Novopharm)*	Tablet: 400, 600, 800mg
Nuprin▲ *(B-M)*	Caplet: 200mg Tablet: 200mg
Pediapropen▲ *(McNeil)*	Suspension: 100mg/5ml
Rufen (Boots)	Tablet: 400, 600mg

ACTION: Antiinflammatory, analgesic, antipyretic activity appears related to inhibition of prostaglandin synthesis. **USE:** Treatment of rheumatoid/osteoarthritis ▪ Relief of mild/moderate pain, primary dysmenorrhea.

PHARMACOKINETICS

PO absorption	Peak	Half-life	Protein binding	Excretion
80%	1-2h	1.8-2h	90%-99%	Via urine primarily as metabolites in 24h

CONTRAINDICATIONS: Hypersensitivity, aspirin/other antiinflammatory agent hypersensitivity.

DOSAGE

Adult *PO*	
Arthritis	400-800mg 3-4 times/d. Do *not* exceed 3.2g/d
Pain	200-400mg q4-6h
Dysmenorrhea	200-400mg q4-6h
Fever	200-400mg q4-6h
Children *PO*	6mo-12y/o
Fever	5mg/kg if <102.5° F. 10mg/kg if >102.5° F. Do *not* exceed maximum dose 40mg/kg/d

SIDE/ADVERSE EFFECTS: CNS: *dizziness*, headache, drowsiness ▪ CV: edema, palpitations, CHF ▪ EENT: tinnitus, ↓ hearing, blurred vision ▪ GI: *abdominal pain, N/V*, constipation, stomatitis ▪ GU: ***glomerular nephritis***, hematuria, ***interstitial nephritis***, nephrotic syndrome ▪ HEM: ***agranulocytosis, aplastic anemia, hemolytic anemia*** ▪ INT: *rash*, alopecia, pruritus, purpura, urticaria ▪ Other: thirst, eosinophilic pneumonia.

DRUG INTERACTIONS: Use c̄ ulcerogenic drugs produces additive effects ▪ Use c̄ PO anticoagulants may ↑ their activity ▪ Aspirin will ↓ ibuprofen plasma levels.

NURSING MANAGEMENT

ADMINISTRATION: Assess for hx of NSAIA hypersensitivity ▪ Avoid administration to individuals c̄ hx of asthma, bleeding disorders, salicylate hypersensitivity ▪ May be administered c̄ food/milk; *best* on empty stomach (1h ac/2h pc); encourage upright position for 15-30m ▪ Avoid exposure to moisture, light in storage ▪ Elderly may require ↓ dosage.

EVALUATION: Monitor hematologic, hepatic, renal status c̄ prolonged use ▪ Monitor pt receiving anticoagulant therapy; may potentiate bleeding ▪ Monitor I&O, daily weight c̄ prolonged use ▪ Assess for edema in extremities ▪ Assess for visual disturbances, skin rash; D/C drug, notify physician.

EDUCATION: Dizziness/drowsiness may occur; use caution in potentially hazardous activities ▪ Take on empty stomach (1h ac/2h pc), c̄ food/milk if GI distress occurs; maintain upright position for 15-30m ▪ Take as ordered by physician; do *not* ↑ dose ▪ Notify physician *immediately* of bleeding, ↑ urine output, swelling of feet/legs, lethargy, GI distress, jaundice, visual disturbance ▪ Avoid taking c̄ aspirin, other NSAIAs ▪ Avoid use c̄ alcohol ▪ Check c̄ physician/pharmacist before taking OTC preparations ▪ Notify physician/dentist of use before treatment ▪ Store in tightly closed container ▪ Full drug effects may require several wks of therapy.

NOTES:

imipenem/cilastatin sodium • (i-mi-pen-em/sye-la-stat-in)

CATEGORY: *Antibiotic combination* Rx; Preg Cat C

BRAND NAME
Primaxin (MSD)

DOSAGE FORMS
IV powder: 250, 500mg vials, infusion bottles

ACTION: Imipenem bactericidal activity due to inhibition of cell wall synthesis in susceptible organisms. Cilastatin sodium inhibits the renal enzyme dipeptidase, which inactivates imipenem, resulting in higher urinary levels of imipenem. Both drugs are present in the IV powder for injection in equivalent amounts (250mg/250mg or 500mg/500mg). **USE:** Treatment of bone, joint, gynecologic, lower respiratory, skin, and UTIs caused by susceptible strains of *Acinetobacter* spp, *Bacteroides* spp, *Bifidobacterium* spp, *Citrobacter* spp, *Clostridium* spp, *Enterobacter* spp, *Escherichia coli, Fusobacterium* spp, *Gardnerella vaginalis*, Groups A, B, D streptococci, *Haemophilus* spp, *Klebsiella* spp, *Peptococcus* spp, *Peptostreptococcus* spp, *Propionibacterium* spp, *Proteus* spp, *Providencia* spp, *Pseudomonas aeruginosa, Serratia marcescens, Staphylococcus* spp ▪ Penicillinase-producing *Staphylococcus* endocarditis.

PHARMACOKINETICS

	Half-life	Protein binding	Excretion
imipenem	1h	20%	Up to 70% of both recovered in urine within 10h
cilastatin	1h	40%	

CONTRAINDICATIONS: Hypersensitivity.

DOSAGE

For normal renal function

Adult *IV*

Mild infections	250-500mg q6h
Moderate/severe infections	500-1g q6h or q8h
UTIs	250mg q6h; 500mg q6h for complicated infections

SIDE/ADVERSE EFFECTS: CNS: dizziness, headache, ***encephalopathy***, paresthesia, psychic disturbances ▪ CV: palpitations, tachycardia, hypotension ▪ EENT: transient

Note: Side/adverse effects: common in *italic;* serious in ***boldface italic.*** *Available in Canada only.

hearing loss, tinnitus ▪ GI: *N/V/D*, ***pseudomembranous and hemorrhagic colitis***, pain, glossitis, ↑ salivation ▪ HEP: ↑ alkaline phosphatase, AST, ALT, LDH ▪ HEM: ***agranulocytosis***, ↓ WBC count ▪ INT: rash, pruritus, urticaria, erythema multiforme ▪ RESP: dyspnea, hyperventilation ▪ Other: ↑ BUN and *local phlebitis*, thrombophlebitis, pain, erythema, asthenia, fever, candidiasis.

DRUG INTERACTIONS: Use c̄ bacteriostatic antibiotics can lead to antibiotic antagonism.

NURSING MANAGEMENT

ADMINISTRATION: Assess for hx of beta-lactam hypersensitivity ▪ Obtain C&S before therapy ▪ Assess renal function; ↓ dosage if impaired ▪ Reconstitute, dilute according to manufacturer's directions ▪ Administer via IV infusion only, over 20-30m period; avoid aminoglycoside administration at same site ▪ Do *not* administer cloudy solutions; yellow-amber color does *not* indicate ↓ potency ▪ Have support equipment available for anaphylaxis ▪ Na^+ content: 0.8mEq (18.8mg)/250mg; calculate in Na^+-restricted diets.

EVALUATION: Monitor VS, esp temperature ▪ Monitor renal, hepatic status ▪ Observe for signs of superinfection (diarrhea, itching, oral ulcers) ▪ May ↑ serum ALT, AST, LDH, alkaline phosphatase, bilirubin, creatinine, BUN; ↓ H&H; (+) Coombs' test ▪ Assess for tremors, seizures; notify physician (may ↓ dose or D/C).

EDUCATION: ↑ Fluid intake (8-10 glasses/d) ▪ Maintain good personal hygiene (esp perineal, oral) ▪ Diarrhea may occur; check c̄ physician before taking any antidiarrheal agents ▪ Notify nurse/physician of symptoms of allergic rx (difficult breathing, rash) ▪ Carry identification (MedicAlert) if beta-lactam allergic.

NOTES:

imipramine hcl/imipramine pamoate/desipramine hcl •

(im-ip-ra-meen/dess-ip-ra-meen)

CATEGORY: *Tricyclic antidepressant* (TCA): mood elevator — Rx; Preg Cat C

BRAND NAMES	DOSAGE FORMS
imipramine hcl	
**Impril (ICN)*	Tablet: 10, 25, 50, 75mg
Janimine (Abbott);	Tablet: 10, 25, 50mg
**Novopramine (Novopharm)*	
Tofranil (Geigy)	Injection (IM): 25mg/2m Tablet: 10, 25, 50mg
imipramine pamoate	
Tofranil-PM (Geigy)	Capsule: 75, 100, 125, 150mg
desipramine hcl	
Norpramin (MMD)	Tablet: 10, 25, 50, 75, 100, 150mg
Pertofrane (RPR)	Capsule: 25, 50mg

ACTION: Antidepressant activity appears related to inhibition of norepinephrine reuptake in central adrenergic neurons; imipramine converted to desipramine in body.

USE: Treatment of endogenous depression ▪ Childhood enuresis (imipramine hcl).

PHARMACOKINETICS

PO absorption	Peak	Half-life	Excretion
Complete	1-2h	8-16h	40% via urine as metabolites in 24h

CONTRAINDICATIONS: Hypersensitivity, MAO-I therapy, myocardial infarction (acute recovery period).

DOSAGE

imipramine hcl

Enuresis *PO*	≥6y/o: 25mg/d 1h before hs >12y/o: up to 75mg/d 1h before hs. Do *not* exceed 75mg/d
Depression	
Adolescent *PO*	30-40mg divided. Do *not* exceed 100mg/d
Adult *PO*	75-200mg/d divided
IM	Up to 100mg/d divided

Geriatric *PO*	30-40mg divided. Do *not* exceed 100mg/d
imipramine pamoate	
Adult *PO*	75-200mg/d divided
desipramine hcl	
Adolescent *PO*	25-100mg/d divided
Adult *PO*	75-300mg/d divided
Geriatric *PO*	25-100mg/d divided

SIDE/ADVERSE EFFECTS: CNS: *drowsiness,* extrapyramidal symptoms, paresthesia (extremities) ▪ CV: ***arrhythmias,*** postural hypotension ▪ EENT: tinnitus ▪ GI: anorexia, N/V, dry mouth, constipation ▪ GU: gynecomastia, urinary hesitancy ▪ HEM: ***agranulocytosis***, eosinophilia, ***thrombocytopenia*** ▪ HEP: cholestatic jaundice ▪ INT: skin rash, photosensitivity, alopecia ▪ PSYCH: delusions, hallucinations, exacerbation of psychosis, confusion.

DRUG INTERACTIONS: Significant depressant effects c̄ alcohol, other CNS depressants ▪ Use c̄ anticholinergics, chlorpromazine may produce ↑ atropinelike effects; paralytic ileus could occur ▪ Significant ↑ in activities c̄ epinephrine, levarterenol, other adrenergic agents ▪ Significant antagonism to effects of reserpine, clonidine, guanethidine-type antihypertensives.

NURSING MANAGEMENT

ADMINISTRATION: Assess for hx of TCA hypersensitivity; glaucoma; prostatic hypertrophy; renal, hepatic disease ▪ PO: administer c̄ food ▪ Parenteral: do *not* administer IV ▪ Institute suicide/safety precautions ▪ ↑ Dosage *slowly* ▪ Avoid abrupt withdrawal.

EVALUATION: Monitor hepatic, renal status; BP, CBC, I&O, weight, constipation ▪ Assess for symptoms of abrupt withdrawal (nausea, headache, malaise) ▪ Assess for actual swallowing of PO forms.

EDUCATION: Dizziness/drowsiness may occur; use caution in potentially hazardous activities ▪ Avoid changing positions (lying/sitting/standing) rapidly ▪ Avoid use c̄ alcohol, CNS depressants for up to 1 wk after end of therapy ▪ Take PO forms c̄ food to ↓ GI irritation ▪ Use sugarless gum/hard candy to diminish dry mouth ▪ Constipation may occur; ↑ fluids, bulk-containing foods ▪ Check c̄ physician/dentist before taking OTC/Rx preparations ▪ Use sunscreen, protective clothing ▪ Notify physician of fever, sore throat, malaise ▪ Full drug effects may require several wks of therapy.

indomethacin/indomethacin sodium trihydrate▲ •

(in-doe-meth-a-sin)

CATEGORY: *Antiinflammatory* Rx; Preg Cat NA

BRAND NAME
Indocin (MSD)
(Indocid in Canada)

DOSAGE FORMS
Capsule: 25, 50, 75mg (SR)
PO suspension: 25mg/5ml
Powder for injection▲ (IV): 1mg/vial
Suppository: 50mg

ACTION: Antiinflammatory activity appears related to inhibition of prostaglandin synthesis. **USE:** Treatment of rheumatoid/osteoarthritis, ankylosing spondylitis, acute gout, acute painful shoulder ▪ Patent ductus arteriosus closure in premature infants (IV).

PHARMACOKINETICS

PO absorption	Peak	Half-life	Protein binding	Excretion
90%	2-4h	4.5h	90%	Via urine (60%), feces (33%) as unchanged drug, metabolites

CONTRAINDICATIONS: Hypersensitivity, aspirin/other antiinflammatory hypersensitivity, proctitis/rectal bleeding (suppositories); IV: infants c̄ infection, hemorrhage, thrombocytopenia, necrotizing enterocolitis, impaired renal function, or congenital heart disease in whom PDA is necessary for adequate pulmonary/systemic blood flow.

DOSAGE

Adults/Children	
>14y/o *PO*	
Arthritis, spondylitis	Start 25mg 2-3 times/d & adjust. Usual range 150-200mg/d divided. Do *not* exceed 200mg/d
Gout	50mg tid. ⬇ to cessation as soon as possible
Painful shoulder	75-150mg/d in 3-4 divided doses. Usual treatment 7-14d
Infants *IV*	Doses at 12-24h intervals based on age: <48h: dose 1, 0.2mg/kg; doses 2 & 3, 0.1mg/kg

Note: Side/adverse effects: common in *italic;* serious in ***boldface italic.*** *Available in Canada only.

2-7d: all 3 doses 0.2mg/kg
>7d: dose 1, 0.2mg/kg; doses 2 & 3, 0.25mg/kg
Second course of 3 doses may be given, c̄ each dose separated 12-24h as described

SIDE/ADVERSE EFFECTS: CNS: *headache, somnolence,* dizziness, tremor, confusion ▪ CV: palpitations, tachycardia, edema ▪ EENT: tinnitus, ↓ hearing, blurred vision, corneal deposits ▪ GI: *dyspepsia,* constipation, N/V, pain, anorexia, flatulence, dry mouth, ***hemorrhage*** ▪ GU: vaginal bleeding ▪ INT: pruritus, rash, urticaria.

DRUG INTERACTIONS: Use c̄ ulcerogenic drugs produces additive effects ▪ Use c̄ PO anticoagulants, thrombolytic agents may ↑ their activity ▪ Use c̄ triamterene will ↓ kidney function.

NURSING MANAGEMENT
ADMINISTRATION: Assess for hx of NSAIA hypersensitivity (incl aspirin) ▪ Avoid administration to pts c̄ hx of asthma, bleeding disorders, salicylate hypersensitivity ▪ Assess renal, hepatic function; use c̄ caution if impaired ▪ PO: administer c̄ food/milk, encourage upright position for 15-30m; shake suspension well before pouring ▪ Administer SR capsules whole ▪ IV: reconstitute c̄ 1-2ml 0.9% NaCl, sterile H_2O for injection (w/out preservatives); use *immediately*; administer direct IV (5-10s), avoid extravasation; discard unused portion ▪ Avoid exposure to moisture, light in storage ▪ Store suppositories in refrigerator; do *not* freeze ▪ Elderly may require ↓ dosage.

EVALUATION: Monitor pt receiving anticoagulant therapy; may potentiate bleeding ▪ Monitor I&O, daily weight ▪ Assess for edema in extremities, visual disturbances; D/C drug, notify physician.

EDUCATION: Dizziness/blurred vision may occur; use caution in potentially hazardous activities ▪ Take c̄ food/milk to ↓ GI distress; maintain upright position for 15-30m ▪ Swallow SR capsules whole ▪ Take as ordered by physician; do *not* ↑ dose ▪ Store in tightly closed, light-resistant container ▪ Notify physician *immediately* of bleeding, rash, flulike symptoms, swelling of feet/legs, GI distress, jaundice, visual disturbances ▪ Avoid use c̄ alcohol, aspirin, other NSAIAs ▪ Check c̄ physician/pharmacist before taking OTC preparations ▪ Keep appointments for blood work/eye exams ▪ Women: avoid breastfeeding.

NOTES:

ipecac syrup • (ip-e-kak)

CATEGORY: *Emetic* OTC; Preg Cat C

AVAILABLE PREPARATION
Syrup; available from various manufacturers/distributors in 1, 2oz bottles

ACTION: Emetic activity due to central stimulation of chemoreceptor trigger zone, local irritation of gastric mucosa.

PHARMACOKINETICS: Normally effective 90% of time w/in 15-20m.

CONTRAINDICATIONS: Semiconsciousness; pregnancy; ingestion of convulsants, corrosive substances, kerosene, strychnine, caustic substances.

DOSAGE

Pediatric *PO*	≤1y/o: usually 5ml. Repeat in 20m if no emesis
	1-12y/o: 10-15ml. Repeat in 20m if no emesis
Adult *PO*	15-30ml. Repeat in 20m if no emesis

SIDE/ADVERSE EFFECTS: No emesis: absorbed alkaloid (emetine) can cause cardiac conduction disturbances ▪ After emesis: GI upset, diarrhea.

DRUG INTERACTIONS: Use c̄ activated charcoal will ↓ chances of emesis; may give activated charcoal after vomiting has occurred.

NURSING MANAGEMENT
ADMINISTRATION: Administer only to conscious pts ▪ Follow administration c̄ H_2O: 1-2 glasses, adult: 1/2-1 glass, child ▪ Avoid concurrent administration c̄ milk, activated charcoal, carbonated beverages ▪ Do *not* administer in cases of corrosive poisoning ▪ Avoid exposure to heat, direct light in storage.

EVALUATION: Monitor VS, esp heart rate (cardiotoxic) ▪ Assess for vomiting; repeat dose in 20-30m if emesis does *not* occur.

EDUCATION: Telephone number for poison control center/emergency room/physician; call before taking drug ▪ Give only to alert/conscious pts ▪ Procedure for home use: take exactly as prescribed on label, follow c̄ H_2O; do *not* use c̄ milk/carbonated beverages; do not take more than 2 doses ▪ *Not* recommended at home for children <1y/o; physician supervision necessary ▪ Store in tightly closed, light-resistant container out of reach of children; check expiration date routinely, replace before expiration.

NOTES:

isoniazid • (eye-soe-nye-a-zid)

CATEGORY: *Antitubercular*

Rx; Preg Cat NA

BRAND NAME
INH (Ciba)
**Isotamine (ICN)*
Laniazid (Lannett)
Nydrazid (Apothecon)

DOSAGE FORMS
Injection (IM): 100mg/ml
Tablet: 50, 100, 300mg

PHARMACOKINETICS

PO absorption	Peak	Half-life	Excretion
Good	1-2h	1-4h	Via urine primarily as unchanged drug

ACTION: Antitubercular activity appears due to inhibition of transaminase activity, other pyridoxine-linked enzymes in actively growing susceptible tubercle bacilli; emergence of mycobacterial strains resistant to isoniazid can be significantly ↓ by combination c̄ other antimycobacterial agents. **USE:** Treatment of all forms of TB as sole agent/in combination c̄ other antitubercular agents ▪ Prophylactic therapy for (listed by priority): (a) household members, other close associates of persons c̄ recently diagnosed TB; (b) positive tuberculin skin test reactors c̄ chest x-ray films consistent c̄ nonprogressive TB, & c̄ neither positive bacteriologic findings nor hx of adequate chemotherapy; (c) newly infected persons; (d) positive tuberculin skin test reactors c̄ prolonged therapy c̄ corticosteroids, immunosuppressive therapy, leukemia, Hodgkin's disease, diabetes, silicosis, recent gastrectomy; (e) other positive tuberculin reactors ≤35y/o.

CONTRAINDICATIONS: Hypersensitivity, hepatic dysfunction.

DOSAGE

Tuberculosis

Pediatric	*PO/Parenteral*	10-20mg/kg/d as single dose
Adult	*PO/Parenteral*	5mg/kg/d as single dose

Prophylaxis

Pediatric	*PO/Parenteral*	10mg/kg/d as single dose
Adult	*PO/Parenteral*	300mg/d as single dose

SIDE/ADVERSE EFFECTS: CNS: peripheral neuropathy, ***toxic encephalopathy, convulsions***, memory impairment, toxic psychosis ▪ EENT: optic neuritis ▪ END: gynecomastia ▪ GI: N/V, epigastric distress, anorexia ▪ EM: ***agranu-***

Note: Side/adverse effects: common in *italic;* serious in ***boldface italic.***

*Available in Canada only.

locytosis; hemolytic, sideroblastic, aplastic anemia; thrombocytopenia ▪ HEP: age-related hepatitis (usually elderly); ↑ in AST, ALT; ***jaundice,*** bilirubinemia ▪ INT: maculopapular or morbilliform rashes, ***exfoliative dermatitis*** ▪ Other: vitamin B_6 deficiency, pellagra, gynecomastia.

DRUG INTERACTIONS: Use c̄ rifampin, cycloserine, ethionamide may produce ↑ CNS toxicity ▪ Use c̄ antacid suspensions may ↓ isoniazid absorption ▪ Use c̄ phenytoin may require dosage adjustments for phenytoin.

NURSING MANAGEMENT

ADMINISTRATION: Assess for hx of hypersensitivity (incl ethionamide, pyrazinamide, niacin) ▪ Obtain C&S before therapy ▪ PO: may administer on empty stomach, or c̄ meals to ↓ GI irritation; administer 1h before antacids ▪ IM: massage site after injection; rotate sites ▪ Avoid exposure to heat, moisture, light in storage ▪ Assess hepatic function; ↓ dose if impaired ▪ Have IV pyridoxine (vitamin B_6) available for OD.

EVALUATION: Monitor VS, esp temperature, BP; hepatic, renal status; serum for ↑ uric acid, AST, ALT ▪ Assess for visual disturbances (ocular toxicity) ▪ Use Clinistix/Tes-Tape for urine test.

EDUCATION: Take as ordered by physician, even if symptom free; do *not* skip doses ▪ May take on empty stomach, or c̄ meals to ↓ GI irritation ▪ Do *not* take antacids for at least 1h after drug ▪ Avoid changing positions rapidly ▪ Keep appointments for eye exams/c̄ physician ▪ Notify physician *immediately* of visual problems, tingling/numbness of hands/feet, jaundice, lethargy, dark urine; D/C drug ▪ Women: avoid pregnancy, breastfeeding ▪ Safety precautions c̄ ↑ activity ▪ Emotional support during long-term therapy ▪ Avoid use of alcohol, tyramine-containing (aged, fermented) foods ▪ Store in tightly closed, light-resistant container ▪ Physician may order vitamin B_6 supplements to alleviate neurotoxic effects ▪ Diabetics: use Clinistix/Tes-Tape to check urine glucose ▪ Full drug effects may require several wks of therapy.

NOTES:

isoproterenol hcl • (eye-soe-proe-ter-e-nole)

CATEGORY: *Sympathomimetic*: beta-adrenergic, bronchodilator — Rx; Preg Cat C

BRAND NAMES	DOSAGE FORMS
Isuprel (Winthrop)	Injection (IV): 0.2mg/ml
	Mistometer: 131µg/spray
	Solution: 0.5%, 1%
	SL tablet (Glossets): 10, 15mg
Medihaler-Iso (3M)	Aerosol: 80µg/spray

ACTION: Sympathomimetic activity selective for beta receptors, c̄ no appreciable alpha receptor activity; $beta_1$ adrenergic activity results in positive inotropic, chronotropic cardiac effect, c̄ ↑ output, stroke volume, oxygen consumption; $beta_2$ adrenergic activity produces bronchial, GI, uterine smooth muscle relaxation. **USE:** Treatment of bronchospasm associated c̄ acute/chronic asthma, pulmonary emphysema, bronchitis, bronchiectasis ▪ Adjunct in treatment of shock ▪ Treatment of cardiac arrest, carotid sinus hypersensitivity, Adams-Stokes syndrome, ventricular arrhythmias due to AV block.

PHARMACOKINETICS: Bronchodilation after inhalation immediate; duration about 1h, 1-2h c̄ SC/sublingual administration; excretion via urine.

CONTRAINDICATIONS: Hypersensitivity, digitalis tachycardia, preexisting cardiac arrhythmias.

DOSAGE

Bronchospasm *Sublingual*	
Pediatric	5-10mg. Do *not* exceed 30mg/d
Adult	10-20mg. Do *not* exceed 60mg/d
Heart block	
Pediatric	1/2 initial adult dose
Adult	10-15mg 4-6 times/d
Asthma/bronchospasm *Inhalation*	1-5 treatments prn
Shock *IV*	0.5-5µg/m. Dosage adjusted to heart rate, BP, urine flow. Doses up to 30µg/m may be required for advanced shock

Heart block/arrhythmias

Intracardiac	0.02mg
IM	Initial dose 0.2mg, subsequent range 0.02-1mg
IV	Initial dose 0.02-0.06mg, subsequent range 0.01-0.2mg
IV infusion	0.05-5μg/m
SC	Initial dose 0.02mg, subsequent range 0.15-0.2mg

SIDE/ADVERSE EFFECTS: CNS: mild tremors, headache, nervousness, dizziness ▪ CV: tachycardia, pulmonary edema, paradoxical Adams-Stokes seizures ▪ Other: flushing of face, sweating.

DRUG INTERACTIONS: Use c̄ MAO-I can produce significant hypertensive crisis ▪ Use c̄ tricyclic antidepressants, epinephrine best avoided ▪ Use c̄ propranolol antagonizes isoproterenol effects.

NURSING MANAGEMENT

ADMINISTRATION: Assess for hx of catecholamine hypersensitivity (incl sulfites) ▪ Avoid concurrent epinephrine administration ▪ SL: have pt dissolve under tongue; do *not* swallow; rinse mouth c̄ H_2O after absorption ▪ Inhalation: consult manufacturer's directions (do *not* inject); excessive use may ↓ effectiveness; rinse mouth c̄ H_2O after administration ▪ Do *not* use discolored/precipitated solution ▪ IV: cardiac monitoring; use infusion pump; have emergency support equipment available ▪ Intracardiac: administer chest compressions to perfuse drug into myocardium ▪ Avoid exposure to heat, direct sunlight in storage ▪ Elderly may require ↓ dosage.

EVALUATION: Monitor VS, esp BP, heart rate (D/C drug if >120) ▪ Monitor hemodynamic status, ABGs (parenteral) ▪ Monitor I&O.

EDUCATION: Take as ordered by physician; do *not* ↑ dose ▪ Take on arising ▪ Notify physician *immediately* of rapid/"skipped" heartbeats, chest pain, tremors; D/C drug ▪ May turn saliva pink/red (SL, inhalation) ▪ Procedure for inhalation/sublingual administration.

NOTES:

isosorbide dinitrate • (eye-soe-sor-bide)

CATEGORY: *Antianginal*: coronary vasodilator Rx; Preg Cat C

BRAND NAMES
**Coronex (Ayerst)*
Dilatrate-SR (R-C)
Iso-Bid (Geriatric)
Isordil (W-A)
**Novosorbide (Noropharm)*
Sorbitrate (ICI)

DOSAGE FORMS
Chewable tablet: 5, 10, 15mg; SL tablet: 2.5, 5, 10mg; SR capsule: 40mg; SR tablet: 40mg; tablet: 5, 10, 20, 30, 40mg

ACTION: Vasodilation due to direct relaxation of smooth muscle blood vessels, esp in coronary circulation; ↑ blood supply to myocardium helps relieve ischemia, thereby reduces anginal pain. **USE:** Treatment/prophylaxis of angina pectoris.

PHARMACOKINETICS

	Onset	Duration	Excretion
SL chewable tablet	1-3m	1-2h	Via urine primarily as metabolites
PO tablet	1h	4-6h	
Extended action forms	0.5-1h	Up to 12h	

CONTRAINDICATIONS: Hypersensitivity to drug, nitrates/nitrites.

DOSAGE

Adult *Chewable/sublingual*	2.5-10mg prn
PO	5-30mg 3-4 times/d or more

SIDE/ADVERSE EFFECTS: CNS: headache, dizziness, restlessness ▪ CV: postural hypotension, cutaneous vasodilation, flushing ▪ GI: N/V ▪ INT: rash, exfoliative dermatitis.

DRUG INTERACTIONS: Use c̄ calcium blockers, alcohol, beta blockers, phenothiazines results in additive hypotensive effects.

NURSING MANAGEMENT
ADMINISTRATION: Assess for hx of nitrate hypersensitivity ▪ Administer 1h ac/2h pc ▪ Chewable tablet: have pt chew well, hold in mouth for 2m before swallowing ▪ SR: have pt swallow whole ▪ SL: administer c̄ pt sitting/lying; avoid talking, drinking, eating, smoking until absorbed ▪ Avoid exposure to heat, moisture in storage.

EVALUATION: Monitor VS, esp BP ▪ Assess for headache; notify physician ▪ Assess for tolerance $\bar{c}$ prolonged use.

EDUCATION: Dizziness may occur; use caution in potentially hazardous activities ▪ Avoid changing positions (lying/sitting/standing) rapidly ▪ Avoid use $\bar{c}$ alcohol ▪ Take 1h ac/2h pc ▪ Swallow SR capsules/tablet whole ▪ Store in cool dry area ▪ Chewable tablet: chew well, hold in mouth for 2m before swallowing ▪ SL: dissolve under tongue; do *not* eat, drink, talk, smoke during use; notify physician/go to emergency room if not relieved w/in 15m ▪ Take prescribed analgesic for headache ▪ Notify physician of any ↓ in drug effect (persistent chest pain) ▪ Avoid ↑ exercise, exposure to temperature extremes ▪ Carry medical identification (MedicAlert).

NOTES:

kanamycin • (kan-a-mye-sin)

CATEGORY: *Aminoglycoside*: antibiotic

Rx; Preg Cat D

BRAND NAMES

**Anamid*

Kantrex (Apothecon)

DOSAGE FORMS

Capsule: 500mg
Injection (IM/IV):
500mg/2ml, 1g/3ml
Pediatric injection: (IM/IV):
75mg/2ml

ACTION: Bactericidal activity due to inhibition of ribosomal protein synthesis in susceptible organisms; toxicity usually limits systemic use to serious gram(-) infection; dosage must be adjusted to pts c̄ impaired renal function.

USE: Treatment (parenteral) of infections caused by susceptible strains of *Enterobacter aerogenes, Escherichia coli, Klebsiella pneumoniae, Mima-Herellea (Acinetobacter), Proteus* spp, *Serratia marcescens* ▪ Alternate for penicillin-resistant staphylococcal infection (parenteral) ▪ Treating cirrhotic pts c̄ hepatic coma caused by nitrogen-producing bacteria (PO) ▪ Intestinal antisepsis (PO).

PHARMACOKINETICS

IM peak	Half-life	Excretion
1h	2-2.5h	50% via urine in 4h, complete w/in 24-48h

CONTRAINDICATIONS: Hypersensitivity, previous hx of serious aminoglycoside toxicity.

DOSAGE

Pediatric/ Adult *IM/IV*	Usual dose 15mg/kg/d in 2 doses. Do *not* exceed 1.5g/d
Adult *PO*	
Hepatic encephalopathy	8-12g/d divided
Intestinal antisepsis	1g q4h for 4 doses, followed by 1g q6h for 36-72h

Note: Side/adverse effects: common in *italic;* serious in ***boldface italic.***

*Available in Canada only.

SIDE/ADVERSE EFFECTS: CNS: headache, paresthesia ▪ EENT: ***ototoxicity*** (auditory, vestibular damage: dizziness, vertigo, tinnitus, roaring in ears, hearing loss) ▪ GU: ***nephrotoxicity*** (casts, proteinuria; ↑ BUN, NPN, serum creatinine) ▪ INT: rash ▪ Other: fever.

DRUG INTERACTIONS: Avoid use c̄ neurotoxic/nephrotoxic drugs (eg, other aminoglycosides, colistin, ethacrynic acid, furosemide, polymyxin B, vancomycin, viomycin) ▪ Dimenhydrinate can mask aminoglycoside ototoxicity ▪ Use c̄ succinylcholine/tubocurarine ↑ their activity; Ca^{++} salts can reverse blockade ▪ PO anticoagulant activity may ↑ due to ↓ intestinal vitamin K synthesis.

NURSING MANAGEMENT

ADMINISTRATION: Assess for hx of aminoglycoside hypersensitivity ▪ Obtain C&S before therapy ▪ Obtain pt weight for dosage calculation ▪ Determine creatinine clearance before administration ▪ IM: administer by *deep, slow* injection into gluteal UOQ ▪ IV: dilute 500mg/vial in 200ml normal saline/5% dextrose (1g vial in 400ml) solution; administer 60-80gtt/m; may mix c̄ dextrose, Ringer injection, normal saline solution ▪ Inhalation: dilute 250mg in 3ml normal saline solution, nebulize ▪ Intraperitoneal: instill 500mg in 20ml sterile distilled H_2O ▪ Do *not* mix c̄ other drugs ▪ Avoid exposure to moisture in storage; store in original container ▪ Darkened color does *not* indicate ↓ potency ▪ Maintain hydration ▪ Elderly may require ↓ dosage.

EVALUATION: Assess for hearing dysfunction ▪ Monitor hepatic, renal, VIII CN function ▪ Monitor VS, esp temperature ▪ Assess for edema in extremities ▪ Assess for neuromuscular blockade, respiratory paralysis, nephrotoxicity ▪ Observe for signs of superinfection (diarrhea, URI, coated tongue) ▪ Assess for hypersensitivity (fever, difficult breathing, rash) ▪ Assess peak (<35μg/ml), trough (<5μg/ml) serum concentrations.

EDUCATION: Report hearing, balance difficulties to physician at once ▪ ↑ Fluid intake (10-12 glasses/d).

NOTES:

kaopectate preparations • (kay-oh-peck-tate)

CATEGORY: *Antidiarrheal* OTC

BRAND NAMES	FORMULAS
Kaopectate Chewable Tablets (Upjohn)	Attapulgite 300mg
Kaopectate Concentrate (Upjohn)	Attapulgite 600mg/15ml
Kaopectate Maximum Strength Tablets (Upjohn)	Attapulgite/pectin 600mg

ACTION: Suspension absorbs bacteria, toxins; helps promote their elimination from GI tract; preparation not absorbed. **USE:** Treatment of mild/moderate diarrhea.

PHARMACOKINETICS: Not applicable.

DOSAGE

Chewable tablets *PO*	
Pediatric	3-6y/o: 1 tablet after each BM 6-12y/o: 2 tablets after each BM
Adult	4 tablets after each BM
Concentrate	
Pediatric	3-6y/o: 7.5ml after each BM 6-12y/o: 15ml after each BM
Adult	30ml after each BM
Maximum Strength Tablets	
Pediatric	6-12y/o: 1 tablet after each BM
Adult	2 tablets after each BM

SIDE/ADVERSE EFFECTS: Essentially none, c̄ occasional constipation.

DRUG INTERACTIONS: Use c̄ PO drugs retards their absorption.

NURSING MANAGEMENT

ADMINISTRATION: Shake well before administering concentrate ▪ Assess for severe abdominal pain; do *not* use if present ▪ *Not* for long-term use (48h maximum).

EVALUATION: Monitor bowel function ▪ Monitor F/E status (esp infants, elderly).

EDUCATION: Take after each loose bowel movement ▪ Shake concentrate well before taking ▪ Do *not* take if experiencing severe abdominal pain ▪ D/C if symptoms persist for longer than 2d ▪ Check c̄ physician/pharmacist before taking other PO drugs (⬇ absorption).

NOTES:

ketoconazole • (key-toe-koe-na-zol)

CATEGORY: *Antifungal* Rx; Preg Cat C

BRAND NAME
Nizoral (Janssen)

DOSAGE FORMS
Cream: 2%; Tablet: 200mg

ACTION: Antifungal activity usually fungistatic, due to inhibition of ergosterol synthesis, a vital fungal cell membrane component; this results in cell membrane permeability changes, inhibition of purine transport; drug not suitable for fungal meningitis. **USE:** Treatment of fungal infection (blastomycosis, candidiasis, chromomycosis, coccidioidomycosis, histoplasmosis, paracoccidioidomycosis) caused by susceptible strains ▪ Treatment of cutaneous dermatophyte infections not responsive to topical therapy ▪ Cream used in the topical treatment of candidiasis, dermatophytes, & tinea versicolor.

PHARMACOKINETICS

PO absorption	Peak	Half-life	Protein binding	Excretion
Variable	1-2h	2h	99%	Via feces primarily as metabolites c̄ some urinary excretion

CONTRAINDICATIONS: Hypersensitivity.

DOSAGE

Pediatric *PO*	>2y/o: 3.3-6.6mg/mg/d as single dose
Adult *PO*	200mg/d as single dose. Serious infections may require 400mg once/d
Cream	Once/d over area of infection

SIDE/ADVERSE EFFECTS: CNS: headache, dizziness, somnolence, photophobia ▪ END: gynecomastia ▪ GI: N/V/D, pain ▪ GU: impotence ▪ HEM: ***thrombocytopenia*** ▪ HEP: hepatocellular toxicity.

DRUG INTERACTIONS: Use c̄ antacids, anticholinergics, H_2 blockers ↓ PO absorption ▪ Use c̄ other hepatotoxic drugs ↑ toxicity ▪ Ketoconazole may ↑ anticoagulant effect of PO anticoagulants.

NURSING MANAGEMENT

ADMINISTRATION: Assess for hx of hypersensitivity ▪ Obtain C&S before therapy ▪ Administer in early AM ▪ Assess hepatic function; ↓ dosage if impaired ▪ Do *not* administer w/in 2h of alkaline substances (requires acid media to dissolve); may be ordered c̄ dilute HCl, sip through glass/plastic straw placed on back of teeth, follow c̄ glass of H_2O.

EVALUATION: Monitor VS, esp temperature ▪ Monitor hepatic function.

EDUCATION: Dizziness/drowsiness may occur; use caution in potentially hazardous activities ▪ Take as ordered by physician at same time each day; do *not* change dose ▪ Take c̄ food ▪ Avoid exposure to bright light; wear sunglasses to ↓ discomfort ▪ May require several wks/mo of treatment; take until lab tests normal ▪ Check c̄ physician/pharmacist before taking OTC drugs ▪ Store in tightly closed container ▪ Women: avoid breastfeeding ▪ Avoid alcohol intake.

NOTES:

ketoprofen • (key-toe-proe-fen)

CATEGORY: *Antiinflammatory:* NSAIA, analgesic — Rx; Preg Cat B

BRAND NAME
Orudis (W-A)

DOSAGE FORMS
Capsules: 25, 50, 75mg

ACTION: Antiinflammatory, analgesic activity appears related to inhibition of prostaglandin synthesis. **USE:** Treatment of rheumatoid/osteoarthritis ▪ Relief of mild/moderate pain, primary dysmenorrhea.

PHARMACOKINETICS

PO absorption	Peak	Half-life	Protein binding	Excretion
Complete	0.5-2h	2-4h	99%	Via urine as conjugate

CONTRAINDICATIONS: Hypersensitivity, aspirin/other antiinflammatory agent hypersensitivity.

DOSAGE
Adult *PO*

Arthritis	150-300mg/d divided in 3 or 4 doses. Total daily dose above 300mg not currently recommended
Pain	25-50mg q6-8h
Dysmenorrhea	25-50mg q6-8h

SIDE/ADVERSE EFFECTS: CNS: dizziness, *headache,* drowsiness ▪ CV: edema, palpitations, **CHF**, hypertension ▪ EENT: tinnitus, visual disturbances, conjunctivitis ▪ GI: *dyspepsia, abdominal pain, nausea,* V/D, stomatitis, *GI bleeding,* constipation, flatulence ▪ GU: symptoms of renal infection, hematuria, ***interstitial nephritis, nephrotic syndrome*** ▪ HEM: anemia, ***agranulocytosis, hemolytic anemia, thrombocytopenia, aplastic anemia*** ▪ INT: rash, erythema, urticaria ▪ Other: asthma, jaundice, gynecomastia.

DRUG INTERACTIONS: Use c̄ ulcerogenic drugs produces additive effects ▪ Use c̄ PO anticoagulants may ↑ their activity ▪ Use c̄ aspirin not currently recommended ▪ Use c̄ methotrexate is best avoided ▪ Use c̄ lithium requires monitoring of lithium levels.

NURSING MANAGEMENT
ADMINISTRATION: Assess for hx of NSAIA, salicylate hypersensitivity ▪ Avoid administration to pts c̄ hx of

asthma, bleeding disorders, salicylate hypersensitivity ▪ Assess GI, renal, hepatic function; use caution if impaired ▪ May be administered c̄ food, milk, antacid; administer c̄ full glass of liquid; capsules may be opened; encourage upright position for 15-30m ▪ Avoid exposure to moisture during storage ▪ Elderly may require ↓ dosage.

EVALUATION: Monitor VS, esp BP ▪ Monitor hepatic, renal status c̄ prolonged use ▪ Monitor pt receiving anticoagulant therapy; may potentiate bleeding ▪ Monitor stool for occult blood ▪ Monitor I&O, daily weight ▪ Assess for edema in extremities ▪ Assess for visual/hearing disturbances; D/C drug, notify physician.

EDUCATION: Dizziness/drowsiness may occur; use caution in potentially hazardous activities ▪ Take c̄ food/milk; take c̄ a full glass of liquid; maintain upright position for 15-30m ▪ Take as ordered by physician; do *not* ↑ dose ▪ Notify physician *immediately* of bleeding, ↓ urine output, swelling of feet/legs, lethargy, GI distress, jaundice, visual/hearing disturbances ▪ Avoid taking c̄ aspirin, other NSAIAs ▪ Avoid use c̄ alcohol ▪ Check c̄ physician/pharmacist before taking OTC preparations ▪ Notify physician/dentist of use before treatment ▪ Women: avoid breastfeeding ▪ Store in tightly closed container ▪ Full drug effects may require several wks of therapy.

NOTES:

ketorolac tromethamine • (key-toe-roe-lack)

CATEGORY: *Analgesic:* antiinflammatory, NSAIA — Rx; Preg Cat C

BRAND NAME
Toradol (Syntext)

DOSAGE FORMS
IM: 15, 30mg/ml
Tablets: 10mg

ACTION: Analgesic activity appears related to inhibition of prostaglandin synthesis. **USE:** Short-term relief of pain (up to 5 days).

CONTRAINDICATIONS: Hypersensitivity, with nasal polyps or aspirin and other NSAIA-induced allergies.

DOSAGE

Adult *PO* — 10mg 4-6hprn. Do *not* exceed 40mg/d. Transition from IM to PO should *not* exceed 120mg on transition day which includes 40mg PO maximum.

IM — Loading dose of 30-60mg followed by half the loading dose q6h

SIDE/ADVERSE EFFECTS: CNS: headache (17%), drowsiness, dizziness, paresthesia, nervousness, convulsions, tremors ▪ CV: hypertension, palpitations, edema ▪ EENT: abnormal taste & vision, tinnitus, hearing loss ▪ GI: nausea (12%), dyspepsia (12%), pain (13%), ulcers, bleeding stomatitis, D/V, pancreatitis ▪ HEM: purpura, leukopenia, eosinophilia ▪ INT: rash, pruritus, exfoliative dermatitis, urticaria, maculopapular rash, Lyell's syndrome, ***Stevens-Johnson syndrome*** ▪ REN: ***acute renal failure,*** azotemia, nephritis, hematuria ▪ RESP: asthma, dyspnea, rhinitis, cough ▪ Other: asthenia, anaphylaxis, fever.

PHARMACOKINETICS

PO absorption	Peak	Half-life	Protein binding	Excretion
Complete	20-60m	2.4-9.2h	99%	Via urine (>90) and feces (6.1%) primarily as metabolite

Note: Side/adverse effects: common in *italic;* serious in ***boldface italic.***

*Available in Canada only.

DRUG INTERACTIONS: Use c̄ ulcerogenic drug produces additive effects ▪ Use c̄ warfarin and other high protein binding drugs can ↑ their activity due to protein displacement ▪ Use c̄ lithium, methotrexate, nondepolarizing muscle relaxants may ↑ their activity ▪ Use c̄ furosemide may ↓ diuretic effect.

NURSING MANAGEMENT

ADMINISTRATION: Assess for hx of NSAIA hypersensitivity ▪ Avoid administration to individuals c̄ hx of asthma, bleeding disorders, salicylate hypersensitivity ▪ PO: may be administered c̄ food/milk; *best* on empty stomach (1h ac/2h pc); encourage upright position for 15-30m ▪ Avoid exposure to moisture, light in storage ▪ Elderly may require ↓ dosage.

EVALUATION: Monitor hematologic, hepatic, renal status c̄ prolonged use ▪ Monitor pt receiving anticoagulant therapy; may potentiate bleeding ▪ Monitor I&O, daily weight c̄ prolonged use ▪ Assess for edema in extremities ▪ Assess for visual disturbances, skin rash; D/C drug, notify physician.

EDUCATION: Dizziness/drowsiness may occur; use caution in potentially hazardous activities ▪ Take on empty stomach (1h ac/2h pc), c̄ food/milk if GI distress occurs; maintain upright position of 15-30m ▪ Take as ordered by physician; do *not* ↑ dose ▪ Notify physician *immediately* of bleeding, ↓ urine output, swelling of feet/legs, lethargy, GI distress, jaundice, visual disturbance ▪ Avoid taking c̄ aspirin, other NSAIAs ▪ Avoid use c̄ alcohol ▪ Check c̄ physician/pharmacist before taking OTC preparations ▪ Notify physician/dentist of use before treatment ▪ Store in tightly closed container ▪ Full drug effects may require several wks of therapy.

NOTES:

labetalol hcl • (la-bet-a-lole)

CATEGORY: *Alpha, beta blocker:* antihypertensive

Rx; Preg Cat C

BRAND NAMES

Brand	Dosage forms
Normodyne (Schering)	Injection (IV): 5mg/ml Tablet: 100, 200, 300mg
Trandate (A-H)	Injection (IV): 5mg/ml Tablet: 100, 200, 300mg

COMBINATION PRODUCTS

Normozide 100/25, 200/25, 300/25 (Schering)	labetalol hcl/Hydrochlorothiazide: 100mg/25mg, 200mg/25mg, 300mg/25mg/tablet

ACTION: Selective alpha$_1$, nonselective beta blockage produces enhanced hypotensive effects. **USE:** Treatment of hypertension as sole agent/in combination c̄ other antihypertensives, esp thiazide or loop diuretic; severe hypertensive states treated IV.

PHARMACOKINETICS

PO absorption	Peak	Half-life	Protein binding	Excretion
Complete	1-2h	6-8h	55%-60%	Via urine, bile, primarily as metabolites

CONTRAINDICATIONS: Hypersensitivity, bronchial asthma, cardiac failure, cardiogenic shock, greater than 1° heart block, severe bradycardia.

DOSAGE

Adult *PO*	Usual starting dose 100mg bid. Usual maintenance dose 200-400mg bid
IV	Repeated injection: 20mg by slow injection. Additional doses 40-80mg may be given at 10m intervals until desired results or total 300mg injected. Usual infusion rate 2mg/m
Normozide	Usual maintenance dose 1 tablet bid

SIDE/ADVERSE EFFECTS: CNS: *dizziness*, drowsiness, paresthesias, headache ▪ CV: edema, *bradycardia*, postural hypotension ▪ EENT: nasal stuffiness, vision disturbance ▪ GI: *N/V/D*, dyspepsia, pain, taste distortion ▪ GU: impotence, ejaculation inhibition, ***acute urinary bladder retention*** ▪ INT: rash ▪ RESP: dyspnea, ***bronchospasm*** ▪ Other: *fatigue*.

DRUG INTERACTIONS: Use c̄ beta adrenergics will antagonize therapeutic effects ▪ Use c̄ halothane ↑ hypotensive effects of IV labetalol ▪ Use c̄ cimetidine will ↑ hypotensive effects due to greater labetalol bioavailability ▪ Use c̄ tricyclic antidepressants ↑ incidence of tremors.

NURSING MANAGEMENT

ADMINISTRATION: Assess for hx of hypersensitivity ▪ Assess apical pulse; if <60/m hold drug, notify physician ▪ Assess respiratory function; do *not* administer if impaired ▪ PO: administer c̄ food ▪ IV: place pt in supine position, maintain for 3h; assess BP; prepare according to manufacturer's directions; administer direct (over 2m), use infusion-control device for continuous infusion ▪ Elderly may require ↓ dosage ▪ Avoid abrupt withdrawal; D/C gradually.

EVALUATION: Monitor VS, esp BP (lying/standing), heart rate (parenteral: q5-15m) ▪ Monitor I&O, daily weight ▪ Assess peripheral circulation ▪ Diabetics: closely monitor blood glucose (hypoglycemia) ▪ Assess for edema in extremities ▪ Monitor hepatic, CV, renal, hemopoietic status c̄ long-term use.

EDUCATION: Dizziness may occur; use caution in potentially hazardous activities ▪ Avoid changing positions (lying/sitting/standing) rapidly ▪ Procedure for checking radial pulse ▪ Check pulse before taking; if <60/m do *not* take drug, notify physician ▪ Take as ordered by physician, even if symptom free; do *not* change dose ▪ Take c̄ food to ↓ GI irritation ▪ Used to control, *not* cure hypertension ▪ Avoid use c̄ alcohol ▪ Avoid ↑ exercise, temperature extremes, smoking ▪ Notify physician of muscle cramps, difficult breathing, cold extremities, leg edema ▪ Keep scheduled appointments c̄ physician; have BP checked regularly ▪ Maintain optimum weight ▪ Avoid high-Na^+ foods (canned soups, lunch meats, cheese) ▪ Check c̄ physician/pharmacist before taking OTC preparations ▪ Notify physician/dentist of use before treatment ▪ Do *not* D/C drug w/out checking c̄ physician ▪ Carry medical identification (Medic-Alert) if hypertensive.

NOTES:

levodopa • (<u>lee</u>-voe-doe-pa)

CATEGORY: *Antiparkinsonian agent*: dopaminergic agonist — Rx; Preg Cat NA

BRAND NAMES
Dopar (Roberts)
Larodopa (Roche)

DOSAGE FORMS
Capsule, tablet 0.1, 0.25, 0.5g

COMBINATION PRODUCTS

Sinemet 10/100, 25/100, 25/250 (Du Pont)	Carbidopa/levodopa: 10mg/100mg, 25mg/100mg, 25mg/250mg

ACTION: Parkinson disease related to ↓ levels of dopamine in corpus striatum. Levodopa enters CNS, is converted into dopamine in basal ganglia; concentration of dopamine ↑, symptoms of Parkinson disease ↓. Carbidopa combined c̄ levodopa inhibits decarboxylation of levodopa; thus ↑ levels of levodopa available for transport to brain. **USE:** Treatment of idiopathic, postencephalitic Parkinson disease ▪ Treatment of symptomatic parkinsonism due to carbon monoxide poisoning, cerebral arteriosclerosis.

PHARMACOKINETICS

PO absorption	CNS transport	Half-life	Excretion
Good	1%	1h	80%-85% via urine w/in 24h

CONTRAINDICATIONS: Hypersensitivity, narrow-angle glaucoma, hx of melanoma/undiagnosed skin lesions, pt receiving MAO-I.

DOSAGE

Adult *PO*	Initial dose: 0.5-1g/d in ≥2 doses. ↑ dose to 0.75g q3-7d as tolerated. Usual optimal dose should *not* exceed 8g
Sinemet 10-100	1 tablet 3-4 times/d. May ↑ to 8 tablets/d prn
Sinemet 25-100	1 tablet tid. May ↑ to 6 tablets/d prn
Sinemet 25-250	1 tablet 3-4 times/d if pt requires 1500mg levodopa/d

SIDE/ADVERSE EFFECTS: CNS: *choreiform, dystonic, other involuntary movements;* headache, dizziness ▪ CV: cardiac irregularities, palpitations, orthostatic hypotension, phlebitis ▪ EENT: blurred vision ▪ HEM: ***hemolytic anemia, agranulocytosis*** ▪ PSYCH: delusions, agitation, anxiety, suicidal/psychotic episodes ▪ Other: dark urine/sweat, hot flashes.

DRUG INTERACTIONS: Use c̄ MAO-I can produce hypertensive crisis ▪ Vitamin B_6 (pyridoxine), phenothiazine will antagonize effects of levodopa ▪ Use c̄ antihypertensives can produce additive hypotensive effects.

NURSING MANAGEMENT

ADMINISTRATION: Assess for hx of hypersensitivity ▪ Administer c̄ food ▪ Avoid exposure to moisture, light in storage ▪ Avoid abrupt withdrawal ▪ Elderly may require ↓ dosage.

EVALUATION: Monitor CV, pulmonary, hepatic, renal status ▪ Monitor serum for ↑ AST, ALT, BUN, LDH, bilirubin, alkaline phosphatase ▪ False (+): Coombs' test ▪ Urine glucose determinations inaccurate ▪ Assess for depression/suicidal tendencies ▪ Monitor VS, esp BP.

EDUCATION: Take exactly as ordered by physician ▪ Full drug effects may require several mos ▪ Dizziness may occur on arising; change positions slowly ▪ Avoid preparations containing vitamin B_6 ▪ May darken urine/sweat ▪ Maintain good personal hygiene (daily bath) ▪ Store in tightly closed, light-resistant container ▪ Take c̄ food ▪ Women: avoid breastfeeding ▪ Safety precautions c̄ ↑ activity.

NOTES:

levothyroxine sodium (T) • (lee-voe-thye-<u>rox</u>-een)

CATEGORY: *Thyroid hormone* Rx; Preg Cat A

BRAND NAMES	DOSAGE FORMS
**Eltroxin (Glaxo)*	Tablet: 50, 100, 150, 200, 300µg
Levothroid (Forest)	Injection (IM/IV): 200, 500 µg/vial Tablet: 25, 50, 75, 100, 125, 150, 175, 200, 300µg
Synthroid (Boots)	Injection (IM/IV): 200, 500µg/vial Tablet: 25, 50, 75, 100, 112, 125, 150, 175, 200, 300µg

ACTION: Thyroid hormones regulate general body metabolism by controlling cellular oxidative process; influence growth, tissue differentiation, maturation. **USE:** Treatment of hypothyroidism.

PHARMACOKINETICS

PO absorption	Half-life	Protein binding	Excretion
Up to 80%	6-7d	99%	Via urine, feces as metabolites

CONTRAINDICATIONS: Thyrotoxicosis, uncorrected adrenocortical deficiency, acute myocardial infarction.

DOSAGE: Must be individualized.

Pediatric *PO* — Suggested starting doses:
0-1y/o: 9µg/kg once/d
1-5y/o: 6µg/kg once/d
6-10y/o: 4µg/kg once/d
11-20y/o: 3µg/kg once/d

Adult *PO* — Usual maintenance dose 50-200µg/d. For geriatric myxedematous infiltration c̄ cardiovascular dysfunction, starting dose 25µg/d suggested, c̄ subsequent ↑ at 3-4wks until desired effect is obtained

SIDE/ADVERSE EFFECTS: Usually limited to overdosage ▪ CNS: headache, insomnia, nervousness, tremors ▪ CV: angina, ***cardiac arrhythmias,*** palpitations, tachycardia ▪ GI: diarrhea ▪ Other: intolerance to heat; sweating, weight loss.

Note: Side/adverse effects: common in *italic;* serious in ***boldface italic.*** *Available in Canada only.

DRUG INTERACTIONS: Use c̄ epinephrine in pts c̄ coronary disease may induce coronary insufficiency ▪ Use c̄ PO anticoagulants will ↑ their activity, requires lower anticoagulant doses ▪ Use c̄ cholestyramine ↓ PO absorption of thyroid preparations ▪ Use in diabetic pts may require ↑ dosage of hypoglycemic agents.

NURSING MANAGEMENT

ADMINISTRATION: Assess for hx of hypersensitivity ▪ Administer daily dose before breakfast ▪ Parenteral: reconstitute c̄ 5ml 0.9% NaCl injection (w/out preservative); shake well to dissolve; do *not* add to other IV fluids; discard unused portion ▪ Avoid exposure to moisture, light in storage ▪ Elderly may require ↓ dosage.

EVALUATION: Monitor VS, esp heart rate ▪ Observe for signs of overdose (chest pain, fever, nervousness, rapid/irregular heartbeat) ▪ Monitor thyroid function tests (T_3, T_4, TSH); evaluate pt use of iodine-containing substances before exam ▪ Diabetics: closely monitor blood glucose (hyperglycemia) ▪ May potentiate anticoagulant effect; assess for bleeding/bruising.

EDUCATION: Take as ordered by physician; do *not* change dose ▪ Avoid high-iodine foods (soybeans, cabbage, shellfish) ▪ Procedure for checking radial pulse ▪ Take pulse on arising qd; notify physician if ↑ /irregular, D/C drug ▪ Keep scheduled appointments for lab work/c̄ physician ▪ Do *not* change brand name preparations ▪ Notify physician *immediately* of difficult breathing, chest pain, rapid/irregular heartbeat; D/C drug ▪ Check c̄ physician/pharmacist before taking OTC preparations ▪ Notify physician/dentist of use before treatment ▪ Store in dry, tightly closed, light-resistant container.

NOTES:

lidocaine hcl • (lye-doe-kane)

CATEGORY: *Antiarrhythmic:* local anesthetic

Rx; Preg Cat B

BRAND NAME
Xylocaine (Astra)

DOSAGE FORMS
Injection (IM): 100mg/ml
Injection (IV): 10, 20, 40, 200mg/ml

Available in a wide array of preparations intended for local anesthesia.

ACTION: Antiarrhythmic effect due to depression of ventricular automaticity, depolarization; drug has no effect on atrial arrhythmias; local anesthetic effect due to reversible blocking of nerve conduction by undetermined mechanism. **USE:** Treatment of acute ventricular arrhythmias occurring during MI/cardiac surgical procedures ▪ Local anesthetic.

CONTRAINDICATIONS: Hypersensitivity to amide-type local anesthetics, Stokes-Adams syndrome, Wolff-Parkinson-White syndrome, severe SA/AV intraventricular block.

DOSAGE

Pediatric *IV*	Suggested bolus dose 0.5-1mg/kg. Usual maintenance infusion rate 10-50μg/kg/m
Adult *IM*	4.3mg/kg; may be repeated after 60-90m
IV	Initial bolus dose 50-100mg. May be repeated in 5m. Do *not* exceed 200-300mg over 1h. Usual maintenance infusion rate 1-4mg/m

PHARMACOKINETICS

Onset		Duration			
IV bolus	IM	IV bolus	IM	Protein binding	Excretion
45-90s	5-15m	10-20m	60-90m	60%-80%	Via urine, 90% as metabolites

SIDE/ADVERSE EFFECTS: CNS: ***twitching convulsions, respiratory depression/arrest***, drowsiness, dizziness, sensation of heat/cold, numbness, disorientation ▪ CV: ***hypotension, bradycardia*** (can induce cardiac arrest/CV collapse) ▪ EENT: blurred vision, tinnitus ▪ GI: vomiting.

DRUG INTERACTIONS: Use c̄ succinylcholine, other surgical muscle relaxants may ↑ neuromuscular blockage ▪ Use c̄ other antiarrhythmics ↑ effects ▪ Use c̄ beta blockers, cimetidine ↑ lidocaine serum levels.

NURSING MANAGEMENT

ADMINISTRATION: Assess for hx of amide-type local anesthetic/tocainide hypersensitivity ▪ IM: inject into deltoid muscle ▪ IV: dilute according to manufacturer's directions; administer bolus dose (over 60s), followed by infusion drip; use infusion control device; cardiac monitoring; do *not* give c̄ epinephrine, preservatives ▪ Do *not* administer discolored/precipitated solutions ▪ Do *not* use solutions c̄ preservatives for spinal anesthesia ▪ Do *not* add to blood product infusions ▪ Discard solutions w/out preservatives after use ▪ Have emergency support equipment available ▪ Topical (PO): have pt swish in mouth, abstain from food for 60m ▪ Elderly may require ↓ dosage.

EVALUATION: Monitor VS, esp BP ▪ Monitor respiratory status; auscultate lungs ▪ Observe for neurotoxic effects (confusion, hallucinations, behavioral changes); notify physician, D/C drug ▪ Monitor serum levels of toxicity ▪ Therapeutic blood levels: 1.5-5μg/ml.

EDUCATION: Notify physician/nurse of abnormal rxs (difficult breathing, rash, tremors, lightheadedness, GI distress, blurred vision) ▪ Procedure for topical application.

NOTES:

liothyronine sodium (T_3) • (lye-oh-thye-roe-neen)

CATEGORY: *Thyroid hormone*

Rx; Preg Cat A

BRAND NAME
Cytomel (SKB)

DOSAGE FORMS
Tablet: 5, 25, 50μg

ACTION: Thyroid hormones regulate general body metabolism by controlling cellular oxidative process; influence growth, tissue differentiation, maturation. **USE:** Treatment of hypothyroidism ▪ Suppression of pituitary TSH in prevention/treatment of various types of goiters ▪ Diagnostic T_3 suppression test for hyperthyroidism.

PHARMACOKINETICS

PO absorption	Half-life	Protein binding	Excretion
95%	2½d	99%	Via urine, feces

CONTRAINDICATIONS: Thyrotoxicosis, uncorrected adrenocortical deficiency, acute myocardial infarction.

DOSAGE: Must be individualized.

Cretinism PO	Start c̄ 5μg/d. ↑ by 5μg increments until desired effect is obtained
Infants	Usually require 20μg/d
1-3y/o	Usually require 50μg/d
>3y/o	May require full adult dose
Adult *PO*	
Mild hypothyroidism	Usual maintenance dose 25-75μg/d
Myxedema	Usual maintenance dose 50-100μg/d
Simple goiter	Usual dose 75μg/d
T_3 suppression test	75-100μg/d for 7d. Repeat
^{131}I uptake test	Hyperthyroidism, no significant change after 24h. Normal function, significant ↓ in ^{131}I uptake
Cretinism	Initial dose 5μg/d. ↑ By 5μg increments q3-4d until desired result obtained

Note: Side/adverse effects: common in *italic;* serious in ***boldface italic.***

*Available in Canada only.

SIDE/ADVERSE EFFECTS: Usually limited to overdosage; same as symptoms of hyperthyroidism ▪ CNS: headache, insomnia, nervousness, tremors ▪ CV: angina, ***cardiac arrhythmias***, palpitations, tachycardia ▪ GI: diarrhea ▪ Other: intolerance to heat; sweating, weight loss.

DRUG INTERACTIONS: Use $\bar{c}$ epinephrine in pts $\bar{c}$ coronary disease may induce coronary insufficiency ▪ Use $\bar{c}$ PO anticoagulants ↑ their activity, requires lower anticoagulant doses ▪ Use $\bar{c}$ cholestyramine ↓ PO absorption of thyroid preparations ▪ Use in diabetic pts may require ↑ dosage of hypoglycemic agents.

NURSING MANAGEMENT

ADMINISTRATION: Assess for hx of hypersensitivity ▪ Administer daily dose before breakfast ▪ Avoid exposure to moisture, light in storage ▪ Elderly may require ↓ dosage.

EVALUATION: Monitor VS, esp heart rate ▪ Observe for signs of overdose (chest pain, fever, nervousness, rapid/irregular heartbeat) ▪ Monitor thyroid function tests (T_3, T_4, TSH); evaluate pt use of iodine-containing substances before exam ▪ Diabetics: closely monitor blood glucose (hyperglycemia) ▪ May potentiate anticoagulant effect; assess for bleeding/bruising.

EDUCATION: Take as ordered by physician; do *not* change dose ▪ Avoid high-iodine foods (soybeans, cabbage, shellfish) ▪ Procedure for checking radial pulse ▪ Take pulse on arising each day; notify physician if ↑/irregular, D/C drug ▪ Keep scheduled appointments for lab work/$\bar{c}$ physician ▪ Do *not* change brand name preparations ▪ Notify physician *immediately* of difficult breathing, chest pain, rapid/irregular heartbeat; D/C drug ▪ Check $\bar{c}$ physician/pharmacist before taking OTC preparations ▪ Notify physician/dentist of use before treatment ▪ Store in dry, tightly closed, light-resistant container.

NOTES:

lisinopril • (lye-sin-oh-pril)

CATEGORY: *Antihypertensive:* angiotensin inhibitor Rx; Preg Cat C/D†

BRAND NAMES
Prinivil (MSD)
Zestril (Stuart)

DOSAGE FORMS
Tablet: 5, 10, 20, 40mg
Tablet: 5, 10, 20mg

COMBINATION PRODUCTS

Prinzide (MSD) 12.5, 25	lisinopril/hydrochlorothiazide per tablet:
Zestoretic (Stuart) 20-12.5, 20-25	20mg/12.5mg, 20mg/25mg

ACTION: Antihypertensive activity appears related to suppression of renin-angiotensin-aldosterone system by competitive inhibition of ACE, which produces angiotensin II from angiotensin I; this results in reduction of peripheral arterial resistance, aldosterone secretion. **USE:** Treatment of hypertension as sole agent or in combination c̄ other antihypertensives.

CONTRAINDICATIONS: Hypersensitivity; hx of angioedema c̄ other ACE inhibitors. D/C during pregnancy as soon as possible.

DOSAGE

Normal renal function	
Adult *PO*	Initial dose of 10mg/d. Usual dosage range 20-40mg as a single dose/d
Combination product	Usual dose 1-2 tablets (20-12.5)/d or 1 tablet (20-25)/d

SIDE/ADVERSE EFFECTS: CNS: *headache, dizziness,* somnolence, paresthesias ▪ CV: hypotension, tachycardia, palpitations, chest pain, edema ▪ GI: N/V/D, pain, dyspepsia, flatulence, anorexia ▪ MET: gout ▪ INT: rash, pruritus ▪ REN: azotemia, acute renal failure ▪ RESP: bron-

PHARMACOKINETICS

PO absorption	Onset	Peak	Half-life	Duration	Excretion
25%	1h	6-7h	12h	24h	As unchanged drug via urine

Note: Side/adverse effects: common in *italic;* serious in ***boldface italic.***

*Available in Canada only.
†1st trimester, C; 2nd & 3rd trimesters, D.

chitis, sinusitis, pharyngeal pain, angioedema, nasal congestion, dyspnea ▪ Other: blurred vision, joint pain, muscle cramps, impotence, *fatigue*.

DRUG INTERACTIONS: Use c̄ diuretics may produce transient hypotension ▪ Indomethacin, other NSAIA may antagonize therapeutic effects ▪ Use K^+-sparing diuretics c̄ caution (hyperkalemia).

NURSING MANAGEMENT

ADMINISTRATION: Assess for hx of hypersensitivity ▪ Assess BP; notify physician of extremes ▪ Assess renal function; may require ↓ dosage if impaired ▪ May crush, administer c̄ liquid; may be administered w/out regard to food ▪ Assess serum Na^+ (normal: 135-145mEq/L); notify physician of abnormalities ▪ Assess for rapid ↓ in BP w/in 3h after administration of 1st dose (occurs c̄ hyponatremia) ▪ SLE, elderly may require ↓ dosage ▪ Avoid abrupt withdrawal; D/C gradually.

EVALUATION: Monitor VS, esp BP ▪ Monitor CBC (esp WBC, differential) periodically during therapy ▪ Monitor electrolyte status (↑ K^+; ↓ Na^+) ▪ Monitor I&O, daily weight ▪ Assess for edema in extremities.

EDUCATION: Dizziness may occur; use caution in potentially hazardous activities ▪ Avoid changing positions (lying/sitting/standing) rapidly ▪ Notify physician of fever, sore throat, bruising/bleeding, swelling of feet/legs ▪ Take as ordered by physician, even if symptom free; do *not* skip doses ▪ May take w/out regard to food ▪ Do *not* D/C w/out notifying physician ▪ Check c̄ physician/pharmacist before taking OTC/Rx preparations ▪ Avoid high-Na^+ foods (canned soups, lunch meats, cheese) ▪ Avoid high-K^+ foods (bananas, citrus fruits, raisins) ▪ Check c̄ physician before using salt substitutes ▪ Avoid ↑ exercise, temperature extremes, smoking ▪ Used to control, *not* cure, hypertension ▪ Maintain optimum weight ▪ Keep scheduled appointments c̄ physician; have BP checked at regular intervals ▪ Women: avoid breastfeeding ▪ Full drug effects may require several wks of therapy.

NOTES:

lithium carbonate/lithium citrate ▲ • (li-thee-um)

CATEGORY: *Antimanic*

Rx; Preg Cat D

BRAND NAMES	DOSAGE FORMS
Cibalith-S (Ciba)▲	Syrup: 8mEq/5ml
ESKalith (SKB)	Capsule: 300mg Controlled-release tablet: 450mg Tablet: 300mg
Lithane (Miles)	Tablet: 300mg
Lithobid (Ciba)	Tablet: 300mg
Lithonate (Solvay)	Slow-release tablet: 300mg
Lithotabs (Solvay)	Capsule: 300mg Tablet: 300mg

ACTION: Antimanic effect not determined; studies indicate that lithium ions alter Na^+ transport in nerve cells, which effects shift in catecholamine metabolism; toxic levels of lithium close to therapeutic levels, tolerance greater during acute manic phase, ↓ when symptoms subside; acute mania usually requires serum level 1.0-1.5mEq/L, desirable long-term maintenance levels 0.6-1.2mEq/L; accurate pt evaluation requires clinical & laboratory analysis. **USE:** Treatment of manic depressive illnesses.

PHARMACOKINETICS

PO absorption	Peak	Half-life	Excretion
95%-100%	0.5-3h	Initial 0.8-1.2h	Via urine

CONTRAINDICATIONS: No current absolute contraindications.

DOSAGE: Must be individualized.

Adult *PO* 600mg tid. Maintenance 900-1200mg/d

SIDE/ADVERSE EFFECTS: Dependent on serum levels; relatively few c̄ <1.5mEq/L; mild-moderate c̄ 1.5-2.5mEq/L; moderate-severe c̄ 2.0-2.5mEq/L ▪ CNS: drowsiness, blackout spells, slurred speech, epileptic-type seizures, psychomotor retardation, choreoathetotic movements ▪ CV: ***cardiac arrhythmias,*** hypotension, peripheral circulatory collapse, inversion of T-waves ▪ END: hypothyroidism ▪ GI: anorexia, N/V/D ▪ INT:

alopecia, dry hair, chronic folliculitis, psoriasis ▪ Other: hyperactive deep tendon reflex.

DRUG INTERACTIONS: Use c̄ haloperidol can produce encephalopathic syndrome c̄ irreversible brain damage ▪ Use c̄ ACE-I, calcium blockers, thiazides ↑ lithium toxicity ▪ Use c̄ NSAIA ↑ lithium serum levels ▪ Use c̄ iodine-containing substances ↑ hypothyroid effect.

NURSING MANAGEMENT

ADMINISTRATION: Assess for hx of hypersensitivity ▪ Administe c̄ meals; do *not* crush extended-release tablets ▪ Monitor optimum fluid intake (2-3L/d), Na^+ intake (6-10g/d) ▪ Do *not* mix/concurrently administer syrup c̄ other drugs ▪ Avoid exposure to heat, direct light in storage ▪ Elderly may require ↓ dosage.

EVALUATION: Monitor VS, esp BP ▪ Monitor WBC, ECG ▪ Monitor renal function (I&O, daily weight, urine specific gravity [normal: 1.005-1.025]) ▪ Assess for edema in extremities ▪ Diabetics: closely monitor blood glucose ▪ Monitor lithium blood levels 2 times/wk during treatment, q2-3mo when stabilized ▪ Therapeutic blood levels: 1.0-1.5mEq/L; maintenance, 0.6-1.2mEq/L.

EDUCATION: Dizziness/drowsiness may occur; use caution in potentially hazardous activities ▪ Take as ordered by physician; do *not* ↑ dose ▪ ↑ Fluid intake (10-12 glasses/d) ▪ Maintain normal Na^+ intake (6-10g/d) ▪ Diabetics: closely monitor blood/urine glucose ▪ Take c̄ meals; swallow extended-release tablets whole ▪ Avoid caffeine beverages, ↑ exercise, hot climates, saunas ▪ Keep scheduled appointments c̄ physician/for blood work ▪ Notify physician of symptoms of toxicity (dizziness, blurred vision, trembling, poor coordination) ▪ Women: avoid breastfeeding ▪ Full drug effects may require several wks of therapy.

NOTES:

lomefloxacin hcl • (loe-meh-flox-a-sin)

CATEGORY: *Synthetic antibacterial*: antiinfective, fluoroquinolone Rx; Preg Cat C

BRAND NAME	**DOSAGE FORM**
Maxaquin (Searle)	Tablet: 400mg

ACTION: Bactericidal activity due to interference c̄ DNA gyrase enzyme (required for DNA synthesis) in susceptible organisms, especially gram-negative bacteria. **USE:** Treatment of lower respiratory and UTI caused by susceptible strains of *Citrobacter diversum, Enterobacter cloacae, Escherichia coli, Haemophilus influenzae, Klebsiella pneumoniae, Moraxella catarrhalis, Proteus mirabilis, Pseudomonas aeruginosa, Staphylococcus saprophyticus.* Prophylaxis of postop transurethral surgical procedures infections.

PHARMACOKINETICS

PO absorption	Peak	Half-life	Protein binding	Excretion
95%-98%	1.5h	8h	10%	Via urine (65%) & feces 10% as unchanged drug

CONTRAINDICATIONS: Hypersensitivity to drug or other quinolones.

DOSAGE: For normal renal function

Adult *PO* 400mg qd for 10d for respiratory infections, uncomplicated UTI, and 400mg qd for 14d for complicated infections; 400mg 2-6h preop when prophylaxis for transurethral procedures is appropriate.

SIDE/ADVERSE EFFECTS: CNS: headache (3.2%), dizziness (2.3%), convulsions, hyperkinesia, paresthesia, tremor, somnolence, anxiety, depression, agitation ▪ CV: angina, arrhythmia, ***cardiac failure, cardiomyopathy,*** edema, BP changes, ***pulmonary embolism,*** phlebitis ▪ EENT: abnormal vision, conjunctivitis, earache, tinnitus, eye pain ▪ GI: nausea (3.7%), diarrhea (1.4%), ***bleeding,*** constipation, dyspepsia, flatulence, inflammation, tongue discoloration, taste changes, dry mouth, anorexia ▪ GU: vaginitis, monilia, leukorrhea, intermenstrual bleeding, epididymitis, dysuria, hematuria, micturition disorder ▪

HEM: lymphadenopathy, ↑ fibrinolysis, ***thrombocytopenia,*** thrombocytopenia purpura ▪ INT: photosensitivity (2.4%), pruritus, eczema, exfoliation, rash, urticaria ▪ RESP: bronchospasm, cough, dyspnea, epistaxis ▪ Other: fatigue, back pain, ↓ heat tolerance, flulike symptoms, arthralgia.

DRUG INTERACTIONS: Al and Mg antacids, multivitamins c̄ Fe or Zn and sucralfate ↓ PO absorption ▪ Use c̄ theophylline may ↑ toxicity ▪ Probenecid ↓ lomefloxacin excretion.

NURSING MANAGEMENT

ADMINISTRATION: Assess for hx of quinolone derivative hypersensitivity ▪ Administer c̄ full glass H_2O 1h ac/2h pc at evenly spaced intervals ▪ Assess for CNS disorders; ↓ dosage if impaired ▪ Delay antacid administration for 2h after dose ▪ Avoid exposure to moisture, heat, light in storage ▪ Maintain hydration.

EVALUATION: Monitor VS, esp temperature ▪ Monitor I&O, hepatic, renal status ▪ Assess for CNS toxicity, crystalluria, nephrotoxicity, visual disturbances; D/C drug, notify physician ▪ May ↑ serum ALT, AST, alkaline phosphatase, creatinine, bilirubin, BUN.

EDUCATION: Dizziness/drowsiness may occur; use caution in potentially hazardous activities ▪ Take on empty stomach c̄ full glass H_2O ▪ Take at equal intervals around the clock to maintain blood levels ▪ Take antacids at least 2h after taking drug ▪ Complete full course of therapy even if symptoms subside ▪ ↑ Fluid intake (8-10 glasses/d) ▪ Avoid exposure to direct sunlight, UV light (sunlamp); use sunscreen, protective clothing ▪ Notify physician *immediately* of visual disturbances; D/C drug ▪ Store in dry, tightly closed, light-resistant container ▪ Discard outdated preparations ▪ May cause mouth discomfort, unpleasant taste ▪ Do *not* administer to infants, children ▪ Women: avoid breastfeeding.

NOTES:

loperamide hcl • (loe-per-a-mide)

CATEGORY: *Antidiarrheal agent*

Rx; Preg Cat B

BRAND NAMES
Imodium (Janssen)
Imodium A-D (McNeil)

DOSAGE FORMS
Capsule: 2mg
Caplet: 2mg
Liquid: 1mg/5ml

ACTION: Antidiarrheal effect due to slowing of intestinal motility by direct effect on muscular peristalsis. **USE:** Adjunct in treatment of acute nonspecific diarrhea, chronic diarrhea associated c̄ inflammatory bowel disease ▪ ↓ Ileostomy discharge volume.

PHARMACOKINETICS

PO absorption	Peak	Half-life	Excretion
Adequate	2.5-5h	9.1-14.4h	Primarily via feces as metabolites

CONTRAINDICATIONS: Hypersensitivity, when constipation is contraindicated.

DOSAGE

Pediatric	2.5y/o: 1mg tid d1, followed by 1mg/10kg only after loose stool 5-8y/o: 2mg bid d1, followed by 1mg/10kg only after loose stool 8-12y/o: 2mg tid d1, followed by 1mg/10kg only after loose stool
Adult *PO*	Initial dose 4mg, followed by 2mg after each unformed stool. Do *not* exceed 16mg/d. Usual maintenance dose in chronic diarrhea 4-8mg/d

SIDE/ADVERSE EFFECTS: CNS: drowsiness, dizziness ▪ GI: *N/V, abdominal pain/*distention, constipation, dry mouth ▪ INT: skin rash ▪ Other: tiredness.

DRUG INTERACTIONS: Use c̄ other drugs ↑ their PO absorption.

NURSING MANAGEMENT

ADMINISTRATION: Assess for hx of hypersensitivity ▪ Assess F/E balance; do *not* administer if severely impaired ▪ Assess hepatic function; ↓ dosage if impaired.

EVALUATION: Monitor bowel function; ↓ dose as diarrhea is controlled ▪ Assess hydration status (I&O, daily weight) ▪ Check for signs of abdominal distention; D/C drug ▪ Monitor children, elderly closely (↑ susceptibility to adverse effects).

EDUCATION: Follow clear liquid/bland diet until diarrhea subsides ▪ Take as directed by physician; do *not* ↑ dose ▪ Dizziness/drowsiness may occur; use caution in potentially hazardous activities ▪ Avoid use $\bar{c}$ alcohol, CNS depressants ▪ Notify physician if diarrhea persists >48h, fever occurs ▪ Maintain fluid intake (6-8 glasses/d) ▪ Use sugarless gum/hard candy to diminish dry mouth.

NOTES:

loracarbef •(loe-rah-kar- behf)

CATEGORY: *Antibiotic*: carbacephem, beta-lactam — Rx; Preg Cat B

BRAND NAME
Lorabid (Lilly)

DOSAGE FORMS
Capsules 200mg, powder for PO suspension 100mg/5ml

ACTION: Bactericidal activity due to inhibition of mucopeptide cell wall synthesis in susceptible organisms. Exhibits good resistance to beta-lactamase produced by various bacterial strains. **USE:** Treatment of respiratory infection including bronchitis (acute secondary bacterial or exacerbation of chronic), pneumonia, pharyngitis, sinusitis and tonsillitis, otitis media, uncomplicated skin/skin structure, uncomplicated pyelonephritis caused by susceptible strains of *Escherichia coli, Haemophlius influenzae, Moraxella catarrhalis, Staphylococcus aureus, Staphylococcus saprophyticus, Streptococcus pyogenes.*

PHARMACOKINETICS

PO absorption	Peak	Half-life	Protein binding	Excretion
90%	0.8-1h	1h	25%	Over 90% unchanged via urine

CONTRAINDICATIONS: Hypersensitivity to drug or cephalosporin type antibiotics.

DOSAGE

Adult *PO* (≥13y/o)	Usual dose 200-400mg q12h for 7-10d. Uncomplicated cystitis 200mg q24h for 7d. Pneumonia and uncomplicated pyelonephritis 400mg q12h for 14d.
Pediatric (6mo-2y/o)	Pharyngitis/tonsillitis, impetigo 15mg/kg/d q12h in divided doses for 7-10d. Acute otitis media 30mg/kg/d q12h in divided doses for 10d.

SIDE/ADVERSE EFFECTS: CNS: headache (2.9%), dizziness, nervousness ▪ GI: diarrhea (4.1%), nausea (1.9%), pain (1.4%), anorexia ▪ GU: vaginitis (1.3%) ▪ INT: ***erythrema multiforme,*** pruritus, urticaria ▪ MET: ↑ in SGPT, SGOT, alkaline phosphate, BUN ▪ Other: vasodilation, transient thrombocytopenia, leuokopenia.

Note: Side/adverse effects: common in *italic;* serious in ***boldface italic.***

*Available in Canada only.

DRUG INTERACTIONS: Bacteriostatic antibiotics can antagonize bactericidal activity ▪ Use c̄ PO anticoagulants may ↑ their activity ▪ Use c̄ probenecid will ↓ renal excretion.

NURSING MANAGEMENT

ADMINISTRATION: Assess for hx of cephalosporin/penicillin hypersensitivity ▪ Obtain C&S before therapy ▪ Assess renal status; ↓ dosage if impaired ▪ Administer 1h ac/2h pc c̄ full glass H_2O at evenly spaced intervals ▪ PO suspension: shake well before using ▪ Use caution c̄ ASA/anticoagulants ▪ Do *not* administer c̄ alcohol-containing substances.

EVALUATION: Monitor VS, esp temperature ▪ Observe for signs of superinfection (diarrhea, perineal itching, oral ulcers) ▪ Assess for bleeding, monitor bleeding time; administer vitamin K as ordered ▪ Monitor CBC, renal function ▪ Urine glucose: false (+) c̄ Clinitest; use Clinistix/Tes-Tape.

EDUCATION: Complete full course of therapy ▪ Take on empty stomach at equal intervals around clock to maintain blood levels ▪ Diarrhea may occur; if prolonged, notify physician ▪ Avoid alcohol intake ▪ Report signs of bleeding *immediately* ▪ PO suspension: refrigerate; shake well before use ▪ Store in dry, tightly closed container ▪ Discard outdated preparations ▪ Maintain good personal hygiene, esp perineal, oral ▪ ↑ Fluid intake (8-10 glasses/d) ▪ Use Clinistix/Tes-Tape for urine testing ▪ Notify physician of symptoms of allergic rx (fever, difficult breathing, rash) ▪ Women: avoid breastfeeding ▪ Carry identification (MedicAlert) if cephalosporin allergic.

NOTES:

lorazepam • (lor-az-e-pam)

CATEGORY: *Benzodiazepine:* antianxiety agent, anxiolytic — Rx C-IV; Preg Cat D

BRAND NAMES

Ativan (W-A)

**Novolorazem (Novopharm)*

DOSAGE FORMS

Injection (IM/IV): 2, 4mg/ml
Tablet: 0.5, 1, 2mg
Tablet: 1, 2mg

ACTION: Anxiolytic activity due to depression of CNS at brainstem formation, limbic, thalamic areas. **USE:** Treatment of anxiety, insomnia ▪ Preop sedation.

PHARMACOKINETICS

PO absorption	Peak	Half-life	Protein binding	Excretion
Rapid	2h	12h	85%	Via urine as metabolites

CONTRAINDICATIONS: Hypersensitivity, narrow-angle glaucoma.

DOSAGE

Adult

Anxiety *PO*	2-3mg 2-3 times/d
Insomnia *PO*	2-4mg hs
Pre-op *IM*	0.6mg/kg to a maximum 4mg
IV	2-4mg

SIDE/ADVERSE EFFECTS: CNS: *drowsiness, fatigue, ataxia* ▪ CV: hypotension ▪ HEM: neutropenia (rare) ▪ PSYCH: paradoxical anxiety, hallucinations, hyperexcited states.

DRUG INTERACTIONS: Use $\bar{c}$ other CNS depressants produces additive effects ▪ Use $\bar{c}$ MAO-I can produce serious toxic effects.

NURSING MANAGEMENT

ADMINISTRATION: Assess for hx of benzodiazepine hypersensitivity ▪ Do *not* mix/dilute parenteral preparations (incompatibility); discard discolored/precipitated solution ▪ IM: inject *deep, slowly* into large muscle mass ▪ IV: assess respirations before each dose; administer

Note: Side/adverse effects: common in *italic;* serious in ***boldface italic.***

*Available in Canada only.

slowly (5mg/1ml); keep pt recumbent for 8h ▪ Avoid exposure to heat, moisture, light in storage; avoid plastic for storage of parenteral preparations ▪ Avoid abrupt withdrawal ▪ Have emergency support measures available ▪ Elderly may require ↓ dosage ▪ Problem discussion, sympathetic listening contributes to relief of anxiety.

EVALUATION: Monitor renal, hepatic status ▪ Assess for symptoms of abrupt withdrawal (tremors, abdominal/muscle cramps, convulsions) c̄ prolonged use ▪ Check for signs of dependence (↑ drug request) ▪ Monitor activity status (safety precautions) ▪ Assess for tolerance to therapeutic dose ▪ Assess for paradoxic rxs (CNS stimulation), esp in elderly ▪ Check for depression; suicide precautions prn.

EDUCATION: Drowsiness may occur; use caution in potentially hazardous activities ▪ Avoid use c̄ alcohol, CNS depressants ▪ Indiscriminate use may lead to dependence ▪ Do *not* keep at bedside ▪ Take as ordered by physician, even if symptom free; do *not* ↑ dose ▪ Women: avoid breastfeeding ▪ Check c̄ physician/pharmacist before taking OTC drugs ▪ Practice relaxation exercises, ventilation of feelings.

NOTES:

lovastatin/pravastatin sodium/simvastatin •

(loe-va-stat-in/pra-va-stat-in/sim-va-stat-in)

CATEGORY: *Antilipemic*: lipid altering agent, HMG-CoA reductase inhibitor

Rx; Preg Cat X

BRAND NAMES

lovastatin
Mevacor (MSD)
pravastatin sodium
Pravachol (Apothecon)
simvastatin
Zocor (MSD)

DOSAGE FORMS

Tablet: 20mg
Tablet: 10, 20mg
Tablet: 5, 10, 20, 40mg

ACTION: Lovastatin, pravastatin, simvastatin are inactive-lactone derivative drugs, converted in body to several active metabolites; principal metabolite a potent inhibitor of enzyme HMG-CoA, involved in early synthesis of cholesterol, c̄ marked reduction in hypercholesterolemia, hyperlipidemia; approximately 5% PO dose available for enzyme inhibition (lovastatin and simvastatin), maximum response usually w/in 4-6 wks. **USE:** Adjunct to diet in management of types IIa, IIB[1] hypercholesterolemia.

CONTRAINDICATIONS: Hypersensitivity, pregnancy/lactation, active liver dysfunction/elevated serum transaminase of unknown cause.

PHARMACOKINETICS

	PO absorption	Peak	Protein binding	Excretion
lovastatin	30%	2-4h	95%	10% via urine, 83% via feces, primarily as metabolites
pravastatin sodium	34%	1-1.5h	50%	47% via urine, 53% via feces, primarily as metabolites
simvastatin	85%	4h	95%	13% via urine, 60% via feces, primarily as metabolites

DOSAGE

Adult *PO*

lovastatin	Initial dose 20mg c̄ PM meal. Usual daily range 20-80mg, maximum 80mg/d
pravastatin sodium	Initial dose 10-20mg/d hs. Usual daily range 10-40mg/d hs
simvastatin	Initial dose 5-10mg c̄ PM meal. Usual daily range 5-40mg, maximum 40mg/d

SIDE/ADVERSE EFFECTS: CNS: headache, dizziness ▪ EENT: blurred vision, lens opacities, ophthalmoplegia ▪ GI: constipation, cramps/pain, flatulence, dyspepsia, N/V/D ▪ INT: alopecia, rash, pruritus ▪ MS: cramps/pain, myalgia ▪ Other: edema, ↑ in serum transaminases, URI, chest pain (pravastatin).

DRUG INTERACTIONS: Use c̄ erythromycin, gemfibrozil, niacin can invoke rare cases of rhabdomyolysis ▪ Use c̄ PO anticoagulants requires prothrombin time monitoring.

NURSING MANAGEMENT

ADMINISTRATION: Assess for hx of hypersensitivity ▪ Assess hepatic function; may require ↓ dosage if impaired ▪ Assess for hx of alcoholism; use c̄ caution ▪ Assess serum cholesterol levels ▪ Administer c̄ meals ▪ Avoid exposure to light in storage.

EVALUATION: Monitor hepatic, renal status ▪ Monitor serum cholesterol levels; notify physician if below targeted range (may ↓ dose) ▪ Assess for visual disturbances c̄ prolonged use.

EDUCATION: Take c̄ meals, as ordered by physician; do *not* change dose ▪ Avoid use c̄ alcohol ▪ Notify physician of muscle pain/tenderness, esp c̄ fever/weakness ▪ Report visual disturbances ▪ Follow low-cholesterol diet; maintain optimum body weight ▪ Keep scheduled appointments c̄ physician/for blood work, eye exams ▪ Women: avoid pregnancy, breastfeeding.

NOTES:

loxapine hcl▲/succinate • (<u>lox</u>-a-peen)

CATEGORY: Antipsychotic: tricyclic antipsychotic, neuroleptic Rx; Preg Cat NA

BRAND NAMES
**Loxapac (Lederle)*
Loxitane (Lederle)
Loxitane *IM*
Loxitane C (Lederle)

DOSAGE FORMS
Tablet: 5, 10, 25, 50mg
Capsule: 5, 10, 25, 50mg
Injection: 50mg/ml▲
PO concentrate ▲: 25mg/ml

ACTION: Antipsychotic mechanism not established.
USE: Treatment of psychotic disorders.

SIDE/ADVERSE EFFECTS: CNS: drowsiness, extrapyramidal rxs, tardive dyskinesia ▪ CV: hypotension, tachycardia, hypertension, syncope ▪ EENT: nasal congestion ▪ GI: dry mouth, constipation ▪ GU: urinary retention ▪ INT: dermatitis, seborrhea, photosensitivity, phototoxicity.

DRUG INTERACTIONS: Use c̄ other CNS depressants produces additive depression.

PHARMACOKINETICS

PO absorption	Onset	Peak	Duration	Half-life	Excretion
Complete	20-30m	1.5-3h	12h	5-19h	50% via urine, feces w/in 24h

CONTRAINDICATIONS: Hypersensitivity, coma, presence of large amounts of CNS depressants.

DOSAGE

Adult *PO* Initial dose 10mg bid. Usual maintenance dose 20-100mg/d. Do *not* exceed 250mg/d

IM 12.5-50mg 4-6h or longer for control

NURSING MANAGEMENT
ADMINISTRATION: Assess for hx of amoxapine hypersensitivity ▪ Assess for VS, esp BP ▪ Assess IOP, renal function ▪ PO concentrate: dilute before administration c̄ >60ml orange/grapefruit juice; use manufacturer's dropper to measure dose ▪ IM: inject *slowly, deep* into UOQ of buttock; keep pt lying down for 1/2h after injection ▪

Avoid SC/IV injection ▪ Discard markedly discolored/precipitated solutions ▪ Avoid exposure to moisture, light in storage; do *not* freeze liquid forms ▪ Avoid abrupt withdrawal; D/C gradually ▪ Maintain hydration ▪ Elderly/debilitated may require ↓ dosage.

EVALUATION: Monitor hepatic, ophthalmic, renal status ▪ Monitor BP, CBC ▪ Monitor fluid retention (I&O, daily weight) ▪ Assess for extrapyramidal symptoms (tics/spasms, trembling, shuffling gait) ▪ Seizure precautions in pts c̄ hx of convulsive disorders ▪ Long-term therapy: assess for jaundice, agranulocytosis ▪ Assess for symptoms of abrupt withdrawal (nausea, dyskinesia, trembling, dizziness) ▪ Assess IOP.

EDUCATION: Dizziness/drowsiness may occur; use caution in potentially hazardous activities ▪ Avoid changing positions (lying/sitting/standing) rapidly ▪ Avoid use c̄ alcohol, CNS depressants ▪ Take PO forms c̄ meals ▪ Store in tightly closed, light-resistant container ▪ Use sugarless gum/hard candy to diminish dry mouth ▪ Maintain fluid intake (6-8 glasses/d) ▪ Avoid exposure to direct sunlight, UV light (sunlamps) ▪ Notify physician of fever, sore throat, bruising/bleeding ▪ Notify physician of extrapyramidal symptoms (tics/spasm, trembling, shuffling gait) ▪ Avoid ↑ exercise, temperature extremes ▪ Take as directed by physician ▪ Avoid smoking ▪ Take antacid/antidiarrheal preparations at least 1h before/after drug ▪ Check c̄ physician/pharmacist before taking OTC preparations ▪ Scheduled periodic eye exams ▪ Procedure for PO concentrate administration.

NOTES:

magnesium hydroxide • (mag-nee-zhum hye-drox-ide)

CATEGORY: *Antacid/laxative* OTC

AVAILABLE PREPARATIONS
Suspension (milk/cream of magnesia): 7%-8% $Mg(OH)_2$
Tablets: 375mg

ACTION: Antacid activity due to chemical neutralization of gastric acidity; cathartic activity may be due to hyperosmotic effects of magnesium. **USE:** Antacid/laxative.

PHARMACOKINETICS: Not applicable.

CONTRAINDICATIONS: Appendicitis symptoms, fecal impaction, intestinal obstruction (laxative), severe renal impairment.

DOSAGE
Suspension (MOM) *PO*

Pediatric	1/4-1/2 adult dose
Adult	
Laxative	20-60ml followed by full glass H_2O
Antacid	Usual range of 5-15ml c̄ small glass H_2O up to qid
Tablet	
Adult	1-4 tablets prn

SIDE/ADVERSE EFFECTS: GI: diarrhea (antacid), cramps (laxative).

DRUG INTERACTIONS: Do *not* use c̄ tetracyclines.

NURSING MANAGEMENT
ADMINISTRATION: Shake well before pouring ▪ Antacid: administer 1h ac, hs; follow c̄ H_2O (to reach stomach) ▪ Laxative: administer in AM, hs on empty stomach c̄ full glass H_2O; do *not* administer PO drugs w/in 2h ▪ Avoid exposure to moisture in storage.

EVALUATION: Monitor bowel function (number, quality of stools) ▪ Monitor serum electrolytes (Mg^{++}) ▪ Assess for hypermagnesemia (⬇ reflexes; N/V; ⬇ BP) ▪ Monitor c̄ prolonged use: blood glucose levels ⬆, serum K^+ ⬇.

EDUCATION: Maintain fluid intake (6-8 glasses/d) ▪ Encourage ventilation of feelings ▪ ⬆ Daily exercise ▪ Do *not* take other medications w/in 2h of drug (milk/antacids w/in 1h) ▪ Establish regular bowel elimination ▪ Laxative abuse potential.

NOTES:

magnesium sulfate (injection) • (mag-nee-zhum sul-fate)

CATEGORY: *Anticonvulsant*

Rx; Preg Cat A

AVAILABLE PREPARATIONS
Magnesium sulfate (various)

DOSAGE FORMS
Injection (IM/IV): 10%, 12.5%, 50%

ACTION: Anticonvulsant activity due to inhibition of peripheral neuromuscular transmission. **USE:** Anticonvulsant for seizures associated c̄ epilepsy, pregnancy-induced hypertension ▪ Treatment of Mg deficiency.

PHARMACOKINETICS

	Onset	Duration	Excretion
IV	Immediate	30m	Via urine
IM	1h	3-4h	Via urine

CONTRAINDICATIONS: Heart block/myocardial damage (parenteral), severe renal impairment.

DOSAGE

Anticonvulsant	
Pediatric *IM*	20-40mg/kg
Adult *IM*	1-5g prn
IV	1-4g
Infusion	4g in 250ml 5% dextrose at ≤3ml/m
Cerebral edema	To 2.5g IV
Mg deficiency	
Pediatric	2-10mEq/d
Adult	4-24mEq/d

SIDE/ADVERSE EFFECTS: CNS: depression of deep tendon reflexes ▪ CV: hypotension, depressed cardiac function, circulatory collapse ▪ GI: diarrhea ▪ INT: sweating, flushing ▪ RESP: respiratory depression.

DRUG INTERACTIONS: Use c̄ CNS depressants may ↑ effects ▪ Use c̄ great caution in dig pts.

NURSING MANAGEMENT

ADMINISTRATION: IM: do *not* exceed 50% solution in adults; 1% procaine may be added to ↓ injection pain; *deep* gluteal injection ▪ IV: do *not* exceed 20% solution, 150mg/m ▪ Assess patellar reflex (knee jerk); hold dose until (+) response obtained ▪ Assess respirations; do *not* administer if <16/m ▪ Institute seizure precautions ▪ Do *not* administer discolored/precipitated solutions ▪ Do *not* leave pt unattended ▪ Place pt in left lateral position if pregnant ▪ Assess urinary output (>25ml/h) ▪ Have emergency support equipment available ▪ Avoid abrupt withdrawal ▪ Provide emotional support.

EVALUATION: Monitor CV, renal status ▪ Monitor BP continuously ▪ Monitor serum Mg^{++} levels ▪ Observe for seizure activity; record details (duration, characteristics, pt response) ▪ Monitor respirations (toxicity: <16/m) ▪ Assess patellar reflex; notify physician if hyporeflexic ▪ Monitor urinary output ▪ Assess neonate for Mg^{++} toxicity ▪ Therapeutic serum Mg^{++} concentration: 4-6mEq/L.

EDUCATION: Explain procedure, rationale to pt, family ▪ Safety precautions ▪ Comfort measures.

OVERDOSE MANAGEMENT: Symptoms: hypotension, ↓ respirations/respiratory paralysis, absence of deep tendon reflexes, ↓ fetal heart rate ▪ Treatment: administer IV 10ml 10% aqueous solution calcium gluconate over 3m; *Warning*—do *not* give to dig pts (arrhythmias may occur) ▪ Emergency artificial ventilation may be necessary.

NOTES:

mannitol • (man-i-tole)

CATEGORY: *Osmotic diuretic:* urogenital irrigant — Rx; Preg Cat C

BRAND NAMES

Osmitrol (Baxter)

Resectisol Irrigation (Kendall McGaw)

DOSAGE FORMS

Injection (IV): 5, 10, 15, 20%

Solution: 5%

ACTION: Diuresis due to ↑ in osmotic pressure of glomerular filtrate, which inhibits tubular reabsorption of H_2O solutes, producing rapid urinary excretion. **USE:** Promotion of diuresis in oliguric phase of acute renal failure ▪ ↓ IOP, vitreous volume before surgery ▪ ↓ Intracranial pressure and treatment of cerebral edema ▪ Forced excretion of toxic substances ▪ GU irrigant for transurethral surgical procedures.

PHARMACOKINETICS

Onset	Duration	Half-life	Excretion
30-60m	3-8h	100m	Via urine primarily as unchanged drug

CONTRAINDICATIONS: Hypersensitivity, anuria, severe dehydration/pulmonary congestion, cerebral hemorrhage, severe cardiac/renal dysfunction after institution of therapy.

DOSAGE: Should be administered at rate to produce satisfactory urine flow.

Adult *IV infusion rates*

Renal failure	50-200g/d
Intraocular pressure	1.5-2g/kg over 30-60m
Intracranial pressure	1.5-2g/kg over 30-60m
Toxic substances	Suggested loading dose 25g followed by infusion rate to produce at least 100ml/h urine flow

SIDE/ADVERSE EFFECTS: CNS: headache, ***convulsions*** ▪ CV: anginalike chest pains, edema, ***thrombocytopenia, F/E imbalance***, tachycardia, hypotension, hypertension ▪ EENT: blurred vision ▪ GI: N/V ▪ RESP: ***pulmonary congestion*** ▪ Other: chills, fever.

Note: Side/adverse effects: common in *italic;* serious in ***boldface italic.***

*Available in Canada only.

DRUG INTERACTIONS: Use c̄ lithium salts may ↑ their urinary excretion.

NURSING MANAGEMENT

ADMINISTRATION: Assess renal function; administer test dose if severely impaired ▪ Use in-line filter for concentrations >15% ▪ Do *not* use crystallized solutions; dissolve according to manufacturer's directions ▪ Do *not* mix c̄ blood components in same IV line ▪ Insert indwelling urinary catheter per physician's order ▪ Follow established guidelines for minimal/maximal rate of infusion, desired urinary output.

EVALUATION: Monitor VS, esp BP, respirations ▪ Monitor I&O, urine specific gravity, CVP qh; daily weight ▪ Monitor serum electrolytes (Na^+, K^+, Cl^-) ▪ Check IV site carefully; avoid extravasation ▪ Monitor for signs of ↑ extracellular fluid volume, esp 8-12h postinfusion for rebound fluid overload.

EDUCATION: Avoid changing positions (lying/sitting/standing) rapidly ▪ Urinary catheter inserted for hourly output determinations.

NOTES:

maprotiline hcl • (ma-proe-ti-leen)

CATEGORY: *Tetracyclic antidepressant:* mood elevator Rx; Preg Cat B

BRAND NAME
Ludiomil (Ciba)

DOSAGE FORMS
Tablet: 25, 50, 75mg

ACTION: Antidepressant activity appears related to inhibition of norepinephrine reuptake in central adrenergic neurons; drug is tetracyclic, extremely close to tricyclic drugs. **USE:** Treatment of depressive neurosis (dysthymic disorder), manic depressive states ▪ Treatment of anxiety associated c̄ depression.

PHARMACOKINETICS

PO absorption	Peak	Half-life	Protein binding	Excretion
Slow but complete	8-24h	51h	88%	60%-70% via urine, 30% via feces as metabolites

CONTRAINDICATIONS: Hypersensitivity, MAO-I therapy, myocardial infarction (acute recovery period), glaucoma.

DOSAGE

Adult *PO*	75-225mg/d
Geriatric *PO*	50-75mg/d

SIDE/ADVERSE EFFECTS: CNS: *drowsiness*, dizziness, headache, incoordination, tremors, extrapyramidal symptoms, paresthesia (extremities), insomnia ▪ CV: ***arrhythmias,*** myocardial infarction, stroke, ***heart block,*** postural hypotension ▪ GI: anorexia, N/V/D, stomatitis, cramps, black tongue, dry mouth, constipation ▪ GU: gynecomastia, testicular swelling, galactorrhea, breast enlargement, urinary hesitancy ▪ HEM: ***agranulocytosis***, eosinophilia, ***thrombocytopenia*** ▪ HEP: cholestatic jaundice ▪ INT: skin rash, photosensitivity, alopecia ▪ PSYCH: disorientation, delusions, hallucinations, exacerbation of psychosis, confusion ▪ Other: parotid swelling.

DRUG INTERACTIONS: Significant depressant effects c̄ alcohol ▪ Use c̄ anticholinergics, chlorpromazine may produce ↑ atropinelike effects; paralytic ileus could occur ▪ Significant ↑ in activity c̄ epinephrine, levarterenol, other adrenergic agents ▪ Significant antagonism to effects of reserpine, clonidine, guanethidine-type antihypertensives ▪ Use c̄ MAO-I best avoided.

NURSING MANAGEMENT

ADMINISTRATION: Assess for hx of tricyclic antidepressant hypersensitivity ▪ Assess for hx of glaucoma, prostatic hypertrophy, renal/hepatic disease; may require ↓ dosage ▪ PO: administer as single dose/d hs c̄ food ▪ Institute safety precautions ▪ Institute suicide precautions ▪ Dosage is ↑ *slowly*; maintenance dose is lowest dose that will maintain remission of depression ▪ Avoid abrupt withdrawal; D/C gradually ▪ Heavy smokers may require ↑ dosage ▪ Elderly may require ↓ dosage.

EVALUATION: Monitor CV, hepatic, renal status ▪ Monitor VS, esp BP ▪ Monitor CBC, esp long-term ▪ Monitor fluid retention (I&O, daily weight), constipation ▪ Assess for symptoms of abrupt withdrawal (nausea, headache, malaise) ▪ Assess for actual swallowing of PO forms.

EDUCATION: Dizziness/drowsiness may occur; use caution in potentially hazardous activities ▪ Avoid changing positions (lying/sitting/standing) rapidly ▪ Avoid use c̄ alcohol, other CNS depressants for up to 1 wk after end of therapy ▪ Take c̄ food to ↓ GI irritation ▪ Take as directed by physician ▪ Use sugarless gum/hard candy to diminish dry mouth ▪ Constipation may occur; ↑ fluids, bulk-containing foods ▪ Check c̄ physician before taking OTC/Rx preparations ▪ May produce peculiar taste ▪ Notify physician/ dentist of use before treatment ▪ Store in tightly closed container ▪ Avoid exposure to direct sunlight, UV light (sunlamps); use sunscreen, protective clothing ▪ Encourage recreational/diversional interests ▪ Notify physician of fever, sore throat, malaise ▪ Keep scheduled appointments c̄ physician ▪ Full drug effects may require several wks of therapy.

NOTES:

medroxyprogesterone acetate • (me-drox-ee-proe-jess-te-rone)

CATEGORY: *Progestational hormone* Rx; Preg Cat X

BRAND NAMES	**DOSAGE FORMS**
Amen (Carmick)	Tablet: 10mg
Cycrin (W-A)	Tablet: 10mg
Provera (Upjohn)	Tablet: 2.5, 5, 10mg

ACTION: Progestational agents affect pituitary gland, uterus, vaginal mucosa, mammary glands; inhibit pituitary gonadotropin, resulting in ovarian suppression; uterine effect incl relaxation of uterine smooth muscle, ↑ secretory phase of endometrial development; vaginal mucosa exhibits ↑ mucification; other effects incl stimulation of mammary tissue growth, progesterone withdrawal resulting in menstruation. **USE:** Amenorrhea ▪ Abnormal uterine bleeding due to hormonal imbalance in absence of organic disease.

PHARMACOKINETICS: Good PO absorption; excreted as conjugated metabolites via urine.

CONTRAINDICATIONS: Hypersensitivity, past hx of thrombophlebitis, thromboembolic disorders, cerebral apoplexy, suspected breast/genital malignancy, liver disease.

DOSAGE

Adult *PO*

Amenorrhea	5-10mg/d for 5-10d. Withdrawal bleeding usually w/in 3-7d after ending therapy
Uterine bleeding	5-10mg/d for 5-10d beginning on calculated d 16 or 21 of menstrual cycle. Withdrawal bleeding usually w/in 3-7d after ending therapy

SIDE/ADVERSE EFFECTS: CV: edema, ***thrombophlebitis, pulmonary embolism*** ▪ END: galactorrhea ▪ GU: breakthrough bleeding, spotting, menstrual flow change, amenorrhea, cervical erosion/secretions ▪ HEP: cholestatic jaundice ▪ INT: acne, alopecia, hirsutism, urticaria, pruritus, rash ▪ PSYCH: depression.

DRUG INTERACTIONS: Possible ↓ in glucose tolerance; accordingly, antidiabetic agents may require dose adjustments.

Note: Side/adverse effects: common in *italic;* serious in ***boldface italic.***

*Available in Canada only.

NURSING MANAGEMENT

ADMINISTRATION: Assess for hx of progestin hypersensitivity ▪ PO: administer c̄ meals ▪ Avoid exposure to light in storage.

EVALUATION: Monitor VS, esp BP, pulse ▪ Monitor hydration status (I&O, daily weight) ▪ Assess emotional status (mental depression) ▪ Monitor hepatic status.

EDUCATION: Review package insert c̄ pt ▪ Take as directed by physician ▪ Avoid exposure to direct sunlight, UV light (sunlamps); use sunscreen ▪ Keep scheduled appointments c̄ physician/for Pap/pelvic exams ▪ Notify physician/dentist of use before therapy ▪ Women: avoid breastfeeding, pregnancy; menstrual changes may occur ▪ Procedure for breast self-exam ▪ Symptoms of thrombotic episodes (sudden shortness of breath, migraine headache, chest pain, diplopia).

NOTES:

melphalan • (mel-fa-lan)

CATEGORY: *Alkylating agent:* antineoplastic — Rx; Preg Cat D

BRAND NAME
Alkeran (B-W)

DOSAGE FORMS
Tablet: 2mg

ACTION: Antineoplastic activity due to alkylating effect on DNA replication. **USE:** Treatment of multiple myeloma, epithelial/ovarian cancer.

PHARMACOKINETICS

PO absorption	Peak	Half-life	Excretion
Incomplete	2h	1.5h	10% unchanged in urine w/in 24h

CONTRAINDICATIONS: Depressed neutrophil/platelet count, recent radiation/similar antineoplastic therapy, hypersensitivity, prior resistance to drug.

DOSAGE

Pediatric/ Adult *PO*	Usual dose 6mg/d for 2-3 wks. D/C drug for up to 4wks. Usual maintenance dose 2mg/d Ovarian cancer: 0.2mg/kg/d for 5d. Can be repeated every 4-5wks

SIDE/ADVERSE EFFECTS: GI: *N/V/D,* oral ulcers ▪ HEM: *dose-related depression of bone marrow resulting in anemia, neutropenia,* ***thrombocytopenia*** ▪ INT: *alopecia,* rash ▪ RESP: ***pulmonary fibrosis***, interstitial pneumonitis.

DRUG INTERACTIONS: Live vaccines contraindicated during therapy ▪ Radiation/other myelosuppressive drugs produce additive bone marrow depression.

Note: Side/adverse effects: common in *italic;* serious in ***boldface italic.***

*Available in Canada only.

NURSING MANAGEMENT

ADMINISTRATION: Assess for hx of hypersensitivity (incl chlorambucil) ▪ Check pt hx for recent course of radiation/antineoplastic therapy; report to physician ▪ Avoid exposure to moisture, light in storage ▪ Administer antiemetic before therapy ▪ Force liquids (3000ml/d) ▪ Provide emotional support.

EVALUATION: Monitor CBC throughout therapy ▪ Assess for infection, bleeding, anemia ▪ Assess for ↑ serum uric acid levels ▪ Monitor hepatic function during therapy ▪ Assess hydration status (I&O, daily weight).

EDUCATION: Store in tightly closed, light-resistant container ▪ ↑ Fluid intake (10-12 glasses/d) ▪ Avoid exposure to infection ▪ Check c̄ physician before immunization (pt, family) ▪ Diet as tolerated; avoid spicy foods ▪ Maintain good oral hygiene; use soft-bristled toothbrush ▪ Notify physician of symptoms of bone marrow depression (fever, sore throat, bruising, bleeding, lethargy) ▪ Loss of hair may occur (reversible) ▪ Compliance c̄ prescribed dosage regimen ▪ Women: avoid breastfeeding ▪ Encourage ventilation of feelings ▪ Use contraception if sexually active.

NOTES:

meperidine hcl • (me-per-i-deen)

CATEGORY: *Narcotic*: synthetic opiate

Rx C-II; Preg Cat NA

BRAND NAME
Demerol HCl (Winthrop)

DOSAGE FORMS
Injection (IM/IV/SC): 25, 50, 75, 100mg/ml; syrup: 50mg/ml; tablet: 50,100mg

ACTION: Narcotics produce analgesia, euphoria, sedation; equianalgesic doses of meperidine, morphine produce same amount of euphoria, respiratory depression, sedation, addiction liability; PO administration significantly less effective; 70mg equivalent to 10mg morphine.
USE: Relief of moderate/severe pain ▪ Preop sedation, postop analgesia, obs analgesia, support of anesthesia.

DOSAGE

Analgesic	
Pediatric *PO/IM/SC*	0.5-0.8mg/lb q3-4h prn
Adult *PO/IM/SC*	50-150mg q3-4h prn
OB *IM/SC*	50-100mg when pain is regular. May be repeated every 1-3h
Anesthesia	Titrated against pt needs by IV injection/continuous infusion
Pre-op	
Pediatric *IM/SC*	0.5-1mg/kg 30-90m before anesthesia
Adult *IM/SC*	50-100mg 30-90m before anesthesia

PHARMACOKINETICS

	Onset	Peak	Duration	Protein binding	Half-life	Excretion
PO	15-20m	60m	2-4h	60%-70%	4-8h	Renal as metabolites, 5% unchanged
IM	10m	40-60m	2-4h	60%-70%	4-8h	
SC	10m	30-50m	2-4h	60%-70%	4-8h	

CONTRAINDICATIONS: Hypersensitivity, $\bar{c}$ MAO-I therapy, nursing mothers.

SIDE/ADVERSE EFFECTS: CNS: *sedation, lightheadedness,* euphoria, dysphoria, weakness, tremor, disorientation, transient hallucinations ▪ CV: hypotension, palpitation, flushing of face, phlebitis after IV administration ▪ GI: *N/V,* dry mouth, biliary tract spasm, constipation ▪ GU: urinary retention ▪ INT: *sweating,* pruritus, urticaria ▪ RESP: respiratory depression ▪ Other: addiction.

DRUG INTERACTIONS: Use c̄ alcohol, antihistamines, barbiturates, benzodiazepines, methotrimeprazine, phenothiazines, depressants can produce additive CNS depression; ↓ dosage may be required.

NURSING MANAGEMENT

ADMINISTRATION: Assess for hx of hypersensitivity ▪ Store under double lock/key; document use accurately ▪ Check compatibility chart for mixing preop IM preparations ▪ Do *not* administer if respirations <12/m ▪ IM: inject *deep* into muscle; rotate sites ▪ IV: dilute; administer *slowly* ▪ Have narcotic antagonist, support measures available ▪ Avoid administration in pts c̄ suspected head injury ▪ Administer *before* pt has intense pain ▪ Utilize + power of suggestion ▪ Avoid abrupt withdrawal c̄ long-term use ▪ Elderly may require ↓ dosage.

EVALUATION: Monitor respirations, circulatory function ▪ Assess bowel function, abdominal distention ▪ Assess renal function, urinary retention ▪ Check for signs of dependence (↑ drug request) ▪ Assess for potentiation of CNS depressant effect ▪ Assess for N/V; administer antiemetic ▪ Assess for signs of overdose (coma, pinpoint pupils, respiratory depression).

EDUCATION: Avoid changing positions (lying/sitting/standing) rapidly ▪ Avoid excessive sensory stimulation ▪ Keep bedrails up when nonambulatory ▪ Obtain assistance prn when ambulatory ▪ Turn, cough, deep-breathe after surgery ▪ Constipation may occur; ↑ fluids, bulk-containing foods ▪ Avoid potentially hazardous activities ▪ Avoid smoking ▪ Indiscriminate use may lead to severe dependence ▪ Avoid use c̄ alcohol, CNS depressants.

OVERDOSE MANAGEMENT: *See* Narcotics.

NOTES:

mephobarbital (methylphenobarbital) • (me-foe-bar-bi-tal)

CATEGORY: *Barbiturate:* anticonvulsant, sedative — Rx C-IV; Preg Cat NA

BRAND NAME
Mebaral (SW)

DOSAGE FORMS
Tablet: 32, 50, 100mg

ACTION: Anticonvulsant activty due to depression of motor cortex; after administration, up to 75% converted to phenobarbital by liver. **USE:** Control of grand mal, petit mal seizures ▪ Sedative.

PHARMACOKINETICS

PO absorption	Onset	Duration	Excretion
50%	30-60m	10-16h	Via urine as metabolites

CONTRAINDICATIONS: Hypersensitivity, severe liver/respiratory impairment, porphyria, addiction.

DOSAGE

Anticonvulsant	
Pediatric *PO*	<5y/o: 16-32 mg 3-4 times/d >5y/o: 32-64mg 3-4 times/d
Adult *PO*	400-600mg/d
Sedative	
Pediatric *PO*	16-32mg 3-4 times/d
Adult *PO*	32-100mg 3-4 times/d

SIDE/ADVERSE EFFECTS: CNS: *drowsiness, lethargy,* headache, dizziness, paradoxical restlessness/excitement, *hangover* ▪ GI: N/V ▪ INT: morbilliform rash, ***Stevens-Johnson syndrome***, urticaria ▪ Other: drug tolerance/ addiction, asthma, angioneurotic edema.

DRUG INTERACTIONS: Use c̄ alcohol, antihistamines, benzodiazepines, methotrimeprazine, narcotics, tranquilizers ↑ depressant effects ▪ Barbiturates are enzyme inducers, can ↓ effect of PO anticoagulants, other drugs ▪ MAO-I ↑ activity of barbiturates ▪ Barbiturates ↓ PO absorption of griseofulvin.

NURSING MANAGEMENT

ADMINISTRATION: Assess for hx of barbiturate hypersensitivity ▪ Do *not* administer if respirations <12/m ▪ Avoid exposure to moisture in storage ▪ Avoid abrupt withdrawal; institute strict seizure precautions if drug abruptly withdrawn ▪ Elderly may require ↓ dosage.

EVALUATION: Monitor hepatic, renal, cardiac, respiratory status ▪ Monitor occurrence/characteristics of seizures ▪ Assess for symptoms of abrupt withdrawal (tremors, abdominal/muscle cramps, convulsions) c̄ prolonged use ▪ Assess for actual swallowing of PO forms ▪ Check for signs of dependence (↑ drug request) ▪ Monitor activity status (safety precautions) ▪ Assess for tolerance/barbiturate cross-tolerance to therapeutic dose ▪ Assess for paradoxic rxs (CNS stimulation), esp in elderly ▪ Observe pt sleep patterns ▪ Check for depression; suicide precautions prn.

EDUCATION: Drowsiness may occur; use caution in potentially hazardous activities ▪ Avoid use c̄ alcohol, other CNS depressants ▪ Indiscriminate use may lead to dependence ▪ Do *not* keep at bedside ▪ Take as ordered by physician; do *not* ↑ dose ▪ Store in tightly closed container ▪ Safety precautions may be instituted (bedrails) ▪ Do *not* smoke after taking drugs ▪ Practice relaxation exercises, ventilation of feelings ▪ Utilize sleep producers (reading, warm milk, soft music) ▪ Women: avoid breastfeeding ▪ Carry medical identification (MedicAlert) ▪ Do *not* omit daily dose.

OVERDOSE MANAGEMENT: Principal symptoms: exaggerated CNS depression ▪ Respiration depressed, pupils may be constricted, shock, coma ▪ Emergency medical treatment: Remove drug by lavage/emesis, maintain respiration; administer IV fluids, vasopressor to maintain BP; force renal excretion c̄ osmotic diuretics; hemodialysis if indicated.

NOTES:

metaproterenol sulfate • (met-a-proe-ter-e-nole)

CATEGORY: *Sympathomimetic:* $beta_2$ adrenergic, bronchodilator Rx; Preg Cat C

BRAND NAMES	DOSAGE FORMS
Alupent (B-I)	Inhaler: 0.65mg/dose Solution: 0.4%, 0.6%, 5% Syrup: 10mg/5ml Tablet: 10, 20mg
Metaprel (Sandoz)	Inhaler: 0.65mg/dose Solution: 5% Syrup: 10mg/5ml Tablet: 10, 20mg

ACTION: Sympathomimetic activity at $beta_2$ adrenergic receptors produces bronchodilation. **USE:** Treatment of bronchial asthma; reversible bronchospasm associated c̄ bronchitis, emphysema.

PHARMACOKINETICS

PO absorption	Onset	Peak	Excretion
Good	15m	1h	Via urine primarily as metabolites

CONTRAINDICATIONS: Hypersensitivity, cardiac arrhythmia associated c̄ tachycardia.

DOSAGE

Pediatric *PO*	6-9y/o: 10mg 3-4 times/d >9y/0: 20mg 3-4 times/d
Adult *PO*	20mg 3-4 times/d
Pediatric/ Adult *Inhalation*	Inhaler: single dose (2-3 inhalations) every 3-4h Bulb nebulizer: 10 inhalations 5% solution: 0.3ml c̄ IPPB

SIDE/ADVERSE EFFECTS: CNS: nervousness, tremors, headache, drowsiness ▪ CV: ↑ heart rate, palpitations ▪ GI: N/V ▪ MS: muscle cramps.

DRUG INTERACTIONS: Use c̄ nonselective beta blockers (eg, propranolol) antagonizes bronchodilation ▪ Use c̄ MAO-I requires supervision ▪ Use c̄ other sympathomimetics best avoided.

Note: Side/adverse effects: common in *italic;* serious in ***boldface italic.***

*Available in Canada only.

NURSING MANAGEMENT

ADMINISTRATION: Assess for hx of catecholamine hypersensitivity (incl sulfites) ▪ Avoid concurrent administration of epinephrine, other sympathomimetic agents ▪ PO: administer c̄ food to ↓ GI upset ▪ Inhalation: consult manufacturer's directions; excessive use may ↓ effectiveness; rinse mouth c̄ H_2O after administration ▪ Avoid exposure to heat, light in storage ▪ Elderly may require ↓ dosage ▪ Administer adrenocorticoid inhalations 15m before this aerosol for ↑ effectiveness (if ordered).

EVALUATION: Monitor VS, esp BP, heart rate; D/C drug if >120 ▪ Monitor respiratory rate, sputum ▪ Monitor I&O.

EDUCATION: Tolerance to drug effect may develop; report to physician ▪ Take as ordered by physician; do *not* ↑ dose ▪ Notify physician *immediately* of rapid/"skipped" heartbeats, chest pain, tremors; D/C drug ▪ Report to physician failure to respond to usual dose (tolerance) ▪ Store in tightly closed, light-resistant container ▪ Procedure for inhalation administration (shake well; exhale via nose; administer while inhaling deeply through mouth; exhale slowly after 10s; wait 2m before next dose) ▪ Inhalation: may produce unpleasant taste; excessive use of aerosol may cause paradoxical (rebound) bronchospasm ▪ Check c̄ physician/pharmacist before using OTC preparations.

NOTES:

metaraminol bitartrate • (met-a-ram-i-nole)

CATEGORY: *Sympathomimetic*: vasopressor — Rx; Preg Cat C

BRAND NAME	DOSAGE FORMS
Aramine (MSD)	Injection (IM/IV/SC): 10mg/ml

ACTION: Adrenergic effect due to alpha, $beta_1$ adrenergic agonist activity, resulting in vasoconstriction, positive inotropic cardiac effect. **USE:** Prevention/treatment of acute hypotension due to spinal anesthesia ▪ Adjunct in hypotension due to drugs, hemorrhage, surgical complications, shock associated c̄ brain damage.

PHARMACOKINETICS: Onset of pressor activity about 10m IM, 5-20m SC, 1-2m IV; excretion via urine.

CONTRAINDICATIONS: Hypersensitivity.

DOSAGE

Adult *IM/SC*	2-10mg. Wait 10m before giving additional dosage
IV infusion	15-100mg in 500ml solution, administered at rate to maintain satisfactory BP. Severe shock may require direct IV injection 0.5-5mg, followed by infusion

SIDE/ADVERSE EFFECTS: CV: ***ventricular tachycardia, other arrhythmias*** ▪ Other: tissue necrosis.

DRUG INTERACTIONS: Avoid use c̄ cyclopropane, halothane, MAO-I, tricyclic antidepressants, reserpine, guanethidine.

NURSING MANAGEMENT

ADMINISTRATION: Assess for hx of catecholamine hypersensitivity (incl sulfites) ▪ Assess circulatory status; do *not* administer SC if impaired ▪ Assess F/E balance; correct deficiencies ▪ IV: infuse into large vein; use microdrip/infusion pump; do *not* mix c̄ other drugs in solution; keep vein open after D/C in case therapy must be reinstituted (↓ BP) ▪ Have atropine (for bradycardia), phentolamine (↓ pressor effect), emergency support equipment available ▪ Do *not* leave pt unattended ▪ Avoid exposure to heat, light ▪ Withdraw drug *gradually*.

EVALUATION: Monitor VS, esp BP (q5m until stable, then q15m) ▪ Monitor I&O q1h ▪ Monitor serum electrolytes (Na^+, K^+) ▪ Cardiac monitoring ▪ Check IV site carefully; avoid extravasation ▪ Continue monitoring BP after D/C; resume if ↓ BP ▪ Diabetics: monitor blood glucose carefully.

EDUCATION: Notify physician/nurse of abnormal rxs (difficult breathing, chest pain, irregular heartbeat).

NOTES:

methadone hcl • (meth-a-doan)

CATEGORY: *Narcotic*: synthetic opiate

Rx C-II; Preg Cat NA

BRAND NAME
Dolophine (Lilly)

DOSAGE FORMS
Injection (IM/SC): 10mg/ml
Tablet: 5, 10mg

DOSAGE
Adult *PO/IM/SC*

Analgesic	2.5-10mg q3-4h
Detoxification	≥40mg once/d. Gradually ↓ dose every few days
Maintenance	≥40-120mg once/d

ACTION: Narcotics produce analgesia, euphoria, sedation; methadone has high misuse potential/addiction liability; very long half-life, which makes it suitable for addiction maintenance programs. **USE:** Relief of severe pain ▪ Detoxification of narcotic addiction ▪ Methadone maintenance of narcotic addiction.

PHARMACOKINETICS

PO absorption	Onset	Duration	Methadone maintenance duration	Protein binding	Excretion
Complete	10-15m	4-6h	22-48h	High	Via urine, feces

CONTRAINDICATIONS: Hypersensitivity; use c̄ extreme caution in head injuries.

SIDE/ADVERSE EFFECTS: CNS: *sedation, lightheadedness*, euphoria, dysphoria, tremors, disorientation, ↓ convulsive threshold ▪ CV: hypotension, palpitations, flushing of face ▪ EENT: miosis ▪ GI: *N/V,* dry mouth, constipation, biliary tract spasm ▪ GU: urine retention ▪ INT: pruritus, urticaria ▪ RESP: ***respiratory depression***.

Note: Side/adverse effects: common in *italic;* serious in ***boldface italic.***

*Available in Canada only.

DRUG INTERACTIONS: Use c̄ alcohol, antihistamines, barbiturates, benzodiazepines, methotrimeprazine, phenothiazines, other CNS depressants produces additive CNS depression; dosage reduction may be required ▪ Use c̄ tricyclic antidepressants may produce additive respiratory depression.

NURSING MANAGEMENT

ADMINISTRATION: Assess for hx of opioid hypersensitivity ▪ Assess quality, intensity, location of pain ▪ Store under double lock/key; document use accurately ▪ Check compatibility for mixing c̄ other drugs in solution ▪ Do *not* administer if respirations are <12/m ▪ IM: inject *deep* into muscle; rotate sites ▪ Have narcotic antagonist (naloxone), support measures available ▪ Avoid administration in pts with suspected head injuries ▪ Administer *before* pt has intense pain ▪ Administer around clock to pt c̄ severe, chronic pain ▪ Utilize + power of suggestion ▪ Avoid abrupt withdrawal c̄ long-term use ▪ Elderly may require ↓ dosage.

EVALUATION: Monitor respirations, circulatory function, esp BP ▪ Assess bowel function, abdominal distention ▪ Assess renal function, urinary retention ▪ Check for signs of dependence (↑ drug request) ▪ Assess for potentiation of CNS depressant effect ▪ Assess for N/V; administer antiemetic ▪ Assess for signs of overdose (coma, pinpoint pupils, respiratory depression) ▪ SC: check for tissue irritation ▪ May produce ↑ CSF pressure.

EDUCATION: Avoid changing positions rapidly ▪ Avoid excessive sensory stimulation ▪ Keep bedrails up when nonambulatory ▪ Turn, cough, deep-breathe after surgery ▪ Constipation may occur; ↑ fluids, bulk-containing foods ▪ Avoid potentially hazardous activities ▪ Avoid smoking ▪ Indiscriminate use may lead to severe dependence ▪ Avoid use c̄ alcohol, other CNS depressants ▪ Women: avoid breastfeeding ▪ Take as ordered by physician; do *not* ↑ dose ▪ Notify physician/dentist of use before treatment.

OVERDOSE MANAGEMENT: *See* Narcotics.

NOTES:

methicillin sodium • (meth-i-sill-in)

CATEGORY: *Penicillinase-resistant penicillin*: antibiotic Rx; Preg Cat B

BRAND NAME
Staphcillin (Squibb)

DOSAGE FORMS
Powder for injection (IM/IV): 1, 4, 6, 10g vial

ACTION: Bacteriostatic activity due to inhibition of mucopeptide cell wall synthesis in susceptible organisms. **USE:** Treatment of infections due to susceptible strains of penicillinase-producing staphylococci.

PHARMACOKINETICS

IM peak	Half-life	Protein binding	Excretion
30-60m	0.5h	40%	Via urine primarily as unchanged drug

CONTRAINDICATIONS: Hypersensitivity to any penicillin.

DOSAGE

Pediatric *IM*	25mg/kg q6h
Adult *IM*	1g q4-6h
IV	1g q6h

SIDE/ADVERSE EFFECTS: CNS: neuropathy usually associated c̄ high parenteral doses ▪ GI: N/V/D, epigastric distress, black hairy tongue, flatulence, smell/taste disturbances ▪ GU: rare instances of ***interstitial nephritis*** usually associated c̄ methicillin ▪ HEM: anemia, eosinophilia, leukopenia, neutropenia, ***thrombocytopenia*** ▪ HEP: ↑ serum levels of AST, ALT, LDH ▪ INT: rash, pruritus, urticaria ▪ MS: arthralgia ▪ Other: *local irritation at injection site*, fever, ***anaphylaxis***.

DRUG INTERACTIONS: Bacteriostatic antibiotics c̄ any penicillin can lead to antibiotic antagonism ▪ PO anticoagulant therapy may require dose adjustments.

NURSING MANAGEMENT

ADMINISTRATION: Assess for hx of penicillin, cephalosporin hypersensitivity ▪ Obtain C&S before therapy ▪ Assess renal function; ↓ dose if impaired (esp neonates) ▪ Maintain blood levels; administer at equal intervals around clock ▪ Reconstitute powder according to manufacturer's directions c̄ sterile H_2O for injection; stable for 24h at room temperature, 4d refrigerated ▪ IM: administer by *deep* intragluteal injection ▪ IV: (direct) dilute each ml c̄ 25ml NaCl injection, inject 10ml/m; (drip) mix c̄ diluent recommended by manufacturer; use only 24-48h because of possibility of thrombophlebitis (esp elderly) ▪ Do *not* administer bacteriostatic agents w/in 1h ▪ Do *not* administer discolored/precipitated solutions ▪ Do *not* mix c̄ other drugs ▪ Na^+ content: 2.9-3.1mEq (67-71mg)/g; calculate in Na^+-restricted diets ▪ Have support equipment available for anaphylaxis.

EVALUATION: Monitor pts c̄ allergies/asthma (high risk for hypersensitivity) ▪ Monitor renal, hepatic, hemopoietic status ▪ Observe for signs of superinfection (diarrhea, perineal itching, oral ulcers) ▪ Monitor VS, esp temperature ▪ Monitor IV site closely (thrombophlebitis); rotate site q48h.

EDUCATION: Diarrhea may occur ▪ Maintain good personal hygiene (esp perineal, oral) ▪ Maintain fluid intake (6-8 glasses/d) ▪ Notify physician of symptoms of allergic rx (fever, difficult breathing, rash) ▪ Carry identification (MedicAlert) if penicillin allergic.

NOTES:

methotrexate/methotrexate sodium▲ (amethopterin, mtx) •

(meth-oh-trex-ate)

CATEGORY: *Antineoplastic*: antimetabolic, folic acid antagonist Rx; Preg Cat X

BRAND NAMES	**DOSAGE FORMS**
Folex, Folex PFS (Adria)	Injection (IM/IV), powder for injection ▲
Methotrexate (Lederle)	Tablet: 2.5mg
Rheumatrex (Lederle)	Dose pack: 2.5mg

ACTION: Antimetabolic activity due to competitive inhibition of dehydrofolate reductase, which inhibits folic acid synthesis. **USE:** Treatment of gestational choriocarcinoma, chorioadenoma destruens, hadatidiform mole, lymphoblastic/meningeal leukemias ▪ Treatment of breast cancer, epidermoid cancer of head/neck, lung cancer ▪ Treatment of Burkitt lymphoma, advanced states (III, IV) of lymphosarcoma, advanced mycosis fungoides, disabling psoriasis.

PHARMACOKINETICS: PO peak 1-2h; excreted unchanged.

CONTRAINDICATIONS: Psoriasis in pregnant pts or pts c̄ preexisting blood dyscrasias, liver, kidney impairment.

DOSAGE: Must be individualized.

Trophoblastic tumor	15-30mg/d *PO/IM* for 5d, repeated 3-5 times c̄ ≥1 rest wk between courses
Lymphoblastic leukemia	3.3mg/m^2 c̄ prednisone 60mg/m^2/d. After remission, 30mg/m^2 *PO/IM* twice/wk or 2.5mg/kg IV q14d
Meningeal leukemia	12mg/m^2 intrathecal q2-5d
Lymphoma	10-25mg/d *PO* for 4-8d for several courses c̄ 7-10d rest period
Mycosis fungoides	2.5-10mg/d *PO* for wks/mo
Psoriasis	10-25mg/wk as single *PO/IM/IV* dose. Do *not* exceed dose of 50mg/wk

SIDE/ADVERSE EFFECTS: CNS: headache, drowsiness, aphasia, paresis, ***convulsions***, blurred vision ▪ GI: *N/V/D*, *abdominal distress*, ***ulcerative stomatitis***, anorexia, gingivitis, ***bleeding, hematemesis*** ▪ GU: ***renal failure***,

Note: Side/adverse effects: common in *italic;* serious in ***boldface italic.***

*Available in Canada only.

azotemia, cystitis, ***hematuria***, menstrual dysfunction, abortion, fetal teratogenesis, severe nephropathy ▪ HEM: ***bone marrow depression,*** *leukopenia*, ***thrombocytopenia,*** anemia, ***hypogammaglobulinemia,*** hemorrhage, septicemia ▪ HEP: hepatic toxicity ▪ INT: erythematous rash, pruritus, urticaria, photosensitivity, depigmentation, alopecia ▪ RESP: ***interstitial pneumonitis, chronic interstitial obstructive pulmonary disease.***

DRUG INTERACTIONS: Use c̄ PO hypoglycemics, phenylbutazone, salicylates, sulfonamide, thiazides can ↑ MTX toxicity due to protein storage site displacement ▪ Use c̄ alcohol, other hepatotoxic drugs ↑ toxic effect ▪ Salicylates, probenecid ↓ MTX renal excretion ▪ Folic acid preparations (vitamins) can antagonize antineoplastic effect ▪ Use c̄ PO anticoagulants may enhance their effects.

NURSING MANAGEMENT

ADMINISTRATION: Check pt hx for recent course of radiation/antineoplastic agents ▪ Assess oral cavity for ulceration ▪ Assess renal function; may require ↓ dosage if impaired ▪ Administer antiemetic before therapy ▪ PO: administer 1h ac/2h pc ▪ Parenteral: dilute according to manufacturer's directions; administer by *slow* IV push ▪ Avoid exposure to moisture, light in storage.

EVALUATION: Monitor CBC; neurologic, hepatic function ▪ Assess for infection, bleeding, anemia ▪ May produce hyperglycemia; monitor diabetics closely ▪ Assess hydration status.

EDUCATION: Store in dry, tightly closed, light-resistant container ▪ ↑ Fluid intake (8-10 glasses/d) ▪ Avoid exposure to infection ▪ Check c̄ physician before immunization ▪ Diet as tolerated; avoid spicy foods ▪ Maintain good oral hygiene; use soft-bristled toothbrush ▪ Notify physician of symptoms of bone marrow depression (fever, sore throat, bruising, bleeding, lethargy) ▪ Avoid exposure to direct sunlight, UV light ▪ Loss of hair may occur (reversible) ▪ Compliance c̄ prescribed dosage regimen ▪ Women: avoid breastfeeding ▪ Check c̄ physician/pharmacist before taking OTC preparations ▪ Avoid alcohol ▪ Use contraception (during & for up to 8 wks after therapy).

NOTES:

methoxamine hcl • (meth-ox-a-meen)

CATEGORY: *Sympathomimetic:* vasopressor

Rx; Preg Cat C

BRAND NAME
Vasoxyl (B-W)

DOSAGE FORMS
Injection (IM/IV): 20mg/ml

ACTION: Adrenergic effect due to alpha agonist activity, resulting in peripheral vasoconstriction w/out ↑ cardiac irritability. **USE:** Maintaining BP during anesthesia ▪ Termination of some episodes of paroxysmal supraventricular tachycardia.

PHARMACOKINETICS: Onset of pressor effects 15-20m IM; duration 1-1.5h.

CONTRAINDICATIONS: Hypersensitivity, hypertension.

DOSAGE

Adult

Spinal anesthesia	*IM*	Usual dose 10-15mg shortly before/at time of spinal anesthesia administration. Subsequent doses may be required
Hypotension	*IV*	3-5mg for emergencies
	IM	Usual dose 10-15mg. Usual postop dose for moderate hypotension 5-10mg
Paroxysmal supraventricular tachycardia	*IV*	10mg

SIDE/ADVERSE EFFECTS: ***Sustained hypertension c̄ headache,*** projectile vomiting, urinary frequency/desire to void, pilomotor response.

Note: Side/adverse effects: common in *italic;* serious in ***boldface italic.***

*Available in Canada only.

DRUG INTERACTIONS: Use c̄ MAO-I, tricyclic antidepressants, vasopressin, ergot alkaloids ↑ pressor effects ▪ Use c̄ halothane, other halogenated general anesthetics can induce cardiac arrhythmias ▪ Use c̄ beta blockers, guanethidine, reserpine may result in significant hypertension.

NURSING MANAGEMENT

ADMINISTRATION: Assess for hx of catecholamine hypersensitivity (incl sulfites) ▪ Assess F/E balance; correct deficiencies ▪ IV: administer via *slow* (2-3m) injection if systolic BP <60mmHg ▪ IM: may administer after IV dose for prolonged effect; doses 15m apart ▪ Do *not* leave pt unattended ▪ Have atropine available for bradycardia ▪ Avoid exposure to light ▪ Elderly may require ↓ dosage.

EVALUATION: Monitor VS, esp BP, heart rate (bradycardia) ▪ Monitor I&O (urinary retention) ▪ Check IV site carefully; avoid extravasation.

EDUCATION: Notify physician/nurse of abnormal rxs (difficult breathing, severe headache, severe faintness/dizziness).

NOTES:

methyldopa/methyldopate hcl ▲ • (meth-ill-doe-pa)

CATEGORY: *Antihypertensive* Rx; Preg Cat B

BRAND NAME
Aldomet (MSD)

DOSAGE FORMS
Injection (IV) ▲: 250mg/vial
PO suspension: 250mg/5ml
Tablet: 125, 250, 500mg

COMBINATION PRODUCTS

Aldoril 15, 25, 30, 50 (MSD)	methyldopa/hydrochlorothiazide per tablet: 250mg/15mg, 250mg/25mg, 500mg/30mg, 500mg/50mg

ACTION: Antihypertensive effect probably due to conversion to α-methylnorepinephrine, which stimulates central inhibitory alpha adrenergic receptors, resulting in ↓ BP.
USE: Treatment of hypertension as sole agent in combination c̄ thiazide diuretic.

PHARMACOKINETICS

PO absorption	Peak	Half-life	Excretion
Up to 50%	3-6h	1.7h	Via urine primarily as metabolites

CONTRAINDICATIONS: Hypersensitivity, active hepatic disease associated c̄ previous therapy.

DOSAGE

Pediatric *PO*	Initial dose 10mg/kg/d in 2-4 doses. Maximum dose 65mg/kg or 3g/d, whichever less
IV	20-40mg/kg/d divided, q6h. Maximum dose 65mg/kg or 3g/d, whichever less
Adult *PO*	Initial dose 250mg 2-3 times/d for 2d. ↑ at intervals of at least 2d. Usual maintenance range 500mg-2g in 2-4 doses/d
IV	250-500mg q6h prn. Do *not* exceed 1g q6h
Aldoril *PO*	1-2 tablets (any combination) 2-3 times/d for 2d. ↑ at intervals of at least 2d until satisfactory response obtained

SIDE/ADVERSE EFFECTS: CNS: *sedation, headache, dizziness,* symptoms of cerebrovascular insufficiency, Parkinson disease, Bell palsy, psychic disturbances ▪ CV: bradycardia, edema, orthostatic hypotension, exacerbation of angina, prolonged carotid sinus hypersensitivity ▪ GI: N/V/D, colitis, *dry mouth,* ***pancreatitis,*** sore/black tongue ▪ HEM: ***hemolytic anemia,*** leukopenia, ***thrombocytopenia*** ▪ HEP: jaundice, ↑ serum AST, ALT, alkaline phosphatase, *hepatitis* ▪ INT: eczema rashes, ***toxic epidermal necrolysis*** ▪ Other: breast enlargement, lactation, gynecomastia, nasal congestion, impotence.

DRUG INTERACTIONS: Use c̄ MAO-I can antagonize antihypertensive effect ▪ Use c̄ levodopa, phenothiazines, tricyclic antidepressants can produce additive hypotensive effects ▪ Use c̄ lithium can produce ↑ lithium toxicity.

NURSING MANAGEMENT

ADMINISTRATION: Assess for hx of hypersensitivity ▪ PO suspension: shake well before pouring ▪ IV: dilute c̄ 5% dextrose solution; administer *slowly* (30-60m) ▪ Do *not* administer SC/IM ▪ Elderly may require ↓ dosage.

EVALUATION: Monitor VS, esp BP ▪ Monitor F/E balance, esp Na^+, K^+, Cl^- ▪ Monitor hepatic, CV, renal, hemopoietic status c̄ long-term use ▪ Monitor I&O, daily weight ▪ Assess for edema in extremities.

EDUCATION: Dizziness/drowsiness may occur; use caution in potentially hazardous activities ▪ Avoid changing positions (lying/sitting/standing) rapidly ▪ Take as ordered by physician, even if symptom free; do *not* change dose ▪ Used to control, *not* cure, hypertension ▪ Avoid use c̄ alcohol, CNS depressants ▪ Avoid ↑ exercise, temperature extremes, smoking ▪ Notify physician of muscle cramps, difficult breathing, cold extremities, fever, prolonged tiredness ▪ Keep scheduled appointments c̄ physician; have BP checked regularly ▪ Maintain optimum weight ▪ Avoid high-Na^+ foods (canned soups, lunch meats, cheese) ▪ Check c̄ physician/pharmacist before taking OTC preparations ▪ Notify physician/dentist of use before treatment ▪ Do *not* D/C drug w/out checking c̄ physician ▪ Carry identification (MedicAlert) if hypertensive ▪ May produce ↓ libido, impotence ▪ May darken urine if left standing.

NOTES:

methylprednisolone/methylprednisolone acetate▲ •

(meth-ill-pred-niss-oh-lone)

CATEGORY: *Glucosteroid:* corticosteroid — Rx; Preg Cat NA

BRAND NAMES	DOSAGE FORMS
Medrol (Upjohn)	ADT Pak, Dosepak, tablet: 2, 4, 8, 24, 32mg; retention enema▲
Depo-Medrol▲ (Upjohn)	Injection suspension: 20, 40, 80mg/ml

ACTION: Glucosteroids cause variety of pharmacologic activity; two major effects are potent antiinflammatory effect, inhibition of immune response. **USE:** Treatment of adrenocortical deficiency, adrenogenital syndrome, other endocrine disorders; allergic states, collagen diseases, dermatologic diseases, GI diseases, hematologic disorders, ophthalmologic diseases; respiratory diseases, rheumatic disorders ▪ Treatment of tuberculous meningitis, neurologic/myocardial involvement associated c̄ trichinosis ▪ Remission of proteinuria in nephrotic syndrome; acute exacerbation of multiple sclerosis ▪ Palliative management of leukemia, lymphomas.

PHARMACOKINETICS: PO administration usually produces peak effect in 1-2h, duration of about 1.5 days.

CONTRAINDICATIONS: Systemic fungal infections.

DOSAGE

Adult	*PO*	2-60mg/d
	Injection/ suspension	10-80mg IM qd. Intraarticular, intralesional; 4-80mg/dose
	Enema	1 enema 3-7 times/wk for ≥ 2 wks. Can be administered by continuous drip

SIDE/ADVERSE EFFECTS: CNS: ***convulsions***, headache, psychic impairment, vertigo, mood swings; pseudotumor cerebri may develop after treatment ▪ CV: edema due to Na^+ retention, CHF, hypertension ▪ EENT: ↑ IOP, glaucoma, posterior subcapsular cataracts, exophthalmos ▪ END: Cushingoid states, growth suppression in children, menstrual irregularities, 2° adrenocortical/pituitary unresponsiveness, hyperglycemia, carbohydrate intolerance ▪ GI: peptic ulcer/***possible perforation, pancreatitis***, abdominal distention, ulcerative esophagitis ▪ INT: poor wound healing, fragile skin, petechiae; ecchymoses, facial erythema, ↑ sweating, urticaria, hirsutism ▪ MET:

negative nitrogen balance, hypokalemic alkalosis ▪ MS: muscle weakness/loss of mass, fracture of long bones, osteoporosis.

DRUG INTERACTIONS: Severe hypokalemia can occur c̄ diuretics (nonpotassium sparing) ▪ Use c̄ ulcerogenic drugs (aspirin, indomethacin) can produce additive effects ▪ Use c̄ antidiabetic agents may require ↑ doses of antidiabetic drugs.

NURSING MANAGEMENT

ADMINISTRATION: Assess for hx of hypersensitivity ▪ Administer single daily/alternate-day dose *before* 9AM; multiple doses at equal intervals ▪ PO: administer c̄ food, milk, antacids ▪ IM: shake well; do *not* freeze; inject into gluteal UOQ (avoid deltoid); rotate sites ▪ IV (succinate salt only): (direct) reconstitute according to manufacturer's directions c̄ compatible diluent, administer *slowly* (1m); (infusion) further dilute c̄ 5% dextrose/normal saline, administer at prescribed rate; stable w/in 48h of reconstitution; do *not* use discolored/precipitated solutions ▪ Rectal: administer via continuous drip or retention enema; shake bottle q30m ▪ Avoid abrupt withdrawal ▪ Avoid exposure to heat in storage ▪ Elderly may require ↓ dosage; monitor BP.

EVALUATION: Monitor VS, esp BP ▪ Diabetics: closely monitor blood, urine glucose ▪ Assess mental/emotional status; avoid tricyclic antidepressants if depression induced ▪ Monitor serum electrolytes (esp CA^{++}, K^+, Na^+) vision /IOP, stools for occult blood c̄ prolonged use ▪ Monitor hydration status (I&O, daily weight).

EDUCATION: Take c̄ food/milk (single daily dose *before* 9AM; multiple doses at equal intervals) ▪ Take as ordered by physician; do *not* ↑ dose/stop taking ▪ Eat foods high in K^+, high in protein; avoid black licorice ▪ Follow diet low in Na^+ ▪ Check c̄ physician before immunization (pt, family) ▪ Avoid exposure to infection ▪ Report following symptoms *immediately* to physician: anorexia, difficult breathing, weakness, dizziness; may appear during periods of ↑ stress/trauma ▪ Notify physician if experiencing black/tarry stools, slow wound healing, blurred vision, bruising/bleeding, weight gain, emotional changes ▪ Diabetics: closely monitor blood/urine glucose ▪ Notify physician/dentist of use before treatment ▪ Keep appointments c̄ physician/blood work/eye exams ▪ Women: avoid breastfeeding ▪ Body image changes may occur c̄ prolonged use (reversible).

NOTES:

methyltestosterone • (meth-ill-tess-toss-te-rone)

CATEGORY: *Androgenic hormone* — Rx; Preg Cat X

BRAND NAME	**DOSAGE FORMS**
Oretron Methyl (Schering)	Buccal tablet, tablet

ACTION: Androgens required for development, maintenance of male reproductive system, 2° sex characteristics; initiate specific RNA, protein synthesis in responsive tissue. **USE:** Treatment of conditions due to androgen deficiency, incl eunuchoidism, eunuchism, male climacteric 2° to androgen deficiency, postpubertal cryptorchidism ▪ Prevention of postpartum breast engorgement ▪ Palliation of androgen-responsive, advancing, inoperable postmenopausal mammary cancer ▪ Treatment of delayed male puberty, impotence.

PHARMACOKINETICS

Peak	Half-life	Excretion
1-2h	1h initially 3.5h after 3-4h	Urine, feces, 10% unchanged

CONTRAINDICATIONS: Known/suspected carcinoma of prostate gland/male breast; prepubertal boys; pregnant/breast-feeding women; cardiac, renal, hepatic decompensation.

DOSAGE: Buccal administration produces effects at half PO dose; PO dose about twice buccal dose.

Buccal

Androgen deficiencies	50-20mg or more qd
Postpartum breast engorgement	40mg/d for 3-5d
Breast cancer	25-100mg/d

SIDE/ADVERSE EFFECTS: END: virilization in women, oligospermia, gynecomastia, priapism, amenorrhea ▪ HEP: hepatocellular neoplasms (rare), peliosis hepatitis ▪ INT: acne, edema, hirsutism, stomatitis c̄ buccal preparations ▪ MET: hypercalcemia.

DRUG INTERACTIONS: Use c̄ PO anticoagulants can significantly ↑ anticoagulant activity.

Note: Side/adverse effects: common in *italic;* serious in ***boldface italic.*** — *Available in Canada only.

NURSING MANAGEMENT

ADMINISTRATION: Assess for pregnancy; do *not* administer ▪ Assess for hx of CV, hepatic, renal dysfunction; notify physician ▪ Avoid administration to tartrazine-sensitive pts (Metandren) ▪ Place buccal tablets in upper/lower buccal pouch between gum, cheek; allow 30m to dissolve ▪ PO: administer $\bar{c}$ food ▪ Avoid exposure to moisture, light in storage.

EVALUATION: Assess CV, hepatic, renal status ▪ Observe for signs of jaundice; D/C drug, notify physician ▪ Observe for edema, weight gain ▪ Assess for hypercalcemia ▪ Diabetics: monitor for hypoglycemia ▪ Assess for stomatitis (buccal).

EDUCATION: Store in tightly closed, light-resistant container ▪ Proper use of buccal tablets; do *not* swallow; avoid eating, drinking, smoking; maintain good oral hygiene ▪ Notify physician immediately of jaundice, edema ▪ Women: masculinizing effects may occur; notify physician ▪ Men: overstimulation of sexual function may occur; notify physician ▪ Exercise regimen (esp for immobilized pts) to ↓ hypercalcemia ▪ Take PO forms $\bar{c}$ meals ▪ Diabetics: monitor blood/urine glucose carefully.

NOTES:

metoclopramide hcl • (met-oh-kloe-pra-mide)

CATEGORY: *GI stimulant:* peristaltic stimulant

Rx; Preg Cat B

BRAND NAMES	DOSAGE FORMS
**Emex (Beecham)*	Tablet: 10mg
**Maxeran (Nordic)*	Injection (IV): 5mg/ml PO solution: 1mg/ml Tablet: 5mg
Maxolon (SKB)	Tablet: 10mg
Octamide PFS (Adria)	Injection (IV): 5mg/ml
Reglan (Robins)	Injection (IV): 5, 10mg/ml Syrup: 5mg/5ml Tablet: 5, 10mg

ACTION: Peristaltic stimulation appears related to upper gut sensitizing to acetylcholine, increasing gastric tone, amplitude contraction, relaxation of pyloric sphincter, resulting in accelerated emptying; drug causes release of prolactin. **USE:** Treatment of symptomatic gastroesophageal reflux not responsive to conventional therapy ▪ Treatment of symptoms associated c̄ acute/recurrent diabetic gastroparesis ▪ Antiemetic for cancer chemotherapy ▪ Facilitation of small bowel intubation ▪ Facilitation of barium removal after radiologic exam.

PHARMACOKINETICS

PO absorption	Peak	Half-life	Protein binding	Excretion
Complete	1-2h	2.5-5h	13%-22%	Via urine, feces, primarily as metabolites

CONTRAINDICATIONS: GI hemorrhage, obstruction, perforation; hypersensitivity, pheochromocytoma, epilepsy, c̄ drugs that induce extrapyramidal symptoms.

DOSAGE

Pediatric	
Intubation *IV*	<6y/o: 0.1mg/kg 6-14y/o: 2.5-5mg
Adult	
Reflux *PO*	10-15mg 30m ac, hs. Single 20mg dose before provoking condition
Diabetic gastroparesis *PO*	10mg 30m ac, hs for 2-8 wks
IV	Severe symptoms: 10mg

Note: Side/adverse effects: common in *italic;* serious in ***boldface italic.***

*Available in Canada only.

Antiemetic

Chemotherapy *IV*	1-2mg/kg
Post-op *IM*	10-20mg
Intubation *IV*	10mg
Barium removal *IV*	10mg

SIDE/ADVERSE EFFECTS: CNS: *drowsiness, restlessness, lassitude,* dizziness, headache, insomnia, extrapyramidal rxs, akathisia, extrapyramidal rxs (rare) ▪ EENT: visual disturbances ▪ END: galactorrhea, amenorrhea, gynecomastia, impotence ▪ GI: nausea, bowel disturbances (diarrhea) ▪ INT: rash ▪ RESP: ***bronchospasm*** ▪ Other: porphyria.

DRUG INTERACTIONS: Use c̄ anticholinergics/narcotics can antagonize stimulant effect ▪ Use c̄ CNS depressants produces additive depression ▪ Insulin adjustment may be required for diabetics ▪ Use c̄ other drugs ↑ their PO absorption from intestine.

NURSING MANAGEMENT

ADMINISTRATION: Assess for hx of hypersensitivity ▪ Assess renal function; may require ↓ dosage if impaired ▪ PO: administer 30m ac, hs ▪ IV: dilute according to manufacturer's directions; administer *slowly* (direct injection 1-2m, infusion >15m); discard unused portions ▪ Avoid exposure to heat, light; cover IV bags c̄ aluminum foil ▪ Na^+ content: 0.14mEq/ml (IV); calculate in Na^+-restricted diets ▪ Elderly may require ↓ dosage.

EVALUATION: Monitor VS, daily weight, I&O ▪ Observe for extrapyramidal symptoms (muscle spasms, tremors, shuffling gait); notify physician ▪ Monitor serum electrolytes (↓ K^+, ↑ Na^+), blood glucose ▪ Observe for potentiation of CNS depressant effect.

EDUCATION: Drowsiness may occur; use caution in potentially hazardous activities ▪ Take on empty stomach (30m ac, hs) ▪ Take as ordered by physician; do *not* ↑ dose ▪ Avoid use c̄ alcohol, other CNS depressants.

NOTES:

metolazone • (me-<u>tole</u>-a-zone)

CATEGORY: *Diuretic:* antihypertensive — Rx; Preg Cat B

BRAND NAMES
Diulo (Searle)
Mykrox† *(Fisons)*
Zaroxolyn (Fisons)

DOSAGE FORMS
Tablet: 2.5, 5, 10mg
Tablet: 0.5mg
Tablet: 2.5, 5, 10mg

ACTION: Diuretic activity due to excretion of H_2O, Na, Cl, other electrolytes by inhibiting tubular reabsorption at cortical diluting site, proximal convoluted tubules. **USE:** Treatment of hypertension as sole agent/in combination c̄ other antihypertensives ▪ Treatment of edema due to renal dysfunction ▪ Adjunct in treatment of edema due to CHF.

DOSAGE

Adult *PO*	2.5-20mg/d

SIDE/ADVERSE EFFECTS: CNS: dizziness, drowsiness, fainting, headache, paresthesia ▪ CV: orthostatic hypotension, ***venous thrombosis***, palpitations ▪ EENT: blurred vision; dry nose/throat ▪ GI: constipation, N/V, anorexia, epigastric distress ▪ HEM: ***aplastic anemia,*** leukopenia, ***agranulocytosis, thrombocytopenia*** ▪ HEP: cholestatic jaundice, hepatitis ▪ INT: urticaria, purpura, necrotizing angiitis ▪ Other: gout attack.

PHARMACOKINETICS

PO absorption	Onset	Peak	Duration	Protein binding	Excretion
Incomplete	1h	2h	12-24h	Approximately 35% >50% bound to RBC	Via urine, primarily as unchanged drug

CONTRAINDICATIONS: Hypersensitivity, hepatic precoma/coma.

Note: Side/adverse effects: common in *italic;* serious in ***boldface italic.***

*Available in Canada only.
†More completely absorbed and not therapeutically equivalent to other formulations. Usual dose 0.5-1mg/d.

DRUG INTERACTIONS: ↑ Dig toxicity due to hypokalemia ▪ Use c̄ corticosteroids produces ↑ hypokalemia ▪ Antidiabetic agents may require dose adjustments ▪ Use c̄ diazoxide can produce significant diabetogenic effects.

NURSING MANAGEMENT

ADMINISTRATION: Assess for hx of hypersensitivity (incl sulfonamides) ▪ Assess renal function; do *not* administer if severely impaired ▪ Administer c̄ food/milk on arising ▪ Assess serum K^+ (normal level: 3.5-5mEq/L) ▪ Elderly may require ↓ dosage.

EVALUATION: Monitor F/E, hepatic, renal status ▪ Monitor VS, esp BP, pulse ▪ Monitor serum for ↑ BUN, creatinine, uric acid; ↓ K^+ ▪ Diabetics: closely monitor blood sugar ▪ Monitor fluid retention (I&O, daily weight) ▪ Monitor digitalized pts closely (↓ K^+: ↑ dig toxicity).

EDUCATION: Expect ↑ urine output; have bathroom facilities easily accessible ▪ May cause weakness, lethargy ▪ Take c̄ food ▪ Take on waking, at same time qd ▪ Take even if symptom free ▪ Used to control, *not* cure, hypertension ▪ Notify physician of signs of hypokalemia (muscle cramps, lethargy, nausea) ▪ Avoid changing positions (lying/sitting/standing) rapidly ▪ Take as directed by physician; do *not* skip doses ▪ Eat foods high in K^+ (bananas, fruit juices, raisins); avoid black licorice ▪ Avoid high-Na^+ foods (canned soups, lunch meats, cheese) ▪ Maintain optimum weight ▪ Diabetics: check blood/urine glucose carefully ▪ Avoid smoking ▪ Use sugarless gum/hard candy to diminish dry mouth.

NOTES:

metoprolol tartrate • (me-toe-proe-lole)

CATEGORY: *Beta-adrenergic blocker*: antihypertensive Rx; Preg Cat B

BRAND NAMES
**Betaloc (ASTRA)*
Lopressor (Geigy)

DOSAGE FORMS
Injection (IV): 5mg/vial, syringe
Tablet: 50, 100mg

COMBINATION PRODUCTS

Lopressor HCT (Geigy)	Metoprolol/hydrochlorothiazide per tablet: 50mg/25mg, 100mg/25mg, 100mg/50mg

ACTION: Blocks access of catecholamine neurotransmitter to $beta_1$ receptors located in heart; antihypertensive effect not determined. **USE:** Treatment of hypertension as sole agent/in combination c̄ other antihypertensives (esp thiazide diuretics) ▪ To ↓ mortality rate in MI.

PHARMACOKINETICS

PO absorption	Peak	Half-life	Protein binding	Excretion
95%	1h	3-7h	12%	95% as metabolites via urine

CONTRAINDICATIONS: Hypersensitivity, cardiogenic shock, heart block >1°, overt cardiac failure, sinus bradycardia.

DOSAGE

Adult	
Hypertension *PO*	100-450mg/d
MI early *IV/PO*	3 bolus injections of 5mg at 2m intervals followed in 15m by 50mg PO q6h for 48h. Thereafter 100mg bid
MI late *PO*	100mg bid
Lopressor HCT	
50/25	2 tablets/d
100/25	1-2 tablets/d
100/50	1 tablet/d

SIDE/ADVERSE EFFECTS: CNS: *tiredness, dizziness,* depression, mental confusion ▪ CV: bradycardia, palpitations, shortness of breath, cold extremities, CHF ▪ GI: D/N, gastric pain, constipation, flatulence ▪ INT: pruritus, rash ▪ Other: wheezing, Peyronie disease (1/100,000).

Note: Side/adverse effects: common in *italic;* serious in ***boldface italic.*** *Available in Canada only.

DRUG INTERACTIONS: Use c̄ reserpine, other catecholamine-depleting drugs can result in serious adrenergic blockage ▪ Nonselective beta adrenergics antagonize therapeutic response.

NURSING MANAGEMENT

ADMINISTRATION: Assess for hx of beta blocker hypersensitivity ▪ Assess BP, apical pulse; if <60/m, hold drug, notify physician ▪ Assess hepatic function, I&O ▪ Do *not* administer in presence of respiratory distress (asthma, CHF, COPD) ▪ PO: administer c̄ food ▪ IV: cardiac monitor ▪ Avoid exposure to heat, moisture, light in storage ▪ Avoid abrupt withdrawal ▪ Elderly may require ↓ dosage.

EVALUATION: Monitor hepatic, renal, respiratory status ▪ Monitor BP, pulse ▪ Monitor CBC, FBS (diabetics) ▪ Assess for depression ▪ May produce alteration in blood glucose levels (hypoglycemia); may mask signs of hypoglycemia.

EDUCATION: Check pulse before taking; if <60/m, do *not* take drug, notify physician ▪ Take as directed by physician; do *not* skip doses ▪ Take c̄ food ▪ Do *not* D/C drug w/out notifying physician ▪ Check c̄ physician/pharmacist before taking OTC/Rx preparations ▪ Dizziness/drowsiness may occur; use caution in potentially hazardous activities ▪ Diabetics: carefully monitor blood/urine glucose ▪ May experience ↑ sensitivity to cold ▪ Notify physician of respiratory distress, leg edema ▪ Notify physician/dentist of beta blocker use before treatment ▪ Maintain optimum weight ▪ Keep scheduled appointments c̄ physician ▪ Follow low-Na^+ diet ▪ Store in tightly closed, light-resistant container ▪ Avoid ↑ exercise, cold, smoking ▪ Women: avoid breastfeeding.

NOTES:

metronidazole/metronidazole hcl ▲ • (me-troe-ni-da-zole)

CATEGORY: *Antiprotozoan:* antibacterial   Rx; Preg Cat B

BRAND NAMES	DOSAGE FORMS
Flagyl (Searle) (Rhone-Poulenc in Canada)	Powder for injection (IV): 500mg/vial ▲ IV; IVRTU: 500mg/100ml ▲ Tablet: 250, 500mg
**Neo-Tric (Neolab)*	Tablet: 250mg Vaginal insert: 500mg
**Novonidazol (Novopharm)*	Tablet: 250mg Vaginal insert: 500mg

ACTION: Antimicrobial activity appears related to inhibition of hydrogen release in metabolic pathways in susceptible organisms. **USE:** Treatment of symptomatic/asymptomatic trichomoniasis ▪ Treatment of amebic dysentery, amebic liver abscesses ▪ Treatment of anaerobic bacterial infections caused by susceptible strains of *Bacteroides* spp, *Clostridium* spp, *Eubacterium* spp, *Fusobacterium* spp, *Peptococcus* spp, *Peptostreptococcus* spp.

PHARMACOKINETICS

PO absorption	Peak	Half-life	Protein binding	Excretion
80%	1-3h	8h	20%	60%-80% via urine as metabolites

CONTRAINDICATIONS: Hypersensitivity, first trimester of pregnancy (trichomoniasis).

DOSAGE

Pediatric *PO*

Amebiasis	30-50mg/kg/d in 3 doses for 10d

Adult

Amebiasis *PO*	750mg tid for 5-10d. Amebic liver abscess: 500 or 750mg tid for 5-10d
Bacterial *PO*	7.5mg/kg q6h for 7-10d. Do *not* exceed 4g/d
IV	Loading dose 15mg/kg infused over 1h, $\bar{c}$ maintenance dose after 6h 7.5 mg/kg infused over 1h q6h. Do *not* exceed 4g/d. Switch to PO when clinically indicated

Note: Side/adverse effects: common in *italic;* serious in ***boldface italic.***

*Available in Canada only.

	For surgical prophylaxis, 15mg/kg infused over 30-60m, completed 1h before surgery. 7.5mg/kg infused over 30-60m at 6h & 12h after initial dose
Trichomoniasis *PO*	2g for 1d or 250mg tid for 7d

SIDE/ADVERSE EFFECTS: CNS: ***convulsive seizures***, peripheral neuropathy, dizziness, incoordination, headache ▪ CV: ECG T-wave flattening ▪ EENT: nasal congestion ▪ GI: anorexia, N/V/D, cramps, metallic taste ▪ GU: dysuria, cystitis, polyuria, dark urine ▪ INT: urticaria, erythematous rash, overgrowth of monilia.

DRUG INTERACTIONS: Use c̄ PO anticoagulants may ↑ PT ▪ Use c̄ alcohol produces abdominal distress, N/V, flushing, headache ▪ Use c̄ phenobarbital/phenytoin ↑ metronidazole metabolism ▪ Use c̄ disulfiram may cause acute psychotic rx ▪ Use c̄ lithium may ↑ its toxicity.

NURSING MANAGEMENT

ADMINISTRATION: Assess for hx of hypersensitivity ▪ Obtain C&S before therapy ▪ PO: administer c̄ food/milk; may crush tablets ▪ Administer at equal intervals around clock to maintain blood levels ▪ Do *not* administer direct IV bolus ▪ IV: avoid contact c̄ aluminum-containing products; do *not* mix c̄ other drugs; do *not* refrigerate neutralized solution.

EVALUATION: Monitor VS, esp temperature; CBC, esp WBCs; stools for amebae (3mo) ▪ Assess for neurotoxic effects (paresthesias, tremors, incoordination); D/C drug.

EDUCATION: Take c̄ food/milk to ↓ GI distress; may crush tablets ▪ Take as ordered by physician even if symptom free ▪ Notify physician *immediately* of tremors, alteration in sensation, incoordination; D/C drug ▪ Avoid alcohol ▪ Trichomoniasis: have partner use condom c̄ sexual intercourse during therapy; identify all sexual contacts for treatment; maintain good perineal hygiene ▪ May turn urine red/brown ▪ Women: avoid breastfeeding ▪ May cause metallic taste.

NOTES:

mexiletine hcl • (mex-ill-e-teen)

CATEGORY: *Antiarrhythmic*

Rx; Preg Cat C

BRAND NAME	DOSAGE FORMS
Mexitil (B-I)	Capsules: 150, 200, 250mg

ACTION: Antiarrhythmic effect due to inhibition of inward Na current, which reduces phase 0 action potential. The drug is a class IB antiarrhythmic and ↓ the effective refractory period in Purkinje fibers. **USE:** Treatment of symptomatic ventricular arrhythmias including frequent PVC, tachycardia, and unifocal and multifocal couplets.

PHARMACOKINETICS

PO absorption	Peak	Half-life	Protein binding	Excretion
90%	2-3h	10-12h	50%-60%	10% as unchanged drug via urine

CONTRAINDICATIONS: Hypersensitivity, cardiogenic shock, preexisting second/third degree AV block (in the absence of a pacemaker).

DOSAGE: Initial dose of 200mg q8h. A minimum of 2-3 days is required between dosage adjustments, which are in 50 or 100mg increments up or down. For rapid control the loading dose is 400mg, followed by 200mg in 8h. Stabilized patients may be put on a q12h schedule, with a maximum dose of 450mg q12h.

SIDE/ADVERSE EFFECTS: CNS: *dizziness, tremor, nervousness, difficult coordination,* sleep irregularities, headache, paresthesias, depression, confusion ▪ CV: palpitations, anginal pain, PVC, hypotension, edema ▪ EENT: tinnitus, blurred vision ▪ GI: *N/V, heartburn,* diarrhea, constipation, dry mouth, changes in appetite ▪ Other: rash, arthralgia, dyspnea, fever, fatigue.

DRUG INTERACTIONS: Use $\bar{c}$ enzyme inducers including phenytoin, rifampin, barbiturates can ↓ mexiletine blood levels ▪ Use $\bar{c}$ cimetidine requires monitoring because of erratic mexiletine blood levels ▪ Renal excretion rates will ↑ $\bar{c}$ acidifiers and ↓ $\bar{c}$ alkalizing agents.

NURSING MANAGEMENT

ADMINISTRATION: Assess for hx of hypersensitivity, incl amide-type anesthetics ▪ Administer c̄ food, milk, antacid to ↓ GI distress ▪ Assess for CHF, hepatic dysfunction; may require ↓ dosage ▪ Administer first dose; 6-12h after quinidine, disopyramide; 3-6h after procainamide; 8-12h after tocainide ▪ ↓ Dose/withdraw lidocaine after starting drug ▪ Assess for hx of seizures; institute precautions ▪ Dosage may be ↑/↓ q2-3d by 50-100mg/dose ▪ Heavy smokers may require ↑ dosage ▪ Avoid exposure to heat, moisture, light in storage.

EVALUATION: Monitor VS, esp BP, heart rate (hypotension, heart block) ▪ Assess neurologic status; notify physician if impaired ▪ Monitor CBC (leukopenia), platelets (thrombocytopenia); notify physician ▪ Monitor I&O, daily weight ▪ May ↑ serum AST; (+) ANA titer.

EDUCATION: Dizziness may occur; use caution in potentially hazardous activities ▪ Take c̄ food, milk, antacids to ↑ GI irritation ▪ Take as ordered by physician, even if symptom free ▪ Notify physician/dentist of use before treatment ▪ Keep scheduled appointments c̄ physician ▪ Notify physician *immediately* of chest pain, difficult breathing, seizures, bleeding/bruising, swelling of legs/feet ▪ Store in dry, tightly closed, light-resistant container ▪ Women: avoid breastfeeding.

NOTES:

mezlocillin sodium • (mez-loe-sill-in)

CATEGORY: *Extended-spectrum penicillin*: antibiotic — Rx; Preg Cat B

BRAND NAME
Mezlin (Miles)

DOSAGE FORMS
Powder for injection (IM/IV): 1, 2, 3, 4g vials

ACTION: Bactericidal activity due to inhibition of mucopeptide cell wall synthesis in susceptible organisms. **USE:** Treatment of infections due to susceptible strains of *Bacteroides* spp, *Escherichia coli,* group A hemolytic streptococci, *Haemophilus influenzae, Klebsiella* spp, *Morganella morganii, Neisseria gonorrhoeae, Peptococcus* spp, *Peptostreptococcus* spp, *Proteus mirabilis, Pseudomonas* spp, *Serratia* spp, *Streptococcus faecalis, Streptococcus pneumoniae* ▪ In combination c̄ aminoglycoside in treating serious *Pseudomonas aeruginosa* infections.

PHARMACOKINETICS

PO absorption	Peak	Half-life	Protein binding	Excretion
65%	45m	1-1.5h	16%-42%	55% via urine in 6h

CONTRAINDICATIONS: Hypersensitivity to any penicillin/cephalosporin.

DOSAGE

Pediatric *IV/IM*	≥1mo: 50mg/kg q4h
Adult *IV/IM*	Usual range 6-18g/d divided given q4-6h. Do *not* exceed 2g/IM injection site. Usual maximum IV dose 24g/d

SIDE/ADVERSE EFFECTS: CNS: ***possible convulsions***, neuromuscular irritability ▪ GI: N/V/D, abnormal taste ▪ HEM: anemia, eosinophilia, leukopenia, neutropenia, ***thrombocytopenia*** ▪ HEP: ↑ serum AST, ALT, bilirubin ▪ INT: rash, pruritus, urticaria ▪ Other: local pain/***thrombophlebitis*** at injection site, ***anaphylactic rxs,*** ↓ K^+ level.

DRUG INTERACTIONS: Use c̄ bacteriostatic antibiotics can lead to antibiotic antagonism ▪ PO anticoagulant therapy may require dose adjustments.

NURSING MANAGEMENT

ADMINISTRATION: Assess for hx of penicillin/cephalosporin hypersensitivity ▪ Obtain C&S before therapy ▪ Have support equipment available for anaphylaxis ▪ Do *not* mix c̄ aminoglycosides, other antibacterial solutions ▪ Reconstitute according to manufacturer's directions ▪ Maintain blood levels; administer at equal intervals around clock ▪ IM: inject *deep, slowly* into gluteal UOQ ▪ IV: administer by *slow* direct injection, IVPB (30m infusion) ▪ Na^+ content: 1.9mEq (43mg)/g; calculate in Na^+-restricted diets.

EVALUATION: Monitor VS, esp temperature ▪ Monitor hepatic, renal status (I&O) ▪ Assess for hypokalemia; may require supplemental K^+ ▪ Observe for signs of superinfection (diarrhea, perineal itching, oral ulcers) ▪ Assess for hypersensitivity rxs (fever, difficult breathing, rash) ▪ Monitor blood cultures, WBC, differential for drug effectiveness.

EDUCATION: Diarrhea may occur ▪ Maintain good personal hygiene (esp perineal, oral) ▪ Maintain fluid intake (6-8 glasses/d) ▪ Avoid concurrent ingestion of highly acidic substances (fruit juices) ▪ Carry identification (MedicAlert) if penicillin allergic.

NOTES:

miconazole/miconazole nitrate ▲ • (mi-kon-a-zole)

CATEGORY: *Antifungal* Rx-OTC; Preg Cat NA

BRAND NAMES	DOSAGE FORMS
Micatin ▲ (Ortho)	OTC topical preparations
Monistat-DERM ▲ (Ortho)	Rx topical preparations
Monistat 7 ▲ (Ortho)	Vaginal cream: 2% Vaginal suppository: 100mg
Monistat 3 ▲ (Ortho)	Vaginal suppository: 200mg
Monistat IV (Janssen)	Injection (IV): 10mg/ml

ACTION: Antifungal activity due to alteration in cell membrane permeability, resulting in leakage of vital intracellular components. **USE:** Treatment of systemic infections caused by susceptible strains of *Candida albicans, Coccidioides immitis, Cryptococcus neoformans, Paracoccidioides brasiliensis, Petriellidium boydii* ▪ Topical treatment of cutaneous/vaginal moniliasis, dermatophytes (tinea infections).

DOSAGE

Pediatric *IV infusion*	20-40mg/kg/d. Do *not* exceed 15mg/kg/infusion
Adult *IV infusion*	
Coccidioidomycosis	1800-3600mg/d
Cryptococcosis	1200-2400mg/d
Candidiasis	600-1800mg/d
Paracoccidioidomycosis	200-1200mg/d
Petriellidiosis	600-3000mg/d
Topical	
Vaginal moniliasis	One applicatorful/suppository into vagina once/d for 3d (Monistat 3) or 7d (Monistat 7)
Dermatophytes/ cutaneous moniliasis	Apply preparation at least twice/d

PHARMACOKINETICS: After IV administration, drug metabolized in liver, excreted as metabolites via urine, feces.

SIDE/ADVERSE EFFECTS: Phlebitis, pruritus, nausea, fever, chills, rash, ***thrombophlebitis;*** local topical application can produce irritation, burning.

CONTRAINDICATIONS: Hypersensitivity.

DRUG INTERACTIONS: Use c̄ PO anticoagulants ↑ their activity, dosage adjustment may be required ▪ Use c̄ amphotericin B may result in antimicrobial antagonism.

NURSING MANAGEMENT

ADMINISTRATION: Assess for hx of hypersensitivity ▪ Obtain C&S before therapy ▪ IV: dilute in 5% dextrose/normal saline solution; stable for 48h at room temperature; administer *slowly* (30-60m); do *not* mix c̄ other IV drugs ▪ Do *not* administer discolored/precipitated solutions ▪ Administer antiemetic/antihistamine as ordered before IV dose (↓ nausea) ▪ Cleanse areas for application well before administration ▪ Shake topical preparations well before administering ▪ Use lotion on skinfold areas (toes, fingers) ▪ Avoid occlusive dressings.

EVALUATION: Monitor VS, esp temperature ▪ Monitor CBC (H&H), serum electrolytes, lipids ▪ Monitor skin, mucous membranes for redness, swelling, irritation ▪ May potentiate anticoagulant effect; assess for bleeding.

EDUCATION: Take as ordered by physician; complete full course of therapy ▪ Keep affected areas dry, exposed to air; avoid occlusive dressings ▪ Maintain good hygiene, esp in affected area; keep towels, personal items separate from those of others to avoid spread of infection ▪ Vaginal: use sanitary napkin to prevent staining of clothing; avoid sexual intercourse during therapy (prevent reinfection) ▪ Avoid contact c̄ eyes ▪ Procedure for topical/vaginal application ▪ Full drug effects may require 1-2 wks.

NOTES:

minoxidil • (mi-nox-i-dill)

CATEGORY: *Antihypertensive* — Rx; Preg Cat C

BRAND NAMES
Loniten (Upjohn)
Rogaine (Upjohn)

DOSAGE FORMS
Tablet: 2.5, 10mg
Topical solution: 2%

ACTION: Antihypertensive effect due to direct peripheral vasodilation, resulting in reduction of peripheral vascular resistance; drug has recently received much publicity for restoring hair growth when applied topically (usually as pharmacy-prepared suspension made from crushed tablets). **USE:** Limited to treatment of severe hypertension that is symptomatic or associated c̄ target organ damage & cannot be controlled c̄ diuretic plus two other antihypertensive drugs c̄ maximum dosage. Topical solution treats male baldness of the scalp (vertex).

PHARMACOKINETICS

PO absorption	Peak	Half-life	Protein binding	Excretion
90%	2-8h	4.2h	None	90% metabolized excreted primarily via urine

CONTRAINDICATIONS: Hypersensitivity, pheochromocytoma.

DOSAGE: *PO*

Pediatric <12/yo	Initial dose 0.2mg/kg as single daily dose. Usual effective maintenance dose 0.25-1mg/kg/d. Do *not* exceed 50mg/d
Adult/ Children >12y/o	Initial dose 5mg as single daily dose. Usual dose 5mg as single daily dose. Usual effective maintenance dose 10-40mg/d. Do *not* exceed 100mg/d
Topical solution	Apply 1ml to scalp and rub in. Do *not* exceed 2ml/d

SIDE/ADVERSE EFFECTS: CV: temporary edema, ***ECG, T wave changes in direction/magnitude, pericardial effusion/tamponade,*** possible exacerbation of angina pectoris ▪ END: breast tenderness ▪ GI: N/V ▪ HEM: leukopenia, ***thrombocytopenia*** ▪ INT: skin rash, *hypertrichosis.*

Note: Side/adverse effects: common in *italic;* serious in ***boldface italic.***

*Available in Canada only.

DRUG INTERACTIONS: Use c̄ guanethidine can result in significant orthostatic effects.

NURSING MANAGEMENT

ADMINISTRATION: Assess for hx of hypersensitivity ▪ Avoid abrupt withdrawal; D/C gradually ▪ Elderly may require ↓ dosage ▪ Topical: Apply to dry hair/scalp, wash hands afterward; do *not* use if scalp is irritated or sunburned.

EVALUATION: Monitor VS, esp BP (sitting/lying/standing), apical pulse ▪ Monitor I&O, daily weight ▪ Monitor CV, hepatic, renal status ▪ Assess for edema; auscultate lungs (rales).

EDUCATION: Review package insert c̄ pt ▪ Take as ordered by physician even if symptom free; do *not* skip/change dose ▪ Do *not* D/C drug w/out notifying physician ▪ Maintain optimum weight ▪ Keep scheduled appointments c̄ physician; have BP checked regularly ▪ Follow low Na^+ diet ▪ Avoid ↑ exercise, temperature extremes, smoking, alcohol ▪ Notify physician *immediately* of shortness of breath, chest pain, fluid retention, dizziness, bruising/bleeding ▪ Used to control, *not* cure, hypertension ▪ Check c̄ physician/pharmacist before taking OTC/Rx preparations ▪ Procedure for checking radial pulse ▪ Take pulse daily; report any ↑ of >20 beats/m to physician *immediately* ▪ Notify physician/dentist of use before treatment ▪ ↑ Body hair growth/darkening may occur several wks after therapy started (reversible); depilatory may be used ▪ Procedure for topical application; full effects may take several mos of therapy.

NOTES:

misoprostol • (mis-oh-prost-ole)

CATEGORY: *Gastric antisecretory*: synthetic prostaglandin E analog Rx; Preg Cat X

BRAND NAME
Cytotic (Searle)

DOSAGE FORMS
Tablet: 100, 200μg

ACTION: Drug is converted in body into prostaglandin F analogs which inhibit gastric acid secretion and ↑ mucus and bicarbonate production in stomach. Stimulation of uterus resulting in contraction is also produced. **USE:** Prevention of gastric ulcers during NSAIA therapy in pts at high risk of developing gastric ulcers.

SIDE/ADVERSE EFFECTS: CNS: headache (2.4%), drowsiness, dizziness, anxiety ▪ CV: chest pain, edema, blood pressure changes ▪ EENT: abnormal vision, conjunctivitis, earache, tinnitus ▪ GI: diarrhea (13%), pain (7%), nausea (3.2%), flatulence (2.9%), dyspepsia (2%), vomiting (1.3%), abnormal taste ▪ GU: cramps, menstrual disorders, spotting, polyuria, dysuria ▪ INT: alopecia, rash, dermatitis ▪ Other: fatigue, fever, URI, bronchospasm, anemia, thrombocytopenia.

PHARMACOKINETICS

PO absorption	Onset	Duration	Half-life	Protein binding	Excretion
Extensive	30m	3h	20-40m	90%	Via urine

CONTRAINDICATIONS: Hypersensitivity, pregnancy.

DOSAGE

Adult *PO* 200 μg qid c̄ meals and hs for duration of NSAIA therapy. A reduced dose of 100μg qid c̄ meals and hs can be used if higher dose cannot be tolerated.

DRUG INTERACTIONS: Use c̄ antacids ↓ misoprostol availability.

NURSING MANAGEMENT

ADMINISTRATION: Assess for hx of prostaglandin hypersensitivity ▪ Assess for pregnancy; do *not* administer ▪ Administer c̄ meals & hs ▪ Use c̄ caution in pts c̄

Note: Side/adverse effects: common in *italic;* serious in ***boldface italic.***

*Available in Canada only.

seizure disorders ▪ Avoid concurrent administration c̄ antacids.

EVALUATION: Monitor VS, esp BP ▪ Monitor GI status; notify physician of abdominal pain.

EDUCATION: Take c̄ meals & hs ▪ Do *not* take antacids w/in 2h of drug; avoid Mg^{++}-containing antacids (diarrhea) ▪ Take as directed by physician, usually not for >4wks ▪ Diarrhea may occur ▪ Women: notify physician of pregnancy possibility; avoid breastfeeding; D/C if pregnant.

NOTES:

morphine sulfate • (mor-feen)

CATEGORY: *Narcotic:* opium alkaloid Rx C-II; Preg Cat C

AVAILABLE PREPARATIONS
Injection (IM/IV/SC): 2, 4, 8, 10, 15mg/ml
PO solution: 10mg/5ml, 20mg/5ml, 20mg/10ml, 20mg/ml
Suppository: 5, 10, 20mg
Tablet: 10, 15, 30mg

ACTION: Narcotics produce analgesia, euphoria, sedation; morphine sulfate has high misuse potential, addiction liability. **USE:** Relief of pain ▪ Sedation, hypnosis when pain is present ▪ Pre/postop sedation/analgesia.

DOSAGE

Pediatric *SC*	0.1-0.2mg/kg/dose. Do *not* exceed single dose 15mg
Adult *PO*	10-30mg q4h
IM	5-20mg q4h
IV	2.5-15mg/dose
SC	5-20mg q4h
Rectal	10-20mg q4h

PHARMACOKINETICS

	Onset	Peak	Duration	Half-life	Protein binding	Excretion
PO	15-20m	60m	4-7h	2.25h	35%	Approximately 90% excreted in urine primarily as metabolites
IM	10m	30-60m	6-7h	2.25h	35%	
IV	1-3m	20m	6-7h	2.25h	35%	
SC	10m	50-90m	6-7h	2.25h	35%	
Rectal	15-20m	60m	6-7h	2.25h	35%	

CONTRAINDICATIONS: Hypersensitivity; use c̄ extreme caution in head injuries.

SIDE/ADVERSE EFFECTS: CNS: *sedation, lightheadedness,* euphoria, dysphoria, tremors, disorientation, ↓ con-

Note: Side/adverse effects: common in *italic;* serious in ***boldface italic.***

*Available in Canada only.

vulsive threshold ▪ CV: hypotension, palpitations, flushing of face, phlebitis of IV site ▪ EENT: miosis ▪ GI: *N/V*, dry mouth, constipation, biliary tract spasm ▪ GU: urine retention ▪ INT: pruritus, urticaria ▪ RESP: ***respiratory depression***.

DRUG INTERACTIONS: Use c̄ alcohol, antihistamines, barbiturates, benzodiazepines, methotrimeprazine, phenothiazines, other CNS depressants produces additive CNS depression; ↓ dosage may be required ▪ Use c̄ tricyclic antidepressants may produce additive respiratory depression.

NURSING MANAGEMENT

ADMINISTRATION: Assess for hx of opioid hypersensitivity ▪ Assess quality, intensity, location of pain ▪ Store under double lock/key; document use accurately ▪ Check compatibility for mixing c̄ other drugs in solution ▪ PO liquid: dilute c̄ juice to mask disagreeable taste ▪ Do *not* administer if respirations are <12/m ▪ IM: inject *deep* into muscle; rotate sites ▪ IV: dilute; administer *slowly* (3-5m); keep pt supine for 2h ▪ Have narcotic antagonist (naloxone), support measures available ▪ Avoid administration in pts with suspected head injury ▪ Administer *before* pt experiences intense pain ▪ Avoid abrupt withdrawal c̄ long-term use ▪ Administer around clock to pts c̄ severe chronic pain ▪ Elderly may require ↓ dosage.

EVALUATION: Monitor respirations, circulatory function, esp BP ▪ Assess bowel function, abdominal distention, renal function, urinary retention ▪ Check for signs of dependence ▪ Assess for potentiation of CNS depressant effect ▪ Assess for N/V; administer antiemetic ▪ Assess for signs of overdose (coma, pinpoint pupils, respiratory depression) ▪ SC: check for tissue irritation.

EDUCATION: Avoid changing positions rapidly ▪ Avoid excessive sensory stimulation ▪ Keep bedrails up when nonambulatory ▪ Turn, cough, deep breathe after surgery ▪ Constipation may occur; ↑ fluids, bulk-containing foods ▪ Avoid potentially hazardous activities ▪ Avoid smoking ▪ Avoid use c̄ alcohol, other CNS depressants ▪ Women: avoid breastfeeding ▪ Take as ordered ▪ PO liquid: may mix c̄ juice; do *not* freeze ▪ Notify physician/dentist of use before treatment.

OVERDOSE MANAGEMENT: *See* Narcotics.

NOTES:

nabumetone • (na-byoo-meh-tone)

CATEGORY: *Antiinflammatory:* NSAIA

Rx; Preg Cat C

BRAND NAME
Relafen (SKB)

DOSAGE FORMS
Tablet: 500, 750mg

ACTION: Drug is converted by hepatic biotransformation into 6-methyoxy-2 napthylacetic acid (6 MNA), a potent inhibitor of prostaglandin synthesis resulting in an antiinflammatory effect. **USE:** Treatment of acute & chronic osteoarthritis, rheumatoid arthritis.

PHARMACOKINETICS

PO absorption	Peak	Half-life	Protein binding	Excretion
Good	2.5-4h	22.5-30h	99%	Via urine & feces as metabolites

CONTRAINDICATIONS: Hypersensitivity, pts c̄ aspirin- or other NSAIA-induced allergies (asthma, urticaria).

DOSAGE

Adult *PO* — Initial dose of 1000mg as a single dose w/out regard to meals c̄ a maximum dose of 2000mg/d.

SIDE/ADVERSE EFFECTS: CNS: Dizziness, headache, fatigue, somnolence, insomnia, asthenia, nightmares ▪ CV: edema, vasculitis ▪ EENT: tinnitus ▪ GI: diarrhea (14%), dyspepsia (13%), abdominal pain (12%), N/V, dry mouth, anorexia, ulcers, bleeding, ↑ appetite, melena ▪ GU: azotemia, dysuria, hematuria, renal stones ▪ HEM: anemia, leukopenia, granulocytopenia, ***thrombocytopenia*** ▪ INT: acne, alopecia, photosensitivity, pruritus, rash, sweating, ***erythema multiforme, Stevens-Johnson syndrome*** ▪ Other: fever, chills, hypokalemia.

DRUG INTERACTIONS: Use c̄ ulcerogenic drugs produces additive effects ▪ Use c̄ warfarin, other high protein binding drugs can ↑ their activity due to protein displacement.

NURSING MANAGEMENT

ADMINISTRATION: Assess for hx of NSAIA hypersensitivity ▪ Avoid administration to individuals c̄ hx of asthma, bleeding disorders, salicylate hypersensitivity ▪ Assess for hepatic, renal status; ↓ dosage if impaired ▪ May be administered c̄ food/milk; encourage upright position for 15-30m ▪ Avoid exposure to moisture, light in storage ▪ Elderly may require ↓ dosage.

EVALUATION: Monitor hematologic, hepatic, renal status c̄ prolonged use ▪ Monitor pt receiving anticoagulant therapy; may potentiate bleeding ▪ Monitor I&O, daily weight c̄ prolonged use ▪ Assess for edema in extremities, GI bleeding ▪ Assess for visual disturbances, skin rash; D/C drug, notify physician.

EDUCATION: Dizziness/drowsiness may occur; use caution in potentially hazardous activities ▪ Take c̄ food/milk; maintain upright position for 15-30m ▪ Take as ordered by physician; do *not* ↑ dose ▪ Notify physician *immediately* of bleeding, ↑ urine output, swelling of feet/legs, lethargy, GI distress, jaundice, visual disturbance ▪ Avoid taking c̄ aspirin, other NSAIAs ▪ Avoid use c̄ alcohol ▪ Check c̄ physician/pharmacist before taking OTC preparations ▪ Notify physician/dentist of use before treatment ▪ Store in tightly closed container ▪ Full drug effects may require several wks of therapy.

NOTES:

nadolol • (nay-doe-lole)

CATEGORY: *Beta-adrenergic blocker*: antianginal, antihypertensive   Rx; Preg Cat C

BRAND NAME	**DOSAGE FORMS**
Corgard (Bristol)	Tablet: 20, 40, 80, 120, 160mg

COMBINATION PRODUCTS

Corzide 40/5, 80/5 (Bristol)	Nadolol/bendroflumethiazide per tablet: 40mg/5mg, 80mg/5mg

ACTION: Blocks access of catecholamines to $beta_1$, $beta_2$ receptors, resulting in bronchial constriction, ↓ heart rate, ↓ myocardial contractility; antihypertensive effect not determined. **USE:** Treatment of angina pectoris ▪ Treatment of hypertension as sole agent/in combination c̄ other antihypertensives (esp thiazide diuretics).

PHARMACOKINETICS

PO absorption	Peak	Half-life	Protein binding	Excretion
30%	3-4h	20-24h	30%	Via urine as unchanged drug

CONTRAINDICATIONS: Hypersensitivity, bronchial asthma, cardiogenic shock, overt cardiac failure, sinus bradycardia, heart block >1°.

DOSAGE

Adult *PO*

Angina	80-240mg/d as single dose
Hypertension	80-320mg/d as single dose. Up to 640mg/d may be required
Corzide 40/5, 80/5	Usual dose one tablet/d

SIDE/ADVERSE EFFECTS: CNS: dizziness, fatigue, paresthesias, sedation, behavioral changes ▪ CV: bradycardia (≤60), hypotension, ***cardiac failure,*** peripheral vascular insufficiency ▪ EENT: dry eyes, nasal congestion, tinnitus, blurred vision ▪ GI: N/D, anorexia, abdominal discomfort, flatulence, dry mouth ▪ GU: impotence ▪ RESP: bronchospasm ▪ Other: weight gain.

DRUG INTERACTIONS: Use c̄ reserpine, other catecholamine-depleting drugs can result in serious adrenergic blockage ▪ Nonselective beta adrenergics antagonize therapeutic response.

NURSING MANAGEMENT

ADMINISTRATION: Assess for hx of beta blocker hypersensitivity ▪ Assess BP, apical pulse; if <60/m, hold drug, notify physician ▪ Assess hepatic function, I&O ▪ Do *not* administer in presence of respiratory distress (asthma, CHF, COPD) ▪ Administer c̄ food ▪ Avoid exposure to heat, moisture, light in storage ▪ Avoid abrupt withdrawal ▪ Elderly may require ↓ dosage.

EVALUATION: Monitor hepatic, renal, respiratory status ▪ Monitor BP, pulse ▪ Monitor CBC, FBS (diabetics) ▪ Assess for depression ▪ May produce alteration in blood glucose levels (hypoglycemia); may mask signs of hypoglycemia.

EDUCATION: Check pulse before taking; if <60/m, do *not* take drug, notify physician ▪ Take as directed by physician; do *not* skip doses ▪ Take c̄ food ▪ Do *not* D/C drug w/out notifying physician ▪ Check c̄ physician/pharmacist before taking OTC/Rx preparations ▪ May cause drowsiness; use caution in potentially hazardous activities ▪ Diabetics: carefully monitor blood/urine glucose ▪ May experience ↑ sensitivity to cold ▪ Notify physician of respiratory distress, leg edema ▪ Notify physician/dentist of beta blocker use before treatment ▪ Maintain optimum weight ▪ Keep scheduled appointments c̄ physician ▪ Follow low-Na^+ diet ▪ Store in tightly closed, light-resistant container ▪ Avoid ↑ exercise, cold, smoking ▪ Women: avoid breastfeeding.

NOTES:

nafcillin sodium • (naf-sill-in)

CATEGORY: *Penicillinase-resistant penicillin*: antibiotic Rx; Preg Cat NA

BRAND NAMES	DOSAGE FORMS
Nafcil (Apothecon)	Powder for injection (IM/IV): 0.5, 1, 2, 10g vial
Unipen (W-A)	Capsule: 250mg Powder for injection (IM/IV): 0.5, 1, 2, 10g vial Powder for PO solution: 250mg/5ml Tablet: 500mg

ACTION: Bactericidal activity due to inhibition of mucopeptide cell wall synthesis in susceptible organisms. **USE:** Treatment of infections due to susceptible strains of penicillinase-producing staphylococci.

PHARMACOKINETICS

PO absorption	Peak	Half-life	Protein binding	Excretion
Adequate	0.5-2h	0.5-1.5h	70%-90%	Via urine as unchanged drug, metabolites

CONTRAINDICATIONS: Hypersensitivity to any penicillin.

DOSAGE

Neonate	*PO*	10mg/kg 3-4 times/d
	IM	10mg/kg bid
Pediatric	*PO*	50mg/kg/d in 4 doses
	IM	25mg/kg bid
Adult	*PO*	250-500mg q4-6h. Severe infections may require 1g q4-6h
	IM	500mg q6h. Severe infections may require 500mg q4h
	IV	500mg q4h. Severe infections may require 1g q4h

SIDE/ADVERSE EFFECTS: CNS: neuropathy usually associated c̄ high parenteral doses ▪ GI: *N/V/D, epigastric distress, black hairy tongue,* flatulence, smell/taste disturbances ▪ GU: ***interstitial nephritis*** (rare) ▪ HEM: anemia, eosinophilia, leukopenia, neutropenia, ***thrombocytopenia*** ▪ HEP: ↑ serum levels of AST, ALT, LDH ▪ INT: rash, pruritus, urticaria ▪ MS: arthralgia ▪ Other: *local irritation at injection site,* fever, ***anaphylaxis.***

DRUG INTERACTIONS: Bacteriostatic antibiotics c̄ any penicillin can lead to antibiotic antagonism ▪ PO anticoagulant therapy may require dose adjustments.

NURSING MANAGEMENT

ADMINISTRATION: Assess for hx of penicillin/cephalosporin hypersensitivity ▪ Obtain C&S ▪ Maintain blood levels; administer at equal intervals around clock ▪ Reconstitute powder according to manufacturer's directions c̄ sterile or bacteriostatic H_2O for injection/0.9% NaCl injection; stable for 3d at room temperature, 7d refrigerated ▪ IM: administer by *deep* intragluteal injection (vastus lateralis <3y/o) ▪ IV: (direct) dilute in 15-30ml sterile H_2O for injection/NaCl injection, administer over 5-10m; (infusion) mix c̄ diluent recommended by manufacturer; use only 24-48h because of possibility of thrombophlebitis (esp elderly) ▪ Do *not* administer bacteriostatic agents w/in 1h ▪ Do *not* administer discolored/precipitated solutions ▪ Have support equipment available for anaphylaxis ▪ Na^+ content: 2.9mEq (67mg)/g; calculate in Na^+-restricted diets.

EVALUATION: Monitor pts c̄ allergies/asthma (high risk for hypersensitivity) ▪ Monitor VS, renal, hepatic, hemopoietic status ▪ Observe for signs of superinfection ▪ Check IV insertion site; rotate q48h.

EDUCATION: Complete full course of therapy (usually 10d) even if symptom free ▪ Take on empty stomach at equal intervals ▪ Take c̄ H_2O, *not* c̄ acidic beverage (orange juice, carbonated beverages) ▪ Diarrhea may occur ▪ Store in dry, tightly closed container ▪ Discard outdated preparations ▪ Maintain good personal hygiene (esp perineal, oral) ▪ Maintain fluid intake (6-8 glasses/d) ▪ Notify physician of symptoms of allergic rx (fever, difficult breathing, rash) ▪ Carry identification (MedicAlert) if penicillin allergic.

NOTES:

nalbuphine hcl • (<u>nal</u>-byoo-feen)

CATEGORY: *Analgesic:* opioid agonist-antagonist   Rx; Preg Cat NA

BRAND NAME
Nubain (Du Pont)

DOSAGE FORMS
Injection (IM/IV/SC): 10, 20mg/ml

ACTION: Analgesic mechanism not determined; possible site of activity may be in subcortical areas of brain; narcotic agonist activity equivalent to morphine (mg/mg); narcotic antagonist activity 1/4 that of nalorphine, 10 times pentazocine. **USE:** Relief of moderate/severe pain ▪ Pre-op sedation, obstetrical analgesia, adjunct to surgical anesthesia.

PHARMACOKINETICS

Onset				
IV	IM/SC	Duration	Half-life	Excretion
2-3m	15m	3-6h	5h	Via urine, feces as unchanged drug, metabolites

CONTRAINDICATIONS: Hypersensitivity.

DOSAGE

Adult *IM/IV/SC* — 10mg/70kg weight, repeat q3-6h. Do *not* exceed single dose 20mg, daily total 160mg in nontolerant pts

SIDE/ADVERSE EFFECTS: CNS: *sedation*, dizziness, vertigo, headache, dreams, depression ▪ CV: hypertension, hypotension, bradycardia, tachycardia ▪ EENT: blurred vision ▪ GI: bitter taste, cramps, dyspepsia, dry mouth ▪ GU: urinary retention ▪ INT: urticaria, rash ▪ Other: autonomic responses (sweating/clammy sensation, flushing, warmth).

DRUG INTERACTIONS: Use c̄ CNS depressants produces additive effects ▪ Use in narcotic-dependent pts can produce withdrawal symptoms.

NURSING MANAGEMENT

ADMINISTRATION: Assess for hx of opioid hypersensitivity ▪ Check compatibility chart for mixing pre-op IM preparations ▪ Do *not* administer if respirations are <12/m ▪ IM: inject *deep* into muscle; rotate sites ▪ IV: dilute;

administer *slowly* ▪ Have narcotic antagonist, support measures available ▪ Avoid administration in pts c̄ suspected head injury ▪ Administer *before* pt has intense pain ▪ Avoid light, freezing in storage ▪ Utilize + power of suggestion ▪ Avoid abrupt withdrawal ▪ Elderly may require ↓ dosage.

EVALUATION: Monitor respirations, circulatory function ▪ Assess bowel function, abdominal distention ▪ Assess renal function, urinary retention ▪ Check for signs of dependence c̄ prolonged use (↑ drug request) ▪ Assess for potentiation of CNS depressant effect ▪ Assess for signs of overdose (coma, pinpoint pupils, respiratory depression).

EDUCATION: Avoid changing positions (lying/sitting/standing) rapidly ▪ Avoid excessive sensory stimulation ▪ Keep bedrails up when nonambulatory ▪ Obtain assistance prn when ambulatory ▪ Turn, cough, deep-breathe after surgery ▪ Constipation may occur; ↑ fluid, bulk-containing foods ▪ Avoid potentially hazardous activities ▪ Avoid smoking while taking drug ▪ Indiscriminate use may lead to dependence ▪ Avoid use c̄ alcohol, other CNS depressants.

OVERDOSE MANAGEMENT: naloxone hcl is specific antidote, in conjunction c̄ support therapy using oxygen, IV fluids, vasopressors.

NOTES:

naloxone hcl • (nal-ox-one)

CATEGORY: *Narcotic antagonist*

Rx; Preg Cat B

BRAND NAME
Narcan (Du Pont)

DOSAGE FORMS
Injection (IM/IV/SC): 0.4, 1mg/ml
Neonatal injection (IM/IV/SC): 0.02mg/ml

ACTION: Narcotic antagonism primarily due to competition c̄ narcotics for CNS receptor sites. **USE:** Induce complete/partial reversal of narcotic depression (incl respiratory) induced by natural/synthetic narcotics, propoxyphene, narcotic agonist/antagonist, nalbuphine, pentazocine, butorphanol ▪ Diagnosis of suspected acute opioid overdosage.

PHARMACOKINETICS: IM/SC onset 2-5m, IV 1-2m; half-life 60-90m in adults, longer in infants; excreted via urine primarily as metabolites.

CONTRAINDICATIONS: Hypersensitivity.

DOSAGE

Pediatric *IM/IV/SC*	
Overdose	0.01mg/kg IV. Subsequent dose 0.1mg/kg may be given IV prn
Post-op	0.005-0.01mg/kg IV. Repeat at 2-3m intervals to desired degree of reversal Neonate: 0.01mg/kg. Repeat at 2-3m intervals to desired degree of reversal
Adult *IM/IV/SC*	
Overdose	0.4-2mg IV. Repeat at 2-3m intervals to desired degree of reversal
Post-op	0.1-0.2mg/kg IV. Repeat at 2-3m intervals to desired degree of reversal

SIDE/ADVERSE EFFECTS: GI: N/V (rare) c̄ high doses post-op ▪ Other: withdrawal symptoms in narcotic-dependent pt.

Note: Side/adverse effects: common in *italic;* serious in ***boldface italic.***

*Available in Canada only.

NURSING MANAGEMENT

ADMINISTRATION: Mix c̄ sterile H_2O for injection prn ▪ Do *not* leave pt unattended ▪ Have emergency support equipment available ▪ Store in original container; avoid exposure to light.

EVALUATION: Monitor VS, esp respirations ▪ Observe for ↓ respirations after treatment, because duration of action of narcotic may be longer than that of naloxone ▪ Observe for signs of narcotic withdrawal (restlessness, muscle spasms, ↑ VS, lacrimation) ▪ Assess for ↑ PTT ▪ Assess ABGs.

EDUCATION: Explain procedure, rationale to pt, family ▪ Safety precautions ▪ Comfort measures.

NOTES:

naproxen/naproxen sodium ▲ • (na-prox-en)

CATEGORY: *Antiinflammatory:* analgesic Rx; Preg Cat B

BRAND NAMES	DOSAGE FORMS
Anaprox ▲ (Syntex)	Tablet: 275mg
Anaprox DS ▲ (Syntex)	Tablet: 550mg
Naprosyn (Syntex)	PO suspension: 125mg/5ml Tablet: 250, 375, 500mg (also 125mg in Canada)
**Naxen (SynCare); *Novonaprox (Novopharm)*	Tablet: 125, 250, 375, 500mg

ACTION: Antiinflammatory, analgesic activity appears related to inhibition of prostaglandin synthesis. **USE:** Treatment of rheumatoid/osteoarthritis, ankylosing spondylitis, acute gout, tendinitis, bursitis ▪ Relief of mild/moderate pain, primary dysmenorrhea.

PHARMACOKINETICS

PO absorption	Peak	Half-life	Protein binding	Excretion
Complete	2-4h	13h	99%	95% via urine primarily as unchanged drug

CONTRAINDICATIONS: Hypersensitivity, aspirin/other antiinflammatory agent hypersensitivity.

DOSAGE

Adult *PO*

Pain, dysmenorrhea, tendinitis, bursitis	Naproxen 500mg followed by 250mg q6-8h, c̄ maximum dose 1.25g/d. Naproxen sodium 550mg followed by 275mg q6-8h, c̄ maximum dose 1.375g/d
Acute gout	Naproxen 750mg followed by 250mg q8h until remission. Naproxen sodium 825mg followed by 275mg q8h until remission
Arthritis, spondylitis	Naproxen 250-375mg bid, adjust, c̄ maximum dose 1g/d. Naproxen sodium 275mg bid, adjust, c̄ maximum dose 1.1g/d

Note: Side/adverse effects: common in *italic;* serious in ***boldface italic.***

*Available in Canada only.

SIDE/ADVERSE EFFECTS: CNS: headache, dizziness, drowsiness ▪ CV: edema, palpitations, CHF ▪ EENT: tinnitus, ↓ hearing, blurred vision ▪ GI: *constipation, abdominal pain, nausea,* vomiting, stomatitis ▪ GU: ***glomerular nephritis,*** hematuria, ***interstitial nephritis,*** nephrotic syndrome ▪ HEM: ***agranulocytosis, aplastic anemia, hemolytic anemia*** ▪ INT: rash, alopecia, pruritus, purpura, urticaria ▪ Other: thirst, eosinophilic pneumonia.

DRUG INTERACTIONS: Use c̄ ulcerogenic drugs produces additive effects ▪ Use c̄ PO anticoagulants may ↑ their activity ▪ Aspirin will ↓ naproxen plasma levels.

NURSING MANAGEMENT

ADMINISTRATION: Assess for hx of NSAIA hypersensitivity ▪ Avoid administration to pts c̄ hx of asthma, bleeding disorders, salicylate hypersensitivity ▪ Assess for hx of peptic ulcer; use c̄ caution ▪ Assess hematologic, renal, hepatic function; use caution if impaired ▪ Administer c̄ food/milk to ↓ GI irritation; encourage upright position for 15-30m ▪ Avoid exposure to moisture in storage ▪ Elderly may require ↓ dosage.

EVALUATION: Monitor hepatic, renal status c̄ prolonged use ▪ Monitor pt receiving anticoagulant therapy; may potentiate bleeding ▪ Monitor I&O, daily weight ▪ Assess for edema in extremities ▪ Assess for visual/hearing disturbances; D/C drug, notify physician.

EDUCATION: Dizziness/drowsiness may occur; use caution in potentially hazardous activities ▪ Take c̄ food/milk to ↓ GI distress; maintain upright position for 15-30m ▪ Take as ordered by physician, do *not* ↑ dose ▪ Notify physician *immediately* of bleeding, ↓ urine output, swelling of feet/legs, lethargy, GI distress, jaundice, visual disturbance ▪ Avoid taking c̄ aspirin/other NSAIAs ▪ Avoid use c̄ alcohol ▪ Check c̄ physician/pharmacist before taking OTC preparations ▪ Notify physician/dentist of use before treatment ▪ Store in tightly closed container ▪ Schedule eye exams c̄ prolonged use ▪ Full drug effects may require several wks of therapy.

NOTES:

neostigmine bromide/neostigmine methylsulfate • (nee-oh-stig-meen)

CATEGORY: *Anticholinesterase*: cholinergic, parasympathomimetic Rx; Preg Cat C

BRAND NAMES	DOSAGE FORMS
Prostigmin bromide (ICN)	Tablet: 15mg
Prostigmin methylsulfate (ICN)	Injection (IM/IV/SC): 0.25, 0.5, 1mg/ml (2.5mg/ml in Canada)

ACTION: Anticholinesterase drugs inhibit acetylcholinesterase enzyme, resulting in higher levels of acetylcholine, producing nicotinic effect at autonomic ganglia, skeletal muscle myoneural junctions, muscarinic effect at postganglionic fibers in parasympathetic nervous system. **USE:** Symptomatic control of myasthenia gravis ▪ Prevention/treatment of postoperative distention, urinary retention ▪ Antidote for tubocurarine-like drugs (nondepolarizing agents).

PHARMACOKINETICS

PO absorption	Peak	Half-life	Protein binding	Excretion
Poor	1-2	42-60m	15%-25%	80% via urine in 24h

CONTRAINDICATIONS: Hypersensitivity, mechanical bowel/urinary tract obstruction, peritonitis.

DOSAGE

Pediatric/ Adult *PO*	Dosage must be individualized for myasthenia gravis, varies from 15-375mg/d
Adult	
Myasthenia gravis *SC/IM*	0.5mg. Subsequent doses dependent on response
Post-op *SC/IM*	0.25mg as soon as possible after surgery. May be repeated q4-6h for 2-3d for prevention of urinary retention
Urinary retention *SC/IM*	0.5mg. If urination does not occur w/in 1h, catheterize. After urine voiding, continue doses of 0.5mg q3h for at least 5 injection
Antidote *IV*	0.5-2mg by slow injection. Recommended that atropine sulfate 0.6-1.2mg also be given IV by separate syringe

SIDE/ADVERSE EFFECTS: CNS: dizziness, drowsiness, headache, ***convulsions*** ▪ CV: bradycardia, tachycardia, ***AV block,*** hypotension ▪ EENT: miosis, vision change ▪ GI: N/V, flatulence, cramps ▪ GU: urinary frequency ▪ INT: rash, urticaria ▪ RESP: ↑ secretion, dyspnea, ***bronchospasm,*** depression ▪ Other: diaphoresis.

DRUG INTERACTIONS: Use c̄ anticholinergics antagonizes cholinergic effects.

NURSING MANAGEMENT

ADMINISTRATION: Assess for hx of hypersensitivity ▪ Do *not* administer c̄ other cholinergic drugs ▪ Largest dose scheduled before periods of ↑ fatigue ▪ PO: administer c̄ food/milk to ↓ GI irritation ▪ Document response after each dose ▪ Have atropine, support equipment available.

EVALUATION: Monitor VS, esp pulse, respirations ▪ Monitor muscle strength ▪ Assess for excessive cholinergic manifestations (↑ sweating, ↑ salivation, muscle tremors) ▪ Monitor GI status (flatus, abdominal distention) ▪ Assess for urinary retention; catheterize if no voiding w/in 1h of first dose.

EDUCATION: Take c̄ food/milk to ↓ GI distress ▪ Take as ordered by physician; do *not* change dose ▪ Space daily activities to ↓ fatigue, conserve energy ▪ Adhere to scheduled cough, deep-breathing, ROM activities ▪ Record high, low points of muscle strength ▪ Rectal tube may be inserted after administration to help expel gas related to post-op abdominal distention ▪ Carry medical identification (MedicAlert) for myasthenia gravis.

NOTES:

netilmicin sulfate • (ne-til-mye-sin)

CATEGORY: *Aminoglycoside:* antibiotic

Rx; Preg Cat D

BRAND NAME
Netromycin (Schering)

DOSAGE FORMS
Injection (IM/IV): 100mg/ml

ACTION: Bactericidal activity due to inhibition of ribosomal protein synthesis in susceptible organisms. **USE:** Indicated for infections caused by susceptible strains of *Citrobacter* spp, *Enterobacter* spp, *Escherichia coli, Klebsiella pneumoniae, Proteus* spp, *Pseudomonas aeruginosa, Serratia* spp ▪ Alternate for penicillin-resistant staphylococcal infections.

PHARMACOKINETICS

IM peak	Half-life	Excretion
0.5-1h	2-2.5h	80% unchanged in urine in 24h

CONTRAINDICATIONS: Hypersensitivity, previous aminoglycoside toxicity (possible).

DOSAGE: *IM/IV.* For pts c̄ impaired renal function, adjust dose according to manufacturer's recommendations.

Neonate <6wks	4-6.5mg/kg/d given as 2-3.25mg/kg q12h
Pediatric 6wks-12y/o	5.5-8mg/kg/d given as 1.8-2.7mg/kg q8h or 2.7-4mg/kg q12h
Adult	3-4mg/kg/d given as 1.5-2mg/kg q8-12h. More serious infection may require 4-6.5mg/kg/d

SIDE/ADVERSE EFFECTS: CNS: paresthesias ▪ CV: palpitations, hypotension ▪ EENT: ***ototoxicity*** (auditory vestibular damage: dizziness, vertigo, tinnitus, roaring in ears, hearing loss), blurred vision ▪ GI: D/V ▪ GU: ***nephrotoxicity*** (casts, proteinuria, ↑ BUN, ↑ serum creatinine) ▪ HEM: anemia, leukopenia, ***thrombocytopenia*** ▪ HEP: ↑ Alkaline phosphatase, bilirubin, AST, ALT ▪ MET: hypokalemia.

DRUG INTERACTIONS: Avoid use c̄ neurotoxic/nephrotoxic drugs (eg, other aminoglycosides, colistin, ethacrynic acid, furosemide, polymyxin B, vancomycin, viomycin) ▪ Dimenhydrinate can mask aminoglycoside ototoxicity ▪ ↑ Succinylcholine/tubocurarine activity; Ca salts can reverse blockade ▪ PO anticoagulant activity may ↑ due to ↓ intestinal vitamin K synthesis.

NURSING MANAGEMENT

ADMINISTRATION: Assess for hx of aminoglycoside hypersensitivity ▪ Obtain C&S before therapy ▪ Obtain pt weight for dosage calculation ▪ Determine creatinine clearance before administration ▪ IV: single dose may be diluted in 50-200ml parenteral solution; infuse over 1/2-1h; use less diluent for pediatric IV ▪ Store solution in glass containers for up to 72h ▪ IM: administer by *deep, slow* injection; rotate sites; avoid inflamed areas ▪ Maintain hydration.

EVALUATION: Assess for hearing dysfunction ▪ Monitor hepatic, renal, VIII CN function during therapy ▪ Assess for edema in extremities ▪ Assess for neuromuscular blockade, respiratory paralysis, nephrotoxicity ▪ Observe for signs of superinfection (diarrhea, URI, coated tongue) ▪ Assess for hypersensitivity rx (fever, difficult breathing, rash) ▪ Assess peak (<16μg/ml), trough (<4μg/ml) serum concentrations.

EDUCATION: Report hearing, balance difficulties to physician at once ▪ ↑ Fluid intake (10-12 glasses/d) ▪ Women: avoid breastfeeding.

NOTES:

nicardipine hcl • (nye-card-i-peen)

CATEGORY: *Calcium blocker:* antianginal, antihypertensive, slow channel blocker Rx; Preg Cat C

BRAND NAME
Cardene (Syntex)

DOSAGE FORMS
Capsule: 20, 30mg

ACTION: Antianginal and antihypertensive effect due to inhibition of extracellular calcium-ion transmembrane migration in cardiac, vascular smooth muscle via slow channel passageway, resulting in coronary dilation; ↑ myocardial oxygen supply, ↓ oxygen consumption. Slow channel effect is greater in vascular smooth muscle. **USE:** Treatment as a sole agent or in combination with a beta blocker for chronic stable angina pectoris; treatment for hypertension as a sole agent or in combination c̄ other antihypertensives.

CONTRAINDICATIONS: Hypersensitivity, advanced aortic stenosis.

DOSAGE: Normal hepatic and renal function
Adult *PO*

Angina/hypertension	20-40mg tid. Dosage ↑ require 3d intervals.

SIDE/ADVERSE EFFECTS: CNS: *headache, dizziness,* tremor, paresthesia, flushing, somnolence ▪ CV: *pedal edema,* palpitations, tachycardia, angina, abnormal ECG ▪ GI: *nausea, dypepsia, dry mouth,* constipation, vomiting ▪ Other: rash, dyspnea, myalgia, malaise, *asthenia.*

PHARMACOKINETICS

PO absorption	Onset	Peak	Half-life	Protein binding	Excretion
Complete	20m	0.5-2h	2-4h	95%	As metabolites via urine (60%), feces (35%)

Note: Side/adverse effects: common in *italic;* serious in ***boldface italic.*** *Available in Canada only.

DRUG INTERACTIONS: Calcium blockers may ↑ dig serum level ▪ Use c̄ beta blockers is well tolerated ▪ Cimetidine ↑ nicardipine serum levels ▪ Nicardipine may ↑ cyclosporine serum levels.

NURSING MANAGEMENT

ADMINISTRATION: Assess for hx of hypersensitivity ▪ Assess for hx of heart failure; use c̄ caution ▪ Assess BP, heart rate; if apical pulse <60/m, hold dose, notify physician ▪ Assess hepatic, renal function; ↓ dosage if impaired ▪ Assess dietary intake (avoid high-fat meals) ▪ Avoid exposure to light, moisture in storage ▪ Elderly may require ↓ dosage.

EVALUATION: Monitor VS, esp BP (2h & 8h after administration), heart rate ▪ Monitor I&O ▪ Assess for CHF (dyspnea, peripheral edema, ↑ weight); notify physician ▪ Monitor hepatic, renal status.

EDUCATION: Dizziness may occur; use caution in potentially hazardous activities ▪ Avoid changing positions (lying/sitting/standing) rapidly ▪ Avoid high-fat meals during therapy ▪ Procedure for checking radial pulse ▪ If pulse slow (<60/m) or irregular, notify physician ▪ Avoid caffeine ▪ Check c̄ physician/pharmacist before taking OTC preparations ▪ Take as ordered by physician; do *not* change dose ▪ Notify physician of difficult breathing, chest pain, swelling of hands/legs ▪ Keep scheduled appointments c̄ physician; have BP checked regularly ▪ Continue to use SL nitroglycerin (if ordered) to relieve sudden chest pain or for prophylaxis before exertion ▪ Avoid use c̄ alcohol ▪ Avoid smoking ▪ Carry identification (MedicAlert) if hypertensive ▪ Women: avoid breastfeeding.

NOTES:

nifedipine • (nye-fed-i-peen)

CATEGORY: *Calcium blocker*: antianginal, slow channel blocker   Rx; Preg Cat C

BRAND NAMES
Adalat (Miles)
Procardia (Pfizer)

DOSAGE FORMS
Capsule 10, 20mg
Capsule, 10, 20mg
XL tablet: 30, 60, 90mg

DOSAGE
Adult *PO*: Initial dose 10mg tid. Usual daily range 10-20mg tid. Do *not* exceed 30mg/dose or 180mg/d
OB (labor) dose is usually 10mg tid as required
XL tablets: start c̄ 30 or 60mg tablet once/d and adjust over 7-14d. Do *not* exceed 120mg/d

ACTION: Antianginal effect due to inhibition of extracellular calcium-ion transmembrane migration in cardiac, vascular smooth muscle via slow channel passageway, resulting in coronary dilation; in addition, ↑ myocardial oxygen supply, ↓ oxygen consumption. **USE:** Treatment of chronic, stable, vasospastic angina pectoris ▪ Nonlabeled OB uses include prophylaxis of preterm labor ▪ Treatment of hypertension as a sole agent or in combination (XL only).

PHARMACOKINETICS

PO absorption	Onset	Peak	Half-life	Protein binding	Excretion
90%	20m	30m	2h	92%-98%	80% via urine as unchanged drug, metabolites

CONTRAINDICATIONS: Hypersensitivity.

SIDE/ADVERSE EFFECTS: CNS: *dizziness*, headache, nervousness ▪ CV: *peripheral edema*, transient hypotension, palpitations ▪ EENT: nasal congestion, sore throat, blurred

Note: Side/adverse effects: common in *italic;* serious in ***boldface italic.***   *Available in Canada only.

vision, gingival hyperplasia (rare) ▪ GI: *nausea*, diarrhea, cramps, flatulence, constipation ▪ HEM: anemia, leukopenia, purpura ▪ INT: urticaria, dermatitis, pruritus ▪ MS: muscle cramps, tremor, joint stiffness ▪ Other: flushing, weakness.

DRUG INTERACTIONS: Use c̄ dig may ↑ dig body levels ▪ Use c̄ antihypertensives may ↑ hypotensive effects ▪ Use c̄ beta blockers may occasionally ↑ possibility of CHF, severe hypotension, angina attacks.

NURSING MANAGEMENT

ADMINISTRATION: Assess for hx of hypersensitivity ▪ Assess for hx of heart failure; use c̄ caution ▪ Assess BP, heart rate; if apical pulse <60, hold dose, notify physician ▪ May puncture capsule c̄ needle, deposit solution sublingually or in buccal pouch for rapid action ▪ Avoid exposure to light, moisture in storage ▪ Elderly may require ↓ dosage.

EVALUATION: Monitor VS, esp BP, heart rate ▪ Monitor I&O ▪ Assess for CHF (dyspnea, peripheral edema, ↑ weight); notify physician ▪ Monitor hepatic, renal status ▪ Diabetics: closely monitor blood glucose ▪ Digitalized pts: assess for dig toxicity (bradycardia, anorexia, palpitations).

EDUCATION: Dizziness occur; use caution in potentially hazardous activities ▪ Avoid changing positions (lying/sitting/standing) rapidly ▪ Procedure for checking radial pulse ▪ If pulse slow (<60) or irregular, do *not* take drug; notify physician ▪ Avoid caffeine ▪ Check c̄ physician/pharmacist before taking OTC preparations ▪ Take as ordered by physician; do *not* change dose ▪ Notify physician of difficult breathing, chest pain, swelling of hands/legs; D/C drug ▪ Keep scheduled appointments c̄ physician ▪ Continue to use SL nitroglycerin (if ordered) to relieve sudden chest pain or for prophylaxis before exertion ▪ Avoid use c̄ alcohol ▪ Avoid smoking ▪ Diabetics: monitor blood or urine glucose carefully; keep scheduled lab appointments.

NOTES:

nitrofurantoin • (nye-troe-fyoor-an-toyn)

CATEGORY: *Antiinfective:* urinary antimicrobial Rx; Preg Cat NA

BRAND NAMES	DOSAGE FORMS
Furadantin (P-G)	Suspension: 25mg/5ml Tablet: 50, 100mg
Furalan (Lannett)	Tablet: 50, 100mg
Macrobid (P-G)	Capsule: 100mg
Macrodantin (P-G)	Capsule: 25, 50, 100mg
**Nephronex (Cortunon)*	Tablet: 50, 100mg
**Novofuran (Novopharm)*	Suspension: 25mg/5ml Tablet: 50, 100mg

ACTION: Bacteriostatic activity due to possible interference c̄ several enzyme systems incl coenzme A in susceptible organisms. **USE:** Treatment of UTIs caused by susceptible strains of *Enterobacter* spp, enterococci, *Escherichia coli, Klebsiella* spp, *Proteus* spp, *Staphylococcus aureus* (not indicated for treatment of associated renal cortical/perinephric abscesses).

PHARMACOKINETICS

PO absorption	Half-life	Protein binding	Excretion
Good	20m	25%-60%	Via urine as unchanged drug, metabolites

CONTRAINDICATIONS: Hypersensitivity, anuria, oliguria, significant renal dysfunction, pregnancy at term, infants <1mo

DOSAGE

Pediatric *PO*	5-7mg/kg/d in 4 equal doses c̄ food
Adult *PO*	50-100mg qid c̄ food

SIDE/ADVERSE EFFECTS: CNS: peripheral neuropathy, headache, dizziness, drowsiness ▪ EENT: nystagmus ▪ GI: *anorexia, N/V/D*, pain, ***pancreatitis*** ▪ HEM: ***hemolytic anemia***, granulocytopenia, ***agranulocytosis***, leukopenia,

*Available in Canada only.

thrombocytopenia, megaloblastic anemia, eosinophilia ▪ HEP: cholestatic jaundice, hepatitis ▪ INT: pruritus, urticaria, maculopapular rash, ***exfoliative dermatitis, erythema multiforme,*** alopecia ▪ MS: arthralgia ▪ RESP: acute, subacute, chronic diffuse ***interstitial pneumonitis/pulmonary fibrosis;*** asthma attack ▪ Other: ***anaphylaxis,*** drug fever.

DRUG INTERACTIONS: Probenecid/sulfinpyrazone ↓ renal excretion, ↑ toxicity ▪ Use c̄ nalidixic acid best avoided ▪ Use c̄ magnesium trisilicate antacid ↓ PO absorption of nitrofurantoin.

NURSING MANAGEMENT

ADMINISTRATION: Assess for hx of nitrofuran hypersensitivity ▪ Assess creatinine clearance; if <40ml/m, do *not* administer ▪ Obtain C&S before therapy ▪ Administer c̄ food/milk to ↓ GI irritation; do *not* crush (may stain teeth); have pt rinse mouth after administration ▪ PO suspension: shake well before pouring ▪ Avoid exposure to light, metals (except stainless steel, aluminum) in storage.

EVALUATION: Monitor VS, esp temperature ▪ Monitor respiratory status ▪ Monitor I&O, CBC, urine pH (acidity ↑ drug effect) ▪ Assess for UTI (cloudy, foul-smelling urine; painful urination) ▪ Urine glucose: false (+) c̄ Clinitest; use Clinistix/Test-Tape.

EDUCATION: Take c̄ food/milk to ↓ GI distress ▪ Take as ordered by physician; Rx will be continued for 3d after sterile urine specimens obtained ▪ Notify physician *immediately* of numbness, tingling, ↓ muscle strength; D/C drug ▪ Use Clinistix/Tes-Tape for urine testing ▪ May turn urine brown ▪ Store in amber glass container ▪ Women: avoid breastfeeding ▪ Check c̄ physician/pharmacist before taking antacids.

NOTES:

nitroglycerin (glyceryl trinitrate) formulations • (nye-troe-gli-ser-in)

CATEGORY: *Antianginal*: coronary vasodilator — Rx; Preg Cat C

FORMULATIONS/BRAND NAMES

Capsule:	Nitro-Bid Plateau (Marion), Nitrocine (Schwartz), Nitrostat (P-D)
IV injection:	Nitrol (Rorer), Nitrobid IV (Marion), Nitrostat (IV) (P-D), Tridil (Du Pont)
Lingual aerosol:	Nitrolingual (RPR)
Tablet:	Nitrong (RPR)
SL tablet:	Nitrostat (P-D), generic (various manufacterers)
Ointment:	Nitro-Bid (Marion), Nitrol (Adria)
Transdermal:	Nitrodisc (Searle), Nitro-Dur (Key), Deponit (Schwartz), Transderm-Nitro (Summit), Minitran (3M)
Transmucosal:	Nitrogard (Forest)

ACTION: Nitrates relax smooth muscle in small blood vessels, dilate arteries/capillaries, esp in coronary circulation, relieving myocardial ischemia & thereby ↓ anginal pain. **USE:** Prevention/treatment of angina pectoris ▪ Control of blood pressure during surgery (IV) ▪ Congestive heart failure associated c̄ acute MI (IV).

PHARMACOKINETICS

	Onset	Duration
SL tablet	2-3m	25-30m
Extended action: Capsule, ointment, transdermal	20-60m	Several h, to maximum 24h depending on dosage, release system

CONTRAINDICATIONS: Hypersensitivity, severe anemia, glaucoma, recent MI, ↑ cranial pressure, uncorrected hypovolemia (IV).

DOSAGE: Must be individualized

Adult *IV*	Non-PVC sets: 5μg/m c̄ 5μg/g increments q3-5m until response obtained. PVC sets require larger doses because drug penetrates plastic
Ointment	A ribbon of 1-5in q8h
PO	2.5-6.5mg q8-12h
Sublingual	0.15-0.6mg
Transdermal	Specific release system selected

(2.5mg/24h, 5mg/24h, 7.5mg/24h, 10mg/24h, 15mg/24h) should produce greatest clinical response c̄ minimum adverse effects

SIDE/ADVERSE EFFECTS: CNS: *transient headache,* dizziness, apprehension ▪ CV: hypotension, tachycardia, flushing ▪ GI: N/V ▪ INT: rash, local contact dermatitis c̄ topical systems.

DRUG INTERACTIONS: Additive hypotensive effects c̄ calcium blockers, alcohol, phenothiazines, beta blockers, other antihypertensives.

NURSING MANAGEMENT

ADMINISTRATION: Assess for hx of nitrate/nitrite hypersensitivity ▪ SL: assess BP; administer c̄/pt sitting/lying; pt should let tablet dissolve under tongue, *not* swallow saliva ▪ Administer extended-release preparations whole ▪ Spray: hold canister vertically, spray on tongue; have pt close mouth *immediately*, not inhale spray ▪ IV: dilute in 5% dextrose/normal saline solution; use special non-PVC tubing; do *not* use in-line filters; administer via infusion pump ▪ Ointment: measure proper dose on special applicator paper; do *not* touch medication; spread on skin via paper in thin, uniform layer ▪ Transdermal: apply to clean, hairless area; rotate sites ▪ Avoid exposure to heat, air, moisture, light in storage.

EVALUATION: Monitor VS, esp BP, heart rate; hemodynamic status (IV) ▪ Assess for transient headache, burning under tongue (SL); indicates potency ▪ Assess angina pain characteristics, duration; effectiveness.

EDUCATION: Dizziness, lightheadness may occur; use caution in potentially hazardous activities ▪ Avoid changing positions (lying/sitting/standing) rapidly ▪ Notify physician *immediately* of dry mouth, blurred vision; D/C drug ▪ SL: use *before* activities known to trigger angina attacks, to relieve acute attacks; burning sensation should occur when SL tablet placed under tongue (indicates potency); if pain *not* relieved c̄ 3 tablets/15m, notify physician/go to emergency room ▪ Transient headache expected ▪ Procedure for administration of various preparations; warn pt (esp c̄ impaired vision, taste)/family of potential for mistaking nitrate ointment for toothpaste ▪ Store in original amber glass container, avoid metal/plastic, remove cotton; replace c̄ fresh supply w/in 3-6mos after opening ▪ Carry medical identification (MedicAlert).

NOTES:

nizatidine • (ni-za-ti-deen)

CATEGORY: *H_2 blocker:* antihistamine — Rx; Preg Cat C

BRAND NAME
Axid (Lilly)

DOSAGE FORMS
Capsule: 150, 300mg

ACTION: H_2 antihistamine activity due to competitive inhibition of histamine at H_2 histamine receptors on parietal cells, resulting in ↓ gastric acid secretions. **USE:** Treatment and/or prophylaxis of active duodenal ulcer ▪ Treatment of erosive and ulcerative esophagitis.

PHARMACOKINETICS

PO absorption	Peak	Half-life	Protein binding	Excretion
Very high	0.5-3h	1-2h	35%	90% via urine in 12h

CONTRAINDICATIONS: Hypersensitivity.

DOSAGE

Normal renal function

Adult *PO* — 300mg daily hs or 150mg bid for active ulcers and gastroesophageal reflux disease. Maintenance dose for healed ulcers is 150mg/d

SIDE/ADVERSE EFFECTS: CNS: *somnolence,* headache, dizziness, rare cases of reversible mental confusion ▪ CV: rare cases of asymptomatic ventricular tachycardia ▪ GI: N/V, abdominal discomfort ▪ GU: hyperuricemia unassociated c̄ gout ▪ HEM: eosinophilia, one case of fatal thrombocytopenia ▪ HEP: ↑ in ALT, AST, alkaline phosphatase ▪ RESP: bronchospasm, laryngeal edema ▪ INT: *rash, urticaria, sweating,* exfoliative dermatitis ▪ Other: rare gynecomastia, impotence.

DRUG INTERACTIONS: None currently reported.

NURSING MANAGEMENT

ADMINISTRATION: Assess for hx of H_2 blocker hypersensitivity ▪ Administer c̄ meals, hs ▪ Avoid exposure to moisture in storage ▪ Elderly may require ↓ dosage.

EVALUATION: Monitor GI, hepatic, neurologic, renal status ▪ Assess for reversible confusion in elderly/debilitated pts ▪ False (+): urobilinogen, urine protein c̄ Multistix (use sulfosalicylic acid) ▪ Monitor serum for ↑ AST, ALT, alkaline phosphatase ▪ Assess for gout symptoms.

EDUCATION: Take c̄ food ▪ Dizziness may occur; use caution in potentially hazardous activities ▪ Avoid smoking ▪ Avoid GI-irritating foods ▪ Check c̄ physician/pharmacist before taking OTC preparations ▪ Avoid anxiety-producing situations ▪ Notify physician of H_2 blocker use before allergy & gastric acid secretion testing ▪ Store in tightly closed container in cool, dry area ▪ Take as ordered by physician; do *not* change or skip dose ▪ Women: avoid breastfeeding.

NOTES:

norepinephrine bitartrate (levarterenol bitartrate) • (nor-ep-i-nef-rin)

CATEGORY: *Sympathomimetic:* vasopressor

Rx; Preg Cat NA

BRAND NAME	**DOSAGE FORM**
Levophed (Winthrop)	Injection (IV): 1mg/ml

ACTION: Adrenergic activity produces powerful vasoconstriction (alpha activity), cardiac stimulation (beta activity), dilation of coronary arteries (beta activity), resulting in ↑ systemic BP, coronary artery circulation. **USE:** Treatment of acute hypotensive states ▪ Adjunct in cardiac arrest.

PHARMACOKINETICS: Duration of activity extremely short; excretion via urine primarily as metabolites.

CONTRAINDICATIONS: Hypotensive states due to deficient blood volume except as emergency measure, mesenteric/peripheral vascular thrombosis unless life threatening, cyclopropane/halothane anesthesia.

DOSAGE

Pediatric *IV*	Usual infusion rate 2μg/m
Adult *IV*	Usual infusion rate 8-12μg/m

SIDE/ADVERSE EFFECTS: Occasional bradycardia, headache.

DRUG INTERACTIONS: Use c̄ alpha, beta blockers will antagonize pressor, cardiac effects of NE ▪ Use c̄ MAO-I, tricyclic antidepressants produces significant hypertension.

NURSING MANAGEMENT

ADMINISTRATION: Assess for hx of catecholamine hypersensitivity (incl sulfites) ▪ Assess F/E balance; correct deficiencies ▪ Administer via infusion pump ▪ Dilute c̄ dextrose/saline solution (do *not* administer in NaCl solution alone); infuse into large vein; avoid use of leg veins, esp in elderly, pts c̄ vascular disease ▪ Do *not* administer SC/IM ▪ Do *not* mix c̄ blood components in same IV line ▪ Do *not* use discolored/precipitated solutions ▪ Avoid exposure to light in storage ▪ Have emergency support equipment available ▪ Do *not* leave pt unattended ▪ Withdraw drug *gradually* ▪ Elderly may require ↓ dosage.

EVALUATION: Monitor VS, esp BP (q2-3m until stable, then q5m) ▪ Monitor I&O q1h ▪ Assess respiratory status, ABGs, circulatory overload ▪ Assess CV status (ECG, heart rate, skin color/temperature) ▪ Check IV site carefully; avoid extravasation.

EDUCATION: Notify physician/nurse of abnormal rxs (difficult breathing, chest pain, irregular heartbeat).

NOTES:

norfloxacin • (nor-flox-a-sin)

CATEGORY: *Synthetic antibacterial*: fluoroquinolone antiinfective Rx; Preg Cat C

BRAND NAME
Noroxin (MSD)

DOSAGE FORM
Tablet: 400mg

ACTION: Bactericidal activity due to interference c̄ DNA gyrase enzyme, which is required for DNA synthesis in susceptible organisms, especially gram-negative bacteria.
USE: Treatment of UTIs caused by susceptible strains of *Citrobacter freundii, Enterobacter cloacae, Escherichia coli*, group D streptococci, *Klebsiella pneumoniae, Proteus* spp, *Pseudomonas aeruginosa, Providencia rettgeri, Staphylococcus* spp.

PHARMACOKINETICS

PO absorption	Peak	Half-life	Protein binding	Excretion
Moderate	2-3h	3-4.5h	10%-15%	Via bile and urine

CONTRAINDICATIONS: Hypersensitivity to drug or other quinolones.

DOSAGE
Normal renal function
Adult *PO* 400mg bid 1h ac or 2h pc for 7-10d and up to 21d for complicated infections

SIDE/ADVERSE EFFECTS: CNS: *headache*, depression, *dizziness*, insomnia, convulsive seizures ▪ GI: *nausea*, pain, flatulence, V/D, dyspepsia, ***pseudomembranous colitis*** ▪ HEM: eosinophilia, neutropenia, ↓ in hematocrit ▪ HEP: ↑ in ALT, AST, alkaline phosphatase, BUN ▪ INT: rash, urticaria, photosensitivity, ***Stevens-Johnson syndrome,*** erythema ▪ Other: fever, visual disorders, arthralgia, fatigue.

DRUG INTERACTIONS: Al and Mg antacids may ↓ PO absorption ▪ Nitrofurantoin can ↓ antibacterial activity ▪ Probenecid will ↓ renal excretion.

NURSING MANAGEMENT
ADMINISTRATION: Assess for hx of quinolone derivative hypersensitivity ▪ Administer c̄ full glass of H_2O 1h

ac/2h pc at evenly spaced intervals ▪ Assess for CNS disorders; use caution if present ▪ Assess hepatic, renal function; ↓ dosage if impaired ▪ Delay antacid administration for 2h after dose ▪ Avoid exposure to moisture, heat, light in storage ▪ Maintain hydration.

EVALUATION: Monitor VS, esp temperature ▪ Monitor I&O, hepatic, renal status ▪ Assess for CNS toxicity, crystalluria, nephrotoxicity, visual disturbances; D/C drug, notify physician ▪ May ↑ serum ALT, AST, LDH, creatinine, BUN; ↓ Hct.

EDUCATION: Dizziness/drowsiness may occur; use caution in potentially hazardous activities ▪ Take on empty stomach c̄ full glass of H_2O ▪ Take at equal intervals around clock to maintain blood levels ▪ Take antacids at least 2h after taking drug ▪ Complete full course of therapy even if symptoms subside ▪ ↑ Fluid intake (8-10 glasses/d) ▪ Avoid exposure to direct sunlight, UV light (sunlamp); use sunscreen, protective clothing ▪ Use sugarless gum/hard candy to diminish dry mouth ▪ Wear sunglasses to ↓ discomfort from bright light ▪ Notify physician *immediately* of visual disturbances; D/C drug ▪ Store in dry, tightly closed, light-resistant container ▪ Discard outdated preparations ▪ May cause mouth discomfort ▪ Do *not* administer to infants, children ▪ Women: avoid breastfeeding.

NOTES:

nystatin • (nye-stat-in)

CATEGORY: *Antibiotic:* antimonilial antibiotic

Rx; Preg Cat NA

BRAND NAMES	DOSAGE FORMS
Mycostatin (Squibb)	Cream, ointment, powder: 100,000U/g PO suspension: 100,000U/ml PO tablets: 500,000U PO troches: 200,000U/pastille Vaginal tablet: 100,000U
**Nadostine (Nadeau)*	PO suspension: 100,000U/ml PO tablet: 500,000U
Nilstat (Lederle)	Cream, ointment: 100,000U/g PO suspension: 100,000U/ml PO tablet: 500,000U Vaginal tablet: 100,000U

ACTION: Antimonilial activity due to drug binding to cell membrane sterols, altering cell membrane permeability & allowing leakage of vital intracellular components; drug exhibits no oral absorption. **USE:** Treatment of cutaneous, mucocutaneous, vulvovaginal, intestinal, oral infections caused by susceptible strains of *Candida* (moniliasis, candidiasis); antibiotic exhibits no appreciable PO absorption.

PHARMACOKINETICS: Not applicable.

CONTRAINDICATIONS: Hypersensitivity.

DOSAGE

Oral candidiasis (thrush) *PO*	
Infants	200,000U (PO suspension) in oral cavity qid
Children/Adult	400,000U (PO suspension) in oral cavity qid
Intestinal candidiasis *PO*	
Adult	0.5-1 million U (tablet) tid
Topical candidiasis	Various dosage forms (cream, etc) applied 2-3 times/d to infected area. Vaginal tablet inserted once/d for 2 wks

SIDE/ADVERSE EFFECTS: GI: large PO doses occasionally cause N/V/D, distress ▪ INT: local irritation $\bar{c}$ topical use.

Note: Side/adverse effects: common in *italic;* serious in ***boldface italic.***

*Available in Canada only.

DRUG INTERACTIONS: None currently reported.

NURSING MANAGEMENT

ADMINISTRATION: Assess for hx of hypersensitivity ▪ Obtain C&S before therapy ▪ PO suspension: instruct pt to retain on each side of mouth for as long as possible ▪ Troche: instruct pt to dissolve in mouth; do *not* chew or swallow ▪ Cleanse areas for application well before administration ▪ Avoid occlusive dressings ▪ Store vaginal tablets in refrigerator ▪ Avoid exposure to heat, moisture, light in storage.

EVALUATION: Monitor VS, esp temperature ▪ Monitor skin, mucous membranes for redness, swelling, irritation ▪ Monitor GI status.

EDUCATION: Contact dermatitis may occur ▪ Keep affected areas dry, exposed to air; avoid occlusive dressings ▪ May require several wks/mos of treatment; take until lab tests normal ▪ Maintain good hygiene; esp in affected area ▪ Avoid use of mouthwash if taking nystatin for oral candidiasis ▪ Avoid reinfection (use condoms, separate laundering, avoid tight clothing).

NOTES:

ofloxacin • (oh-flox-a-sin)

CATEGORY: *Synthetic antibacterial:* fluoroquinolone antiinfective Rx; Preg Cat C

BRAND NAME	**DOSAGE FORMS**
Floxin (Ortho)	Tablet: 200, 300, 400mg IV injection: 200, 400mg/container

ACTION: Bactericidal activity due to interference c̄ DNA gyrase enzyme (which is required for DNA synthesis) in susceptible organisms, esp gram-negative bacteria. **USE:** Treatment of lower respiratory, skin, venereal infections, and UTIs caused by susceptible strains of *Chlamydia trachomatis, Citrobacter diverus, Enterobacter aerogenes, Escherichia coli, Haemophilus influenzae, Klebsiella pneumoniae, Neisseria gonorrhoeae, Proteus mirabilis, Pseudomonas aeruginosa, Staphylococcus aureus, Streptococcus pneumoniae, Streptococcus pyogenes* ▪ Prostatis due to *Escherichia coli.*

PHARMACOKINETICS

PO absorption	Peak	Half-life	Protein binding	Excretion
98%	1-2h	9h	32%	70%-80% via urine as unchanged drug

CONTRAINDICATIONS: Hypersensitivity to drug or other quinolones.

DOSAGE: For normal renal function

Adult	*PO*	400mg q12h for 10d for respiratory, skin infection; 200-300mg q12h for 3-10d for renal infection; 400mg single dose for uncomplicated gonorrhea. 300mg q12h for 7-10d for chlamydial sexual disease. 300mg q12h for 6 wks for prostatitis;
	IV	200-400mg q12h by infusion

SIDE/ADVERSE EFFECTS: CNS: dizziness, headache, insomnia, anxiety, hallucinations, euphoria, nightmares ▪ CV: edema, hypertension, palpitation, vasodilation ▪ EENT: photophobia, loss of hearing acuity ▪ GI: nausea, constipation, dyspepsia ▪ GU: vaginitis, dysmenorrhea, menorrhagia, metrorrhagia, dysuria, glycosuria, proteinuria, hematuria ▪ HEM: leukocytosis, lymphocytopenia ▪ HEP: ↑ SGPT ▪ INT: diaphoresis, vasculitis ▪ Other: arthralgia, myalgia, cough.

DRUG INTERACTIONS: Al and Mg antacids, multivitamins with Fe, Zn, sucralfate ↓ PO absorption ▪ Use c̄ theophylline may ↑ theophylline toxicity.

NURSING MANAGEMENT

ADMINISTRATION: Assess for hx of quinolone derivative hypersensitivity ▪ Obtain C&S before therapy ▪ Administer c̄ full glass of H_2O 1h ac/2h pc at evenly spaced intervals ▪ Assess for CNS disorders; ↓ dosage if impaired ▪ Delay antacid administration for 2h after dose ▪ Avoid exposure to moisture, heat, light in storage ▪ Maintain hydration.

EVALUATION: Monitor VS, esp temperature ▪ Monitor I&O, hepatic, renal status ▪ Assess for CNS toxicity, crystalluria, nephrotoxicity, visual disturbances; D/C drug, notify physician ▪ May ↑ serum ALT, AST; ↑ or ↓ serum glucose ▪ Institute seizure precautions in pts c̄ hx of convulsive disorders.

EDUCATION: Dizziness/drowsiness may occur; use caution in potentially hazardous activities ▪ Take on empty stomach c̄ full glass of H_2O ▪ Take at equal intervals around clock to maintain blood levels ▪ Take antacids at least 2h after taking drug ▪ Complete full course of therapy even if symptom free ▪ ↑ Fluid intake (8-10 glasses/d) ▪ Avoid exposure to direct sunlight, UV light (sunlamps); use sunscreen, protective clothing ▪ Notify physician *immediately* of visual disturbances; D/C drug ▪ Store in dry, tightly closed, light-resistant container ▪ Discard outdated preparations ▪ May cause mouth discomfort, unpleasant taste ▪ Do *not* administer to infants, children ▪ Women: avoid breastfeeding.

NOTES:

olsalazine sodium• (ole-sal-a-zeen)

CATEGORY: *Salicylate:* colon antiinflammatory Rx; Preg Cat C

BRAND NAME	**DOSAGE FORM**
Dipentum (Pharmacia)	Capsules: 250mg

ACTION: Drug is converted by colon bacteria into active metabolite mesalamine (5-aminosalicylic acid; 5-ASA) where it exerts a topical antiinflammatory effect in ulcerative colitis. **USE:** Maintenance of ulcerative colitis remission in pts unable to take sulfasalazine.

PHARMACOKINETICS

PO absorption	Peak	Half-life	Protein binding	Excretion
Poor	1h	0.9h	99%	1% in urine

CONTRAINDICATIONS: Salicylate hypersensitivity.

DOSAGE

Adult *PO* Usual maintenance dose is 1g/d in 2 divided doses

SIDE/ADVERSE EFFECTS: CNS: headache (5%), drowsiness, lethargy, fatigue, depression, dizziness, insomnia ▪ GI: diarrhea (11%), pain/cramps (10%), N/V, dyspepsia, anorexia, stomatitis ▪ INT: rash, itching ▪ Other: arthralgia, URI.

DRUG INTERACTIONS: None currently reported.

NURSING MANAGEMENT

ADMINISTRATION: Assess for hx of salicylate hypersensitivity ▪ Assess renal status; ↓ dosage if impaired ▪ Administer c̄ food at evenly spaced intervals ▪ Assess abdominal pain, characteristics of stools.

EVALUATION: Monitor renal status ▪ Assess for rash, fever; D/C drug, notify physician ▪ May ↑ serum ALT, AST.

EDUCATION: Take c̄ food ▪ Take at evenly spaced intervals around the clock ▪ Take as directed by physician ▪ Diarrhea may occur; notify physician ▪ Keep scheduled appointments c̄ physician for proctoscopy/sigmoidoscopy.

NOTES:

omeprazole • (oh-mep-ra-zol)

CATEGORY: *Antisecretory*: gastric acid pump inhibitor   Rx; Preg Cat C

BRAND NAME
Prilosec (MSD)

DOSAGE FORM
Delayed capsule: 20mg

ACTION: Antisecretory activity due to blockage of final metabolic step of gastric acid synthesis (gastric acid pump inhibitor) by specific inhibition of the H^+ - K^+ ATPase enzyme system within the gastric mucosa (secretory surface of gastric parietal cells). Drug exhibits no anticholinergic or H_2 blocking activity. **USE:** Short-term treatment of active duodenal ulcer ▪ Short-term treatment of severe erosive esophagitis (grade 2 or above) diagnosed by endoscopy ▪ Short-term treatment of esophagitis that does not respond well to H_2 blocker therapy ▪ Long-term treatment of Zollinger-Ellison syndrome, multiple endocrine adenomas, systemic mastocytosis (pathologic hypersecretory conditions).

PHARMACOKINETICS

PO absorption	Peak	Half-life	Protein binding	Excretion
Rapid	0.5-3.5h	0.5-1h	95%	77% via urine and feces as metabolites

CONTRAINDICATIONS: Hypersensitivity.

DOSAGE

Adult *PO*

Active duodenal ulcer	20mg/d for 4-8 wks
Esophagitis	20mg/d for 4-8 wks
Hypersecretory condition	Individualized dosage starting 60mg once/d. Doses ↑ than 80mg/d should be given in divided doses. Doses up to 120mg tid may be required.

SIDE/ADVERSE EFFECTS: CNS: anxiety, dream disorders, apathy, vertigo, insomnia, paresthesia ▪ CV: bradycardia, chest pain, tachycardia, peripheral edema ▪ EENT: taste perversion, tinnitus ▪ GI: anorexia, dry mouth, fecal discoloration, tongue mucosal atrophy ▪ GU: proteinuria, hematuria, glycosuria, testicular pain ▪ HEM: anemia, neutropenia, pancytopenia, ***thrombocytopenia*** ▪ INT: alopecia, dry skin, hyperhidrosis, pruritus, urticaria ▪ RESP: epistaxis, pharyngeal pain ▪ Other: fever, pain, abdominal swelling, weight gain.

DRUG INTERACTIONS: Use c̄ diazepam, phenytoin, warfarin may ↑ their effects.

NURSING MANAGEMENT

ADMINISTRATION: Assess for hx of hypersensitivity ▪ Avoid exposure to moisture, light in storage ▪ Take in AM ac; swallow capsule whole, do *not* open ▪ May administer w/out regard to antacids.

EVALUATION: Monitor GI, hepatic, neurologic, renal status ▪ Monitor serum for ↑ creatinine, AST, ALT, alkaline phosphatase, total bilirubin ▪ Assess for reversible confusion in elderly/debilitated pts.

EDUCATION: Take in AM ac; swallow capsule whole ▪ Dizziness may occur; use caution in potentially hazardous activities ▪ Women: avoid breastfeeding ▪ Men: breast enlargement may occur ▪ Avoid smoking ▪ Avoid GI-irritating foods ▪ Check c̄ physician/pharmacist before taking OTC preparations ▪ Avoid anxiety-producing situations ▪ Take as ordered by physician ▪ Store in tightly closed, light-resistant container ▪ Notify physician *immediately* if experiencing diarrhea, black tarry stools, abdominal pain.

NOTES:

oxacillin sodium • (ox-a-sill-in)

CATEGORY: *Penicillinase-resistant penicillin*: antibiotic　　Rx; Preg Cat B

BRAND NAMES	DOSAGE FORMS
Bactocill (SKB)	Capsule: 250, 500mg Powder for injection (IM/IV): 0.5, 1, 2, 4, 10g vial
Prostaphlin (Apothecon)	Capsule: 250, 500mg Powder for injection (IV/IV): 0.25, 0.5, 1, 2, 4, 10g vial Powder for PO solution: 250mg/5ml

ACTION: Bactericidal activity due to inhibition of mucopeptide cell wall synthesis in susceptible organisms. **USE:** Treatment of infections due to susceptible strains of penicillinase-producing staphylococci.

PHARMACOKINETICS

PO absorption	Peak	Half-life	Protein binding	Excretion
30%-35%	30-60m	20-48m	92%-96%	Via urine as unchanged drug, metabolites

CONTRAINDICATIONS: Hypersensitivity to any penicillin.

DOSAGE

Premature/Neonate *IM/IV*	25mg/kg/d divided
Pediatric (<40g) *PO/IM/IV*	50mg/kg/d divided q4h. Severe infections 100mg/kg/d divided q4-6h
Adult *PO*	500mg q4-6h. Severe infections 1g q4-6h
IM/IV	250-500mg q4-6h. Severe infections 1g q4-6h

SIDE/ADVERSE EFFECTS: CNS: neuropathy usually associated c̄ high parenteral doses ▪ GI: PO incl *N/V/D, epigastric distress*, black hairy tongue, flatulence, smell/taste disturbances ▪ GU: ***interstitial nephritis*** (rare) ▪ HEM: anemia, eosinophilia, leukopenia, neutropenia, ***thrombocytopenia*** ▪ HEP: ↑ serum levels of AST, ALT, LDH ▪ INT: rash, pruritus, urticaria ▪ MS: arthralgia ▪ Other: *local irritation at injection site*, fever, ***anaphylaxis***.

DRUG INTERACTIONS: Bacteriostatic antibiotics c̄ any penicillin can lead to antibiotic antagonism ▪ PO anticoagulant therapy may require dose adjustments ▪ Probenecid inhibits tubular secretion of penicillin.

NURSING MANAGEMENT

ADMINISTRATION: Assess for hx of penicillin/cephalosporin hypersensitivity ▪ Obtain C&S before therapy ▪ Maintain blood levels; administer at equal intervals around clock ▪ PO: administer 1h ac/2h pc ▪ Avoid exposure to moisture in storage ▪ Reconstitute powder according to manufacturer's directions c̄ sterile H_2O for injection; shake well; do *not* administer discolored/precipitated solutions; check product information for stability (parenteral/PO solution) ▪ IM: administer by *deep* intragluteal injection ▪ IV: (direct) dilute according to manufacturer's directions; administer *slowly* (10m); (infusion) mix c̄ diluent recommended by manufacturer ▪ Do *not* administer bacteriostatic agents w/in 1h or mix c̄ aminoglycosides ▪ Have support equipment available for anaphylaxis ▪ Na^+ content: 2.8-3.1mEq (64-71mg)/g; calculate in Na^+-restricted diets.

EVALUATION: Monitor pts c̄ allergies/asthma (high risk for hypersensitivity) ▪ Observe for signs of superinfection (diarrhea, perineal itching, oral ulcers) ▪ Monitor VS, esp temperature; renal, hepatic, hematologic status ▪ Check IV insertion site; rotate q48h.

EDUCATION: Complete full course of therapy (usually 10d) even if symptom free ▪ Take on empty stomach ▪ Take c̄ H_2O, *not* c̄ acidic beverage (orange juice, carbonated beverage) ▪ Take at equal intervals ▪ Diarrhea may occur ▪ Store in dry, tightly closed container ▪ Discard outdated preparations ▪ Maintain good personal hygiene (esp perineal, oral) ▪ Maintain fluid intake (6-8 glasses/d) ▪ Notify physician of symptoms of allergic rx (fever, difficult breathing, rash) ▪ Women: avoid breastfeeding ▪ Carry identification (MedicAlert) if penicillin allergic.

NOTES:

oxazepam • (ox-az-e-pam)

CATEGORY: *Benzodiazepine*: antianxiety agent, anxiolytic   Rx C-IV; Preg Cat NA

BRAND NAMES	DOSAGE FORMS
**Ox-Pam (ICN)*	Tablet: 10, 15, 30mg
Serax (Wyeth)	Capsule: 10, 15, 30mg
	Tablet: 15mg
**Zapex (Riva)*	Tablet: 10, 15, 30mg

ACTION: Anxiolytic activity due to depression of CNS at brainstem formation, limbic thalamic areas. **USE:** Treatment of anxiety, alcohol withdrawal.

PHARMACOKINETICS: Half-life 4-20h; excretion via urine primarily as conjugated metabolites.

CONTRAINDICATIONS: Hypersensitivity.

DOSAGE: *PO*

Adult	
Alcoholism	15-30mg 3-4 times/d
Anxiety	10-15mg 3/4 times/d. Severe cases 15-30mg 3-4 times/d
Geriatric	10mg tid. May ↑ to 15mg 3-4 times/d

SIDE/ADVERSE EFFECTS: CNS: *drowsiness, fatigue, ataxia* ▪ CV: hypotension ▪ HEM: neutropenia (rare) ▪ PSYCH: paradoxical anxiety, hallucinations, hyperexcited states.

DRUG INTERACTIONS: Use c̄ other CNS depressants produces additive effects ▪ Use c̄ MAO-I can produce serious toxic effects.

NURSING MANAGEMENT

ADMINISTRATION: Assess for hx of benzodiazepine hypersensitivity ▪ Avoid exposure to heat, moisture, light in storage ▪ Avoid abrupt withdrawal ▪ Have emergency support measures available ▪ Elderly may require ↓ dosage ▪ Problem discussion, sympathetic listening contribute to relief of anxiety.

EVALUATION: Monitor renal, hepatic status ▪ Assess for symptoms of abrupt withdrawal (tremors, abdominal/muscle cramps, convulsions) c̄ prolonged use ▪ Check for signs of dependence (↑ drug request) ▪ Assess for tolerance to therapeutic dose ▪ Assess for paradoxic rxs (CNS stimulation), esp in elderly ▪ Check for depression; suicide precautions prn.

Note: Side/adverse effects: common in *italic;* serious in ***boldface italic.***   *Available in Canada only.

EDUCATION: Drowsiness may occur; use caution in potentially hazardous activities ▪ Avoid use c̄ alcohol, CNS depressants ▪ Indiscriminate use may lead to dependence ▪ Do *not* keep at bedside ▪ Take as ordered by physician; do *not* ↑ dose ▪ Women: avoid breastfeeding ▪ Check c̄ physician/pharmacist before taking OTC preparations ▪ Practice relaxation exercises, ventilation of feelings.

NOTES:

oxycodone hcl • (ox-i-koe-doan)

CATEGORY: *Narcotic:* semisynthetic opiate

Rx C-II; Preg Cat C

BRAND NAMES
Oxycodone HCl (various)

DOSAGE FORMS
PO solution: 5mg/5ml
Tablet: 5mg

COMBINATION PRODUCTS Rx C-II

Percocet (Du Pont)	oxycodone hcl/acetaminophen per tablet: 5mg/325mg
Percodan (Du Pont)	oxycodone/aspirin per tablet: 4.88 mg/325mg
Percodan-Demi (Du Pont)	oxycodone/aspirin per tablet: 2.44mg/325mg
Tylox (McNeil)	oxycodone hcl/acetaminophen per capsule: 5mg/500mg

ACTION: Narcotics produce analgesia, euphoria, sedation. **USE:** Relief of moderate/severe pain.

PHARMACOKINETICS: Good PO absorption c̄ onset at 10-15m, peak about 1h, duration 4-6h; excretion via urine.

CONTRAINDICATIONS: Hypersensitivity; use c̄ extreme caution in head injuries.

DOSAGE

Adult *PO*	5mg q6h. All fixed combination products, usual dose 1 tablet/capsule q6-8h

SIDE/ADVERSE EFFECTS: CNS: *sedation, lightheadedness,* euphoria, dysphoria, tremors, disorientation, ↓ convulsive threshold ▪ CV: hypotension, palpitations, flushing of face ▪ EENT: miosis ▪ GI: *N/V*, dry mouth, constipation, biliary tract spasm ▪ GU: urine retention ▪ INT: pruritus, urticaria ▪ RESP: ***respiratory depression***.

DRUG INTERACTIONS: Use c̄ alcohol, antihistamines, barbiturates, benzodiazepines, methotrimeprazine, phenothiazines, other CNS depressants produces additive CNS depression; ↓ dosage may be required ▪ Use c̄ tricyclic antidepressants may produce additive respiratory depression.

NURSING MANAGEMENT

ADMINISTRATION: Assess for hx of opioid hypersensitivity ▪ Assess quality, intensity, location of pain ▪ Store under double lock/key; document use accurately ▪ Assess hepatic function; may require ↓ dosage if impaired ▪ Do *not* administer if respirations are <12/m ▪ Have narcotic antagonist (naloxone), support measures available ▪ Avoid administration in pts c̄ suspected head injury ▪ Administer *before* pt has intense pain ▪ Administer around clock to pts c̄ severe, chronic pain ▪ Administer c̄ food/milk ▪ PO liquid: may mix c̄ juices; avoid freezing ▪ Utilize + power of suggestion ▪ Avoid abrupt withdrawal c̄ long-term use; D/C gradually ▪ Elderly may require ↓ dosage.

EVALUATION: Monitor respirations, circulatory function, esp BP ▪ Assess bowel function, abdominal distention ▪ Assess renal function, urinary retention ▪ Check for signs of dependence (↑ drug request) ▪ Assess for potentiation of CNS depressant effect ▪ Assess for N/V; administer antiemetic ▪ Assess for signs of overdose (coma, pinpoint pupils, respiratory depression) ▪ May produce ↑ CSF pressure.

EDUCATION: Avoid changing positions (lying/sitting/standing) rapidly ▪ Avoid excessive sensory stimulation ▪ Keep bedrails up when nonambulatory ▪ Turn, cough, deep breathe after surgery ▪ Constipation may occur; ↑ fluids, bulk-containing foods ▪ Avoid potentially hazardous activities ▪ Avoid smoking ▪ Indiscriminate use may lead to severe dependence ▪ Avoid use c̄ alcohol, other CNS depressants ▪ Take as ordered by physician; do *not* ↑ dose ▪ PO liquid: may mix c̄ juice; do *not* freeze ▪ Notify physician/dentist of use before treatment.

OVERDOSE MANAGEMENT: Principal symptoms are respiratory depression, stupor/coma ▪ Acute overdose results in apnea, circulatory collapse, cardiac arrest, possible death ▪ Emergency treatment: maintain respiration; remove drug by gastric lavage; administer naloxone hcl 0.01mg/kg IV; administer IV fluids to maintain adequate BP; because narcotics ↓ convulsive threshold, use of stimulants should be avoided.

NOTES:

oxytocin • (ox-i-toe-sin)

CATEGORY: *Oxytoxic* Rx; Preg Cat NA

BRAND NAMES

Pitocin (P-D)

Syntocinon (Sandoz) (Sandoz Pharma in Canada)

DOSAGE FORMS

Injection (IM/IV): 5U/0.5ml, 10U/ml

Injection (IM/IV): 10U/ml

Nasal spray: 40U/ml (2, 5ml bottle)

ACTION: Oxytoxic effect due to ↑ sodium ion permeability in uterine smooth muscle cells, which ↑ number of contracting myofibrils, enables uterus to contract; uterine sensitivity to oxytocin gradually ↑ during pregnancy, reaching peak before parturition. **USE:** Antepartum: initiation/augmentation of uterine contractions ▪ Stimulate uterine contractions during stage 3 of labor, control postpartum hemorrhage ▪ Initiate milk let-down reflex (spray).

PHARMACOKINETICS

IM absorption	Onset	Duration	Excretion
Excellent	3-5m	2-3h	Via urine primarily as metabolites

CONTRAINDICATIONS: Hypersensitivity, cephalopelvic disproportion, unfavorable fetal position, obstetrical emergencies that favor surgical intervention, fetal distress when delivery not imminent, prolonged use in uterine inertia/severe toxemia, hypertonic uterine patterns, when vaginal delivery is contraindicated; nasal spray during pregnancy.

DOSAGE

Adult *IM/IV*

Antepartum	Start c̄ infusion rate 1-2mU/m. Slowly ↑ until contractions reach desired rate, intensity
Postpartum	10-40U in 100ml, infused at sufficient rate to control uterine atony. 3-10U after delivery of placenta
Nasal spray	1 spray in one/both nostrils 2-3m before nursing/pumping breasts

SIDE/ADVERSE EFFECTS: CV: ***cardiac arrhythmia,*** postpartum hemorrhage, fetal bradycardia ▪ GI: N/V ▪ GU: pelvic hematoma; uterine hypertonicity, spasms, tetanic contractions, rupture.

DRUG INTERACTIONS: Use $\bar{c}$ vasopressors can produce severe hypertension.

NOTES:

NURSING MANAGEMENT

ADMINISTRATION: Fetal monitoring: assess fetal maturity, position ▪ Administer by only *one* route, *not* simultaneous routes ▪ IV: use infusion pump; do *not* give IV push ▪ Place pt in left lateral position ▪ Do *not* leave pt unattended ▪ Have emergency support equipment available ▪ Avoid overstimulation of uterus ▪ Do *not* administer discolored/precipitated solutions ▪ Parenteral: store in original container, avoid freezing.

EVALUATION: Monitor BP, pulse q15m ▪ Monitor fetal heart rate, intrauterine pressure ▪ Assess uterine rupture, fetal distress ▪ Monitor uterine contractions; stop if very frequent (<q2m)/prolonged ▪ Monitor I&O; assess hydration status (continuous infusion, PO fluids can lead to H_2O intoxication) ▪ Postpartum: monitor fundal height/tone.

EDUCATION: Explain procedure, rationale to pt, family ▪ Occurrence of contractions ▪ Relaxation techniques ▪ Comfort measures ▪ Procedure for use of nasal spray.

penicillin g benzathine/penicillin g procaine • (pen-i-sill-in)

CATEGORY: *Natural repository penicillin*: antibiotic   Rx; Preg Cat NA

BRAND NAMES	**DOSAGE FORMS**
pen g benzathine	Suspension (IM)
Bicillin LA, CR, CR 900/300 (Wyeth), Permapen (Roerig)	
pen g procaine	Suspension (IM)
Crysticillin AS (Apothecon)	
Pfizerpen AS (Roerig)	
Wycillin (W-A)	

ACTION: Bactericidal activity due to inhibition of mucopeptide cell wall synthesis in susceptible organisms; sterile aqueous suspension after deep IM injection produces tissue repository from which drug slowly absorbed. **USE:** *See* penicillin g potassium.

PHARMACOKINETICS

PO absorption	Peak	Protein binding	Excretion
Very slow	Varies up to 24h	45%-68%	Via urine by tubular excretion

CONTRAINDICATIONS: Hypersensitivity to any penicillin.

DOSAGE: Variable due to severity of infection

pen g benzathine *IM*	
Pediatric	600,000-1.2 million U usually as single dose
Adult	1.2-2.4 million U usually as single dose
pen g procaine *IM*	
Pediatric	500,000-1 million U/d
Adult	600,000-1.2 million U/d

SIDE/ADVERSE EFFECTS: GI: N/V/D, epigastric distress, black hairy tongue ▪ HEM: ***hemolytic anemia,*** leukopenia, ***thrombocytopenia*** ▪ HEP: ↑ serum AST, bilirubin ▪ INT: maculopapular rash, urticaria, ***exfoliative dermatitis*** ▪ Other: Jarrisch-Herxheimer syndrome (arthralgia, chills, fever, headache, sore throat, sweating, altered BP), local pain at injection site, ***anaphylaxis,*** overgrowth of nonsusceptible organisms.

Note: Side/adverse effects: common in *italic;* serious in ***boldface italic.***   *Available in Canada only.

DRUG INTERACTIONS: Use c̄ bacteriostatic antibiotics can produce antibiotic antagonism ▪ Antacid, antidiarrheal suspension ↓ PO absorption ▪ Probenecid delays penicillin excretion ▪ Avoid administration c̄ strong acidic/alkaline substances (can inactivate penicillin).

NURSING MANAGEMENT

ADMINISTRATION: Assess for hx of penicillin/cephalosporin hypersensitivity (incl procaine) ▪ Obtain C&S before therapy ▪ IM: dilute according to manufacturer's directions; shake well; inject *slowly* into gluteal UOQ ▪ Refrigerate parenteral preparations ▪ Do *not* administer w/in 1h of bacteriostatic agents ▪ Avoid exposure to moisture in storage ▪ Have support equipment available for anaphylaxis.

EVALUATION: Monitor pt c̄ allergies/asthma (high risk for hypersensitivity) ▪ Monitor renal, hepatic, hematologic status ▪ Observe for signs of superinfection (diarrhea, perineal itching, oral ulcers) ▪ Monitor VS, esp temperature.

EDUCATION: Diarrhea may occur ▪ Maintain good personal hygiene (esp perineal, oral) ▪ Maintain fluid intake (6-8 glasses/d) ▪ Women: avoid breastfeeding ▪ Notify physician of symptoms of allergic rx (fever, difficult breathing, rash) ▪ Carry identification (MedicAlert) if penicillin allergic ▪ IM injection may be painful.

NOTES:

penicillin g potassium/penicillin v potassium • (pen-i-sill-in)

CATEGORY: *Natural penicillin*: antibiotic Rx; Preg Cat NA

BRAND NAMES

penicillin g potassium
Pentids (Squibb)
Pfizerpen (Roerig)
penicillin v potassium
Beepen VK (SKB)
Betapen VK (Apothecon)
Ledercillin VK (Lederle)
Pen Vee K (W-A)
Robicillia VK (Robins)
V-Cillin K (Lilly)
Veetids (Apothecon)

DOSAGE FORMS: An array of oral and parenteral dosage forms including many nonproprietary preparations.

ACTION: Bactericidal activity due to inhibition of mucopeptide cell wall synthesis in susceptible organisms; PO preparations limited to microorganisms c̄ sensitivity to penicillin v potassium w/in range of serum levels attainable by PO administration. The severity of infection dictates PO administration (V) or parenteral IM (G-procaine) or IV (G-potassium). **USE:** penicillin g/v drug of choice for most strains of *Actinomyces*, α-hemolytic streptococci, *Bacillus anthracis, Bacteroides* (except *B. fragilis*), *Clostridium perfringens, Clostridium tetani* (c̄ antitoxin), *Corynebacterium diphtheriae* (c̄ antitoxins), *Erysipelothrix rhusiopathiae, Fusobacterium* (Vincent angina), group A β-hemolytic streptococci, *Neisseria gonorrhoeae, Neisseria meningitidis, Pasteurella multocida,* staphylococci (nonpenicillinase producing), *Streptobacillus moniliformis*, streptococci (groups C, G, H, L, M), *Streptococcus pneumoniae, Treponema pallidum* (syphilis), *Treponema pertenue* (yaws) ▪ Prophylaxis of group A strep infections in pts c̄ rheumatic fever, prevention of recurrence ▪ Prevention of bacterial endocarditis in pts c̄ congenital/rheumatic heart lesions who require dental procedure, upper respiratory tract surgery, instrumentation ▪ Prevention of bacteremia after tooth extraction.

CONTRAINDICATIONS: Hypersensitivity to any penicillin.

Pharmacokinetics: Pen g poorly absorbed PO and acid labile. Use pen v for PO use.

DOSAGE: Highly variable due to severity of infection
Pen G
Pediatric *PO* 25,000-90,000 U/kg in 3-6 doses

IM/IV	300,000-1.2 million U/d. Up to 10 million U/d may be required. Usual dose for premature/full-term infants 30,000 U/kg bid
Adult *IM/IV*	300,000-8 million U/d. Up to 60 million U/d may be required
Pen V	
Pediatric *PO*	<12y/o: 15-50mg/kg/d in 3-6 doses
Adult *PO*	250-500mg 3-4 times/d

SIDE/ADVERSE EFFECTS: GI: N/V/D, epigastric distress, black hair tongue ▪ HEM: ***hemolytic anemia***, leukopenia, ***thrombocytopenia*** ▪ HEP: ↑ serum AST, bilirubin ▪ INT: maculopapular rash, urticaria, ***exfoliative dermatitis*** ▪ Other: Jarrisch-Herxheimer syndrome (arthralgia, chills, fever, headache, sore throat, sweating, alterations in BP); local pain at injection site; anaphylaxis, overgrowth of nonsusceptible organisms.

DRUG INTERACTIONS: Use c̄ bacteriostatic antibiotics can produce antibiotic antagonism ▪ Antacid/antidiarrheal suspension ↓ PO absorption ▪ Probenecid delays penicillin excretion ▪ Avoid PO administration c̄ strong acidic/alkaline substances (can inactivate penicillin).

NURSING MANAGEMENT

ADMINISTRATION: Assess for hx of penicillin/cephalosporin hypersensitivity ▪ Obtain C&S before therapy ▪ PO: administer on empty stomach (1h ac/2h pc); avoid citrus juices, carbonated beverages ▪ IV: dilute according to manufacturer's directions; administer by *slow* direct infusion/IVBP ▪ IM: dilute according to manufacturer's directions; shake well; inject *slowly* into gluteal UOQ ▪ Refrigerate parenteral preparations ▪ Do *not* administer w/in 1h of bacteriostatic agents ▪ Avoid exposure to moisture in storage ▪ Have support equipment available for anaphylaxis ▪ Na^+ content: 0.3mEq (6.9mg)/1 million U; calculate in Na^+-restricted diet.

EVALUATION: Monitor pt c̄ allergies/asthma (high risk for hypersensitivity) ▪ Monitor renal, hepatic, hemopoietic status ▪ Observe for signs of superinfection (diarrhea, itching, coated tongue) ▪ Monitor VS, esp temperature.

EDUCATION: Take at equal intervals around clock to maintain blood levels ▪ Diarrhea may occur ▪ Maintain good personal hygiene (esp perineal, oral) ▪ Maintain fluid intake (6-8 glasses/d) ▪ Women: avoid breastfeeding ▪ Notify physician of symptoms of allergic rx (fever, difficult breathing, rash) ▪ Carry identification (MedicAlert) if penicillin allergic ▪ IM injection may be painful.

NOTES:

pentamidine isethionate • (pen-tam-i-deen eye-seh-thy-oh-nate)

CATEGORY: *Antiprotozoan agent* Rx; Preg Cat C

BRAND NAMES	DOSAGE FORMS
Pentam 300 (Fujisawa)	Powder for injection (IM/IV) 300mg vials
NebuPent (Fujisawa)	300mg aerosol vials

ACTION: Antiprotozoan activity not established. The drug may inhibit protein and nucleic acid synthesis in susceptible organisms. **USE:** Treatment of *Pneumocystis carinii* pneumonia (PCP). Has been used to treat African sleeping sickness (trypanosomiasis) and visceral leishmaniasis (not FDA approved).

PHARMACOKINETICS: Few studies have been done. A daily dose of 4mg/kg over 12 days produced a plasma concentration of 0.3-0.5µg/ml. Complete excretion via the urine required 6-8 wks after the drug was withdrawn.

CONTRAINDICATIONS: Hypersensitivity, especially to inhalation therapy.

DOSAGE

Pediatric/Adult

IM/IV	4mg/kg once/d for 14d. Infuse IV dose over 60m
Inhalation	300mg administered until nebulizer is empty (30-45m) q4wks

SIDE/ADVERSE EFFECTS: CNS: confusion/hallucinations, dizziness ▪ CV: ***fatal episodes of cardiac arrhythmias*** *and hypotension* ▪ GI: *N/V/D*, bad taste, *anorexia* ▪ HEM: severe leukopenia and ***thrombocytopenia,*** anemia ▪ INT: *rash,* ***Stevens-Johnsons syndrome*** ▪ Renal: nephrotoxicity (25%) is most common, ***acute renal failure*** ▪ Other: local phlebitis, hypoglycemia, ↑ AST (SGOT) and ALT (SGPT) levels, hypocalcemia, bronchospasm (inhalation administration), fever.

DRUG INTERACTIONS: Use c̄ nephrotoxic drugs, including aminoglycosides, amphotericin B, colistin, and vancomycin, can result in significant toxicity.

NURSING MANAGEMENT

ADMINISTRATION: Assess for hx of hypersensitivity ▪ Obtain C&S before therapy ▪ Assess renal function; may require ↓ dosage if impaired ▪ Administer by deep IM injection c̄ pt lying down (hypotension); monitor BP afterward q5-15m until stable ▪ IM: add 3ml sterile H_2O for injection to each 300mg vial; rotate injection sites ▪ IV: add 3-5ml sterile H_2O for injection or D_5W injection to each 300mg vial; dilute in 50-250ml D_5W injection, administer over 60m period; stable for 24h (room temperature); discard unused portion.

EVALUATION: Monitor VS, CBC ▪ Avoid extravasation; assess for pain, redness at site ▪ Diabetics: monitor blood glucose (hypo/hyperglycemia) ▪ Monitor renal function (nephrotoxicity); notify physician ▪ Monitor ECG throughout therapy (arrhythmias) ▪ May ↑ serum ALT, AST, creatinine, K^+; ↓ Ca^{++}.

EDUCATION: Dizziness/drowsiness may occur; use caution in potentially hazardous activities ▪ Complete full course of therapy as directed by physician ▪ Notify nurse/physician of pain, redness at IV injection site ▪ Notify physician *immediately* of bleeding/bruising, difficult breathing, rash, severe GI distress ▪ Maintain good personal hygiene ▪ May produce unpleasant, metallic taste.

NOTES:

pentazocine lactate▲/pentazocine hcl • (pen-taz-oh-seen)

CATEGORY: *Analgesic:* opioid agonist-antagonist

Rx C-IV; Preg Cat NA

BRAND NAME
Talwin (S-W)

DOSAGE FORMS
Injection (IM/IV/SC) ▲: 30mg/ml

COMBINATION PRODUCTS

Talwin Compound (S-W)	pentazocine hcl/aspirin per tablet: 12.5mg/325mg
Talwin NX (S-W)	pentazocine hcl/naloxone per tablet: 50mg/0.5mg

ACTION: Analgesic mechanism not determined; possible site of activity may be in subcortical areas of brain; narcotic agonist activity in 30mg dose equivalent to 10mg morphine, 75mg meperidine; narcotic antagonist activity equivalent to 1/50 that of nalorphine; drug has low misuse potential, weak addiction liability. **USE:** Relief of moderate/severe pain ▪ Preop sedation, obstetrical analgesia, adjunct to surgical anesthesia.

CONTRAINDICATIONS: Hypersensitivity.

DOSAGE

Adult *IM/IV/SC*

Analgesic	30mg q3-4h. Do *not* exceed 60mg IM/SC, 30mg IV. Do *not* exceed 360mg/d
Obstetric	30mg IM, 20mg IV
Talwin Compound	2 tablets PO 3-4 times/d
Talwin NX	1-2 tablets PO q3-4h. Do *not* exceed 12 tablets/d

PHARMACOKINETICS

Onset IV	Onset IM/SC	Duration	Half-life	Protein binding	Excretion
2-3m	15m	1-2h	2-3h	60%	Via urine, feces as unchanged drug, metabolites

Note: Side/adverse effects: common in *italic;* serious in ***boldface italic.***

*Available in Canada only.

SIDE/ADVERSE EFFECTS: CNS: *dizziness, lightheadedness, euphoria,* mood change, sedation, depression ▪ CV: tachycardia, edema of face ▪ EENT: blurred vision, nystagmus, miosis ▪ GI: *vomiting,* dry mouth, constipation ▪ GU: urinary retention ▪ INT: soft tissue induration, nodules, cutaneous depression at injection site, multiple-dose sclerosis of tissue, ***toxic epidermal necrolysis.***

DRUG INTERACTIONS: Use c̄ CNS depressants produces additive effects ▪ Use in narcotic-dependent pts can produce withdrawal symptoms ▪ Use c̄ MAO-I can result in severe excitation, rigidity, hypertension.

NURSING MANAGEMENT

ADMINISTRATION: Assess for hx of opioid hypersensitivity ▪ Check compatibility chart for mixing pre-op preparations ▪ Do *not* administer if respirations are <12/m ▪ IM: inject *deep* into muscle; rotate sites ▪ IV: dilute; administer *slowly* ▪ Have narcotic antagonist, support measures available ▪ Avoid administration in pts c̄ suspected head injury ▪ Administer *before* pt has intense pain ▪ Avoid light, freezing in storage ▪ Utilize (+) power of suggestion ▪ Avoid abrupt withdrawal ▪ Elderly may require ↓ dosage.

EVALUATION: Monitor respirations, circulatory function ▪ Assess bowel function, abdominal distention ▪ Assess renal function, urinary retention ▪ Check for signs of dependence (↑ drug request) ▪ Assess for potentiation of CNS depressant effect ▪ Check for signs of overdosage (coma, pinpoint pupils, respiratory depression).

EDUCATION: Avoid changing positions (lying/sitting/standing) rapidly ▪ Avoid excessive sensory stimulation ▪ Keep bedrails up when nonambulatory ▪ Obtain assistance prn when ambulatory ▪ Turn, cough, deep-breathe after surgery ▪ Constipation may occur; ↑ fluid, bulk-containing foods ▪ Avoid potentially hazardous activities ▪ Avoid smoking while taking drug ▪ Indiscriminate use may lead to dependence ▪ Avoid use c̄ alcohol, other CNS depressants.

NOTES:

pentobarbital/pentobarbital sodium▲ • (pen-toe-<u>bar</u>-bi-tal)

CATEGORY: *Barbiturate*

Rx C-II; Preg Cat D

BRAND NAMES

Nembutal (Abbott)
Nembutal Sodium▲ *(Abbott)*
**Novopentobarb*
**Pentogen*

DOSAGE FORMS

Elixir
Capsule, injection (IM/IV)
suppository

DOSAGE

Pediatric	*IM*	2-6mg/kg. Do *not* exceed 100mg
	PO	2-6mg/kg/24h divided
	Rectal	2mos-1y/o: 30mg hs 1-4y/o: 30-60mg hs 5-12y/o: 60mg hs 12-24y/o: 60-120mg hs
Adult	*IM*	150-200mg
	IV	150mg/70kg weight suggested
	PO	100-200mg hs
	Rectal	120-200mg hs

ACTION: Sedative, hypnotic activity due to depression of midbrain reticular formation; anticonvulsant properties due to depression of motor cortex. **USE:** Sedative, hypnotic ▪ Treatment of acute convulsive conditions.

PHARMACOKINETICS

PO absorption	Onset	Duration	Half-life	Protein binding	Excretion
90%-95%	10-15m	3-4h	4h	35%-45%	98%-99% in urine as metabolites

CONTRAINDICATIONS: Hypersensitivity, severe liver/respiratory impairment, porphyria, addiction.

Note: Side/adverse effects: common in *italic;* serious in ***boldface italic.***

*Available in Canada only.

SIDE/ADVERSE EFFECTS: CNS: *drowsiness, lethargy, hangover*, headache, dizziness, paradoxical restlessness/excitement ▪ GI: N/V ▪ INT: morbilliform rash, ***Stevens-Johnson syndrome***, urticaria ▪ Other: drug tolerance/addiction, asthma, angioneurotic edema.

DRUG INTERACTIONS: Use c̄ alcohol, antihistamines, benzodiazepines, methotrimeprazine, narcotics, tranquilizers produces ↑ depressant effects ▪ Barbiturates are enzyme inducers, can ↓ effect of PO anticoagulants, other drugs ▪ MAO-I ↑ activity of barbiturates ▪ Barbiturates ↓ PO absorption of griseofulvin.

NURSING MANAGEMENT

ADMINISTRATION: Assess for hx of barbiturate hypersensitivity ▪ Administer PO hypnotic dose 15-30m before hs ▪ IM: inject *deeply, slowly* into large muscle mass ▪ IV: inject *slowly*, wait 1m for full effect; additional small increments may be given to total 200-500mg in normal adults ▪ Avoid abrupt withdrawal ▪ Elderly may require ↓ dosage.

EVALUATION: IV: observe for coughing, chest wall spasm, hiccoughs, laryngospasm, pain at injection site, excessive CNS depression, thrombophlebitis ▪ Monitor hepatic, renal, cardiac, respiratory status ▪ Assess for symptoms of abrupt withdrawal (tremors, abdominal/muscle cramps, convulsions) c̄ prolonged use ▪ Assess for actual swallowing of PO forms ▪ Check for signs of dependence (↑ drug request) ▪ Monitor activity status (safety precautions) ▪ Assess for tolerance/barbiturate cross-tolerance to therapeutic dose ▪ Assess for paradoxic rxs (CNS stimulation), esp in elderly ▪ Observe pt sleep patterns ▪ Check for depression; suicide precautions prn.

EDUCATION: Drowsiness may occur; use caution in potentially hazardous activities ▪ Avoid use c̄ alcohol, other CNS depressants ▪ Indiscriminate use may lead to dependence ▪ Do *not* keep at bedside ▪ Take as ordered by physician ▪ Do *not* smoke after taking drug ▪ Women: avoid breastfeeding.

OVERDOSE MANAGEMENT: *See* Barbiturates.

NOTES:

pentoxifylline • (pen-tox-if-i-lin)

CATEGORY: : *Hemorrheologic agent* Rx; Preg Cat C

BRAND NAME
Trental (H-R)

DOSAGE FORM
Controlled-release tablet: 400mg

ACTION: Hemorrheologic effect due to ↓ blood viscosity, enhancement of erythrocyte flexibility, resulting in significant ↑ in tissue oxygen levels in pts c̄ peripheral arterial disease. **USE:** Symptomatic treatment of intermittent claudication associated c̄ peripheral arterial disease ▪ Investigational agent for symptomatic treatment of acute/chronic cerebrovascular insufficiency.

PHARMACOKINETICS

PO absorption	Peak	Half-life	Excretion
Almost complete	1h	0.4-0.8h	Primarily via urine as metabolites

CONTRAINDICATIONS: Intolerance to drug/methylxanthines (caffeine, theophylline, theobromine).

DOSAGE
Adult *PO* 400mg tid c̄ meals

SIDE/ADVERSE EFFECTS: CNS: *dizziness,* drowsiness, headache, tremor ▪ CV: anginal chest pain ▪ EENT: blurred vision ▪ GI: dyspepsia, N/V, bloating, flatulence ▪ HEM: leukopenia ▪ INT: pruritus, rash, urticaria ▪ Other: flulike symptoms.

DRUG INTERACTIONS: Use c̄ PO anticoagulants may ↑ PT.

NURSING MANAGEMENT
ADMINISTRATION: Assess for hx of xanthine hypersensitivity ▪ Administer c̄ food to ↓ GI irritation; swallow tablet whole ▪ Assess renal function; ↑ dose if impaired ▪ Avoid exposure to heat, moisture in storage.

EVALUATION: Monitor VS, esp BP ▪ Monitor renal status ▪ Observe for CNS effects (drowsiness, flushing, fainting), notify physician *immediately.*

EDUCATION: Drowsiness/dizziness may occur, use caution in potentially hazardous activities ▪ Take $\bar{c}$ meals; do *not* crush/chew tablets; swallow whole ▪ Notify physician of drowsiness, flushing, fainting ▪ Avoid smoking ▪ May require several wks for therapeutic effect; do *not* D/C.

NOTES:

perphenazine • (per-<u>fen</u>-a-zeen)

CATEGORY: *Phenothiazine*: antipsychotic, neuroleptic — Rx; Preg Cat NA

BRAND NAMES
**Phenazine (ICN)*
Trilafon (Schering)

DOSAGE FORMS
Tablet: 2, 4, 8, 16mg
Injection (IM/IV): 5mg/ml
PO concentrate: 16mg/5ml
Tablet: 2, 4, 8, 16mg

COMBINATION PRODUCTS
*Etrafon (Schering), *PMS Levazine (Pharmascience), Triavil (MSD)* — *See* perphenazine/amitriptyline hcl

ACTION: Antipsychotic activity associated c̄ a ↓ in central dopamine dependent pathways, which results in a tranquilizing effect: drug exhibits anti-alpha-adrenergic, anticholinergic, antiemetic, antiserotonin, ganglionic blocking activity.

PHARMACOKINETICS: Drug has good PO absorption, exhibits high protein binding, and is excreted via the urine as metabolites.

CONTRAINDICATIONS: Hypersensitivity, comatose states, bone marrow depression, presence of large amounts of CNS depressants, subcortical brain damage.

DOSAGE

Psychiatric	
Adult *PO*	6-64mg/d divided
IM	5-10mg. Do *not* exceed 30mg/d
Nausea/vomiting	
Adult *PO*	8-16mg/d divided
IM	5-10mg for rapid control.
IV	Do *not* exceed 5mg/dose for severe symptoms

SIDE/ADVERSE EFFECTS: CNS: drowsiness, extrapyramidal rxs, tardive dyskinesia, ***seizures*** ▪ CV: postural hypotension, tachycardia, ECG changes ▪ EENT: blurred vision, corneal/lenticular changes, pigmentary retinopathy ▪ END: lactation, moderate breast enlargement in women ▪ HEM: ***agranulocytosis,*** leukopenia ▪ HEP: cholestatic jaundice ▪ INT: urticaria, photosensitivity, exfoliative dermatitis ▪ PSYCH: adverse behavioral changes incl catatonic-like states ▪ Other: fever, hemolytic anemia, hypothermia.

Note: Side/adverse effects: common in *italic;* serious in ***boldface italic.***

*Available in Canada only.

DRUG INTERACTIONS: Al/Mg antacid preparations ↓ absorption ▪ Use c̄ narcotics, barbiturates, other CNS depressants ↑ CNS depression ▪ Guanethidine, other related antihypertensives antagonized.

NURSING MANAGEMENT

ADMINISTRATION: Assess for hx of phenothiazine hypersensitivity ▪ PO: administer c̄ food; do *not* crush/break SR tablets ▪ PO concentrate: dilute before administration c̄ >60ml fluid ▪ IM: inject *slowly*, deep into UOQ of buttock; keep pt lying down for 30m after injection ▪ IV: dilute according to manufacturer's directions; administer 1mg/injection at 1-2m intervals; monitor BP; maintain pt supine for 30m ▪ Avoid skin contact c̄ liquid forms (contact dermatitis) ▪ Position vomiting pt to avoid aspiration ▪ Avoid abrupt withdrawal ▪ Heavy smokers may require ↑ dosage ▪ Elderly/debilitated may require ↓ dosage.

EVALUATION: Monitor hepatic, ophthalmic, renal status; BP, CBC, I&O, weight, constipation ▪ Assess for extrapyramidal symptoms (tics/spasms, trembling, shuffling gait) ▪ Seizure precautions in pts c̄ hx of convulsive disorders ▪ Long-term therapy: assess for jaundice, agranulocytosis ▪ Assess for symptoms of abrupt withdrawal (nausea, dyskinesia, trembling, dizziness).

EDUCATION: Use caution in potentially hazardous activities ▪ Avoid changing positions rapidly ▪ Avoid use of alcohol, other CNS depressants ▪ Store in tightly closed, light-resistant container ▪ Use sugarless gum/hard candy to diminish dry mouth ▪ Constipation may occur; ↑ fluids, bulk-containing foods ▪ May turn urine pink/red/brown ▪ Avoid contact c̄ liquid forms ▪ Take PO forms c̄ meals; swallow SR tablets whole ▪ Use sunscreen, protective clothing ▪ Notify physician of fever, sore throat, bruising/bleeding, extrapyramidal symptoms ▪ Take as directed by physician ▪ Avoid smoking ▪ Check c̄ physician before taking OTC preparations ▪ Do *not* take antacids/antidiarrheals w/in 2h of drug ▪ Full drug effects may require several wks.

OVERDOSE MANAGEMENT: *See* Phenothiazines.

NOTES:

perphenazine/amitriptyline hcl • (per-fen-a-zeen/a-mee-trip-ti-leen)

CATEGORY: *Fixed-combination antidepressant/antipsychotic* Rx; Preg Cat NA

BRAND NAMES	DOSAGE FORMS
Etrafon (Schering)	perphenazine/amitriptyline per tablet: 2mg/10mg, 2mg/25mg, 4mg/10mg (A), 4mg/25mg (Forte)
Triavil (MSD)	perphenazine/amitriptyline per tablet: 2mg/10mg, 2mg/25mg, 4mg/10mg, 4mg/25mg, 4mg/50mg

ACTION: *See* amitriptyline hcl; perphenazine. **USE:** Treatment of moderate/severe depression ▪ Agitation, depressed mood ▪ Depression c̄ severe anxiety/agitation ▪ Depression, anxiety c̄ chronic physical disease.

DOSAGE

Adult *PO* Suggested starting dose, one 2/25 or 4/25mg tablet 3-4 times/d or one 4/25mg bid. Dosage must be adjusted to needs of pt. Full therapeutic response may require several wks.

NURSING MANAGEMENT

ADMINISTRATION: Assess for hx of phenothiazine/tricyclic antidepressant hypersensitivity ▪ Assess for hx of hepatic disease; may require ↓ dosage ▪ Assess VS, esp BP ▪ Administer c̄ food ▪ Avoid abrupt withdrawal; D/C gradually ▪ Maintain hydration ▪ Heavy smokers may require dosage evaluation ▪ Elderly/debilitated may require ↓ dosage.

EVALUATION: Monitor hepatic, ophthalmic, renal status ▪ Monitor BP, CBC ▪ Assess for extrapyramidal symptoms (tics/spasms, trembling, shuffling gait) ▪ Assess for symptoms of abrupt withdrawal (nausea, dyskinesia, trembling, dizziness, headache, malaise) ▪ Assess for actual swallowing of PO forms.

EDUCATION: Dizziness/drowsiness may occur; use caution in potentially hazardous activities ▪ Avoid changing positions (lying/sitting/standing) rapidly ▪ Avoid use of alcohol, other CNS depressants ▪ Take c̄ meals to ↓ GI irritation ▪ Store in tightly closed, light-resistant container

▪ Use sugarless gum/hard candy to diminish dry mouth ▪ Constipation may occur; ↑ fluids, bulk-containing foods ▪ May turn urine pink/red/brown ▪ Women: avoid breast-feeding ▪ Notify physician/dentist of use before treatment ▪ Avoid exposure to direct sunlight, UV light (sunlamps); use sunscreen, protective clothing ▪ Notify physician of fever, sore throat, bruising/bleeding, headache, malaise ▪ Notify physician of extrapyramidal symptoms (tics/spasms, trembling, shuffling gait) ▪ Avoid ↑ exercise, temperature extremes ▪ Take as directed by physician; do *not* ↑ dose ▪ Check c̄ physician before taking OTC/Rx preparations ▪ Do *not* take antacids/antidiarrheals w/in 2h of drug ▪ Keep scheduled appointments c̄ physician ▪ Full drug effects may require several wks.

NOTES:

phenazopyridine hcl • (fen-az-oh-peer-i-deen)

CATEGORY: *Urinary analgesic* Rx; Preg Cat B

BRAND NAMES
**Phenazo (ICN)*
Phenazodine (Lannett)
Pyridium (P-D)
**Pyronium (ProDoc)*

DOSAGE FORMS
Tablet: 100mg
Tablet: 100mg
Tablet: 100, 200mg

COMBINATION PRODUCTS: Preg Cat C
Pyridium Plus (P-D)
phenazopyridine hcl 150mg, hyoscyamine HBr 0.3mg, butabarbital 15mg per tablet

ACTION: Urinary analgesic mechanism not determined.
USE: Symptomatic treatment of pain, burning, urgency, frequency, other discomfort arising from irritation of lower urinary tract associated c̄ endoscopic procedures, infection, passage of sounds/catheters, surgery, trauma.

PHARMACOKINETICS: Not applicable.

CONTRAINDICATIONS: Hypersensitivity, renal insufficiency.

DOSAGE: *PO*

Pediatric	4mg/kg tid pc
Adult	200mg tid pc
Pyridium Plus	1 tablet qid pc and hs

SIDE/ADVERSE EFFECTS: GI: GI disturbances ▪ GU: renal toxicity ▪ HEM: ***hemolytic anemia,*** methemoglobinemia ▪ HEP: hepatic toxicity.

DRUG INTERACTIONS: None currently reported.

NURSING MANAGEMENT
ADMINISTRATION: Assess for hx of hypersensitivity ▪ Assess renal function; do *not* administer if impaired ▪ Administer pc.

EVALUATION: Monitor renal status ▪ Assess for jaundice; D/C drug, notify physician ▪ Urine glucose: may produce false (+) c̄ Clinistix/Tes-Tape; use Clinitest ▪ May interfere c̄ excretion, urine tests ▪ Diabetics: closely monitor blood/urine glucose, ketones.

Note: Side/adverse effects: common in *italic;* serious in ***boldface italic.*** *Available in Canada only.

EDUCATION: Take pc ▪ Discolors urine orange/red; may stain clothing ▪ Notify physician *immediately* of yellow skin/eyeballs; D/C drug ▪ D/C when pain, other symptoms disappear ▪ Diabetics: use Clinitest for urine testing ▪ Do *not* use tablets for future symptoms w/out checking c̄ physician.

NOTES:

phenobarbital/phenobarbital sodium▲ • (fee-noe-bar-bi-tal)

CATEGORY: *Barbiturate*

Rx C-IV; Preg Cat D

BRAND NAMES
**Gardenal*
Luminal, Luminal Sodium▲ *(Winthrop)*
Solfoton (Poythress)

DOSAGE FORMS
Capsule, elixir, injection (IM/IV), tablet

ACTION: Sedative, hypnotic activity due to depression of midbrain reticular formation; anticonvulsant properties due to depression of motor cortex. **USE:** Sedative, hypnotic ▪ Anticonvulsant for grand mal, status epilepticus, fever-, drug-, tetanus-induced convulsions ▪ Treatment of hyperbilirubinemia in neonates, Gilbert syndrome.

DOSAGE

Pediatric	
Anticonvulsant *PO*	15-50mg 2-3 times/d
IM/IV	3-5mg/kg
Sedative *PO*	2mg/kg tid
IM/IV	2mg/kg
Adult	
Anticonvulsant *PO*	50-100mg 2-3 times/d
IM/IV	200-300mg
Sedative *IM/IV*	100-130mg
Hypnotic *PO*	100-320mg hs
IM/IV	130-200mg hs

PHARMACOKINETICS

PO absorption	Onset	Duration	Half-life	Protein binding	Excretion
75%-90%	24-40m	6-8h	2-6d	20%-45%	75% in urine as metabolites

CONTRAINDICATIONS: Hypersensitivity, severe liver/respiratory impairment, porphyria, addiction.

SIDE/ADVERSE EFFECTS: CNS: *drowsiness, lethargy, hangover,* dizziness, paradoxical restlessness/excitement ▪ GI: N/V ▪ INT: morbilliform rash, ***Stevens-Johnson syndrome,*** urticaria ▪ Other: drug tolerance/addiction, asthma, angioneurotic edema.

DRUG INTERACTIONS: Use c̄ alcohol, antihistamines, benzodiazepines, methotrimeprazine, narcotics, tranquilizers ↑ depressant effects ▪ Barbiturates are enzyme inducers, can ↓ effect of PO anticoagulants, other drugs ▪ MAO-I ↑ activity of barbiturates ▪ Barbiturates ↓ PO absorption of griseofulvin.

NURSING MANAGEMENT

ADMINISTRATION: Assess for hx of barbiturate hypersensitivity ▪ Do *not* administer if respirations <12/m ▪ Administer hypnotic dose 1h before hs ▪ Avoid exposure to moisture, light (elixir) in storage ▪ Avoid abrupt withdrawal ▪ Elderly may require ↓ dosage ▪ ↓ Environmental stimuli.

EVALUATION: Monitor hepatic, renal, cardiac, respiratory status ▪ Assess for symptoms of abrupt withdrawal (tremors, abdominal/muscle cramps, convulsions) c̄ prolonged use ▪ Assess for actual swallowing of PO forms ▪ Check for signs of dependence (↑ drug request) ▪ Monitor serum concentrations; therapeutic blood levels: 10-40μg/ml ▪ Monitor activity status (safety precautions) ▪ Assess for tolerance/barbiturate cross-tolerance to therapeutic dose ▪ Assess for paradoxic rxs (CNS stimulation), esp in elderly ▪ Observe pt sleep patterns ▪ Check for depression; suicide precautions prn.

EDUCATION: Drowsiness may occur; use caution in potentially hazardous activities ▪ Avoid use c̄ alcohol, other CNS depressants ▪ Indiscriminate use may lead to dependence ▪ Do *not* keep at bedside ▪ Take as ordered by physician ▪ Store in tightly closed, light-resistant container (elixir) ▪ Safety precautions may be instituted (bedrails) ▪ Do *not* smoke after taking drug ▪ Women: avoid breastfeeding ▪ Practice relaxation exercises, ventilation of feelings ▪ Utilize sleep producers (reading, warm milk, soft music).

OVERDOSE MANAGEMENT: Principal symptoms: ↑ CNS depression ▪ Respiration depressed, pupils may be constricted, shock, coma ▪ Emergency medical treatment: remove drug by lavage/emesis, maintain respiration; administer IV fluids, vasopressor to maintain BP; diuresis beneficial c̄ normal renal function; hemodialysis if indicated (anuria, shock).

NOTES:

phenoxybenzamine hcl • (fen-ox-se-ben-za-meen)

CATEGORY: *Alpha-adrenergic blocker*: antihypertensive, sympatholytic   Rx; Preg Cat C

BRAND NAME
Dibenzyline (SKB)

DOSAGE FORM
Capsule: 10mg

ACTION: Antihypertensive effect due to noncompetitive blocking of alpha adrenergic receptors, resulting in ↓ peripheral vascular resistance, reflex tachycardia. **USE:** Treatment of hypertensive episodes due to pheochromocytoma ▪ Possibly effective for vasospastic peripheral vascular disorders, incl Raynaud's syndrome, acrocyanosis, frostbite sequelae.

PHARMACOKINETICS

Half-life	Duration	Excretion
24h	3-4d after single dose	Up to 50% in 12h, 80% in 24h; in urine, bile

CONTRAINDICATIONS: Any condition in which ↓ BP may be undesirable.

DOSAGE

Adult *PO* — Start c̄ 10mg bid. May be ↑ by 10mg qod, usually to 20-40mg 2-3 times/d

SIDE/ADVERSE EFFECTS: CV: postural hypotension, tachycardia ▪ EENT: nasal congestion, miosis ▪ GI: GI irritation ▪ GU: inhibition of ejaculation.

DRUG INTERACTIONS: Use c̄ nonselective adrenergic agents may produce significant hypotension, tachycardia.

NURSING MANAGEMENT

ADMINISTRATION: Assess BP ▪ Avoid exposure to moisture in storage ▪ Prevent postural hypotension ▪ Elderly may require ↓ dosage.

EVALUATION: Monitor BP; observe for hypotension ▪ Observe pt for at least 4d before each dose ↑ ▪ Assess peripheral circulation (skin color, temperature, pulse) ▪ Assess renal, respiratory status.

Note: Side/adverse effects: common in *italic;* serious in ***boldface italic.***

*Available in Canada only.

EDUCATION: Avoid changing positions (lying/sitting/standing) rapidly ▪ Dizziness, lightheadedness may occur; use caution in potentially hazardous activities ▪ Avoid smoking ▪ Compliance c̄ prescribed drug regimen ▪ Store in tightly closed container ▪ Men: disturbance of sexual function may occur ▪ Avoid use c̄ alcohol, constrictive clothing, extremely hot objects ▪ Check c̄ physician before taking OTC cold/cough/allergy preparations ▪ Nasal stuffiness may occur ▪ Avoid positions that may impair peripheral circulation ▪ Use sugarless gum/hard candy to diminish dry mouth ▪ Full therapeutic effect requires several wks.

NOTES:

phentolamine mesylate • (fen-tole-a-meen)

CATEGORY: *Alpha-adrenergic blocker*: antihypertensive, sympatholytic Rx; Preg Cat C

BRAND NAMES
Regitine (Ciba)
**Rogitine (Ciba)*

DOSAGE FORMS
Powder for injection (IM/IV): 5mg/vial

ACTION: Antihypertensive effect due to competitive blocking of alpha adrenoreceptors, resulting in ↓ peripheral vascular resistance; drug also produces beta adrenergic activity, resulting in positive inotropic, chronotropic cardiac effect. **USE:** Control of hypertensive crisis before/during surgery for pheochromocytoma ▪ Treatment of dermal necrosis after norepinephrine administration ▪ Dx of pheochromocytoma.

PHARMACOKINETICS

Half-life	Excretion
19m	Up to 13%, unchanged in urine

CONTRAINDICATIONS: Hypersensitivity, myocardial infarction, coronary artery disease.

DOSAGE

Pediatric/Adult

Surgery	Pre-op: 1mg 1-2h in children, 5mg 1-2h in adults. Repeat prn Surgery: 1mg prn in children, 50mg prn in adults
Necrosis	Prevention: 10mg/L of norepinephrine Treatment: 5-10mg into extravasation area w/in 12h
Hypertensive crisis	5-30mg
Pheochromocytoma dx	1mg in children, 5mg in adults. Inject, record BP at 30s intervals for 3m, 60s intervals for next 7m

SIDE/ADVERSE EFFECTS: CV: hypotension, tachycardia, ***cardiac arrhythmias***, orthostatic hypotension ▪ EENT: nasal stuffiness.

DRUG INTERACTIONS: Use in pediatric diabetics may result in ↑ antidiabetic effects.

Note: Side/adverse effects: common in *italic;* serious in ***boldface italic.***

*Available in Canada only.

NURSING MANAGEMENT

ADMINISTRATION: Assess for hx of hypersensitivity ▪ Assess BP ▪ Avoid exposure to moisture, light in storage ▪ Prevent postural hypotension ▪ Assess for hx of coronary artery disease; use c̄ caution ▪ Avoid CNS depressants 24h before pheochromocytoma dx test ▪ Have norepinephrine, support equipment available.

EVALUATION: Monitor BP; observe for hypotension ▪ Monitor heart rate ▪ Monitor serum for ↑ catecholamine, ↓ glucose ▪ (+) Pheochromocytoma dx: severe hypotension.

EDUCATION: Explain procedure for pheochromocytoma dx test ▪ Avoid changing positions (lying/sitting/standing) rapidly ▪ Dizziness, lightheadedness may occur ▪ Nasal stuffiness may occur ▪ Avoid smoking ▪ Avoid positions that may impair peripheral circulation.

NOTES:

phenylephrine hcl • (fen-ill-ef-rin)

CATEGORY: *Sympathomimetic:* decongestant, vasopressor — Rx/OTC; Preg Cat C

BRAND NAMES
**Mydfrin (Alcon)*
Neo-Synephrine (Winthrop) (Sterling in Canada)

DOSAGE FORMS
Ophthalmic solution
Injection (IM/IV/SC), ophthalmic solution, viscous ophthalmic solution
OTC: jelly, nasal drops, spray

ACTION: Sympathomimetic effect primarily alpha response, producing peripheral vasoconstriction, ↓ heart rate, ↑ BP; no beta-adrenergic effect on heart at normal doses. **USE:** Maintain BP during spinal/inhalation anesthesia; prolong spinal anesthesia ▪ Treatment of hypotension due to drugs, hypersensitivity, shock ▪ Ophthalmic, nasal decongestant.

PHARMACOKINETICS

IM/SC absorption	IM/SC onset	Duration	Excretion
Good	10-15m	1-2h	Probably via urine

CONTRAINDICATIONS: Hypersensitivity, ophthalmic solutions in narrow-angle glaucoma, 10% solution c̄ aneurysms or in infants, parenteral use c̄ hypertension or ventricular tachycardia may be contraindicated.

DOSAGE

Injection

Hypotension	Usual dose 2-5mg IM/SC. Usual range 1-10mg. Do *not* exceed initial dose 5mg
Severe hypotension	Add 10mg to 100ml infusion solution. For rapid response start infusion at 100-180 gtt/m. Maintenance rate 40-60 gtt/m
Spinal anesthesia	3mg, or 2mg for lower anesthesia levels, SC/IM 3-4m before administration of anesthetic. For hypotensive emergencies, 0.2mg IV recommended. Subsequent doses should *not* exceed previous dose by >0.1-0.2mg, c̄ single maximum dose 0.5mg

Indication	Dose
Paroxysmal supraventricular tachycardia	Initial dose up to 0.5mg by rapid IV injection (15-20s). Subsequent doses should *not* exceed previous dose by >0.1-0.2mg, $\bar{c}$ single maximum dose 1mg
Topical ophthalmic	
Vasoconstriction, pupil dilation	1 gtt suitable topical anesthetic followed by 1 gtt 10% ophthalmic solution on upper limbus. May be repeated in 1h
Surgery	Apply 2.5%/10% solution 30-60m before surgery
Ophthalmic exam	1 gtt 2.5% solution in each eye
Topical nasal	Apply 1-2 gtt/spray or small amount of jelly in each nostril q2-4h

SIDE/ADVERSE EFFECTS: CNS: headache, excitement, restlessness ▪ CV: ***arrhythmias*** (rare) ▪ INT: local irritation (topical preparations).

DRUG INTERACTIONS: Concurrent/sequential use $\bar{c}$ MAO-I produces significant hypertension ▪ Use $\bar{c}$ halothane can cause arrhythmias ▪ Use $\bar{c}$ oxytoxic drugs can cause persistent hypertension.

NURSING MANAGEMENT

ADMINISTRATION: Assess for hx of sympathomimetic, sulfite hypersensitivity ▪ Ophthalmic: place pressure on lacrimal sacs for 1m after administration ▪ IV: dilute according to manufacturer's directions; do *not* freeze, expose to light; titrate according to findings following physician's guidelines; use infusion pump; avoid abrupt withdrawal, D/C gradually ▪ Do *not* use discolored/precipitated solutions ▪ Have phentolamine available for OD (parenteral preparations) ▪ Elderly may require ↓ dosage.

EVALUATION: Monitor VS, esp BP (IV: q2-3m, then q5m when stable) ▪ IV: monitor ECG, heart rate, respirations ▪ Check IV insertion site carefully; avoid extravasation.

EDUCATION: Take as ordered by physician; do *not* ↑ dose ▪ Ophthalmic: blurred vision may occur; use caution in potentially hazardous activities; wear dark glasses ▪ Notify physician *immediately* of rapid/irregular heart rate, numbness/tingling of arms and legs, headache ▪ Procedure for ophthalmic, intranasal administration.

NOTES:

phenytoin/phenytoin sodium▲ • (fen-i-toyn)

CATEGORY: *Anticonvulsant*: antiepileptic

Rx; Preg Cat NA

BRAND NAME
Dilantin (P-D)

DOSAGE FORMS
Capsules, Infatabs, injection (IM/IV), PO suspension.

ACTION: Anticonvulsant activity due to inhibition of seizure activity in motor cortex; drug tends to stabilize threshold against hyperexcitability caused by excessive stimulation/environmental changes; ↓ maximal activity of brain for tonic phase of grand mal seizures; phenytoin exhibits antiarrhythmic activity, esp due to dig toxicity.
USE: Treatment of grand mal, psychomotor seizures ▪ Prevention/treatment of seizures during neurosurgery ▪ Pain associated c̄ trigeminal neuralgia, migraine.

PHARMACOKINETICS

PO absorption	Peak: Prompt	Peak: Extended	Half-life	Excretion
Complete	1.5-3h	4-12h	22h	Via urine, feces

CONTRAINDICATIONS: Hypersensitivity, IV use in sinus bradycardia, sinoatrial block, Adams-Stokes syndrome, 2°/3° AV block.

DOSAGE

Pediatric *PO*	Initial dose 5mg/kg/d in 2-3 doses. Usual maintenance range 4-8mg/kg/d
Adult *PO*	Initial dose 100mg tid, then individualize dose. Usual maintenance range 300-400mg/d, c̄ maximum dose 600mg
Status epilepticus	
Pediatric	15-20mg/kg by slow IV injection. Do *not* exceed 1-3mg/kg/m
Adult	10-15mg/kg by slow IV injection. Do *not* exceed 50mg/m
Arrhythmias	100mg IV at 5m intervals until satisfactory response or total 1g given
Neurosurgery	100-200mg IM at 4h intervals, continued during postop period

SIDE/ADVERSE EFFECTS: CNS: headache, ataxis, nystagmus, ↓ coordination, mental confusion, slurred speech, dizziness, insomnia, sensory peripheral polyneuropathy c̄ long-term treatment ▪ CV: ***atrial, ventricular conduction depression*** ▪ GI: constipation ▪ HEM: ***agranulocytosis,*** leukopenia, ***thrombocytopenia***, pancytopenia, ***megaloblastic anemia*** ▪ INT: morbilliform rash, ***exfoliative dermatitis, lupus erythematosus, Stevens-Johnson syndrome*** ▪ Other: gingival hyperplasia, enlargement of lips, local/injection site irritation.

DRUG INTERACTIONS: Use c̄ dicumarol is best avoided ▪ Disulfiram, isoniazid, valproic acid, many other drugs can inhibit phenytoin metabolism, resulting in ↑ phenytoin toxicity ▪ Use c̄ tricyclic antidepressants can induce seizures.

NURSING MANAGEMENT

ADMINISTRATION: Assess for hx of hydantoin hypersensitivity ▪ Assess hepatic, hemopoietic, renal function; use caution if impaired ▪ PO: may crush tablet/empty capsule, mix c̄ food/liquid ▪ PO suspension: shake well before pouring ▪ IV: preferred parenteral route; administer *slowly* (<50mg/m); flush c̄ 0.9% NaCl solution; do *not* administer cloudy solutions; do *not* mix c̄ 5% dextrose solutions; do *not* mix c̄ other IV infusions ▪ Maintain seizure precautions ▪ Have emergency support equipment available ▪ Avoid abrupt withdrawal ▪ Elderly may require ↓ dosage ▪ Therapeutic blood levels: 10-20µg/ml.

EVALUATION: Monitor occurrence/characteristics of seizures ▪ Monitor BP; hepatic, renal, hematologic status; activity ▪ Assess oral cavity for gingival hyperplasia ▪ Assess for skin rash; D/C drug, notify physician ▪ Check IV insertion site carefully; avoid extravasation.

EDUCATION: Drowsiness may occur ▪ Maintain good oral hygiene (overgrowth of gum tissue) ▪ Take at equal intervals; do *not* omit doses ▪ Take c̄ /immediately after meals ▪ May color urine pink/red/brown ▪ Avoid use c̄ alcohol ▪ Notify physician/dentist of use before treatment ▪ Use sugarless gum/hard candy to diminish dry mouth ▪ Keep appointments for dental exams/c̄ physician ▪ Avoid changing generic-name preparations ▪ Do *not* D/C drug w/out checking c̄ physician ▪ Carry medical identification (MedicAlert).

NOTES:

pilocarpine hcl • (pye-loe-kar-peen)

CATEGORY: *Parasympathomimetic*: cholinergic, muscarinic Rx; Preg Cat C

BRAND NAMES
*Absorbocarpine (Alcon), Akarpine (Akorn), *Carpine Nitrate (Allergan), Isopto-Carpine (Alcon), *Minims (Sandu), *Miocarpine (Cooper Vision), Ocusert Pilo (Alza), Pilocar (Cooper Vision), Pilopine HS (Alcon), Piloptic (Optopics)*

AVAILABLE PREPARATIONS
Sterile ophthalmic solutions 0.25%-10%, ocular therapeutic systems (Ocusert)

ACTION: Direct-acting parasympathomimetic produces ↑ GI motility, profuse sweating/secretions, contractions of pupils/ciliary muscle, causing ↓ IOP. **USE:** Main therapeutic use is to treat glaucoma by producing miosis, reduction of IOP by topical application.

PHARMACOKINETICS: After instillation of 1% solution, onset is about 10-30m, usual duration 4-10h.

CONTRAINDICATIONS: Hypersensitivity, undesirable papillary constriction (eg, acute inflammatory disease of anterior segment of eye).

DOSAGE: Must be individualized to clinical needs of pt.

SIDE/ADVERSE EFFECTS: Contact allergy/follicles in conjunctiva after prolonged use, ciliary spasm.

DRUG INTERACTIONS: Anticholinergics, antihistamines, hydroxyzine, tricyclic antidepressants can antagonize therapeutic effects.

NURSING MANAGEMENT
ADMINISTRATION: Assess for hx of hypersensitivity ▪ Wash hands thoroughly before administration ▪ Carefully check label ("For ophthalmic use"), % of solution ▪ Avoid contamination of solution, dropper tip ▪ Apply pressure to lacrimal sac 1-2m after instillation; instruct pt to keep eyes closed for 3-5m after insertion of gtt ▪ Store ocular system in refrigerator ▪ Avoid exposure to moisture, light in storage.

EVALUATION: Monitor IOP ▪ Assess for systemic cholinergic manifestations (↑ sweating, ↑ salivation, muscle tremors) ▪ Assess for altered mental status, esp in pts c̄ dementia ▪ Assess for signs of contact allergy.

EDUCATION: Will produce blurred vision, ↓ night/distance vision; avoid potentially hazardous activities ▪ Take as ordered by physician; do *not* ↑ dose ▪ Notify physician *immediately* of eye irritation; D/C drug ▪ Keep scheduled appointments c̄ ophthalmologist ▪ Procedure for ocular system insertion; store in refrigerator ▪ Tolerance may develop to brow pain.

NOTES:

pimozide • (pim-oh-zide)

CATEGORY: *Antipsychotic*

Rx; Preg Cat C

BRAND NAME
Orap (Gate)

DOSAGE FORM
Tablet: 2mg

ACTION: Suppression of motor, phonic tics appears related to blockage of CNS dopamenergic receptors.
USE: Suppression of motor tics associated c̄ Tourette's disorder that is unresponsive to standard treatment.

PHARMACOKINETICS

PO absorption	Peak	Half-life	Excretion
>50%	4-12h	55h	Via urine primarily as metatolites

CONTRAINDICATIONS: Hypersensitivity, pts c̄ cardiac arrhythmias or congenital long QT syndrome or taking drugs that prolong QT interval of ECG, tics not associated c̄ Tourette's disorder, severe toxic CNS depression or any comatose state.

DOSAGE

Adult/children *PO*

12y/o	Starting dose of 1-2mg/d in divided doses c̄ subsequent increase qod. Usual maintenance dose <0.2mg/kg/d. Do *not* exceed 0.2mg/kg/d or 10mg/d

SIDE/ADVERSE EFFECTS: CNS: drowsiness, extrapyramidal rxs, tardexic dyskinesia, ***neuroleptic malignant syndrome,*** akathisia, dizziness ▪ CV: postural hypotension, tachycardia, ECG changes in Q, T waves ▪ EENT: blurred vision, cataracts ▪ GI: dry mouth, N/V/D ▪ GU: impotence, urinary frequency, nocturia ▪ HEM: *hemolytic anemia* ▪ INT: rash, sweating ▪ PSYCH: adverse behavioral changes ▪ Other: asthenia, chest pain, muscle cramps, weight changes.

DRUG INTERACTIONS: Use c̄ other CNS depressants produce additive depression ▪ Use c̄ drugs (phenothiazines, antiarrhythmics) that prolong the Q-T interval is best avoided ▪ Use c̄ anticholinergics can produce additive effects ▪ Use c̄ anticonvulsants can ↓ their effect.

NURSING MANAGEMENT

ADMINISTRATION: Assess for hx of neuroleptic agent hypersensitivity ▪ Assess VS, esp BP ▪ Obtain baseline ECG ▪ Administer c̄ food ▪ Assess hepatic, renal status; ↓ dosage if impaired ▪ Avoid exposure to moisture, light in storage ▪ Avoid abrupt withdrawal (c̄ long-term therapy); D/C gradually ▪ Maintain hydration ▪ Elderly/debilitated may require ↓ dosage.

EVALUATION: Monitor hepatic, renal status ▪ Monitor BP, CBC, fluid retention (I&O, daily weight), constipation, ECG ▪ Assess for extrapyramidal rx (difficulty swallowing, muscle spasms) ▪ Seizure precautions in pts c̄ hx of convulsive disorders ▪ Long-term therapy: assess for jaundice, agranulocytosis ▪ Assess for symptoms of abrupt withdrawal (nausea, dyskinesia, trembling, dizziness if on long-term therapy) ▪ Assess for neuroleptic malignant syndrome (NMS) (fever, convulsions, muscle rigidity, sweating); D/C drug, notify physician.

EDUCATION: Dizziness/drowsiness may occur; use caution in potentially hazardous activities ▪ Avoid changing positions (lying/sitting/standing) rapidly ▪ Avoid use c̄ alcohol, other CNS depressants ▪ Take as directed by physician ▪ Take c̄ meals ▪ Store in tightly closed, light-resistant container ▪ Use sugarless gum/hard candy to diminish dry mouth ▪ Maintain fluid intake (6-8 glasses/d) ▪ Avoid exposure to direct sunlight, UV light (sunlamps); use sunscreen, protective clothing ▪ Notify physician of fever, sore throat, bruising/bleeding ▪ Notify physician of extrapyramidal symptoms (tics/spasms, trembling, shuffling gait) ▪ Avoid ↑ exercise, temperature extremes ▪ Avoid smoking ▪ Check c̄ physician/pharmacist before taking OTC preparations ▪ Do *not* take antacids/antidiarrheals w/in 2h of drug ▪ Full drug effects may require several wks.

NOTES:

piperacillin sodium • (pi-per-a-sill-in)

CATEGORY: *Extended-spectrum penicillin:* antibiotic — Rx; Preg Cat B

BRAND NAME
Pipracil (Lederle)

DOSAGE FORMS
Powder for injection (IM/IV): 2, 3, 4g vial

ACTION: Bactericidal activity due to inhibition of mucopeptide cell wall synthesis in susceptible organisms. **USE:** Treatment of infections due to susceptible strains of *Acinetobacter, Bacteroides, Clostridium* spp, *Enterobacter* spp, *Escherichia coli, Haemophilus influenzae, Klebsiella* spp, *Neisseria gonorrhoeae, Pseudomonas aeruginosa, Proteus* spp, *Serratia* spp, *Streptococcus pneumoniae* ▪ In combination c̄ aminoglycoside, esp in pts c̄ impaired immune response.

PHARMACOKINETICS

IM absorption	Peak	Half-life	Protein binding	Excretion
70%-80%	30m	0.5-1.1h	16%-22%	60%-80% via urine in 24h as unchanged drug

CONTRAINDICATIONS: Hypersensitivity to any penicillin/cephalosporin.

DOSAGE

Adult *IM/IV*	Usual range 6-18g divided Gonorrhea: usual dose 2g IM c̄ 1g probenecid PO Do *not* exceed 2g/IM injection site

SIDE/ADVERSE EFFECTS: CNS: dizziness, headache ▪ GI: N/V/D, ***pseudomembranous colitis*** ▪ HEM: eosinophilia, leukopenia, neutropenia, ***thrombocytopenia*** ▪ HEP: cholestatic hepatitis, ↑ serum AST, ALT, LDH ▪ INT: rash, pruritus, vesicular eruptions ▪ Other: local pain/***thrombophlebitis*** at injection site, ***anaphylactic rxs.***

DRUG INTERACTIONS: Use c̄ bacteriostatic antibiotics can lead to antibiotic antagonism ▪ PO anticoagulant therapy may require dose adjustment.

NURSING MANAGEMENT

ADMINISTRATION: Assess for hx of penicillin/cephalosporin hypersensitivity ▪ Obtain C&S before therapy ▪ Have support equipment available for anaphylaxis ▪ Do *not* mix c̄ aminoglycosides, other antibacterial solutions ▪ Reconstitute according to manufacturer's directions ▪ Maintain blood levels; administer at equal intervals around clock ▪ IM: inject *deep, slowly* into gluteal UOQ ▪ IV: administer by *slow* direct injection, IVPB (30m infusion) ▪ Na^+ content: 1.98mEq (45.5mg)/g; calculate in Na^+-restricted diets.

EVALUATION: Monitor VS, esp temperature ▪ Monitor hepatic, renal status (I&O) ▪ Assess for hypokalemia; may require supplemental K^+ ▪ Observe for signs of superinfection (diarrhea, perineal itching, oral ulcers) ▪ Assess for hypersensitivity rxs (fever, difficult breathing, rash) ▪ Monitor blood cultures, WBC, differential for drug effectiveness.

EDUCATION: Diarrhea may occur ▪ Maintain good personal hygiene (esp perineal, oral) ▪ Maintain fluid intake (6-8 glasses/d) ▪ Carry identification (MedicAlert) if penicillin allergic.

NOTES:

piroxicam • (peer-ox-i-kam)

CATEGORY: *Antiinflammatory* Rx; Preg Cat NA

BRAND NAME
Feldene (Pfizer)

DOSAGE FORMS
Capsule: 10, 20mg

ACTION: Antiinflammatory activity appears related to inhibition of prostaglandin synthesis. **USE:** Treatment of rheumatoid/osteoarthritis.

PHARMACOKINETICS

PO absorption	Peak	Half-life	Excretion
Good	3-5h	50h	Via urine, feces as metabolites (95%)

CONTRAINDICATIONS: Hypersensitivity; aspirin, other antiinflammatory agent hypersensitivity.

DOSAGE

Adult *PO* Initial dosage 20mg/d as single daily dose or divided. Adjust according to response

SIDE/ADVERSE EFFECTS: CNS: dizziness, drowsiness, vertigo, confusion, dream abnormalities ▪ CV: edema, ***exacerbation of CHF,*** angina ▪ EENT: tinnitus, blurred vision, eye irritations ▪ GI: N/V/D, anorexia, constipation, flatulence, abdominal pain ▪ GU: hematuria, ***interstitial nephritis, nephrotic syndrome,*** dysuria ▪ HEM: ↓ hemoglobin/hematocrit, anemia, eosinophilia, leukopenia ▪ INT: photosensitivity ▪ MET: hypoglycemia, hyperglycemia ▪ Other: positive ANA, ***anaphylaxis.***

DRUG INTERACTIONS: Use c̄ aspirin ↓ plasma levels ▪ Use c̄ lithium may ↑ its plasma levels ▪ May displace/be displaced by other drugs that are highly protein bound (eg, anticoagulants, sulfonamides); dosage adjustment may be required.

NURSING MANAGEMENT

ADMINISTRATION: Assess for hx of NSAIA hypersensitivity ▪ Avoid administration in pts c̄ hx of asthma, bleeding disorders, salicylate hypersensitivity ▪ Assess renal, hepatic function; use c̄ caution if impaired ▪ Administer c̄ food/milk, at same time qd; encourage upright position for 15-30m ▪ Avoid exposure to moisture, light in storage ▪ Elderly may require ↓ dosage.

EVALUATION: Monitor hematologic, hepatic, renal status c̄ prolonged use ▪ Monitor serum for ↑ BUN, creatinine, K^+; hold drug, notify physician ▪ Monitor pt receiving anticoagulant therapy; may potentiate bleeding ▪ Monitor I&O, daily weight ▪ Assess for edema in extremities ▪ Assess for visual, hearing disturbances; D/C drug, notify physician.

EDUCATION: Dizziness/blurred vision may occur; use caution in potentially hazardous activities ▪ Take c̄ food/milk to ↓ GI distress; maintain upright position for 15-30m ▪ Take as ordered by physician; do *not* skip dose ▪ Store in tightly closed, light-resistant container ▪ Avoid exposure to direct sunlight, UV light (sunlamps); use sunscreen, protective clothing ▪ Notify physician *immediately* of bleeding, rash, flulike symptoms, swelling of feet/legs, GI distress, jaundice, visual/hearing disturbance ▪ Avoid taking c̄ aspirin, other NSAIAs ▪ Avoid use c̄ alcohol ▪ Check c̄ physician/pharmacist before taking OTC preparations ▪ Keep scheduled appointments c̄ physician/for blood work/eye exams ▪ Women: avoid breastfeeding ▪ Full drug effects may require several wks.

NOTES:

potassium chloride

CATEGORY: *Electrolyte:* mineral

Rx; Preg Cat C

BRAND NAMES

Kaon (Adria)
K-Lease (Adria)
K-Lor (Abbott)
Klorvess (Sandoz)
Klotrix (Bristol)
K-Lyte (Apothecon)
K-Tab (Abbott)
Micro-K Extentabs (Robins)
Rum-K (Fleming)
Slow-K (Summit)

DOSAGE FORMS

Capsule, injection (IV), pediatric injection (IV), PO solution, powder for PO solution, tablet (enteric-coated, extended-release)

ACTION: Potassium is essential electrolyte required for nerve transmission, contraction of muscle tissue, gastric secretion, carbohydrate metabolism, acid-base balance; main intracellular cation; potassium chloride has 13.4mEq K^+/g. **USE:** Prevention/treatment of K^+ deficiency ▪ Treatment of dig-induced cardiac arrhythmias.

PHARMACOKINETICS: Well absorbed PO; excreted primarily via urine.

CONTRAINDICATIONS: Existing conditions that result in ↑ K^+ levels, eg, renal impairment of potassium excretion, untreated Addison's disease, acute dehydration, heat cramps, conditions that result in extensive tissue necrosis.

DOSAGE: Must be individualized. Normal daily adult requirement 40-80mEq. Usual daily supplemental dose 20mEq; 40-100mEq for potassium depletion.

SIDE/ADVERSE EFFECTS: GI: N/V/D, abdominal discomfort, ulceration, ***hemorrhage*** ▪ Other: tissue necrosis, phlebitis, vasospasm at parenteral injection site.

DRUG INTERACTIONS: Use c̄ potassium-sparing diuretics may result in severe hyperkalemia.

NURSING MANAGEMENT

ADMINISTRATION: Assess renal function; do *not* administer if impaired ▪ Assess ECG, serum electrolytes, esp K^+ (normal levels: 3.5-5mEq/L); notify physician of abnormalities ▪ PO: do *not* crush/chew tablets; do *not* remove foil wrapper until ready to use; administer c̄ pt in upright position, c̄ full glass of liquid or c̄ food ▪ IV: dilute according to manufacturer's directions; infuse *slowly* (10-20mEq/L); do *not* exceed 40mEq/L ▪ Do *not* administer discolored/precipitated solutions ▪ Do *not* administer IM or IV push ▪ Chloride salt is preferred salt.

EVALUATION: Monitor VS, esp heart rate ▪ Monitor I&O, GI status ▪ Monitor serum electrolytes (K^+ levels) ▪ Monitor ECG for U waves (hypokalemia), tented T waves (hyperkalemia) ▪ Assess for symptoms of hypokalemia (muscle cramps, lethargy, nausea), hyperkalemia (difficult breathing, tingling in extremities, nervousness, irregular heartbeat) ▪ Check IV insertion site carefully (phlebitis); avoid extravasation.

EDUCATION: Take as ordered by physician; do *not* skip doses ▪ Swallow tablets whole; do *not* crush; take c̄ food/full glass of liquid ▪ Dilute liquid, powder preparations c̄ H_2O; sip slowly when eating ▪ Notify physician *immediately* of ↓ muscle strength, restlessness, irregular heart rate ▪ Avoid using c̄ salt substitutes, low-Na^+ milk (↑ K^+) ▪ Check c̄ physician/pharmacist before taking OTC preparations ▪ Use caution c̄ OTC laxatives (hypokalemia) ▪ Notify physician/dentist of use before treatment ▪ Avoid changing brand-name preparations ▪ Keep scheduled appointments c̄ physician/for blood work.

NOTES:

prazepam • (praz-e-pam)

CATEGORY: *Benzodiazepine:* antianxiety agent, anxiolytic — Rx C-IV; Preg Cat NA

BRAND NAME
Centrax (P-D)

DOSAGE FORMS
Capsule: 5, 10, 20mg
Tablet: 10mg

ACTION: Anxiolytic activity due to depression of CNS at brainstem formation, limbic, thalamic areas. **USE:** Treatment of anxiety.

PHARMACOKINETICS: Drug exhibits slow PO absorption, peaks in 6h (metabolites) and is excreted via urine.

CONTRAINDICATIONS: Hypersensitivity, narrow-angle glaucoma.

DOSAGE: *PO*

Adult	20-60mg/d divided
Geriatric	10-15mg/d

SIDE/ADVERSE EFFECTS: CNS: *drowsiness, fatigue, ataxia* ▪ CV: hypotension ▪ HEM: neutropenia (rare) ▪ PSYCH: paradoxical anxiety, hallucinations, hyperexcited states.

DRUG INTERACTIONS: Use c̄ other CNS depressants produces additive effects ▪ Use c̄ MAO-I can produce serious toxic effects.

NURSING MANAGEMENT

ADMINISTRATION: Assess for hx of benzodiazepine hypersensitivity ▪ Administer as single daily dose at hs ▪ Avoid exposure to heat, moisture, light in storage ▪ Avoid abrupt withdrawal ▪ Elderly may require ↓ dosage ▪ Problem discussion, sympathetic listening contribute to relief of anxiety.

EVALUATION: Monitor renal, hepatic status ▪ Assess for symptoms of abrupt withdrawal (tremors, abdominal/muscle cramps, convulsions) c̄ prolonged use ▪ Check for signs of dependence (↑ drug request) ▪ Monitor activity status (safety precautions) ▪ Assess for tolerance to therapeutic dose ▪ Assess for paradoxic rxs (CNS stimulation), esp in elderly ▪ Check for depression; suicide precautions prn.

EDUCATION: Drowsiness may occur; use caution in potentially hazardous activities ▪ Avoid use $\bar{c}$ alcohol, other CNS depressants ▪ Indiscriminate use may lead to dependence ▪ Do *not* keep at bedside ▪ Take as ordered by physician; do *not* ↑ dose ▪ Women: avoid breastfeeding ▪ Check $\bar{c}$ physician/pharmacist before taking OTC preparations ▪ Practice relaxation exercises, ventilation of feelings.

NOTES:

prazosin hcl • (pra-zoe-sin)

CATEGORY: *Antihypertensive:* α , blocker

Rx; Preg Cat C

BRAND NAME

Minipress (Pfizer)

DOSAGE FORMS

Capsule: 1, 2, 5mg

COMBINATION PRODUCTS

Minizide 1, 2, 5, (Pfizer) prazosin hcl/polythiazide per capsule: 1mg/0.5mg, 2mg/0.5mg, 5mg/0.5mg

ACTION: Antihypertensive effect possibly due to alpha adrenergic blockade, resulting in ↓ peripheral vascular resistance. **USE:** Treatment of hypertension as sole agent/in combination c̄ other antihypertensives, esp thiazides.

PHARMACOKINETICS

PO absorption	Peak	Half-life	Protein binding	Excretion
Good	2-3h	2-4h	95%-97%	Via urine, feces as unchanged drug, metabolites

CONTRAINDICATIONS: Hypersensitivity.

DOSAGE

Adult *PO*	Initial dose 1mg 2-3 times/d, may ↑ to total 20mg/d. Usual maintenance range 6-15mg/d
Minizide	Usual dosage 1 capsule (1, 2, 5) 2-3 times/d

SIDE/ADVERSE EFFECTS: CNS: *dizziness, headache, drowsiness,* depression, nervousness, paresthesia ▪ CV: edema, tachycardia ▪ EENT: blurred vision, tinnitus, nasal congestion, reddened sclera ▪ GI: N/V/D, discomfort, ***pancreatitis,*** pain ▪ GU: priapism, urinary frequency ▪ INT: rash, pruritus, alopecia, lichen planus ▪ RESP: dyspnea ▪ Other: diaphoresis.

DRUG INTERACTIONS: Use c̄ beta blockers produces additive hypotension.

NURSING MANAGEMENT

ADMINISTRATION: Assess for hx of hypersensitivity ▪ Assess BP before administration ▪ Assess renal function; may require ↓ dose if impaired ▪ Administer c̄ food ▪ Elderly may require ↓ dosage.

EVALUATION: Monitor VS, esp BP ▪ Monitor for first-dose phenomenon (syncope) ▪ Monitor I&O, daily weight ▪ Assess peripheral circulation ▪ Assess for edema in extremities ▪ Monitor CV, renal status.

EDUCATION: Dizziness may occur; use caution in potentially hazardous activities ▪ Avoid changing positions (lying/sitting/standing) rapidly ▪ Take as ordered by physician; do *not* change dose ▪ Used to control, *not* cure, hypertension ▪ Avoid use c̄ alcohol ▪ Avoid ↑ exercise, temperature extremes, smoking ▪ Maintain optimum weight ▪ Avoid high-Na^+ foods (canned soups, lunch meats, cheese) ▪ Check c̄ physician/pharmacist before taking OTC preparations ▪ Notify physician/dentist of use before treatment ▪ Do *not* D/C drug w/out checking c̄ physician ▪ Keep scheduled appointments c̄ physician; have BP checked regularly ▪ Carry identification (MedicAlert) if hypertensive.

NOTES:

prednisone • (pred-ni-sone)

CATEGORY: *Glucosteroid:* corticosteroid

Rx; Preg Cat NA

BRAND NAMES	**DOSAGE FORMS**
Deltasone (Upjohn)	Tablet: 2.5, 5, 10, 20, 50mg
Liquid Pred (Muro)	Syrup: 5mg/5ml
Meticorten (Schering)	Tablet: 1mg
Orasone (Solvay)	Tablet: 1, 5, 10, 20, 50mg

ACTION: Glucosteroids cause wide variety of pharmacologic activity; two major effects are potent antiinflammatory effect, inhibition of immune response. **USE:** Treatment of adrenocortical deficiency, adrenogenital syndrome, other endocrine disorders, allergic states, collagen diseases, dermatologic diseases, GI diseases, hematologic disorders, ophthalmologic diseases, respiratory diseases, rheumatic disorders ▪ Treatment of tuberculous meningitis, neurologic/myocardial involvement associated c̄ trichinosis ▪ Remission of proteinuria in nephrotic syndrome, acute exacerbation of multiple sclerosis ▪ Palliative management of leukemias, lymphomas.

PHARMACOKINETICS: PO administration usually produces peak effect in 1-2h, duration about 1.5d.

CONTRAINDICATIONS: Systemic fungal infection.

DOSAGE

Pediatric *PO*	0.1-0.15mg/kg/d
Adult *PO*	5-60mg/d, c̄ high 250mg if needed

SIDE/ADVERSE EFFECTS: CNS: ***convulsions,*** headache, psychic impairment, vertigo, mood swings; pseudotumor cerebri may develop after treatment ▪ CV: edema due to Na^+ retention, CHF, hypertension ▪ EENT: ↑ IOP, glaucoma, posterior subcapsular cataracts, exophthalmos ▪ END: cushingoid states, growth suppression in children, menstrual irregularities, 2° adrenocortical/pituitary unresponsiveness, hyperglycemia, carbohydrate intolerance ▪ GI: peptic ulcer/***possible perforation, pancreatitis***, abdominal distention, ulcerative esophagitis ▪ INT: poor wound healing, fragile skin, petechiae/ecchymoses, facial erythema, ↑ sweating, urticaria, hirsutism ▪ MET: negative nitrogen balance, hypokalemic alkalosis ▪ MS: muscle weakness/loss of mass, pathologic fracture of long bones, osteoporosis.

Note: Side/adverse effects: common in *italic;* serious in ***boldface italic.***

*Available in Canada only.

DRUG INTERACTIONS: Severe hypokalemia can occur $\bar{c}$ diuretics (non-potassium sparing) ▪ Use $\bar{c}$ ulcerogenic drugs (eg, aspirin, indomethacin) can produce additive effects ▪ Use $\bar{c}$ antidiabetic agents may require ↑ doses of antidiabetic drugs.

NURSING MANAGEMENT

ADMINISTRATION: Assess for hx of hypersensitivity ▪ Administer single daily/alternate-day dose *before* 9 AM; multiple doses at equal intervals ▪ Administer $\bar{c}$ food ▪ Avoid abrupt withdrawal; ↓ gradually ▪ Avoid exposure to heat, light in storage; do *not* freeze ▪ Elderly may require ↓ dosage; monitor BP.

EVALUATION: Monitor VS, esp BP ▪ Diabetics: closely monitor blood, urine glucose (hyperglycemia) ▪ Assess mental/emotional status; avoid tricyclic antidepressants if depression induced ▪ Monitor serum electrolytes (esp K^+, Na^+), ophthalmologic exams, stools for occult blood $\bar{c}$ prolonged use ▪ Monitor hydration status (I&O, daily weight).

EDUCATION: Take $\bar{c}$ food/milk (single daily dose *before* 9 AM; multiple doses at equal intervals) ▪ Take as ordered by physician; do *not* ↑ dose/D/C drug ▪ Eat foods high in K^+, protein; avoid black licorice ▪ Follow diet low in Na^+ ▪ Check $\bar{c}$ physician before immunization (pt, family) ▪ Avoid exposure to infection ▪ Report following symptoms *immediately* to physician: anorexia, difficult breathing, weakness, dizziness; may appear during periods of ↑ stress/trauma ▪ Notify physician of black/tarry stools, slow wound healing, blurred vision, bruising/bleeding, emotional changes ▪ Diabetics: carefully monitor blood/urine glucose ▪ Store in tightly closed, light-resistant container ▪ Keep scheduled appointments $\bar{c}$ physician/blood work/eye exams ▪ Women: avoid breastfeeding ▪ Body image changes (full face, ↑ facial hair, ↑ fat deposit) may occur $\bar{c}$ prolonged use (reversible).

NOTES:

probenecid • (proe-ben-e-sid)

CATEGORY: *Antigout agent*: uricosuric Rx; Preg Cat NA

BRAND NAMES	DOSAGE FORMS
Benemid (MSD)	Tablet: 0.5g
**Benuryl (ICN)*	Tablet: 0.5g
Probalan (Lannett)	Tablet: 0.5g

COMBINATION PRODUCTS

ColBENEMID (MSD)	probenecid/colchicine per tablet: 500mg/0.5mg

ACTION: Uricosuric activity due to inhibition of tubular urate reabsorption in kidney; drug used in combination c̄ penicillins because it inhibits tubular penicillin excretion.
USE: Treatment of hyperuricemia associated c̄ gout, gouty arthritis ▪ Adjunct to penicillin therapy.

PHARMACOKINETICS

PO absorption	Peak	Half-life	Protein binding	Excretion
Complete	2-4h	4-17h	75%	Via urine primarily as metabolites

CONTRAINDICATIONS: Hypersensitivity, known blood dyscrasias, uric acid kidney stones, children <2y/o; do not start therapy until acute gouty attack subsides.

DOSAGE: *PO*

Adult	250mg bid for 1wk. Subsequent dose 500mg bid thereafter or suitable dose to maintain normal uric acid level
Adjunct to penicillin/ cephalosporin therapy	
Pediatric	
2-14y/o	25mg/kg, maintenance dose of 40mg/kg/d in 4 doses; >50kg: 1-2g/d
Adult/Children >50kg	1-2g/d

SIDE/ADVERSE EFFECTS: CNS: headache, dizziness ▪ GI: sore gums, anorexia, N/V ▪ GU: nephrotic syndrome, exacerbation of uric acid stones, hematuria, renal colic ▪ HEM: ***hemolytic anemia,*** aplastic anemia ▪ INT: dermatitis, pruritus ▪ Other: exacerbation of gout, fever, flushing, ***anaphylaxis***.

Note: Side/adverse effects: common in *italic;* serious in ***boldface italic.***

*Available in Canada only.

DRUG INTERACTIONS: Salicylates, pyrazinamide antagonize uricosuric activity ▪ Use c̄ methotrexate may ↑ methotrexate toxicity ▪ Probenecid inhibits renal excretion of penicillins, indomethacin, cephalosporins, sulfonamides, sulfonylureas.

NURSING MANAGEMENT

ADMINISTRATION: Assess for hx of hypersensitivity ▪ Administer c̄ food/milk/antacid ▪ Force liquids (3000 ml/d) ▪ Avoid exposure to moisture in storage ▪ Normal serum uric acid: 2.5-6.0mg/dl ▪ Start only after initial gout attack subsides.

EVALUATION: Monitor hepatic, renal status ▪ Monitor CBC, serum uric acid, I&O ▪ Assess joint, mobility status ▪ Diabetics: monitor blood glucose closely (hypoglycemia) ▪ Use Clinistix/Tes-Tape for urine testing.

EDUCATION: Take as directed by physician ▪ ↑ Fluid intake (8-10 glasses/d) ▪ Avoid alcohol intake ▪ Avoid aspirin-containing products (may take acetaminophen) ▪ Store in tightly closed container ▪ Notify physician of bruising/bleeding, lethargy, jaundice, sore throat ▪ Keep scheduled appointments for serum uric acid determinations ▪ ↓ Intake of high-purine foods (organ meats, legumes) ▪ Check c̄ physician/pharmacist before taking OTC preparations.

NOTES:

procainamide hcl • (proe-kane-a-mide)

CATEGORY: *Antiarrhythmic*

Rx; Preg Cat C

BRAND NAMES
Procan-SR (P-D)

Pronestyl (Princeton Pharm)

DOSAGE FORMS
SR tablet: 250, 500, 750mg, 1g
Capsule: 250, 375, 500mg
Injection (IM/IV): 100, 500mg/ml
SR tablets: 500mg
Tablet: 250, 375, 500mg

ACTION: Antiarrhythmic activity due to depression of cardiac automaticity, excitability, conductivity, resulting in widening QRS complex; P-R, Q-T intervals prolonged; exhibits anticholinergic activity, produces effects similar to quinidine. **USE:** Treatment of arrhythmias incl atrial flutter, fibrillation, paroxysmal atrial tachycardia, PVCs, ventricular tachycardia ▪ Arrhythmias associated c̄ surgery.

PHARMACOKINETICS

PO absorption	Peak	Half-life	Protein binding	Excretion
75%-95%	90-120m	2.5-7.5h	15%-30%	Via urine

CONTRAINDICATIONS: Hypersensitivity, hypersensitivity to procainelike anesthetics, complete heart block, lupus erythematosus, 2°/3° heart block w/out pacemaker.

DOSAGE

Adult *PO*

Atrial arrhythmia	Loading dose 1.25g, followed by 0.75g in 1h. Additional doses 0.5-1g may be given until satisfactory response/tolerance limit reached. Usual maintenance dose 0.5-1g q4-6h
PVCs	50mg/kg/d divided q3h, then adjusted
Ventricular tachycardia	Loading dose 1g, followed by total daily dose 50mg/kg divided q3h, then adjusted. Extended-action tablets should be used for maintenance therapy only
IM	0.5-1g q4-8h for arrhythmias, 100-500mg for arrhythmias during surgery

IV 25-50mg/m
IV infusion 500-600mg over 30m, followed by maintenance infusion rate 2-6mg/m

SIDE/ADVERSE EFFECTS: CNS: dizziness, mental depression, rare psychosis episodes ▪ CV: hypotension, ***ventricular arrhythmias*** (IV), **2° *heart block*** ▪ GI: N/V/D, anorexia, bitter taste ▪ HEM: neutropenia, ***hemolytic anemia, thrombocytopenia, agranulocytosis*** (rare) ▪ INT: *pruritus, urticaria,* maculopapular rash ▪ Other: ***SLE,*** angioneurotic edema.

DRUG INTERACTIONS: Use c̄ anticholinergics, antihypertensives, antiarrhythmics produces additive effects ▪ Use c̄ surgical neuromuscular blocking agents ↑ their effects ▪ Use in pts c̄ myasthenia gravis is best avoided; drug antagonizes therapeutic response.

NURSING MANAGEMENT

ADMINISTRATION: Assess for hx of hypersensitivity ▪ Assess cardiac, renal function; may require ↓ dosage ▪ May be administered c̄ food; *best* on empty stomach; tablets may be crushed/capsules opened; administer SR tablets whole ▪ Avoid exposure to moisture in storage ▪ Maintain blood levels; administer at equal intervals ▪ Have emergency support equipment available ▪ Solution may be clear/pale yellow ▪ IV: (direct) dilute 100mg c̄ 10ml 5% dextrose for injection; use cardiac monitoring; administer *slowly* (25-50mg/m); keep pt recumbent; (infusion) mix 1g in 250-500ml 5% dextrose; infuse 2-6mg/m via infusion control device; monitor BP q5-15m.

EVALUATION: Monitor VS, esp BP, heart rate & ECG (IV); notify physician of BP ↓ >15mmHg ▪ Monitor CBC, blood levels, I&O, daily weight ▪ Assess for SLE c̄ prolonged use; D/C drug, notify physician ▪ Assess for edema in extremities ▪ Therapeutic blood levels: 4-8μg/ml.

EDUCATION: Dizziness may occur; use caution in potentially hazardous activities ▪ May take c̄ food to ↓ GI irritation; *best* on empty stomach; swallow SR tablets whole ▪ Take as ordered by physician at equal intervals around clock ▪ Avoid caffeine ▪ Procedure for checking radial pulse ▪ Notify physician *immediately* of lethargy, fever, sore throat, swelling of feet/legs, irregular/changed pulse, bruising/bleeding ▪ Notify physician/dentist of use before treatment.

NOTES:

prochlorperazine▲/edisylate△/maleate◆ • (proe-klor-pair-a-zeen)

CATEGORY: *Phenothiazine*: antiemetic, antipsychotic Rx; Preg Cat NA

BRAND NAMES

Compazine (SKB)

**Stenetil (Rhone-Poulenc)*

DOSAGE FORMS

Compazine (SKB):
Injection (IM)△: 5mg/ml
Spansule◆: 10, 15, 30mg
Suppository▲: 2.5, 5, 25mg
Syrup△: 5mg/5ml
Tablet◆: 5, 10, 25mg

*Stenetil (Rhone-Poulenc):
Injection (IM)△: 5mg/ml
Suppository▲: 10mg
Tablet◆: 5, 10mg

ACTION: Antipsychotic activity associated c̄ a ↓ in central dopamine dependent pathways, which results in a tranquilizing effect; exhibits good antiemetic properties.

PHARMACOKINETICS

PO absorption	Onset	Duration	Excretion
Good	30-40m	10-12h	Via urine

CONTRAINDICATIONS: Hypersensitivity; comatose states, bone marrow depression, presence of large amounts of CNS depressants, pediatric surgery.

DOSAGE

Psychiatric	
Pediatric *PO/Rectal*	2.5mg 2-3 times/d. ↑ According to response 2-5y/o: Do *not* exceed 20mg/d 6-12y/o: Do *not* exceed 25mg/d
IM	0.6mg/lb for control
Adult *PO*	15-150mg/d divided
IM	10-20mg repeated q2-4h prn
Nausea/Vomiting	
Pediatric *PO/Rectal*	20-29lb: 2.5mg 1-2 times/d. Do *not* exceed 7.5mg/d 30-39lb: 2.5mg 2-3 times/d. Do *not* exceed 10mg/d 40-85lb: 2.5mg tid/5mg bid. Do *not* exceed 15mg/d
IM	0.6mg/lb
Adult *PO*	5-10mg 3-4 times/d
Rectal	25mg bid
IM	5-10mg q3-4h. Do *not* exceed 40mg/d

Note: Side/adverse effects: common in *italic;* serious in ***boldface italic.***

*Available in Canada only.

SIDE/ADVERSE EFFECTS: CNS: drowsiness, extrapyramidal rxs, tardive dyskinesia ▪ CV: postural hypotension, tachycardia, ECG changes ▪ EENT: blurred vision, lens opacity, nasal congestion ▪ END: amenorrhea, galactorrhea ▪ GI: dry mouth, constipation ▪ HEM: ***agranulocytosis***, leukopenia ▪ HEP: cholestatic jaundice ▪ INT: urticaria, photosensitivity, skin pigmentation ▪ PSYCH: adverse behavior changes ▪ Other: fever, hyperpyrexia, neuroleptic malignant syndrome.

DRUG INTERACTIONS: Antacids ↓ absorption ▪ Use c̄ narcotics, barbiturates, other CNS depressants ↑ CNS depression ▪ Guanethidine, related antihypertensives will be antagonized.

NURSING MANAGEMENT

ADMINISTRATION: Assess for hx of phenothiazine hypersensitivity ▪ PO: administer c̄ food; do *not* crush/break SR capsules ▪ IM: inject *slow, deep* into UOQ of buttock; keep pt lying down for 30m after injection ▪ Do *not* mix c̄ other drugs in same syringe ▪ Avoid SC injection ▪ IV: add to infusion solution 15-30m before administration ▪ Avoid skin contact c̄ liquid forms (contact dermatitis) ▪ Avoid abrupt withdrawal ▪ Heavy smokers may require ↑ dosage ▪ Elderly/debilitated may require ↓ dosage.

EVALUATION: Monitor hepatic, renal status; BP, CBC; I&O, weight, constipation ▪ Seizure precautions in pts c̄ hx of convulsive disorders ▪ Long-term therapy: assess for jaundice, agranulocytosis ▪ Assess for symptoms of abrupt withdrawal (nausea, dyskinesia, trembling, dizziness).

EDUCATION: Use caution in potentially hazardous activities ▪ Avoid changing positions rapidly ▪ Avoid use c̄ alcohol, other CNS depressants ▪ Use sugarless gum/hard candy to diminish dry mouth ▪ Constipation may occur; ↑ fluids, bulk-containing foods ▪ May turn urine pink/red/brown ▪ Avoid skin contact c̄ liquid forms ▪ Take PO forms c̄ meals; swallow SR capsules whole ▪ Use sunscreen, protective clothing ▪ Notify physician of fever, sore throat, bruising/bleeding, extrapyramidal symptoms ▪ Check c̄ physician before taking OTC preparations ▪ Do *not* take antacids/antidiarrheals w/in 2h of drug ▪ Full drug effects may require several wks.

OVERDOSE MANAGEMENT: *See* Phenothiazines.

NOTES:

promethazine hcl • (proe-meth-a-zeen)

CATEGORY: *Antihistamine:* H_1 blocker

Rx; Preg Cat C

BRAND NAMES

**Histanil*
Phenergan (W-A)
**Rhinaris*
**Secaris*

DOSAGE FORMS: Injection, suppository, syrup, tablet.

ACTION: H_1 antihistaminic activity due to competitive inhibition of histamine at H_1 histamine receptors on peripheral cells; drug exhibits good anticholinergic, antiemetic, antipruritic, sedative properties. **USE:** Symptomatic treatment of allergic disorders mediated by histamine ▪ Treatment of N/V, motion sickness ▪ Sedation for obstetrics, surgery ▪ Adjunct c̄ epinephrine in anaphylactic rxs, c̄ narcotics for post-op pain.

PHARMACOKINETICS

PO absorption	Onset PO	Onset IV	Duration	Excretion
Almost complete	20m	3-5m	4-6h	Via urine mainly as metabolites

CONTRAINDICATIONS: Hypersensitivity, neonates, nursing mothers, lower respiratory tract symptoms.

DOSAGE

Allergy	
Pediatric *PO/IM/IV*	6.25-12.5mg tid. 25mg hs
Adult *PO*	12.5-25mg tid. 25mg hs
IM/IV	25mg, repeat in 2h prn
Motion sickness *PO*	
Pediatric	12.5-25mg 1/2h before travel
Adult	25mg 1/2h before travel
Sedation *PO/IM/Rectal*	
Pediatric	12.5-25mg hs
Adult	25-50mg hs
Nausea/Vomiting *PO/IM/Rectal*	
Pediatric	12.5-25mg q4-6h prn
Adult	25mg q4-6h prn
Obstetric *IM*	Early labor, 50mg Labor, 25-75mg
Pre-op *PO/IM/IV*	
Pediatric	0.5mg/kg
Adult	25-50mg

SIDE/ADVERSE EFFECTS: CNS: *drowsiness*, dizziness, fatigue, euphoria, blurred vision ▪ CV: hypotension, palpitations, tachycardia, extrasystole ▪ GI: N/V ▪ HEM: ***agranulocytosis, thrombocytopenia*** ▪ INT: drug rash, photosensitivity ▪ Other: anticholinergic effects, thickening of bronchial secretions.

DRUG INTERACTIONS: Use c̄ anticholinergics, CNS depressants, tricyclic antidepressants produces additive effects ▪ MAO-I can ↑ anticholinergic effects of antihistamines.

NURSING MANAGEMENT

ADMINISTRATION: Use caution in pts c̄ peptic ulcer, open-angle glaucoma, bladder obstruction, prostatic hypertrophy ▪ PO: administer c̄ food ▪ IM: preferred parenteral route; inject *deep* into large muscle mass ▪ IV: avoid concentrations >25mg/ml; administer *slowly* (<25mg/m); avoid perivascular extravasation, intraarterial injection; protect from light c̄ foil covering ▪ Do *not* use discolored/precipitated solutions ▪ Avoid SC administration ▪ Incompatible c̄ strong alkaline drugs ▪ Have support equipment available for anaphylaxis ▪ Avoid exposure to moisture, light in storage ▪ Maintain hydration.

EVALUATION: Monitor VS, esp BP; serum for ↑ ALT, AST, bilirubin ▪ Assess for excessive drowsiness, dizziness, weakness ▪ False(+)/(-): pregnancy test ▪ May ↑ glucose tolerance ▪ Assess for athetoid-like movements of arms in pts c̄ acute pain after parenteral administration; additional analgesics may be required ▪ Monitor children for paradoxic rxs (CNS stimulation) ▪ Assess for tolerance to therapeutic dose.

EDUCATION: Dizziness, drowsiness, lightheadedness may occur ▪ Avoid alcohol, other CNS depressants ▪ Take PO forms c̄ meals ▪ Store in tightly closed, light-resistant container ▪ Use sugarless gum/hard candy to diminish dry mouth ▪ ↑ Fluid intake (8-10 glasses/d) ▪ Notify physician of symptoms of allergic rx (fever, difficult breathing, rash) ▪ Carry identification (MedicAlert) if allergic ▪ Women: avoid breastfeeding ▪ Avoid prolonged exposure to direct sunlight, UV light ▪ May discolor urine.

NOTES:

propantheline bromide • (proe-pan-the-leen)

CATEGORY: *Anticholinergic*: antimuscarinic, parasympatholytic — Rx; Preg Cat C

BRAND NAMES	DOSAGE FORMS
**Banlin (Technilab)*	
**Novopropanthil (Novopharm)*	
Pro-Banthine (S-S)	Tablet: 7.5, 15mg

ACTION: Anticholinergic activity due to competition c̄ acetylcholine for muscarinic receptors at postganglionic parasympathetic fibers; drug has poor CNS activity, produces main effect on peripheral muscarinic receptors.
USE: Adjunct in treatment of peptic ulcers.

PHARMACOKINETICS

Peak	Half-life	Excretion
1h	1.6h	70% as metabolites via urine

CONTRAINDICATIONS: Hypersensitivity, obstructive GI/renal conditions, intestinal atony, ulcerative colitis, myasthenia gravis, acute hemorrhage c̄ unstable CV adjustment.

DOSAGE

Adult *PO*	15mg tid and 30mg hs

SIDE/ADVERSE EFFECTS: CNS: mental confusion ▪ CV: tachycardia, palpitations ▪ EENT: blurred vision, cycloplegia, mydriasis, ↑ ocular tension, photophobia ▪ GI: N/V, constipation, loss of taste, dysphagia ▪ GU: urinary retention ▪ INT: urticaria, skin rash ▪ Other: suppression of lactation, body secretions.

DRUG INTERACTIONS: ↑ Anticholinergic effect c̄ antihistamines, phenothiazines, tricyclic antidepressants, meperidine, quinidine, disopyramide ▪ MAO-I ↑ activity by ↓ biotransformation ▪ Antacids ↓ PO absorption.

NURSING MANAGEMENT

ADMINISTRATION: Administer tablets 30m before meals ▪ Avoid exposure to moisture in storage ▪ Elderly may require ↓ dosage.

EVALUATION: Monitor VS ▪ Observe for ↑ anticholinergic effects ▪ Monitor I&O; assess for urinary retention.

EDUCATION: Advise pt of expected anticholinergic side effects (dry mouth, photophobia, constipation) ▪ Avoid concurrent antacid administration ▪ Avoid strenuous work/exercise during hot, humid weather ▪ Use sugarless gum/hard candy to diminish dry mouth ▪ Avoid OTC cough/hay fever preparations ▪ Drowsiness, blurred vision may occur; use caution in potentially hazardous activities ▪ Store in original, tightly closed container ▪ Frequent oral hygiene ▪ ↑ Fluid intake (8-10 glasses/d) ▪ Avoid use $\bar{c}$ alcohol.

NOTES:

propoxyphene hcl/napsylate▲ • (proe-pox-i-feen)

CATEGORY: *Analgesic*

Rx C-IV; Preg Cat NA

BRAND NAMES

Brand	Dosage Forms
Dolene (Lederle)	Capsule: 65mg
Darvon (Lilly)	Capsule: 65mg
Darvon-N▲ (Lilly)	PO suspension: 50mg/ml Tablet: 100mg
**Novopropoxyn (Novopharm)*	Capsule: 65mg
**642 (Frosst)*	Tablet: 65mg

COMBINATION PRODUCTS

Darvocet-N 50, 100 (Lilly)	propoxyphene napsylate/acetaminophen per tablet: 50mg/325mg, 100mg/650mg
Darvon Compound-65 (Lilly)	propoxyphene hcl/aspirin/caffeine per capsule: 65mg/389mg/32.4mg

ACTION: Propoxyphene raises pain threshold by undetermined centrally acting mechanism; drug has no antiinflammatory/antipyretic activity; low schedule rating for misuse potential, addiction liability. **USE:** Relief of mild/moderate pain.

PHARMACOKINETICS

PO absorption	Peak	Duration	Half-life	Excretion
Good	2-3h	4-6h	6-12h	Via urine as metabolites, unchanged drug

CONTRAINDICATIONS: Hypersensitivity to drug, aspirin, caffeine.

DOSAGE FORMS

Adult *PO*	65mg q4h prn. Do *not* exceed 390mg/d. Dose for napsylate salt 100mg q4h c̄ a maximum of 600mg/d
Darvocet-N	One tablet (50 or 100) q4h prn
Darvon Compound 65	One capsule q4h prn

SIDE/ADVERSE EFFECTS: CNS: *dizziness, sedation,* euphoria ▪ EENT: minor visual disturbances ▪ GI: *N/V,* constipation, abdominal pain ▪ INT: skin rashes.

Note: Side/adverse effects: common in *italic;* serious in ***boldface italic.***

*Available in Canada only.

DRUG INTERACTIONS: Use c̄ CNS depressants produces additive sedation.

NURSING MANAGEMENT

ADMINISTRATION: Assess for hx of hypersensitivity ▪ Assess quality, intensity, location of pain ▪ Assess emotional status; do *not* use in pts c̄ suicidal tendencies ▪ Administer c̄ food if GI irritation occurs; capsules may be opened, mixed c̄ food/liquid ▪ Administer *before* pt has intense pain ▪ Utilize + power of suggestion ▪ Avoid abrupt withdrawal c̄ prolonged use; D/C gradually ▪ Elderly may require ↓ dosage.

EVALUATION: Monitor respirations, circulatory function ▪ Assess bowel function, abdominal distention ▪ Assess renal function, urinary retention ▪ Check for signs of dependence (↑ drug request) ▪ Assess for potentiation of CNS depressant effect ▪ Assess for N/V; administer antiemetic ▪ Assess for signs of overdose (coma, pinpoint pupils, respiratory depression).

EDUCATION: Dizziness/drowsiness may occur; use caution in potentially hazardous activities ▪ Avoid changing positions (lying/sitting/standing) rapidly ▪ Avoid excessive sensory stimulation ▪ Keep bedrails up when nonambulatory ▪ Turn, cough, deep breathe after surgery ▪ Constipation may occur; ↑ fluids, bulk-containing foods ▪ Avoid smoking ▪ Indiscriminate use may lead to severe dependence ▪ Avoid use c̄ alcohol, other CNS depressants ▪ Women: avoid breastfeeding ▪ Take as ordered by physician; do *not* ↑ dose ▪ Notify physician/dentist of use before treatment.

NOTES:

propranolol hcl • (proe-pran-oh-lole)

CATEGORY: *Beta-adrenergic blocker* Rx; Preg Cat C

BRAND NAMES

**Detensol (Desbergers)*
Inderal (W-A)

DOSAGE FORMS

LA capsule: 60, 80, 120, 160mg
Injection (IV): 1mg/ml
Tablet: 10, 20, 40, 60, 80mg

COMBINATION PRODUCTS

Inderide (W-A)	propranolol hcl/hydrochlorothiazide combinations: 40/25, 80/25 tablet and 80/50, 120/50, 160/50 LA capsule

ACTION: Blocks access of catecholamines to $beta_1$, $beta_2$ receptors, resulting in bronchial constriction, ↓ heart rate, myocardial contractility ▪ Antihypertensive effect not determined. **USE:** Treatment of angina pectoris ▪ Treatment of hypertension ▪ Treatment of cardiac arrhythmias incl paroxysmal atrial tachycardia, atrial flutter/fibrillation, ventricular tachycardia, dig intoxication ▪ To ↓ mortality rate in stable pts after MI ▪ Management of hypertrophic subaortic stenosis and essential tremor ▪ Migraine prophylaxis ▪ Adjunct in pheochromocytoma.

PHARMACOKINETICS

PO absorption	Peak	Half-life	Protein binding	Excretion
90%	1-1½h	3.5-6h	90%	Via urine, feces

CONTRAINDICATIONS: Hypersensitivity, cardiogenic shock, bronchial asthma, sinus bradycardia, heart block, CHF unless secondary to tachyarrhythmia treatable c̄ propranolol.

DOSAGE FORMS

Adult *PO*

Angina	Initial dose 10-20mg 3-4 times/d. Usual effective dose 160mg/d. Do *not* exceed 320mg/d
Hypertension	Initial dose 80mg/d divided, may ↑ until desired effect is obtained. Usual range 120-240mg/d, c̄ doses up to 650mg
Arrhythmia	10-30mg 3-5 times/d
MI prevention	180-240mg/d divided

Note: Side/adverse effects: common in *italic;* serious in ***boldface italic.***

*Available in Canada only.

Hypertrophic subaortic stenosis	20-40mg 3-4 times/d
Essential tremor	120-320mg/d
Migraine	160-240mg/d divided
Pheochromocytoma	60mg/d divided, for 3d before surgery, $\bar{c}$ alpha adrenergic blocking agent
IV	1-3mg for serious arrhythmia
Inderide	Dosage usually 1 LA formulation/d or 1-2 tablet formulations/d

SIDE/ADVERSE EFFECTS: CNS: dizziness, mental depression, fatigue, hallucinations ▪ CV: bradycardia, CHF, hypotension, peripheral vascular insufficiency, heart block ▪ EENT: dry mouth/eyes, visual disturbances ▪ GI: N/V/D, constipation, ischemic colitis ▪ GU: impotence ▪ HEM: ***agranulocytosis,*** thrombocytopenic purpura ▪ INT: alopecia ▪ RESP: bronchospasm.

DRUG INTERACTIONS: Use $\bar{c}$ reserpine, other catecholamine-depleting drugs can result in serious adrenergic blockage ▪ Nonselective beta adrenergics antagonize therapeutic effects ▪ Usually contraindicated $\bar{c}$ furazolidone, general anesthetics, MAO-I.

NURSING MANAGEMENT

ADMINISTRATION: Assess for hx of hypersensitivity ▪ Assess apical pulse: if <60/m hold drug, notify physician ▪ PO: administration ac, hs; may crush tablet; do *not* crush SR capsule, administer whole ▪ IV: inject *slowly* (direct, 1mg/m; infusion, 1mg/10-15m); use cardiac monitoring ▪ Avoid abrupt withdrawal ▪ Elderly may require ↓ dosage.

EVALUATION: Monitor VS, esp BP, heart rate; I&O, weight, blood glucose in diabetics (hypoglycemia).

EDUCATION: Use caution in potentially hazardous activities ▪ Avoid changing positions rapidly ▪ Take ac, hs; swallow SR capsules whole ▪ Take as ordered by physician even if symptom free; do *not* change dose/D/C ▪ Check pulse before taking: if <60/m do *not* take drug, notify physician ▪ Do *not* abstain from food for >12h (low blood sugar) ▪ Avoid use $\bar{c}$ alcohol ▪ Notify physician of muscle cramps, difficult breathing, cold extremities, leg edema ▪ Avoid high-Na^+ foods ▪ Check $\bar{c}$ physician/pharmacist before taking OTC preparations ▪ Diabetics: monitor blood/urine glucose; observe for symptoms of hypoglycemia (headache, ↑ sweating, hunger, weakness) ▪ Notify physician/dentist of use before treatment ▪ Carry identification (MedicAlert) if taking propranolol.

propylthiouracil • (proe-pill-thye-oh-yoor-a-sill)

CATEGORY: *Antithyroid* Rx; Preg Cat D

AVAILABLE PREPARATIONS

Tablet: 50mg (also 100mg in Canada).

ACTION: Antithyroid activity due to interference c̄ oxidation of iodide to active iodine & by inhibition of coupling of iodotyrosines, resulting in ↓ thyroid hormone synthesis; drug does not inactivate existing thyroid hormones. **USE:** Treatment of hyperthyroidism ▪ Amelioration of hyperthyroidism in preparation for subtotal thyroidectomy, radioactive iodine therapy.

PHARMACOKINETICS

PO absorption	Peak	Excretion
Rapid	1-1.5h	35% of dose excreted via urine in 24h as metabolites, unchanged drug

CONTRAINDICATIONS: Hypersensitivity, nursing mothers.

DOSAGE: *PO*

Pediatric	6-10y/o: Starting dose 50-150mg/d. Maintenance dose dependent on response >12y/o: Starting dose 150-300mg/d. Maintenance dose dependent on response
Adult	Starting dose 300mg/d. Severe cases may require 600-900mg/d. Usual maintenance dose 100-150mg/d

SIDE/ADVERSE EFFECTS: CNS: headache, neuritis, paresthesias ▪ GI: N/V, epigastric distress ▪ GU: nephritis ▪ HEM: ***agranulocytosis*** ▪ HEP: hepatitis ▪ INT: urticaria, pruritus, skin pigmentation ▪ MS: arthralgia ▪ Other: fever.

DRUG INTERACTIONS: Use c̄ bone marrow depressants can ↑ development of agranulocytosis ▪ Use c̄ PO anticoagulants may ↑ their activity.

NURSING MANAGEMENT

ADMINISTRATION: Assess for hx of hypersensitivity ▪ Administer c̄ meals at equal intervals around clock ▪ Physician may order concurrent administration of Lugol's (iodine) solution 1-1½ wks before thyroid surgery to ↓ vascularity of gland ▪ Avoid exposure to light in storage.

EVALUATION: Monitor CBC throughout therapy ▪ Monitor thyroid function tests ▪ Assess for signs of hypothyroidism (N/V/D, muscle spasms, weight gain, cold sensation); D/C drug, notify physician ▪ Monitor pt receiving anticoagulant therapy; may potentiate bleeding.

EDUCATION: Take c̄ meals ▪ Take as ordered by physician ▪ Notify physician of fever, sore throat, bruising/bleeding ▪ Procedure for checking radial pulse ▪ Check radial pulse, weight 2-3 times/wk ▪ Check c̄ physician/pharmacist before taking OTC preparations ▪ Women: avoid breastfeeding ▪ Store in light-resistant container ▪ Notify physician *immediately* of skin rash, swollen neck glands; D/C drug ▪ Check c̄ physician before using iodized salt, eating shellfish ▪ Keep scheduled appointments c̄ physician/for blood work ▪ Notify physician/dentist of use before treatment ▪ Full drug effect may require several ds.

NOTES:

protamine sulfate • (proe-ta-meen)

CATEGORY: *Antiheparin agent:* haparin antagonist Rx; Preg Cat C

BRAND NAME
Protamine Sulfate (Lilly)

DOSAGE FORMS
Injection (IV): 50mg of activity/5ml vial, 250mg of activity/25ml vial

ACTION: Interacts c̄ heparin to form inactive complex w/in 5m of IV administration. **USE:** Treatment of heparin overdose.

PHARMACOKINETICS: Neutralization of heparin occurs within 5m after IV administration. Metabolic rate not determined.

CONTRAINDICATIONS: Hx of previous intolerance.

DOSAGE: *IV:* dosage must be individualized; 1mg protamine sulfate neutralizes 90 USP units heparin derived from lung tissue, 110 USP units of heparin derived from intestinal tissue; specific dose depends on heparin origin and severity of heparin overdose.

SIDE/ADVERSE EFFECTS: CV: bradycardia, hypotension (sudden) ▪ RESP: dyspnea ▪ Other: possible cross-allergenicity in pts allergic to fish.

DRUG INTERACTIONS: Possible heparin rebound.

NURSING MANAGEMENT
ADMINISTRATION: Assess for hypersensitivity to fish ▪ Administer by *slow* IV injection; do *not* exceed 50mg in any 10m ▪ Store in refrigerator; avoid freezing.

EVALUATION: Monitor VS, esp BP ▪ Monitor APTT, coagulation studies.

EDUCATION: Report bleeding/bruising *immediately.*

NOTES:

protamine sulfate

quinidine salts • (kwin-i-deen)

CATEGORY: *Antiarrhythmic*

Rx; Preg Cat C

BRAND NAME
Quinidine gluconate:
Quinaglute (Berlex), Quinalan (Lannett)
Quinidine polygalacturonate: Cardioquin (P-F)
Quinidine sulfate: Quinidex (Robins)

DOSAGE FORMS: Capsule, injection (IM/IV), tablets.

ACTION: Main antiarrhythmic effect appears related to prolongation of effective refractory period, ↑ action potential duration in cardiac muscle, His-Purkinje system; drug anticholinergic activity also contributes to cardiac effects. **USE:** Treatment of atrial flutter, established atrial fibrillation, after electrical conversion of atrial flutter/fibrillation; paroxysmal atrial fibrillation, atrial tachycardia, atrioventricular junction rhythm, ventricular tachycardia not associated c̄ complete heart block; premature atrial/ventricular contraction.

PHARMACOKINETICS

PO absorption	Peak	Half-life	Protein binding	Excretion
Almost complete	1-2h	3-16h	80%	Via urine, feces

CONTRAINDICATIONS: Hypersensitivity, thrombocytopenic purpura associated c̄ previous therapy, intraventricular conduction defects, AV block/aberrant impulses, abnormal rhythms due to escape mechanisms.

DOSAGE FORMS

Adult

Gluconate *PO*	324-648mg q8-12h
Gluconate *IM*	Initial dose 600mg. Subsequent doses 400mg can be repeated as often as q2h
IV	≤330mg for most cases, c̄ maximum 500-700mg
Polygalacturonate *PO*	Initial dose 275-825mg. Usual maintenance dose 275mg 3-4 times/d

Sulfate *PO*	
Atrial flutter	Dosage individualized after pt digitalization
Conversion of atrial fibrillation	0.2g q2-3h for 5-8 doses, c̄ subsequent daily dose ↑ until sinus rhythm restored or toxic effects occur
Premature atrial/ ventricular contractions	0.2-0.3g 3-4 times/d
Paroxysmal supraventricular tachycardia	0.4-0.6g q2-3h until paroxysm stops

SIDE/ADVERSE EFFECTS: CNS: headache, dizziness ▪ CV: ***widening of QRS complex, cardiac asystole, ventricular ectopic beats, paradoxical tachycardia, atrial embolism*** ▪ EENT: blurred vision, tinnitus, optic neuritis ▪ GI: *N/V/D,* abdominal pain ▪ HEM: ***acute hemolytic anemia, hypothrombinemia, thrombocytopenic purpura, agranulocytosis*** ▪ INT: pruritus.

DRUG INTERACTIONS: Use c̄ PO anticoagulants may require anticoagulant dosage adjustment ▪ Use c̄ urinary alkalizes may inhibit quinidine excretion, which can ↑ toxicity ▪ Use c̄ verapamil can produce significant hypotensive effects ▪ Use c̄ anticholinergics can produce additive vagolytic effect ▪ Use c̄ dig glycosides can result in cardiac toxicity.

NURSING MANAGEMENT

ADMINISTRATION: Assess for hx of hypersensitivity ▪ Assess BP, apical pulse; notify physician, D/C drug if abnormal ▪ Test dose may be administered; check c̄ physician ▪ PO: administer c̄ full glass H_2O 1h ac/2h pc; may administer c̄ food to ↓ GI irritation ▪ Administer SR tablets whole ▪ Do *not* use discolored/precipitated solution.

EVALUATION: Monitor VS, esp BP; apical pulse; F/E, renal, hepatic, hematologic status ▪ Cardiac monitoring; report ventricular abnormalities to physician (widened QRS, PVCs) ▪ Observe for diarrhea ▪ Monitor blood levels for toxicity ▪ Therapeutic blood levels: 3-6μg/ml.

EDUCATION: Dizziness may occur; use caution in potentially hazardous activities ▪ Avoid changing positions rapidly ▪ Take as ordered by physician ▪ May take c̄ food to ↓ GI distress ▪ Do *not* crush/chew SR tablets ▪ Notify physician of shortness of breath, chest pain, "skipped" heartbeats, sensory disturbances; D/C drug ▪ Check c̄ physician/pharmacist before taking OTC preparations ▪ Avoid alcohol, caffeine ▪ Keep appointments c̄ physician/for lab work ▪ Carry medical identification (MedicAlert).

NOTES:

ranitidine hcl • (ra-nit-te-deen)

CATEGORY: H_2 *blocker*: antihistamine

Rx; Preg Cat B

BRAND NAME

Zantac (Glaxo)

DOSAGE FORMS

Injection (IM/IV): 25mg/ml
Syrup: 16.8mg/ml
Tablet: 150, 300mg

ACTION: H_2 antihistamine activity due to competitive inhibition of histamine at H_2 histamine receptors on parietal cells, resulting in ↓ gastric acid secretions. **USE:** Short-term treatment of benign gastric/duodenal ulcers, and gastroesophageal reflux disease (GERD) ▪ Treatment of pathologic hypersecretory conditions, eg, Zollinger-Ellison syndrome, systemic mastocytosis ▪ Maintenance of healed acute duodenal ulcers.

PHARMACOKINETICS

PO absorption	Peak	Half-life	Protein binding	Excretion
50%	2-3h	2.5-3h	10%-20%	30% unchanged in urine in 24h

CONTRAINDICATIONS: Hypersensitivity.

DOSAGE

Adult *PO*	150mg bid for all indications
IV	50mg q6-8h
IM	50mg diluted to 20ml q6-8h administered ≥5m
Infusion	50mg q6-8h administered 15-20 mg. Do *not* exceed 400mg/d

SIDE/ADVERSE EFFECTS: CNS: dizziness, somnolence, mental confusion, agitation ▪ CV: rare tachycardia, bradycardia ▪ GI: N/V/D ▪ HEM: leukopenia, granulocytopenia, ***thrombocytopenia*** ▪ HEP: ↑ serum ALT, reversible hepatitis ▪ INT: rash ▪ MS: muscular pain ▪ Other: fever, gynecomastia.

DRUG INTERACTIONS: Selected inhibition of metabolism of other drugs, incl acetaminophen.

NURSING MANAGEMENT

ADMINISTRATION: Assess for hx of hypersensitivity (incl cimetidine) ▪ IM: dilution *not* required; may be painful ▪ IV injection: dilute to total volume 20ml; inject over at least 5m ▪ IV intermittent infusion: dilute to total volume 100ml; infuse over 15-20m period ▪ May mix c̄ 0.9% NaCl injection, 5%/10% dextrose, lactated Ringer solution, 5% Na bicarbonate injection for direct IV injection/intermittent IV infusion ▪ Diluted injection stable for 48h at room temperature ▪ Avoid exposure to moisture, light in storage ▪ Stable in hyperalimentation solutions.

EVALUATION: Monitor GI, hepatic, neurologic, renal status ▪ Monitor serum for ↑ creatinine, AST, ALT, alkaline phosphatase, LDH, total bilirubin ▪ False (+): urine protein c̄ Multistix (use sulfosalicylic acid) ▪ Assess for reversible confusion in elderly/debilitated pts.

EDUCATION: May be taken w/out regard to meals/antacids ▪ Dizziness may occur; use caution in potentially hazardous activities ▪ Women: avoid breastfeeding ▪ Men: breast enlargement may occur ▪ Avoid smoking ▪ Avoid GI-irritating foods ▪ Check c̄ physician/pharmacist before taking OTC preparations ▪ Avoid anxiety-producing situations ▪ Take as directed by physician ▪ Store in tightly closed, light-resistant container.

NOTES:

Rh_o (D) immune globulin

CATEGORY: *Immunosuppressant*: biological

Rx; Preg Cat C

BRAND NAMES

Standard dose	Microdose
Gamulin Rh (Armour)	*Mini-Gamulin Rh*
HypRho-D (Cutter)	*HypRho-D Minidose*
RhoGAM (Johnson & Johnson)	*MICRhoGAM*
**WinRho (Winn Rh Institute)*	

ACTION: Sterile solution of immunoglobulin [IgG anti-Rh_o (D)] obtained from fractionated human plasma, used to suppress immune response in nonsensitized pts c̄ Rh− blood who receive Rh+ blood cells because of fetomaternal hemorrhage, transfusion accident. **USE:** Microdose preparation: Used to suppress antibody formation in women c̄ Rh− blood after abortion/pregnancy termination up to and incl week 12 of gestation unless father has Rh− blood. Standard preparation: Used to suppress antibody formation in women c̄ Rh− blood after delivery, abortion/pregnancy termination, abdominal trauma during pregnancy ▪ Used to suppress antibody formation after transfusion accident.

PHARMACOKINETICS: Not applicable.

CONTRAINDICATIONS: Hypersensitivity, previously sensitized individuals; micropreparation for genetic amniocentesis at wk 15-18, antepartum prophylaxis at wk 28.

DOSAGE

OB	IM injection of total contents of single vial w/in 72h. Multiple dose required when fetomaternal hemorrhaging >30ml
Transfusion	IM injection of total contents of single vial(s) w/in ≤3 d. Specific dose dependent on volume of Rh^+ blood transfused

SIDE/ADVERSE EFFECTS: CNS: lethargy ▪ MS: myalgia, localized stiffness/tenderness at injection site ▪ Other: limited allergic rxs including anaphylaxis.

NURSING MANAGEMENT

ADMINISTRATION: Assess for hx of hypersensitivity ▪ Preadministration criteria (type, cross-match, neonatal cord blood): mother must be Rh_o (D)−, D^u−; mother should *not* have been previously sensitized to Rh_o factor:

Note: Side/adverse effects: common in *italic;* serious in ***boldface italic.***

*Available in Canada only.

infant must be Rh_o (D) +, D^u +, direct Coombs−; verify that lot numbers are same for cross-match solution, preparation to be administered ▪ Cross-match 5% suspension of mother's RBCs $\bar{c}$ 2gtt cross-match solution ▪ Administer w/in 72h after Rh-incompatible delivery, terminated incomplete pregnancy, blood transfusions ▪ Administer IM (deltoid); do *not* administer IV ▪ Check preparation $\bar{c}$ another nurse ▪ Do *not* administer to infant ▪ Do *not* administer discolored/precipitated solutions ▪ Store in refrigerator ▪ Provide emotional support.

EVALUATION: Assess for tenderness at injection site ▪ Assess for ↑ body temperature ▪ Assess for lethargy, myalgia if >1 dose administered.

EDUCATION: Explain procedure, rationale to pt, family ▪ Importance of screening both parents for Rh incompatibility.

NOTES:

rifampin • (rif-am-pin)

CATEGORY: *Antitubercular antibiotic*

Rx; Preg Cat NA

BRAND NAMES
Rifadin (MMD)
Rimactane (Ciba)

DOSAGE FORMS
Capsules: 150, 300mg
Capsules: 300mg
Injection (IV): 600mg/vial

COMBINATION PRODUCT
Rifamate (MMD) — 300mg rifampin, 150mg INH per capsule

PHARMACOKINETICS

PO absorption	Peak	Half-life	Protein binding	Excretion
Good	2-4h	3h	85%-91%	Via bile (60%) and urine as unchanged drug and metabolites

CONTRAINDICATIONS: Hypersensitivity.

ACTION: Antimycobacterial activity due to inhibition of DNA-dependent RNA polymerase activity in susceptible organisms. Rapid emergence of resistant strains can occur. The drug is present in breast milk and colors the urine red. **USE:** Treatment of pulmonary tuberculosis in combination c̄ isoniazid, ethambutol, or other effective antimycobacterial agents ▪ Treatment of asymptomatic carriers of *Neisseria meningitidis* (meningococci).

DOSAGE: *PO/IV*

Pulmonary TB
- Pediatric: 10-20mg/kg. Do *not* exceed 600mg/d
- Adult: 600mg in a single daily dose

Meningococcal carriers
- Pediatric: 10-20mg/kg/d for 4d. Do *not* exceed 600mg/d. CDC recommends for 3m-1y/o a dose of 5mg/kg bid for 2d and for 1-12 y/o a dose of 10mg/kg bid for 2d

Adult	600mg once/d for 3d. CDC recommends a dose of 600mg bid for 2d
Rifamate	2 capsules once/d pc

SIDE/ADVERSE EFFECTS: CNS: headache, drowsiness, dizziness, visual disturbances, inability to concentrate ▪ GI: *anorexia, N/V/D, gas, cramps,* sore mouth, heartburn, rare cases of ***pseudomembranous colitis*** ▪ HEM: ***hemolytic anemia,*** transient leukopenia, thrombocytopenia, eosinophilis ▪ INT: urticaria, rash, pruritus, ***pemphigus,*** acneform lesions ▪ Other: flulike symptoms, exudative conjunctivitis, muscular weakness, pain in the extremities, menstrual disturbances.

DRUG INTERACTIONS: Oral contraceptives may lose significant activity during rifampin therapy ▪ Therapy may necessitate dosage adjustment for PO anticoagulants, corticosteroids, dapsone, dig glycosides, PO hypoglycemics, quinidine ▪ Methadone maintenance pts may experience significant withdrawal symptoms, and higher doses of methadone may be required.

NURSING MANAGEMENT

ADMINISTRATION: Assess for hx of hypersensitivity ▪ Assess hepatic function; ↓ dosage if impaired ▪ Assess resistance to *Mycobacterium* ▪ May administer c̄ food to ↓ GI irritation; *best* on empty stomach (1h ac/2h pc); may open capsules & mix content c̄ food ▪ Avoid exposure to heat, moisture, light in storage.

EVALUATION: Monitor VS, esp temperature ▪ Monitor respiratory status (breath sounds, sputum) ▪ Monitor CBC, UA, resistance to *Mycobacterium* ▪ May ↑ serum ALT, AST, alkaline phosphatase, bilirubin, uric acid, BUN.

EDUCATION: Drowsiness may occur; use caution in potentially hazardous activities ▪ Take as ordered by physician even if symptom free; complete full course of therapy ▪ Take on empty stomach; may take c̄ food if GI irritation occurs ▪ Red-brown discoloration of body secretions (tears, urine, saliva) may occur; permanent soft-contact-lens discoloration ▪ Notify physician *immediately* if experiencing vomiting, ↓ appetite, lethargy, yellow eyes/skin, bleeding/bruising, chills, headache ▪ May cause mouth discomfort ▪ Avoid use of alcohol ▪ Women: use alternate form of contraception (*not* oral estrogens) while taking drug ▪ Keep scheduled appointments c̄ physician/for blood work ▪ Store in tightly closed, light-resistant container in cool, dry area.

NOTES:

ritodrine hcl • (ri-toe-dreen)

CATEGORY: *Sympathomimetic:* $beta_2$ adrenergic, uterine relaxant   Rx; Preg Cat B

BRAND NAMES

Yutopar (Astra) (Bristol in Canada)

DOSAGE FORMS

Injection (IV): 10mg/ml
Tablet: 10mg

ACTION: Sympathomimetic activity selective for beta receptors, esp $beta_2$ adrenoreceptors of bronchial tree, peripheral vascular beds, uterus; predominant beta-mimetic effect on uterine smooth muscle, which ↓ intensity, frequency of contractions; placental drug transfer occurs, limited $beta_1$ activity results in transitory ↑ in maternal, fetal heart rates. **USE:** Management of preterm labor in suitable pts.

PHARMACOKINETICS

PO availability	Peak	Half-life	Protein binding	Excretion
30%	30-60m	1.3-20h	32%	Via urine as unchanged drug, metabolites

CONTRAINDICATIONS: Before wk 20 of pregnancy, conditions in which continuation of pregnancy is hazardous, incl antepartum hemorrhage requiring immediate delivery; chorioamnionitis; eclampsia, severe preeclampsia; intrauterine fetal death; maternal cardiac disease, hyperthyroidism, controlled diabetes; pulmonary hypertension ▪ Preexisting maternal medical conditions seriously affected by ritodrine beta-mimetic activity, incl asthma already treated c̄ beta adrenergics/steroids; cardiac arrhythmias associated c̄ tachycardia/drug toxicity; hypovolemia; pheochromocytoma; ritodrine hypersensitivity; uncontrolled hypertension.

DOSAGE

IV infusion	Usual starting dose 50-100µg/m, ↑ q10m by 50µg/m until desired effect obtained. Usual effective range 150-350µg/m. Treatment should continue for at least 12h after uterine contractions cease

PO maintenance	10mg 30m before termination of IV therapy. Usual dosage for first 24h 10mg q2h. Usual maintenance dose 10-20mg q4-6h. Do *not* exceed 120mg/d

SIDE/ADVERSE EFFECTS: CNS: nervousness, anxiety, emotional upset, tremor, headache ▪ CV: dose-related changes in maternal BP; maternal, fetal heart rates; pulmonary edema ▪ GI: N/V/D, epigastric distress, constipation ▪ Other: rash, dyspnea, hyperventilation, lactic acidosis ▪ Fetal: hypoglycemia, ileus.

DRUG INTERACTIONS: Use c̄ corticosteroids can produce pulmonary edema ▪ Use c̄ beta blockers antagonizes therapeutic effects ▪ Use c̄ anesthetics can ↑ hypotensive effects ▪ Use c̄ sympathomimetics produces additive effects.

NURSING MANAGEMENT

ADMINISTRATION: Assess VS ▪ Do *not* use saline diluents unless dextrose undesirable (diabetics) ▪ Use solution w/in 48h of preparation ▪ Do *not* administer discolored/precipitated solution ▪ Place pt in left lateral position ▪ IV: use infusion control device ▪ Restrict fluids per physician's order ▪ Store parenteral form at room temperature; do *not* freeze ▪ Provide emotional support.

EVALUATION: Monitor I&O ▪ Monitor VS, esp BP, respiratory rate (labored breathing) ▪ Monitor uterine contractions, fetal heart rate ▪ Observe for pulmonary edema; D/C drug if present ▪ Assess for ↑ serum glucose, esp diabetics.

EDUCATION: Explain procedure, rationale to pt, family ▪ Relaxation techniques ▪ Comfort measures ▪ Check c̄ physician before using OTC preparations ▪ Notify physician of contractions, rupture of membranes.

NOTES:

scopolamine/scopolamine hcl • (skoe-pol-a-meen)

CATEGORY: *Anticholinergic*: antimuscarinic, parasympatholytic Rx; Preg Cat C

BRAND NAMES
Scopolamine HBr (various)
Transderm-Scop (Ciba)

DOSAGE FORMS
Capsule, injection
Transdermal disc (1.5mg)

ACTION: Anticholinergic activity due to competition c̄ acetylcholine for muscarinic receptors at postganglionic fiber of parasympathetic nervous system; sedative/tranquilizing effect on CNS. **USE:** Prevention of N/V from motion sickness (transdermal disc should be applied to skin in postauricular area) ▪ Preanesthetic medication; induction of obstetrical amnesia, in conjunction c̄ barbiturate/sedative analgesic ▪ May be used (obsolete) as antispasmodic, antiparkinsonian, cycloplegic, mydriatic, sedative.

PHARMACOKINETICS

Route	Peak	Excretion
PO	1-2h	Liver metabolites via urine
IM	1-2h	Liver metabolites via urine

CONTRAINDICATIONS: Hypersensitivity, narrow-angle glaucoma, prostatic hypertrophy/pyloric obstruction, impaired hepatic/renal function.

DOSAGE

Pediatric *IM/IV/SC*	0.006mg/kg
Adult *PO*	0.4-0.8mg
IM/IV/SC	0.32-0.65mg
Disc	1 q3d (delivers 0.5 mg drug at constant rate over 3d)

SIDE/ADVERSE EFFECTS: CNS: mental confusion, psychotic signs, somnolence ▪ CV: tachycardia ▪ EENT: blurred vision, cycloplegia, mydriasis, ↑ ocular tension, photophobia ▪ GU: urinary retention ▪ INT: skin rash.

DRUG INTERACTIONS: Use c̄ antihistamines, phenothiazines, tricyclic antidepressants produces ↑ anticholinergic effects ▪ MAO-I ↑ activity by ↓ anticholinergic biotransformation.

NURSING MANAGEMENT

ADMINISTRATION: Assess for hx of belladonna alkaloid hypersensitivity ▪ Administer tablets 1h before motion-producing event ▪ Avoid exposure to moisture, light in storage ▪ Wash hands after application of transdermal disc; apply to dry area behind ear ▪ Elderly may require ↓ dosage.

EVALUATION: Monitor VS, esp heart rate ▪ Observe for exaggerated anticholinergic effects ▪ Monitor neurologic status (amnesia, confusion) ▪ Monitor I&O; assess for urinary retention.

EDUCATION: Advise pt of expected anticholinergic side effects (dry mouth, photophobia, constipation) ▪ D/C drug, notify physician *immediately* on appearance of skin rash, flushing of skin, eye pain ▪ Avoid concurrent antacid administration ▪ Avoid strenuous work/exercise during hot, humid weather ▪ Use sugarless gum/hard candy to diminish dry mouth ▪ Avoid OTC cough/cold/allergy preparations ▪ Drowsiness, blurred vision may occur; avoid potentially hazardous activities ▪ Store in original, tightly closed, light-resistant container ▪ Frequent oral hygiene ▪ Take capsules 1h before motion-producing event ▪ Procedure for application of transdermal disc; wash hands after applying transdermal disc.

NOTES:

sertraline hcl •(sir-trah-leen)

CATEGORY: *Antidepressant* Rx; Preg Cat B

BRAND NAME
Zoloft (Roerig)

DOSAGE FORMS
Tablet: 50, 100mg

ACTION: Antidepressant activity appears related to selective inhibition of serotonin (5 hydroxytryptamine) reuptake c̄ little effect on norepinephrine & dopamine reuptake in CNS. **USE:** Treatment of depression. Use for >16 wks not currently evaluated.

PHARMACOKINETICS

PO absorption	Peak	Half-life	Protein binding	Excretion
Good	4-5-8.4h	26h	98%	Via urine & feces primarily as metabolites

DOSAGE

Adult *PO* — Initial dose of 50mg c̄ range of 50-200mg/d taken once/d

SIDE/ADVERSE EFFECTS: CNS: headache (20.3%), insomnia (61.4%), somnolence (13.4%), dizziness (11.7%), tremor (10.7%), paresthesia (2%) ▪ CV: palpitations (3.5%), chest pain ▪ EENT: abnormal vision (4.2%), tinnitus, pharyngitis ▪ GI: nausea (26.1%), diarrhea (17.7%), dry mouth (16.3%), constipation (8.4%), dyspepsia (6%), vomiting (3.0%), flatulence (3.3%), anorexia, abdominal pain ▪ GU: Male (15.5%) and female (1.7%) dysfunction, menstrual disorders, urinary disorders ▪ INT: skin rash ▪ Other: fatigue (10.6%), sweating (8.4%), hot flashes, back pain, fever.

DRUG INTERACTIONS: Use c̄ other highly protein bound drugs, such as digitoxin, warfarin, may ↑ their activity by protein displacement ▪ Use c̄ MAO-I or within 1d of D/C MAO-I use not recommended ▪ Use c̄ PO hypoglycemics may ↑ their effects ▪ Use c̄ diazepam can ↓ its excretion ▪ Use c̄ alcohol not recommended.

NURSING MANAGEMENT

ADMINISTRATION: Assess for hx of hypersensitivity ▪ Assess for hx of seizures; use caution ▪ Assess hepatic, renal status; ↓ dosage if impaired ▪ Administer consistently c̄ or w/out food in AM or PM ▪ Institute safety, seizure precautions ▪ Institute suicide precautions ▪

Avoid abrupt withdrawal; D/C gradually ▪ Avoid moisture, heat, direct light in storage ▪ Elderly may require ↓ dosage.

EVALUATION: Monitor CV, hepatic, renal status ▪ Monitor fluid retention (I&O, daily weight), constipation ▪ Assess for weight loss (anorectic effect) ▪ Assess for symptoms of abrupt withdrawal (nausea, headache, malaise) ▪ Assess for actual swallowing of PO forms ▪ Assess for skin rash, hives; notify physician, D/C drug ▪ Diabetics: monitor blood glucose (hypoglycemia).

EDUCATION: Dizziness/drowsiness may occur; use caution in potentially hazardous activities ▪ Avoid changing positions (lying/sitting/standing) rapidly ▪ Avoid use c̄ alcohol, other CNS depressants for up to 1 wk after end of therapy ▪ Take consistently c̄ or w/out food ▪ Take as directed by physician ▪ Use sugarless gum/hard candy to diminish dry mouth ▪ Constipation may occur; ↑ fluids, bulk-containing foods ▪ Notify physician of skin rash, hives; D/C drug ▪ Check c̄ physician/pharmacist before taking OTC/Rx preparations ▪ Notify physician/dentist of use before treatment ▪ Store in tightly closed, light-resistant container ▪ Encourage recreational/diversional interests ▪ Notify physician of weight loss, fever, sore throat, malaise ▪ Keep scheduled appointments c̄ physician ▪ Women: notify physician of possibility of pregnancy; avoid breastfeeding ▪ Full drug effects may require several wks of therapy.

NOTES:

sodium bicarbonate

CATEGORY: *Alkalinizing agent* OTC/Rx*; Preg Cat C

DOSAGE FORMS
Injection (IV)*, PO powder, tablet

ACTION: Chemical correction of acidic conditions; 1g sodium bicarbonate provides 11.9mEq sodium, 11.9mEq bicarbonate. **USE:** Treatment of metabolic acidosis ▪ Antacid ▪ Urinary alkalinizer for selected drug overdose management ▪ Prophylaxis of renal calculi.

PHARMACOKINETICS: Not applicable.

CONTRAINDICATIONS: Alkalosis, chloride loss, hypocalcemia.

DOSAGE

Pediatric *PO*	6-12y/o: Usual dose 520mg repeated once in 30m as antacid
IV	Same as for adults
Adult *PO*	0.3-2g 1-4 times/d as antacid. Usual dose for alkalinization of urine, 4g followed by 1-2g q4h. Do *not* exceed total 16g/d
IV	Cardiac arrest: 1mEq/kg followed by 0.5mEq/kg, repeated every 10m of continued arrest Less urgent metabolic acidosis/urinary alkalinizer: 2-5mEq/kg over 4-8h

SIDE/ADVERSE EFFECTS: CNS: nervousness, headache ▪ CV: ***irregular heartbeat,*** edema ▪ GI: N/V, loss of appetite ▪ MET: alkalosis.

DRUG INTERACTIONS: Use c̄ methenamine best avoided ▪ Use c̄ corticosteroids can produce hypernatremia ▪ Use c̄ *basic* drugs will ↑ their effects by ↓ urinary excretion.

Note: Side/adverse effects: common in *italic;* serious in ***boldface italic.***

*Available in Canada only.

NURSING MANAGEMENT

ADMINISTRATION: Assess ABGs ▪ PO: chew thoroughly; take c̄ full glass H_2O; do *not* administer w/in 2h of milk, other PO drugs ▪ Effervescent tablet: dissolve completely before administering ▪ IV: dilute according to manufacturer's directions; flush lines before, after use ▪ Do *not* administer discolored/precipitated solutions ▪ Do *not* mix c̄ catecholamines in solution.

EVALUATION: Monitor VS, esp BP ▪ Monitor ABGs, F/E status (hypokalemia, hypernatremia) ▪ Cardiac monitoring (parenteral) ▪ Check IV site closely; avoid extravasation.

EDUCATION: Notify physician *immediately* of "skipped" heartbeats, tremors, muscle cramps, lethargy; D/C drug ▪ Effervescent tablet: wait until bubbling stops before taking ▪ Do *not* take for >2wks w/out checking c̄ physician ▪ Avoid taking c̄ milk products/enteric-coated preparations ▪ Check c̄ physician/pharmacist before taking OTC drugs.

NOTES:

spectinomycin hcl • (spek-tin-oh-mye-sin)

CATEGORY: *Antibiotic* Rx; Preg Cat NA

BRAND NAME
Trobicin (Upjohn)

DOSAGE FORMS
Powder for IM injection: 2g vial with 3.2ml of diluent, 4g vial with 6.2ml of diluent

ACTION: Bacteriostatic activity due to inhibition of ribosomal protein synthesis in susceptible organisms. **USE:** Treatment of gonorrhea. However, the drug is usually used only in cases that are resistant (PPNG) to the penicillins or in patients who are hypersensitive to the penicillins, cephalosporins, or other suitable drugs.

PHARMACOKINETICS

IM peak	Half-life	Protein binding	Excretion
1-2h	1.2-2.8h	Very low	70%-100% in 48h via urine

CONTRAINDICATIONS: Hypersensitivity.

DOSAGE: *IM*

Pediatric	CDC recommends 40mg/kg as a single dose
Adult	2g as a single dose, or 4g as a single dose for cases occurring or pts living in geographic areas where penicillin resistance is prevalent

SIDE/ADVERSE EFFECTS: Local: *soreness at injection site* ▪ MET: ↑ in alkaline phosphatase, BUN, ALT (SGPT) ▪ Other: anaphylaxis, chills, dizziness, fever, insomnia, urticaria, N/V, rash.

DRUG INTERACTIONS: No significant interactions reported.

NURSING MANAGEMENT
ADMINISTRATION: Assess for hx of hypersensitivity ▪ Obtain C&S before therapy ▪ Administer deep IM injection ▪ Maintain hydration.

EVALUATION: Monitor VS, esp temperature ▪ Monitor renal function (nephrotoxicity); notify physician.

EDUCATION: Dizziness may occur; use caution in potentially hazardous activities ▪ May experience pain at injection site ▪ ↑ Fluid intake (8-10 glasses/d) ▪ Notify physician *immediately* of fever, chills, difficult breathing, ↓ urination, rash ▪ Identify all sexual contacts for treatment; maintain good perineal hygiene.

NOTES:

spironolactone • (speer-on-oh-lak-tone)

CATEGORY: *Diuretic:* aldosterone antagonist, potassium-sparing diuretic Rx; Preg Cat NA

BRAND NAME
Aldactone (Searle)

DOSAGE FORMS
Tablet: 25, 50, 100mg

COMBINATION PRODUCTS

Aldactazide 25/25; 50/50 (Searle)	spironolactone/hydrochlorothiazide per tablet: 25mg/25mg; 50mg/50mg

ACTION: spironolactone is a competitive antagonist of aldosterone; displaces it from sodium-potassium exchange receptors in distal convoluted tubules, resulting in potassium retention, excretion of H_2O, sodium; drug also exhibits antihypertensive activity. **USE:** Diagnosis of 1° hyperaldosteronism ▪ Short-term pre-op treatment of primary hyperaldosteronism ▪ Maintenance in pts c̄ discrete aldosterone-producing adrenal adenomas, bilateral micro/macronodular adrenal hyperplasia (idiopathic hyperaldosteronism) ▪ Treatment/prevention of hypokalemia when other methods are inadequate ▪ Treatment of nephrosis in pts not suitable to other methods ▪ Adjunct in treating hypertension, edema due to CHF/cirrhosis of liver.

PHARMACOKINETICS

PO absorption	Peak	Half-life	Protein binding	Excretion
90%	2-4h as metabolites	13-24h as metabolites	90%	Via urine as metabolites

CONTRAINDICATIONS: Hypersensitivity, anuria, significant renal insufficiency, hyperkalemia.

DOSAGE

Pediatric *PO*	1.5mg/lb/d divided for edema
Adult *PO*	
Edema	100mg/d for at least 5d. Adjust according to response
Hyperaldosteronism	
Short diagnostic test	400mg/d for 4d
Long diagnostic test	400mg/d for 3-4wks
Maintenance	Lowest effective dose
Pre-op preparation	100-400mg/d

Hypertension	50-100mg/d divided, for at least 2 wks. Adjust according to response
Hypokalemia	Aldactazide 25/25, 50/50 Usual maintenance dose is 1-4 tablets for edema and 2-4 tablets for hypertension/d

SIDE/ADVERSE EFFFECTS: CNS: drowsiness, headache, lethargy, confusion ▪ GI: *cramps,* diarrhea ▪ GU: amenorrhea/irregular menses, postmenopausal bleeding, impotence ▪ INT: urticaria, drug fever, skin rash, hirsutism ▪ MET: hyperkalemia ▪ Other: gynecomastia, carcinoma of breast (no cause/effect relationship established), deepening of voice.

DRUG INTERACTIONS: Use c̄ digoxin/lithium may ↑ toxicity ▪ Use c̄ ganglionic blocking agents ↑ their activity; ↓ dosage may be required.

NURSING MANAGEMENT

ADMINISTRATION: Assess for hx of hypersensitivity, F/E balance; normal serum K^+ level: 3.5-5mEq/L; do *not* administer if hyperkalemic; notify physician ▪ Assess renal function; do *not* administer if impaired ▪ Administer c̄ food/milk on arising; may crush tablets ▪ Avoid exposure to moisture, light in storage ▪ Elderly may require ↓ dosage.

EVALUATION: Monitor F/E, hepatic, renal status ▪ Monitor VS, esp BP, pulse; serum for ↑ BUN, creatinine, uric acid ▪ Assess for hyperkalemia; notify physician ▪ Monitor fluid retention.

EDUCATION: Expect ↑ urine output ▪ May cause weakness, lethargy ▪ Take c̄ food/milk on rising, at same time each day, even if symptom free; may crush tablets ▪ Take as directed; do *not* skip doses ▪ Notify physician of signs of hyperkalemia (weakness, tingling/numbness, irregular heartbeat) ▪ Avoid changing positions (lying/sitting/standing) rapidly ▪ Avoid high-Na^+/K^+ foods ▪ Check c̄ physician before using salt substitutes ▪ Check c̄ physician before taking OTC preparations ▪ Store in tightly closed, light-resistant container ▪ Keep appointments c̄ physician; have BP checked regularly ▪ Full drug effect may require several wks.

NOTES:

streptomycin sulfate • (strep-toe-<u>mye</u>-sin)

CATEGORY: *Aminoglycoside:* antibiotic

Rx; Preg Cat NA

BRAND NAME
Streptomycin Sulfate (various)

DOSAGE FORMS
Injection (IM), powder for injection (IM)

ACTION: Bactericidal activity due to inhibition of ribosomal protein synthesis in susceptible organisms. **USE:** Indicated in treatment of infections caused by *Calymmatobacterium granulomatis* (granuloma inguinale), *Francisella tularensis* (tularemia), *Yersinia pestis* (plague) ▪ In combined therapy for tuberculosis ▪ In combined therapy (c̄ penicillin) for enterococcal, α-, nonhemolytic streptococcal endocarditis.

PHARMACOKINETICS

IM peak	Half-life	Protein binding	Excretion
1h	2-3h	35%	29%-89% unchanged in urine in 24h

CONTRAINDICATIONS: Hypersensitivity, previous hx of serious aminoglycoside toxicity.

DOSAGE: For pts c̄ normal renal function

Pediatric *IM*	Neonates: 20-30mg/kg/d in 2 doses Children: 40mg/kg/d in 2 doses
Adult *IM*	
Tularemia	1-2g/d divided, for 7-10d until patient is afebrile for 5-7d
Plague	2-4g/d divided until patient is afebrile 3d
TB	1g/d c̄ 200-300mg isoniazid, 5g PAS tid
Enterococcal endocarditis	0.5-1g bid for 4wks in combination c̄ penicillin
α-, nonhemolytic strep endocarditis	1g bid for 1wk, 0.5g bid for 2nd wk, in combination c̄ penicillin

SIDE/ADVERSE EFFECTS: CNS: peripheral paresthesia, amblyopia ▪ CV: myocarditis ▪ EENT: ***ototoxicity*** (auditory, vestibular damage), dizziness, vertigo, tinnitus, roaring in ears, hearing loss ▪ HEM: ***agranulocytosis, aplastic anemia,*** eosinophilia, leukopenia, pancytopenia, ***thrombocytopenia*** ▪ HEP: hepatic necrosis ▪ INT: ***exfoliative dermatitis*** ▪ Other: neuromuscular blockade c̄ high doses, esp in young children.

DRUG INTERACTIONS: Avoid use c̄ neurotoxic/nephrotoxic drugs such as other aminoglycosides, colistin, ethacrynic acid, furosemide, polymyxin B, vancomycin, viomycin ▪ Dimenhydrinate can mask aminoglycoside ototoxicity ▪ Use c̄ succinylcholine/tubocurarine ↑ their activity; Ca salts can reverse blockade ▪ PO anticoagulant activity may ↑ due to ↓ intestinal vitamin K synthesis.

NURSING MANAGEMENT

ADMINISTRATION: Assess for hx of aminoglycoside hypersensitivity ▪ Obtain C&S before therapy ▪ Obtain pt weight for dosage calculation ▪ Determine creatinine clearance before administration ▪ Dissolve sterile powder in sterile H_2O for injection or normal saline solution according to manufacturer's directions; avoid contact c̄ solution ▪ Use reconstituted solution w/in 2d at room temperature, w/in 14d refrigerated ▪ Store in original container; darkened vial does *not* affect potency ▪ Administer slowly by *deep* IM injection; rotate sites; avoid inflamed areas ▪ Avoid solutions stronger than 500mg/ml ▪ Do *not* add preservatives to intrathecal preparations ▪ Avoid topical/inhalation administration (↑ risk of sensitization) ▪ Maintain hydration ▪ Elderly may require ↓ dosage.

EVALUATION: Assess for hearing dysfunction ▪ Monitor hepatic, renal, VIII CN function ▪ Monitor VS, esp temperature ▪ Assess for edema in extremities ▪ Assess for neuromuscular blockade, respiratory paralysis, nephrotoxicity ▪ Observe for signs of superinfection (diarrhea, URI, coated tongue) ▪ Assess for hypersensitivity rx (fever, difficult breathing, rash) ▪ Monitor TB pts for changes in sputum.

EDUCATION: Report hearing, balance difficulties to physician at once ▪ ↑ Fluid intake (10-12 glasses/d).

NOTES:

sucralfate • (soo-kral-fate)

CATEGORY: *Antiulcer agent* Rx; Preg Cat B

BRAND NAME	**DOSAGE FORM**
Carafate (MMD)	Tablet: 1g

ACTION: Antiulcer activity due to formulation of complex that covers ulcer, protects from acid, pepsin, bile, facilitates healing process at ulcer site; ulcer-adherent complex formed between drug, proteinaceous exudates from ulcer site; drug minimally absorbed. **USE:** Short-term treatment of duodenal ulcers.

PHARMACOKINETICS: Not applicable.

CONTRAINDICATIONS: None currently known.

DOSAGE

Adult *PO* 1g qid ac, hs. Usual maintenance dose 1g bid

SIDE/ADVERSE EFFECTS: CNS: dizziness, sleepiness ▪ GI: *constipation*, N/D, gastric upset, dry mouth ▪ INT: rash.

DRUG INTERACTIONS: Use c̄ cimetidine, phenytoin, tetracycline ↓ PO absorption; give 2h before/after sucralfate.

NURSING MANAGEMENT

ADMINISTRATION: Administer 1h ac, hs c̄ full glass H_2O; do *not* chew tablets ▪ Do *not* administer antacids w/in 1/2h of drug ▪ Have pharmacist prepare solution for NG tube administration ▪ For short-term use only (<8wks).

EVALUATION: Monitor GI status (constipation).

EDUCATION: Take on empty stomach ▪ Take as ordered by physician; do *not* change dose ▪ Constipation may occur; ↑ fluid intake (8-10 glasses/d), bulk in diet ▪ Avoid smoking.

NOTES:

sucralfate

sulfamethoxazole • (sul-fa-meth-ox-a-zole)

CATEGORY: *Sulfonamide:* antibacterial, antiinfective   Rx; Preg Cat C

BRAND NAME	DOSAGE FORMS
Gantanol (Roche)	PO suspension: 500mg/5ml Tablet: 500mg

COMBINATION PRODUCTS

Azo Gantanol (Roche)	sulfamethoxazole/phenazopyridine hcl per tablet: 0.5g/100mg
Bactrim (B-W), Septra (Roche)	Trimethoprim/sulfamethoxazole: see Co-Triamoxazole

ACTION: Bacteriostatic activity due to inhibition of folic acid synthesis in susceptible microorganisms; addition of phenazopyridine (urinary analgesic) helps to ↓ dysuria. **USE:** Treatment of UTIs caused by susceptible strains of *Enterobacter* spp, *Escherichia coli, Klebsiella* spp, *Proteus mirabilis, Proteus vulgaris, Staphylococcus aureus* ▪ Drug of choice for nocardiosis ▪ Adjunct in treatment of malaria, toxoplasmosis.

PHARMACOKINETICS

PO absorption	Peak	Half-life	Protein binding	Excretion
Incomplete	3-4h	7-12h	50%-70%	25%-70% via urine in 24h

CONTRAINDICATIONS: Hypersensitivity, pregnancy at term, nursing mothers, infants <2mo (except in treatment of congenital toxoplasmosis).

DOSAGE

Neonatal (>2mo)/ Pediatric *PO*	50-60mg/kg loading dose followed by 25-30mg/kg q12h. Do *not* exceed 75mg/kg/d
Adult *PO*	2g loading dose followed by 1-2g 2-3 times/d
Azo Gantanol	Same as adult. Do *not* exceed 2d of treatment

SIDE/ADVERSE EFFECTS: CNS: headache, peripheral neuritis, depression, ataxis, ***convulsions*** ▪ GI: N/V/D, anorexia, abdominal pain, ***pancreatitis,*** stomatitis ▪ GU: crystalluria, toxic nephrosis ▪ HEM: ***agranulocytosis, aplastic anemia, hemolytic anemia, thrombocytopenia,*** purpura, methemoglobinemia, hypoprothrombinemia, leukopenia ▪ INT: maculopapuar/bullous eruptions, ***Stevens-Johnson syndrome, epidermal necrolysis, exfoliative dermatitis,*** urticaria, photosensitization ▪ MS: arthralgia ▪ Other: serum sickness, allergic myocarditis, periorbital edema.

DRUG INTERACTIONS: Use c̄ urinary acidifiers absolutely contraindicated because of high probability of crystalluria ▪ Avoid p-aminobenzoic preparations during therapy ▪ Use c̄ PO anticoagulant may require dosage adjustment due to ↓ vitamin K synthesis in GI tract ▪ Sulfonamides can enhance activity of PO hypoglycemics, methotrexate.

NURSING MANAGEMENT

ADMINISTRATION: Assess for hx of sulfonamide hypersensitivity; furosemide, thiazide diuretics ▪ Obtain C&S before therapy ▪ Administer 1h ac/2h pc c̄ full glass H_2O ▪ PO suspension: shake well before using ▪ Avoid use in group A β-hemolytic streptococcal infections ▪ Maintain hydration ▪ Avoid exposure to moisture, light in storage.

EVALUATION: Monitor VS, esp temperature; CBC, UA; I&O, hepatic, renal status.

EDUCATION: Complete full course of therapy (usually 10d) even if symptoms subside ▪ Take on empty stomach c̄ full glass H_2O ▪ Take at equal intervals to maintain blood levels ▪ Store in tightly closed, light-resistant container ▪ Maintain good personal hygiene (esp perineal, oral) ▪ Maintain fluid intake (6-8 glasses/d) ▪ Avoid exposure to direct sunlight, UV light (sunlamps); use sunscreen, protective clothing ▪ Use calibrated measuring device for PO liquid forms ▪ Women: avoid breastfeeding ▪ Notify physician/dentist of sulfonamide use before general anesthesia ▪ Notify physician of fever, sore throat, difficult breathing, rash, bruising/bleeding.

NOTES:

sulfisoxazole • (sul-fi-sox-a-zole)

CATEGORY: *Sulfonamide:* antibacterial, antiinfective — Rx; Preg Cat C

BRAND NAMES	DOSAGE FORMS
Sulfisoxazole	
Gantrisin (Roche)	Tablet: 500mg
Sulfisoxazole acetyl	
Gantrisin (Roche)	Pediatric suspension: 500mg/ml Syrup: 500mg/5ml
Sulfisoxazole diolamine	
Gantrisin (Roche)	Ophthalmic ointment, solution

COMBINATION PRODUCT

Azo-Gantrisin (Roche)	sulfisoxazole/phenazopyridine hcl per tablet: 0.5g/50mg

ACTION: Bacteriostatic activity due to inhibition of folic acid synthesis in susceptible microorganisms; addition of phenazopyridine (urinary analgesic) helps to ⬇ dysuria.

USE: Treatment of UTIs caused by susceptible strains of *Enterobacter* spp, *Escherichia coli, Klebsiella* spp, *Proteus mirabilis, Proteus vulgaris, Staphylococcus aureus* ▪ Drug of choice for nocardiosis ▪ Adjunct in treatment of malaria, toxoplasmosis ▪ Treatment of ocular infections.

PHARMACOKINETICS

PO absorption	Peak	Half-life	Protein binding	Excretion
Rapid	2-4h	4-8h	85%	95% via urine in 24h

CONTRAINDICATIONS: Hypersensitivity, pregnancy at term, nursing mothers, infants <2mo of age (except in treatment of congenital toxoplasmosis).

DOSAGE

Neonatal (>2mo)/ Pediatric *PO*	75mg/kg loading dose followed by 150mg/kg/d in 4-6 doses. Emulsion dosage 60-75mg/kg loading dose followed by 60-75mg/kg bid. Do *not* exceed 6g/d
Adult *PO*	2-4g loading dose followed by 4-8g/d in 4-6 doses. Emulsion dosage 4-5g q12h

Ophthalmic	Ointment: Apply small amount tid, hs Solution: 2-3 drops ≥3 times/d
Azo-Gantrisin	Same as adult. Do *not* exceed 2d of treatment

SIDE/ADVERSE EFFECTS: CNS: headache, peripheral neuritis, depression, ataxia, ***convulsions*** ▪ GI: N/V/D, anorexia, abdominal pain, ***pancreatitis,*** stomatitis ▪ GU: crystalluria, toxic nephrosis ▪ HEM: ***agranulocytosis, aplastic anemia, hemolytic anemia, thrombocytopenia,*** purpura, methemoglobinemia, hypoprothrombinemia, leukopenia ▪ INT: maculopapular/bullous eruptions, ***Stevens-Johnson syndrome, epidermal necrolysis, exfoliative dermatitis,*** urticaria, photosensitivity ▪ Other: serum sickness, allergic myocarditis, periorbital edema.

DRUG INTERACTIONS: Use c̄ urinary acidifiers absolutely contraindicated because of high probability of crystalluria ▪ Avoid *p*-aminobenzoic preparations during therapy ▪ Use c̄ PO anticoagulant may require dosage adjustment due to ↓ vitamin K synthesis in GI tract ▪ Sulfonamides can ↑ activity of PO hypoglycemics, methotrexate.

NURSING MANAGEMENT

ADMINISTRATION: Assess for hx of hypersensitivity to sulfonamides, furosemide, thiazide diuretics ▪ Obtain C&S ▪ Avoid exposure to moisture, light in storage ▪ Administer 1h ac/2h pc c̄ full glass H_2O ▪ PO suspension: shake well before using ▪ Ophthalmic: administer into lower conjunctival sac.

EVALUATION: Monitor VS, esp temperature; I&O; CBC, UA; hepatic, renal status.

EDUCATION: Complete full course of therapy (usually 10d) even if symptoms subside ▪ Take on empty stomach c̄ full glass H_2O at equal intervals ▪ Store in tightly closed, light-resistant container ▪ Maintain good personal hygiene (esp perineal, oral) ▪ ↑ Fluid intake (8-10 glasses/d) ▪ Avoid exposure to direct sunlight, UV light (sunlamps); use sunscreen, protective clothing ▪ Women: avoid breastfeeding ▪ Notify physician of fever, sore throat, difficult breathing, rash, bruising/bleeding; physician/dentist of sulfonamide use before general anesthesia ▪ Procedure for ophthalmic application.

NOTES:

sulindac • (sul-in-dak)

CATEGORY: *Antiinflammatory*

Rx; Preg Cat NA

BRAND NAME

Clinoril (MSD) (Frosst in Canada)

DOSAGE FORMS

Tablet: 150, 200mg

ACTION: Antiinflammatory activity appears related to inhibition of prostaglandin synthesis. **USE:** Treatment of rheumatoid/osteoarthritis, ankylosing spondylitis, acute gout, acute painful shoulder.

PHARMACOKINETICS

PO absorption	Peak	Half-life	Protein binding	Excretion
90%	2-4h	7.8h	93%	Via urine, feces as unchanged drug, metabolites

CONTRAINDICATIONS: Hypersensitivity, aspirin/other antiinflammatory agent hypersensitivity.

DOSAGE

Adult *PO*

Arthritis, spondylitis	150mg bid, then adjust. Do *not* exceed 400mg/d
Painful shoulder, gout	200mg bid. ↓ Dosage after improvement, usually 7-14d for painful shoulder, 7d for gout

SIDE/ADVERSE EFFECTS: CNS: headache, dizziness, drowsiness ▪ CV: edema, palpitations, CHF ▪ EENT: tinnitus, ↓ hearing, blurred vision ▪ GI: *abdominal pain,* constipation, N/V, stomatitis ▪ GU: ***glomerular nephritis,*** hematuria, ***interstitial nephritis,*** nephrotic syndrome ▪ HEM: ***agranulocytosis, aplastic anemia, hemolytic anemia*** ▪ INT: rash, alopecia, pruritus, purpura, urticaria.

DRUG INTERACTIONS: Use $\bar{c}$ ulcerogenic drugs produces additive effects ▪ Use $\bar{c}$ PO anticoagulants may ↑ their activity ▪ Aspirin ↓ sulindac plasma levels.

NURSING MANAGEMENT

ADMINISTRATION: Assess for hx of NSAIA hypersensitivity ▪ Avoid administration to pts c̄ hx of asthma, bleeding disorders, salicylate hypersensitivity ▪ Assess for hx of peptic ulcer; use c̄ caution ▪ Assess renal function; may require ↓ dosage if impaired ▪ Administer on arising & hs, c̄ food/milk/antacids to ↓ GI irritation; tablets may be crushed; encourage upright position for 15-30m ▪ Avoid exposure to moisture in storage ▪ Elderly may require ↓ dosage.

EVALUATION: Monitor hematologic, hepatic, renal status c̄ prolonged use ▪ Monitor I&O, daily weight c̄ prolonged use ▪ Assess for edema in extremities ▪ Assess for visual disturbances; D/C drug, notify physician.

EDUCATION: Dizziness/drowsiness may occur; use caution in potentially hazardous activities ▪ Take c̄ food/milk to ↓ GI distress; maintain upright position for 15-30m ▪ Take as ordered by physician; do *not* ↑ dose ▪ Notify physician *immediately* of bleeding, ↓ urine output, swelling of feet/legs, lethargy, GI distress, jaundice, visual disturbance ▪ Avoid taking c̄ aspirin/other NSAIAs ▪ Avoid use c̄ alcohol ▪ Check c̄ physician/pharmacist before taking OTC preparations ▪ Notify physician/dentist of use before treatment ▪ Store in tightly closed container ▪ Full drug effect may require several wks.

NOTES:

temazepam/triazolam • (tem-az-e-pam/trye-ay-zoe-lam)

CATEGORY: *Benzodiazepine:* hypnotic

Rx C-IV; Preg Cat X

BRAND NAMES

BRAND NAMES	DOSAGE FORMS
temazepam	
Restoril (Sandoz)	Capsule: 15, 30mg
triazolam	
Halcion (Upjohn)	Tablet: 0.125, 0.025mg

ACTION: Hypnotic activity improves total sleep time, ↓ number of nocturnal awakenings; REM sleep *not* affected. **USE:** Short-term use as hypnotic.

DOSAGE: *PO*

temazepam	
Adult	15-30mg 30m before hs
triazolam	
Adult	0.25-0.5mg hs
Geriatric	0.125-0.25mg hs

DRUG INTERACTIONS: Use c̄ other CNS depressants produces additive effects ▪ Use c̄ MAO-I can produce serious toxic effects.

PHARMACOKINETICS

	PO absorption	Onset	Peak	Half-life	Protein binding	Excretion
temazepam	Very good	30-40m	2-3h	10h	96%	Via urine as metabolites
triazolam	Readily	—	1.3h	1.6-5.1h	—	Via urine as metabolites & unchanged drug

CONTRAINDICATIONS: Hypersensitivity, narrow-angle glaucoma, pregnancy.

NURSING MANAGEMENT

ADMINISTRATION: Assess for hx of benzodiazepine hypersensitivity ▪ Use c̄ caution in hepatic disease ▪

Avoid exposure to heat, moisture, light in storage ▪ Avoid abrupt withdrawal ▪ Elderly may require ↓ dosage ▪ ↓ Environmental stimuli.

EVALUATION: Monitor renal, hepatic status ▪ Assess for symptoms of abrupt withdrawal (tremors, abdominal/muscle cramps, convulsions) c̄ prolonged use ▪ Check for signs of dependence (↑ drug request) ▪ Monitor activity status (safety precautions) ▪ Assess for tolerance to therapeutic dose ▪ Assess for paradoxic rxs (CNS stimulation), esp elderly ▪ Check for depression; suicide precautions prn ▪ Assess pt sleep patterns.

EDUCATION: Drowsiness may occur; use caution in potentially hazardous activities ▪ Avoid use c̄ alcohol, other CNS depressants ▪ Indiscriminate use may lead to dependence ▪ Do *not* smoke after taking drug ▪ Do *not* keep at bedside ▪ Take as ordered by physician; do *not* ↑ dose ▪ Women: avoid breastfeeding ▪ Check c̄ physician/pharmacist before taking OTC drugs ▪ Practice relaxation exercises, ventilation of feelings ▪ Utilize sleep producers (reading, warm milk, soft music).

NOTES:

terbutaline sulfate • (ter-byoo-ta-leen)

CATEGORY: *Sympathomimetic*: $beta_2$ adrenergic, bronchodilator — Rx; Preg Cat B

BRAND NAMES	DOSAGE FORMS
Brethaire (Geigy)	Aerosol: 0.2mg/dose
Brethine (Geigy)	Injection (SC): 1mg/ml Tablet: 2.5, 5mg
Bricanyl (MMD)	Injection (SC): 1mg/ml Tablet: 2.5, 5mg

ACTION: Sympathomimetic activity at $beta_2$ receptors produces bronchodilation. **USE:** Treatment of bronchial asthma, reversible bronchospasm associated c̄ bronchitis/emphysema.

PHARMACOKINETICS

PO absorption	Onset	Peak	Excretion
35%-50%	30m	1-2h	Via urine primarily as unchanged drug

CONTRAINDICATIONS: Hypersensitivity.

DOSAGE

Adolescent *PO* 12-15y/o		2.5mg q6h tid. Do *not* exceed 7.5mg/d
	Aerosol	2 inhalations q4-6h
Adult *PO*		5mg q6h tid. Do *not* exceed 15mg/d
	SC	0.25mg. Repeat if no improvement w/in 15-30m. Do *not* exceed 0.5mg/4h
	Aerosol	2 inhalations q4-6h

SIDE/ADVERSE EFFECTS: CNS: nervousness, tremor, headache, drowsiness ▪ CV: ↑ heart rate; palpitations ▪ GI: N/V ▪ MS: muscle cramps.

DRUG INTERACTIONS: Use c̄ nonselective beta blockers (eg, propranolol) will antagonize bronchodilation ▪ Use c̄ MAO-I contraindicated ▪ Use c̄ other sympathomimetics best avoided.

NURSING MANAGEMENT

ADMINISTRATION: Assess for hx of catecholamine hypersensitivity ▪ Assess BP, pulse before administration ▪ Administer c̄ food to ↓ GI irritation; may crush tablets ▪ Check dosages c̄ another RN.

EVALUATION: Monitor VS, esp heart rate ▪ Monitor I&O ▪ Diabetics: closely monitor blood glucose (hyperglycemia).

EDUCATION: Take c̄ food to ↓ GI distress; may crush tablets ▪ Take as ordered by physician; do *not* ↑ dose ▪ Procedure for radial pulse determination ▪ Keep scheduled appointments c̄ physician ▪ Check c̄ physician/pharmacist before taking OTC preparations ▪ Procedure for inhalation administration (do *not* puncture/incinerate aerosol container).

NOTES:

terfenadine • (ter-fen-a-deen)

CATEGORY: *Antihistamine:* H_1 blocker — Rx; Preg Cat C

BRAND NAME — *Seldane (MMD)*

DOSAGE FORM — Tablet: 60mg

COMBINATION PRODUCT

Seldane-D (MMD) — terfenadine 60mg/pseudoephrine 10mg/tablet

ACTION: H_1 antihistaminic activity due to competitive inhibition of histamine at H_1 histamine receptors on peripheral cells; drug lacks anticholinergic activity, does not cross blood-brain barrier well. **USE:** Symptomatic treatment of seasonal allergic rhinitis.

PHARMACOKINETICS

PO absorption	Onset	Peak	Duration	Protein binding	Excretion
Almost complete	1-2h	3-4h	12h	97%	60% in feces, 40% in urine

CONTRAINDICATIONS: Hypersensitivity.

DOSAGE

Pediatric (>12y/o)/ Adult *PO*	60mg bid
Seldane-D	1 tablet in AM & PM

SIDE/ADVERSE EFFECTS: CNS: *drowsiness, headache,* fatigue, dizziness, weakness ▪ EENT: cough, sore throat, epistaxis ▪ GI: N/V ▪ INT: pruritus.

DRUG INTERACTIONS: Use c̄ CNS depressants may produce additive effects.

NURSING MANAGEMENT

ADMINISTRATION: Assess for hx of antihistamine hypersensitivity ▪ Administer c̄ food ▪ Avoid exposure to heat, moisture, light in storage ▪ Maintain hydration.

EVALUATION: Monitor VS, esp BP ▪ Assess for tolerance to therapeutic dose ▪ Closely monitor asthmatic pts (anticholinergic effect).

EDUCATION: Drowsiness may occur; use caution in potentially hazardous activities ▪ Take c̄ meals ▪ Use sugarless gum/hard candy to diminish dry mouth ▪ ↑ Fluid intake (8-10 glasses/d) ▪ Notify physician of symptoms of allergic rx (fever, difficult breathing, rash) ▪ Carry identification (MedicAlert) if antihistamine allergic ▪ Notify physician of antihistamine use before allergy testing ▪ Expect symptom relief in 1h ▪ Store in tightly closed, light-resistant container in cool, dry area ▪ Take only as needed; do *not* exceed prescribed dose ▪ Do *not* administer to children under 12y/o.

NOTES:

tetracycline hcl • (te-tra-sye-kleen)

CATEGORY: *Tetracycline*: broad-spectrum antibiotic Rx; Preg Cat NA

BRAND NAMES

Achromycin V (Lederle)
Panmycin (Upjohn)
Robitet (Robins)
Sumycin (Apothecon)
Tetracyn (Pfizer)

DOSAGE FORMS: Capsule, IM injection, IV injection, syrup, tablets

ACTION: Bacteriostatic effect due to inhibition of ribosomal protein synthesis. **USE:** Tetracyclines are the drug(s) of choice for chlamydial, mycoplasmal, rickettsial infections; acne control, balantidiasis, brucellosis, chancroid, cholera, granuloma inguinale, shigellosis, spirochetal relapsing fever ▪ Alternative in penicillin allergy/infections when bacteriologic testing indicates good activity.

CONTRAINDICATIONS: Hypersensitivity, pregnancy, nursing mothers, children <8y/o.

DOSAGE

Pediatric *PO*	20-50mg/kg/d divided
IM	15-25mg/kg/d divided
IV	10-20mg/kg/d divided
Adult *PO*	250-500mg qid
IM	250-300mg qd
IV	250-500mg bid

SIDE/ADVERSE EFFECTS: GI: *gastric upset, diarrhea,* bleeding, enterocolitis ▪ GU: dose-related ↑ BUN ▪ HEM: *hemolytic anemia, thrombocytopenia* ▪ INT: *monilial overgrowth,* maculopapular rashes, exacerbation of systemic LE, photosensitivity ▪ MS: bulging fontanels in neonates (reversible), fetal skeletal retardation.

PHARMACOKINETICS

PO absorption		Peak			
No food	Food	No food	Half-life	Protein binding	Excretion
60%-80%	10%-30%	2-4h	6-12h	20%-65%	60% excreted unchanged in urine

Note: Side/adverse effects: common in *italic;* serious in ***boldface italic.*** *Available in Canada only.

DRUG INTERACTIONS: Do *not* use c̄ antacids, antidiarrheals, bactericidal antibiotics, dairy products, methoxyflurane ▪ PO anticoagulants may require ↓ dose, esp during extended antibiotic therapy.

NURSING MANAGEMENT

ADMINISTRATION: Assess for allergy before administration ▪ Obtain C&S before therapy ▪ Administer PO dose 1h ac/2h pc ▪ Avoid PO administration c̄ milk, dairy products, antacids ▪ Shake PO suspensions well before pouring ▪ IM: inject *deep* into muscle; contains local anesthetic, can lead to CV collapse if injected into vasculature ▪ IV: dilute; administer *slowly* ▪ Discard parenteral preparations after 24h ▪ Avoid exposure to heat, moisture, light in storage ▪ Do *not* administer to pregnant women, neonates, children <8y/o (may cause permanent discoloration of teeth).

EVALUATION: Monitor patients receiving anticoagulant therapy; may potentiate bleeding ▪ Assess renal, hepatic status ▪ Monitor VS, esp temperature ▪ Observe for signs of superinfection (diarrhea, perineal itching, oral ulcers) ▪ Urine glucose: false (+) c̄ Clinitest; false (-) c̄ Clinistix/Tes-Tape.

EDUCATION: Complete full course of therapy (usually 10 ds) even if symptoms subside ▪ Avoid prolonged exposure to direct sunlight, UV light (sunlamps); use sunscreen, protective clothing ▪ Take c̄ full glass H_2O on empty stomach; do *not* take w/in 1h of hs ▪ Diarrhea may occur ▪ Store in dry, opaque container ▪ Avoid products containing Al^{+++}, Mg^{++}, Ca^{++}, Fe^{++}, Zn^{++} ▪ Discard outdated, unused preparations.

NOTES:

theophylline • (thee-off-i-lin)

CATEGORY: *Bronchodilator:* xanthine drug

Rx; Preg Cat C

BRAND NAMES

Accurbron (MMD)
Aerolate (Fleming)
Bronkodyl (Winthrop)
Constant-T (Geigy)
Elixophyllin (Forest) (Pentagone in Canada)
**Pulmophylline (Riva)*
Quibron-T (Bristol)
**Quibron-T/SR (Bristol)*
Respbid (B-I)
Slo-Bid Gyrocaps (RPR)
Slo-Phyllin Gyrocaps (RPR)
Sustaire (Pfizer)
Theo-24 (Searle)
Theobid (Russ)
Theo-Dur (Key) (Astra in Canada)
Theolair (3M Riker)

DOSAGE FORMS: Capsule (regular, extended release), elixir, syrup, tablet (regular, extended release).

ACTION: Bronchodilation due to direct relaxation of respiratory smooth muscle; drug stimulates CNS, produces diuresis, has positive chronotropic/inotropic cardiac effect. **USE:** Treatment of asthma, reversible bronchospasm associated c̄ chronic bronchitis, emphysema.

PHARMACOKINETICS

PO absorption	Peak	Half-life	Protein binding	Excretion
Usually complete	1-2h	7-9h	56%	Via urine as metabolites, unchanged drug

CONTRAINDICATIONS: Hypersensitivity.

DOSAGE: Must be individualized.

Pediatric *PO*	Usual dose 2.5mg/kg q6h
Adult *PO*	Usual dose 160mg q6h

SIDE/ADVERSE EFFECTS: CNS: *headache*, reflex hyperexcitability, ***clonic/tonic generalized convulsions***, insomnia, *nervousness* ▪ CV: hypotension, tachycardia, ***ventricular arrhythmias,*** palpitations ▪ GI: N/V/D, epigastric pain ▪ GU: albuminuria, diuresis ▪ RESP: tachypnea.

DRUG INTERACTIONS: ↑ Serum levels c̄ cimetidine, allopurinol, erythromycin, oral contraceptives, flu vaccine ▪ ↑ Excretion of lithium, ↓ propranolol effects ▪ Use c̄ adrenergic drugs ↑ CNS stimulation.

Note: Side/adverse effects: common in *italic;* serious in ***boldface italic.***

*Available in Canada only.

NURSING MANAGEMENT

ADMINISTRATION: Assess for hx of xanthine hypersensitivity ▪ PO: may administer after meals c̄ full glass H_2O; *best* on empty stomach; do *not* crush enteric-coated SR preparations, administer whole ▪ PO suspension: shake well before pouring ▪ Parenteral: use cardiac monitoring ▪ Do *not* administer discolored/precipitated solutions ▪ Check compatibility chart for IV administration ▪ Maintain hydration (2000ml/d) ▪ Elderly may require ↓ dosage.

EVALUATION: Monitor VS, esp heart rate ▪ Monitor I&O ▪ Monitor respiratory status (breath sounds, sputum) ▪ Parenteral: monitor ABGs, electrolytes ▪ Therapeutic blood levels: 10-20μg/ml.

EDUCATION: Dizziness may occur; use caution in potentially hazardous activities ▪ Take c̄ meals/full glass H_2O to ↓ GI irritation ▪ Swallow enteric-coated/SR preparations whole; do *not* break, crush, chew ▪ Take as ordered by physician; do *not* ↑ dose ▪ Notify physician of irritability, GI distress, palpitations; D/C drug ▪ ↑ Fluid intake (8-10 glasses/d) ▪ Avoid smoking, caffeine-containing substances ▪ Women: avoid breastfeeding ▪ Do *not* substitute brand-name preparations ▪ Check c̄ physician/pharmacist before taking OTC preparations.

OVERDOSE MANAGEMENT: Symptoms incl anorexia, nausea, restlessness, hyperthermia, convulsions, cardiac arrhythmias ▪ Emergency treatment: maintain respiration c̄ oxygen; give 5% dextrose for dehydration; control convulsions c̄ IV diazepam/short-acting barbiturates.

NOTES:

thiopental sodium • (thye-oh-pen-tal)

CATEGORY: *Barbiturate:* anesthetic

Rx C-III; Preg Cat C

BRAND NAME
Pentothal (Abbott)

DOSAGE FORMS
Injection (IV)
Rectal suspension

ACTION: Hypnotic activity due to depression of midbrain reticular formation. **USE:** Anesthetic agent for short surgical procedures ▪ Anesthesia induction, supplement for regional anesthesia ▪ Narcoanalysis, narcosynthesis, treatment of acute convulsive conditions ▪ Neurosurgical pts c̄ ↑ ICP c̄ adequate ventilation.

PHARMACOKINETICS: Produces hypnosis in 30-40s IV; half-life 3-8h; protein binding 80%.

CONTRAINDICATIONS: Hypersensitivity, status asthmaticus, porphyria; relative contraindications incl severe CV disease, hypotension, shock, conditions in which hypnotic effect may be prolonged/potentiated.

DOSAGE: Dose required must be titrated according to surgical requirement, pt age, sex, weight

Anesthesia	50-75mg at 20-40s intervals. After anesthesia obtained, additional dose 25-50mg can be given whenever pt moves
Convulsions	75-125mg. Convulsions due to local anesthetics may require 125-250mg
Neurosurgical	1.5-2.5mg/kg
Psychiatric	100mg/m. D/C when pt becomes confused (usually indicated by failure to correctly count backward), before sleep produced

SIDE/ADVERSE EFFECTS: CV: myocardial depression ▪ RESP: respiratory depression, bronchospasm ▪ Other: laryngospasm.

DRUG INTERACTIONS: Use c̄ CNS depressants may ↑ effect of ultra-short-acting barbiturates.

NURSING MANAGEMENT

ADMINISTRATION: Assess for hx of barbiturate hypersensitivity ▪ Do *not* mix any drugs into infusion solutions ▪ Follow manufacturer's directions for specific mg/ml dilutions ▪ Discard unused dilutions after 24h ▪ Do *not* administer discolored/precipitated solution ▪ Have emergency support equipment available ▪ IV: inject test dose (25-75mg), observe pt for 1m; inject *slowly* ▪ Rectal: administer cleansing enema only in cases of fecal impaction.

EVALUATION: Monitor hepatic, renal, cardiac, respiratory status ▪ Assess for paradoxic rxs (CNS stimulation), esp in elderly ▪ Monitor VS, esp BP, q5m.

EDUCATION: Safety precautions may be instituted (bedrails, restraints).

OVERDOSE MANAGEMENT: Principal symptom: exaggerated CNS depression ▪ Respiration depressed, pupils may be constricted, shock, coma ▪ Emergency medical treatment: administer IV fluids, vasopressor to maintain BP; force renal excretion $\bar{c}$ osmotic diuretics.

NOTES:

thyroid • (thye-roid)

CATEGORY: *Thyroid hormone:* desiccated thyroid Rx; Preg Cat A

BRAND NAME
Thyroid (various)

DOSAGE FORMS
Capsule (in oil): 65, 130, 195, 325mg
Tablet: 16, 32, 65, 98, 130, 195, 260, 325mg

ACTION: Thyroid hormones regulate general body metabolism by controlling cellular oxidative process; influence growth, tissue differentiation, maturation. **USE:** Treatment of hypothyroidism.

PHARMACOKINETICS: Natural thyroid preparations exhibit adequate (but variable) PO absorption, full therapeutic effect usually requires 1-3 wks, excretion via feces and urine.

CONTRAINDICATIONS: Thyrotoxicosis, uncorrected adrenocortical deficiency, acute MI.

DOSAGE FORMS: Must be individualized.

Pediatric/Adult *PO*	Usual maintenance dose 65-195mg/d

SIDE/ADVERSE EFFECTS: Usually limited to overdose ▪ CNS: headache, insomnia, nervousness, tremors ▪ CV: angina, ***cardiac arrhythmias,*** palpitations, tachycardia ▪ GI: diarrhea ▪ Other: intolerance to heat; sweating, weight loss.

DRUG INTERACTIONS: Use c̄ epinephrine in pts c̄ coronary disease may induce coronary insufficiency ▪ Use c̄ PO anticoagulants ↑ their activity, requires ↓ anticoagulant doses ▪ Use c̄ cholestyramine ↓ PO absorption of thyroid preparations ▪ Use in diabetic pts may require ↑ dosage of hypoglycemic agents.

NURSING MANAGEMENT

ADMINISTRATION: Assess for hx of hypersensitivity ▪ Administer daily dose before breakfast ▪ Avoid exposure to moisture in storage ▪ Elderly may require ↓ dosage.

EVALUATION: Monitor VS, esp heart rate ▪ Observe for signs of overdose (chest pain, fever, nervousness, rapid/irregular heartbeat) ▪ Monitor thyroid function tests (T_3, T_4, TSH); evaluate pt use of iodine-containing substances before exam ▪ Diabetics: closely monitor blood glucose (hyperglycemia) ▪ May potentiate anticoagulant effect; assess for bleeding/bruising.

EDUCATION: Take as ordered by physician; do *not* change dose ▪ Avoid high-iodine foods (soybeans, cabbage, shellfish) ▪ Procedure for checking radial pulse ▪ Take pulse on arising each day; notify physician if ↑ or irregular, D/C drug ▪ Keep scheduled appointments $\bar{c}$ physician/for lab work ▪ Do *not* change brand name preparations ▪ Notify physician *immediately* of difficult breathing, chest pain, rapid/irregular heartbeat; D/C drug ▪ Check $\bar{c}$ physician/pharmacist before taking OTC preparations ▪ Notify physician/dentist of use before therapy.

NOTES:

ticarcillin disodium • (tye-kar-sill-in)

CATEGORY: *Extended-spectrum penicillin*

Rx; Preg Cat NA

BRAND NAME
Ticar (SKB)

DOSAGE FORMS
Powder for injection (IM/IV): 1, 3, 6g vial; 3g IVPB; 20, 30g bulk

COMBINATION PRODUCTS

Timentin (Beecham)	ticarcillin disodium/clavulanic acid per vial: 3g/100mg, 3g/200mg

ACTION: Bactericidal activity due to inhibition of mucopeptide cell wall synthesis in susceptible organisms; addition of clavulanic acid helps protect ticarcillin from actin of penicillinase, if present. **USE:** Treatment of infections due to susceptible strains of *Enterobacter* spp, *Escherichia coli, Morganella morganii, Proteus* spp, *Pseudomonas aeruginosa* ▪ In combination c̄ aminoglycoside (eg, gentamicin sulfate) in treatment of selected strains of *P. aeruginosa.*

PHARMACOKINETICS

IM absorption	Peak	Protein binding	Excretion
Rapid	30-75m	45%-65%	80%-93% via tubular secretion, glomerular filtration w/in 24h

CONTRAINDICATIONS: Hypersensitivity to any penicillin.

DOSAGE

Neonatal *IM/IV*	<2000g: 75mg/kg/12h for first 7d. After 7d of age, 75mg/kg/8h >2000g: 75mg/kg/8h for first 7d. After 7d of age, 100mg/kg/8h
Pediatric *IM/IV*	>40kg: same as adult
Adult *IM/IV*	150-300mg/kg/d divided, q3h, 4h, or 6h

SIDE/ADVERSE EFFECTS: CNS: possible ***convulsions,*** neuromuscular irritability c̄ extremely high doses ▪ GI:

Note: Side/adverse effects: common in *italic;* serious in ***boldface italic.***

*Available in Canada only.

N/V/D ▪ HEM: anemia, eosinophilia, leukopenia, neutropenia, ***thrombocytopenia*** ▪ HEP: ↑ Serum AST, ALT ▪ INT: rash, pruritus, urticaria ▪ Other: local discomfort at site of injection; induration usually not present; fever, ***anaphylaxis.***

DRUG INTERACTIONS: Bacteriostatic antibiotics c̄ any penicillin can lead to antibiotic antagonism ▪ PO anticoagulant therapy may require dose adjustment.

NURSING MANAGEMENT

ADMINISTRATION: Assess for hx of penicillin hypersensitivity ▪ Obtain C&S before therapy ▪ IM: reconstitute 1g/2ml sterile H_2O for injection (1g dose equals 2.5ml solution); inject in UOQ of buttock or midlateral thigh (children); do *not* exceed 2g/injection site ▪ IV: reconstitute 1g/4ml sterile H_2O for injection; administer *slowly*; may be added to 5% dextrose, 10% invert sugar, normal saline, Ringer/lactated Ringer injection; rotate sites q48h ▪ IVPB: use at least 1g/10ml diluent ▪ Have support equipment available for anaphylaxis ▪ Reconstituted solutions are stable for 24h at room temperature, 72h refrigerated.

EVALUATION: Monitor hepatic, neuromuscular, renal status ▪ Monitor VS, esp temperature ▪ Monitor bleeding time, serum K^+, Na^+ ▪ Monitor I&O ▪ Monitor CBC ▪ Observe for signs of superinfection (diarrhea, perineal itching, oral ulcers) ▪ Assess for hypersensitivity rx (fever, difficult breathing, rash) ▪ Check IV insertion site carefully (phlebitis).

EDUCATION: Diarrhea may occur ▪ Maintain good personal hygiene (esp perineal, oral) ▪ Maintain fluid intake (6-8 glasses/d) ▪ Notify physician of symptoms of allergic rx (fever, difficult breathing, rash) ▪ Carry identification (MedicAlert) if penicillin allergic.

NOTES:

timolol maleate • (tim-oh-lole)

CATEGORY: *Beta-adrenergic blocker*

Rx; Preg Cat C

BRAND NAMES

Blocadren (MSD)
Timoptic (MSD)

DOSAGE FORMS

Tablet: 5, 10, 20mg
Ophthalmic solution: 0.25%, 0.5%
Occudose (unit dose container): 0.25%, 0.5%

COMBINATION PRODUCTS

Timolide (MSD) 10-25	timolol maleate/hydrochlorothiazide per tablet: 10mg/25mg

ACTION: Blocks access of catecholamines to β_1, β_2 receptors, resulting in bronchial constriction, ↓ heart rate, myocardial contractility; antihypertensive effect not determined; drug applied topically to treat glaucoma. **USE:** Treatment of hypertension as sole agent/in combination c̄ other antihypertensive drugs, esp thiazide diuretic ▪ To ↓ mortality in stable pts after MI ▪ Treatment of chronic open-angle glaucoma, aphakic glaucoma, secondary glaucoma ▪ Migraine prophylaxis.

PHARMACOKINETICS

PO absorption	Peak	Half-life	Protein binding	Excretion
90%	1-2h	4h	10%	Via urine, feces

CONTRAINDICATIONS: Hypersensitivity, bronchial asthma, cardiogenic shock, sinus bradycardia, heart block >1°, cardiac failure.

DOSAGE

Adult *PO*

Hypertension	Initial dose 10mg bid. Usual range 20-40mg divided, to maximum 60mg/d
MI prevention	10mg bid
Glaucoma	Initial dose 1gtt 0.25% or 0.5% solution bid
Migraine	10-30mg/d
Timolide	Initial dose 1 tablet/d, then adjust

SIDE/ADVERSE EFFECTS: CNS: *dizziness,* mental depression, fatigue, hallucinations ▪ CV: *bradycardia,* CHF, hypotension, peripheral vascular insufficiency, ***exacerbation of AV block*** ▪ EENT: dry mouth/eyes, visual disturbances ▪ GI: *N/V/D*, cramps, constipation, ischemic colitis ▪ GU: impotence ▪ HEM: ***agranulocytosis, thrombocytopenia,*** purpura ▪ INT: alopecia ▪ RESP: bronchospasm.

DRUG INTERACTIONS: Use c̄ reserpine, other catecholamine-depleting drugs can result in serious adrenergic blockage ▪ Nonselective beta-adrenergics antagonize therapeutic effects ▪ Usually contraindicated c̄ furazolidone, general anesthetics, MAO-I.

NURSING MANAGEMENT

ADMINISTRATION: Assess for hx of hypersensitivity; apical pulse (if <60/m, hold drug, notify physician); respiratory function (do *not* administer if impaired) ▪ PO: may crush, administer c̄ liquid ▪ Ophthalmic: place pressure on lacrimal sacs for 1m ▪ Avoid abrupt withdrawal ▪ Elderly may require ↓ dosage.

EVALUATION: Monitor VS, esp BP, heart rate; I&O; IOP ▪ Diabetics: closely monitor blood glucose ▪ Assess for edema in extremities; peripheral circulation ▪ Monitor hepatic, CV, renal, hemopoietic status c̄ long-term use.

EDUCATION: Dizziness may occur; use caution in potentially hazardous activities ▪ Avoid changing positions rapidly ▪ Take as ordered by physician; do *not* change dose ▪ Procedure for checking radial pulse ▪ Check pulse before taking; if <60/m, do *not* take drug; notify physician ▪ Do *not* abstain from food for >12h (low blood sugar) ▪ Used to control, *not* cure, hypertension ▪ Avoid ↑ exercise, temperature extremes, smoking, alcohol ▪ Maintain optimum weight ▪ Avoid high-Na^+ foods ▪ Check c̄ physician/pharmacist before taking OTC preparations ▪ Notify physician/dentist of use before treatment ▪ Do *not* D/C drug w/out checking c̄ physician ▪ Carry identification (MedicAlert) if taking timolol ▪ Diabetics: carefully monitor blood/urine glucose; observe for symptoms of hypoglycemia ▪ Keep scheduled appointments for eye exams ▪ Procedure for ophthalmic administration.

NOTES:

tobramycin sulfate • (toe-bra-mye-sin)

CATEGORY: *Aminoglycoside:* antibiotic

Rx; Preg Cat D

BRAND NAME
Nebcin (Lilly)

DOSAGE FORMS
Injection (IM/IV): 60mg/1.5ml, 60mg/6ml, 80mg/2ml, 80mg/8ml, 1.2g/30ml; Pediatric: 20mg/2ml

ACTION: Bactericidal activity due to inhibition of ribosomal protein synthesis in susceptible organisms. **USE:** Indicated for infections caused by susceptible strains of *Citrobacter* spp, *Enterobacter* spp, *Escherichia coli, Klebsiella-Enterobacter* grp, *Proteus* spp (indole +/-), *Providencia* spp, *Pseudomonas aeruginosa, Serratia* spp ▪ Alternate for penicillin-resistant staphylococcal infections.

PHARMACOKINETICS

IM peak	Half-life	Excretion
0.5-1.5h	2h	85% unchanged in urine in 8h

CONTRAINDICATIONS: Hypersensitivity, previous hx of serious aminoglycoside toxicity.

DOSAGE: For pts c̄ normal renal function. Treatment usually 7-10d.

Pediatric *IM/IV*	<1wk old: Up to 4mg/kg/d in 2 equal doses, q12h Children: 6-7.5mg/kg/d in 3-4 equal doses. More serious infections may require 5mg/kg/d in 3-4 equal doses
Adult *IM/IV*	3mg/kg/d in 3 equal doses, q8h. ↓ Dosage as soon as clinically indicated

SIDE/ADVERSE EFFECTS: CNS: headache, paresthesia ▪ EENT: ***ototoxicity*** (auditory, vestibular damage), dizziness, vertigo, tinnitus, roaring in ears, hearing loss ▪ GU: ***nephrotoxicity:*** casts, proteinuria, ↑ BUN, NPN, serum creatinine ▪ INT: rash ▪ Other: fever.

DRUG INTERACTIONS: Avoid use c̄ neurotoxic/nephrotoxic drugs such as other aminoglycosides, colistin, ethacrynic acid, furosemide, polymyxin B, vancomycin, viomycin ▪ Dimenhydrinate can mask aminoglycoside ototoxicity ▪ Use c̄ succinylcholine/tubocurarine ↑

their activity; Ca salts can reverse blockade ▪ PO anticoagulant activity may ↑ due to ↓ intestinal vitamin K synthesis.

NURSING MANAGEMENT

ADMINISTRATION: Assess for hx of aminoglycoside hypersensitivity ▪ Obtain C&S before therapy ▪ Obtain pt weight for dosage calculation ▪ Determine creatinine clearance before administration ▪ IV: single dose may be diluted in 50-100ml sterile normal saline, 5% dextrose; infuse over 20-60m; use less diluent for pediatric IV; may mix c̄ dextrose, Ringer/lactated Ringer injection, normal saline solution ▪ Do *not* mix c̄ other drugs, incl penicillin ▪ Store in original container; avoid exposure to heat ▪ IM: administer by *deep, slow* injection; rotate sites; avoid inflamed areas ▪ Maintain hydration ▪ Elderly may require ↓ dosage.

EVALUATION: Assess for hearing dysfunction ▪ Monitor hepatic, renal, VIII CN function ▪ Monitor VS, esp temperature ▪ Assess for edema in extremities ▪ Assess for neuromuscular blockade, respiratory paralysis, nephrotoxicity ▪ Observe for signs of superinfection (diarrhea, URI, coated tongue) ▪ Assess for hypersensitivity rx (fever, difficult breathing, rash) ▪ Assess peak (<12µg/ml), trough (<2µg/ml) serum concentrations.

EDUCATION: Report hearing, balance difficulties to physician at once ▪ ↑ Fluid intake (10-12 glasses/d).

NOTES:

tocainide hcl • (toe-kay-nide)

CATEGORY: *Antiarrhythmic*

Rx; Preg Cat C

BRAND NAME
Tonocard (MSD)
(Astra in Canada)

DOSAGE FORMS
Tablet: 400, 600mg

ACTION: Antiarrhythmic effect due to depression of ventricular automaticity, depolarization during diastole; drug has no appreciable effect on atrial arrrhythmias, produces effects similar to lidocaine (group IB antiarrhythmic). **USE:** Treatment of life-threatening ventricular arrhythmias incl PVCs, uni-multifocal couplets, ventricular tachycardia.

PHARMACOKINETICS

PO absorption	Peak	Half-life	Protein binding	Excretion
Almost complete	0.5-2h	15h	10%-20%	80% via urine in 72h primarily as metabolites

CONTRAINDICATIONS: Hypersensitivity to drug/local anesthetics of amide type, 2°/3° AV block w/out pacemaker.

DOSAGE

Adult *PO* — Initial dose 400mg q8h, c̄ daily range 1200-1800mg in 3 doses; dosage can be as high as ≥2400mg/d

SIDE/ADVERSE EFFECTS: CNS: *dizziness*, paresthesia, tremor, confusion, restlessness ▪ CV: hypotension, bradycardia, palpitations, chest pain, ***left ventricular failure*** ▪ EENT: blurred vision, nystagmus, tinnitus, hearing loss ▪ GI: *N/V/D*, anorexia ▪ HEM: ***agranulocytosis,*** leukopenia, ***thrombocytopenia,*** hypoplastic anemia ▪ INT: lupus, rash ▪ MS: arthralgia ▪ RESP: ***pulmonary fibrosis, interstitial pneumonitis***, edema ▪ Other: night sweats, ***LE syndrome.***

DRUG INTERACTIONS: Use c̄ metoprolol may produce additive effects.

NURSING MANAGEMENT

ADMINISTRATION: Assess for hx of hypersensitivity (incl amide-type local anesthetics) ▪ Assess hepatic, renal function; may require ↓ dosage if impaired ▪ Administer c̄ food ▪ Assess serum K^+ levels (normal range: 3.5-

5mEq/L); correct imbalances before administration ▪ Maintain blood levels; administer at equal intervals around clock ▪ If switching from lidocaine, administer tocainide 6h *before* stopping lidocaine ▪ Elderly may require ↓ dosage.

EVALUATION: Monitor VS, esp heart rate, BP ▪ Assess for CHF (dyspnea, peripheral edema, ↑ weight); notify physician ▪ Monitor serum for ↑ alkaline phosphatase c̄ prolonged use ▪ Monitor ECG, CBC, blood levels throughout therapy ▪ Assess for tremors (signifies maximum dose) ▪ Therapeutic blood levels: 3.5-10μg/ml.

EDUCATION: Dizziness may occur; use caution in potentially hazardous activities ▪ Avoid changing positions (lying/sitting/standing) rapidly ▪ Take as ordered by physician; do *not* skip doses ▪ Take at equal intervals around clock, c̄ food to ↓ GI irritation ▪ Procedure for checking radial pulse ▪ Notify physician *immediately* of irregular pulse, lethargy, fever, sore throat, bruising/bleeding ▪ Keep scheduled appointments c̄ physician ▪ Notify physician/dentist of use before treatment ▪ Full drug effect may require several ds.

NOTES:

tolazamide/tolbutamide/tolbutamide sodium ▲ • (tole-byoo-ta-mide)

CATEGORY: *Oral hypoglycemic*: antidiabetic, sulfonylurea | Rx; Preg Cat C

BRAND NAME	DOSAGE FORMS
tolazamide	
Tolinase (Upjohn)	Tablet: 100, 250, 500mg
tolbutamide	
**Mobanol (Horner)*	Tablet: 500mg
**Novobutamide (Novopharm)*	
Orinase (Upjohn)	Powder for diagnostic injection (IV)▲: 1g vial c̄ diluent Tablet: 250, 500mg

ACTION: Antidiabetic activity due to stimulation of insulin release from functioning beta cells of pancreas.

USE: Management of type II (non-insulin-dependent) diabetes that cannot be controlled by diet alone.

CONTRAINDICATIONS: Hypersensitivity, diabetic ketoacidosis c̄, w/out coma.

DOSAGE

Adult *PO*	Must be individualized
tolazamide	Usual maintenance dose 100mg-1g/d
tolbutamide	Usual maintenance dose 0.2-2g/d
IV	Usual IV diagnostic test dose 1g as single dose

SIDE/ADVERSE EFFECTS: GI: *nausea, epigastric fullness,* heartburn ▪ HEM: ***aplastic anemia, agranulocytosis,*** leukopenia, ***hemolytic anemia,*** pancytopenia, ***thrombocytopenia*** ▪ INT: erythema, morbilliform/maculopapular eruptions, photosensitivity ▪ MET: hypoglycemia.

PHARMACOKINETICS

PO absorption	Onset	Peak	Duration	Half-life	Excretion
tolbutamide-rapid	1h	3-5h	6-12h	4-7h	75% via urine
tolazamide-rapid	2-4h	2-6h	10h	7h	85% via urine

Note: Side/adverse effects: common in *italic;* serious in ***boldface italic.***

*Available in Canada only.

DRUG INTERACTIONS: Use c̄ alcohol, MAO-I, phenylbutazones, beta blockers can significantly ↑ hypoglycemic effects ▪ Use c̄ anabolic steroids, chloramphenicol, guanethidine, PO anticoagulants, probenecid, salicylates, sulfinpyrazone, sulfonamides ↑ hypoglycemic effects ▪ Use c̄ adrenergics, corticosteroids, phenytoin, thiazides, thyroid preparations ↓ hypoglycemic effects ▪ Use c̄ NSAIA(s) can ↑ hypoglycemic effects.

NURSING MANAGEMENT

ADMINISTRATION: Assess for hx of hypersensitivity ▪ Administer as single AM dose/d c̄ breakfast/divided doses c̄ meals ▪ Avoid exposure to moisture in storage ▪ Elderly may require ↓ dosage.

EVALUATION: Monitor hepatic, renal, hematologic status ▪ Monitor FBS ▪ Evaluate pt closely during first wk to assess effectiveness ▪ Monitor for signs of hypo/hyperglycemia.

EDUCATION: Compliance c̄ special diet therapy ▪ Blood/urine glucose/ketone testing procedure ▪ Symptoms of hypoglycemia (anxiety, headache, fatigue, nausea, sweating); notify physician immediately ▪ Always carry lump of sugar/candy for quick use in hypoglycemia ▪ Avoid alcohol ▪ Check c̄ physician before taking OTC preparations ▪ Symptoms of hyperglycemia (excessive hunger, thirst, urination; rapid pulse, sweet-smelling breath, weight loss); notify physician immediately ▪ Need for good personal hygiene ▪ Carry identification (MedicAlert) ▪ Store in tightly closed container ▪ Keep scheduled appointments c̄ physician/for blood glucose determinations ▪ Schedule periodic eye exams ▪ Maintain optimum body weight ▪ Avoid prolonged exposure to direct sunlight; use sunscreen, protective clothing ▪ Women: avoid breastfeeding ▪ PO hypoglycemic needs may change c̄ ↑ stress, ↑ exercise, ↓ appetite; notify physician.

NOTES:

tolazoline hcl • (tole-az-oh-leen)

CATEGORY: *Alpha-adrenergic blocker:* peripheral vasodilator, sympatholytic

BRAND NAME	DOSAGE FORM
Priscoline (Ciba)	Injection (IV): 25mg/ml

ACTION: Antihypertensive effect due to direct peripheral activity & moderate competitive blocking of alpha adrenoreceptors ↓ pulmonary arterial BP, vascular resistance. **USE:** Treatment of persistent neonatal pulmonary hypertension when systemic arterial oxygenation cannot be maintained by usual supportive care.

PHARMACOKINETICS

Half-life	Excretion
3-10h	Rapidly in urine as unchanged drug

CONTRAINDICATIONS: Hypersensitivity.

DOSAGE FORMS

Neonatal *IV*	1-2mg/kg via scalp vein, followed by infusion 1-2mg/kg/h

SIDE/ADVERSE EFFECTS: CV: hypertension, hypotension, tachycardia, ***cardiac arrhythmias, pulmonary hemorrhage,*** edema ▪ GI: hemorrhage, N/V/D ▪ GU: oliguria, hematuria ▪ HEM: ***thrombocytopenia,*** leukopenia.

DRUG INTERACTIONS: Use c̄ alcohol can cause toxic disulfiram reaction, an interaction not possible c̄ neonate ▪ Use c̄ norepinephrine/epinephrine may cause severe hypotension followed by sudden rebound in BP.

NURSING MANAGEMENT

ADMINISTRATION: Assess for hx of hypersensitivity ▪ Assess BP; do *not* administer if systolic BP <40mmHg ▪ Have support equipment available.

EVALUATION: Monitor BP; observe for hypotension ▪ Assess peripheral circulation (skin color, temperature, pulses) ▪ Monitor for ↑ gastric juice acidity, pepsin; ↓ RBC, WBC, platelet count ▪ Monitor fluid/electrolyte, acid/base status ▪ Monitor VS, ABGs.

Note: Side/adverse effects: common in *italic;* serious in ***boldface italic.***

*Available in Canada only.

EDUCATION: Avoid changing positions (horizontal/vertical) rapidly ▪ Avoid use of alcohol-containing substances ▪ Keep pt warm; avoid extremely hot objects ▪ Avoid positions that may impair peripheral circulation.

NOTES:

tolmetin sodium • (<u>tole</u>-met-in)

CATEGORY: *Antiinflammatory*

Rx; Preg Cat C

BRAND NAMES
Tolectin (McNeil)
Tolectin DS (McNeil)

DOSAGE FORMS
Tablet: 200, 600mg
Double-strength (DS) capsule: 400mg

ACTION: Antiinflammatory activity appears related to inhibition of prostaglandin synthesis. **USE:** Treatment of rheumatoid/osteo-/juvenile arthritis.

PHARMACOKINETICS

PO absorption	Peak	Half-life	Protein binding	Excretion
Complete	30-60m	1h	99%	Via urine in 24h primarily as metabolites

CONTRAINDICATIONS: Hypersensitivity, aspirin/other nonsteroidal antiinflammatory agent hypersensitivity.

DOSAGE FORMS

Pediatric *PO*	20mg/kg/d divided. Usual range 15-30mg/kg/d. Do *not* exceed 30mg/kg/d
Adult *PO*	400mg tid, then adjust. Usual range 600-1800mg/d in 3-4 equal doses, c̄ maximum 2g/d

SIDE/ADVERSE EFFECTS: CNS: *headache, dizziness,* drowsiness ▪ CV: edema, CHF, ↑ BP ▪ EENT: tinnitus, blurred vision, retinal/macular changes ▪ GI: *abdominal pain, nausea,* constipation, flatulence, vomiting, stomatitis ▪ GU: hematuria, proteinuria, dysuria ▪ HEM: ***agranulocytosis*** (rare), ***hemolytic anemia,*** granulocytopenia ▪ INT: purpura, urticaria, skin irritation, ***erythema multiforme*** ▪ Other: weight gain; loss, fever, ***anaphylactoid rxs.***

DRUG INTERACTIONS: Use c̄ ulcerogenic drugs produces additive effects ▪ Use c̄ PO anticoagulants may ↑ their activity ▪ Aspirin ↓ tolmetin plasma levels.

Note: Side/adverse effects: common in *italic;* serious in ***boldface italic.***

*Available in Canada only.

NURSING MANAGEMENT

ADMINISTRATION: Assess for hx of NSAIA hypersensitivity ▪ Avoid administration in pts c̄ hx of asthma, bleeding disorders, salicylate hypersensitivity ▪ Assess for hx of peptic ulcer; use c̄ caution ▪ Assess renal function; may require ↓ dosage if impaired ▪ Administer on arising & hs, c̄ food/milk/antacids to ↓ GI irritation; tablets may be crushed/capsules opened; encourage upright position for 15-30m ▪ Avoid exposure to moisture in storage ▪ Elderly may require ↓ dosage.

EVALUATION: Monitor renal status c̄ prolonged use ▪ Monitor I&O, daily weight c̄ prolonged use ▪ Assess for edema in extremities ▪ Assess for visual/hearing disturbances; D/C drug, notify physician.

EDUCATION: Dizziness/drowsiness may occur; use caution in potentially hazardous activities ▪ Take c̄ food/milk/antacid to ↓ GI distress; maintain upright position for 15-30m ▪ Take as ordered by physician; do *not* ↑ dose ▪ Notify physician *immediately* of bleeding, ↓ urine output, swelling of feet/legs, lethargy, GI distress, jaundice, visual disturbances ▪ Avoid taking c̄ aspirin/other NSAIAs ▪ Avoid use c̄ alcohol ▪ Check c̄ physician/pharmacist before taking OTC preparations ▪ Notify physician/dentist of use before treatment ▪ Store in tightly closed container ▪ Avoid exposure to direct sunlight, UV light (sunlamps); use sunscreen, protective clothing ▪ Full drug effects may require several wks.

NOTES:

trazodone hcl • (tray-zoe-doan)

CATEGORY: *Antidepressant* Rx; Preg Cat C

BRAND NAME
Desyrel (MJP)

DOSAGE FORMS
Tablet: 50, 100, 150mg

ACTION: Antidepressant activity appears related to inhibition of serotonin reuptake in CNS. **USE:** Treatment of depression that closely resembles DSM-III category of major depressive disorder.

PHARMACOKINETICS

PO absorption	Peak	Half-life	Excretion
Good	1-2h	3-9h	Via urine & feces as metabolites

CONTRAINDICATIONS: Hypersensitivity.

DOSAGE
Adult *PO* Initial dose of 150mg/d in divided doses, ↑ by 50mg/d q3-4ds. Do *not* exceed 400mg/d for outpts and 600mg/d for inpts.

SIDE/ADVERSE EFFECTS: CNS: drowsiness, dizziness, nervousness, headache, insomnia, incoordination, confusion, anger, hostility, impaired memory ▪ CV: hypotension, hypertension, palpitations, edema ▪ EENT: blurred vision. tinnitus, nasal congestion, red eyes ▪ GI: dry mouth, constipation, N/V, diarrhea, pain, decreased appetite ▪ Other: muscle pain, malaise, sweating.

DRUG INTERACTIONS: Use $\bar{c}$ CNS depressants produce additive drowsiness ▪ Use $\bar{c}$ digoxin, phenytoin ↑ their effects.

NURSING MANAGEMENT
ADMINISTRATION: Assess for hx of hypersensitivity ▪ Assess for hx of seizures; use caution ▪ Assess hepatic, renal status; ↓ dosage if impaired ▪ Administer pc ▪ Institute safety, seizure precautions ▪ Institute suicide precautions ▪ Avoid abrupt withdrawal; D/C gradually ▪ Avoid moisture, heat, direct light in storage ▪ Elderly may require ↓ dosage.

EVALUATION: Monitor BP (hypertension $\bar{c}$ antihypertensive therapy) ▪ Monitor CV, hepatic, renal status ▪ Monitor fluid retention (I&O, daily weight), constipation ▪ Assess for weight loss (anorectic effect) ▪ Assess for symptoms of abrupt withdrawal (nausea, headache, malaise) ▪ Assess for actual swallowing of PO forms ▪ Assess for skin rash, hives; notify physician, D/C drug.

EDUCATION: Dizziness/drowsiness may occur; use caution in potentially hazardous activities ▪ Avoid changing positions (lying/sitting/standing) rapidly ▪ Avoid use $\bar{c}$ alcohol, other CNS depressants for up to 1wk after end of therapy ▪ Take shortly after meals ▪ Take as directed by physician ▪ Use sugarless gum/hard candy to diminish dry mouth ▪ Constipation may occur; ↑ fluids, bulk-containing foods ▪ Notify physician of skin rash, hives; D/C drug ▪ Check $\bar{c}$ physician/pharmacist before taking OTC/Rx preparations ▪ Notify physician/dentist of use before treatment ▪ Store in tightly closed, light-resistant container ▪ Encourage recreational/diversional interests ▪ Notify physician of weight loss, fever, sore throat, malaise ▪ Keep scheduled appointments $\bar{c}$ physician ▪ Women: notify physician of pregnancy possibility; avoid breastfeeding ▪ Full drug effects may require several wks of therapy.

NOTES:

triamcinolone/triamcinolone acetonide ▲/ triamcinolone diacetate△ • (trye-am-sin-oh-lone)

CATEGORY: *Glucosteroid:* corticosteroid

Rx; Preg Cat NA

BRAND NAMES
Aristocort (Fujisawa)
Kenacort (Apothecon)
Kenalog (Squibb) ▲

AVAILABLE PREPARATIONS
Injection suspension,△ syrup,△ tablets, various topical preparations

DOSAGE

Adult *PO*	6-60mg/d
Diacetate injection	40mg IM wk; 5-40mg intraarticular/intrasynovial. Intralesional/sublesional 5-48mg, c̄ maximum 12.5mg/injection site
Acetonide injection	40-80mg IM; 2.5-60mg intraarticular/intrabursal

ACTION: Glucosteroids cause wide variety of pharmacologic activity; two major effects are potent antiinflammatory effect, inhibition of immune response. **USE:** Treatment of adrenocortical deficiency, adrenogenital syndrome, other endocrine disorders; allergic states, collagen diseases, dermatologic diseases, GI diseases, hematologic disorders, ophthalmologic diseases, respiratory diseases, rheumatic disorders ▪ Treatment of tuberculous meningitis; neurologic/myocardial involvement associated c̄ trichinosis ▪ Remission of proteinuria in nephrotic syndrome, acute exacerbation of multiple sclerosis ▪ Palliative management of leukemias/lymphomas.

PHARMACOKINETICS: PO administration usually produces peak effect in 1-2h, c̄ duration about 2.25d.

CONTRAINDICATIONS: Systemic fungal infections.

SIDE/ADVERSE EFFECTS: CNS: ***convulsions,*** headache, psychic impairment, vertigo, mood swings; pseudotumor cerebri may develop after treatment ▪ CV: edema due to Na^+ retention, CHF, hypertension ▪ EENT: ↑ IOP, glaucoma, posterior subcapsular cataracts, exophthalmos ▪ END: cushingoid states, growth suppression in children, menstrual irregularities, 2° adrenocortical/pituitary unresponsiveness, hyperglycemia, carbohydrate intolerance ▪ GI: peptic ulcer/***possible perforation, pancreatitis,*** abdominal distention, ulcerative esophagitis ▪ INT: poor wound healing, fragile skin, petechiae/ecchymoses, facial erythema, ↑ sweating, urticaria, hirsutism ▪ MET:

negative nitrogen balance, hypokalemic alkalosis ▪ MS: muscle weakness/loss of mass, fracture of long bones, osteoporosis.

DRUG INTERACTIONS: Severe hypokalemia can occur c̄ diuretics (non-potassium sparing) ▪ Use c̄ ulcerogenic drugs (eg, aspirin, indomethacin) can produce additive effects ▪ Use c̄ antidiabetic agents may require higher doses of antidiabetic drugs.

NURSING MANAGEMENT

ADMINISTRATION: Assess for hx of hypersensitivity ▪ Administer single daily dose *before* 9AM; multiple doses at equal intervals ▪ PO: administer c̄ food/milk/antacids ▪ Do *not* administer IV ▪ IM: shake well; do *not* mix, dilute, freeze; inject *deep* into gluteal UOQ (avoid deltoid); rotate sites ▪ Avoid abrupt withdrawal; ↓ dose gradually ▪ Avoid exposure to heat, light in storage ▪ Elderly may require ↓ dosage; monitor BP.

EVALUATION: Monitor VS, esp BP; hydration status (I&O, daily weight) ▪ Diabetics: closely monitor blood/urine glucose (hyperglycemia) ▪ Assess mental/emotional status; avoid tricyclic antidepressants if depression is induced ▪ Monitor serum electrolytes (esp K^+, Na^+), vision/IOP, stools for occult blood c̄ prolonged use ▪ Assess for ↓ appetite.

EDUCATION: Avoid changing positions rapidly ▪ Take c̄ food/milk (single dose *before* 9AM; multiple doses at equal intervals) ▪ Take as ordered by physician; do *not* ↑ dose/D/C ▪ Eat foods high in K^+, high in protein; avoid black licorice ▪ Follow diet low in Na^+ ▪ Check c̄ physician before immunization (pt, family) ▪ Avoid exposure to infection ▪ Report following symptoms *immediately* to physician: anorexia, difficult breathing, weakness, dizziness; may appear during periods of ↑ stress/trauma ▪ Notify physician of black/tarry stools, slow wound healing, blurred vision, bruising/bleeding, weight gain, emotional changes ▪ Diabetics: closely monitor blood or urine glucose ▪ Store in tightly closed, light-resistant container ▪ Keep scheduled appointments c̄ physician/for blood work/eye exams ▪ Women: avoid breastfeeding ▪ Body image changes may occur c̄ prolonged therapy (reversible).

NOTES:

triamterene • (trye-am-ter-een)

CATEGORY: *Diuretic:* potassium-sparing diuretic Rx; Preg Cat B

BRAND NAME	DOSAGE FORMS
Dyrenium (SKB)	Capsule: 50, 100mg

COMBINATION PRODUCTS

Dyazide (SKB)	triamterene/hydrochlorothiazide per capsule: 50mg/25mg
Maxizide (Lederle)	triamterene/hydrochlorothiazide per tablet: 75mg/50mg
Maxizide-25 MG	triamterene/hydrochlorothiazide per tablet: 37.5mg/25mg
**Novotriamide (Novopharm)*	triamterene/hydrochlorothiazide per tablet: 50mg/25mg

ACTION: Triamterene acts directly at portion of distal tubule under control of mineralosteroids (esp aldosterone) to inhibit reabsorption of sodium ions in exchange for potassium, hydrogen ions; drug has no appreciable antihypertensive activity. **USE:** Edema associated c̄ CHF, cirrhosis of liver, nephrotic syndrome ▪ Steroid-induced edema, idiopathic edema, edema due to 2° hyperaldosteronism ▪ Combination products are employed as antihypertensives (due to HCT content).

PHARMACOKINETICS

PO absorption	Onset	Duration	Protein binding	Excretion
Good	2-4h	7-9h	67%	Via urine as metabolites, unchanged, drug

CONTRAINDICATIONS: Hypersensitivity, anuria, significant renal insufficiency, hyperkalemia.

DOSAGE

Adult *PO*	Usual dose 100mg bid pc. Do *not* exceed 300mg/d
Dyazide	Usual adult dose 1-2 capsules bid pc
Maxizide	Usual adult dose 1 tablet/d
Maxizide-25 MG	Usual adult dose 1-2 tablets/d as single dose

SIDE/ADVERSE EFFECTS: CNS: headache, weakness, dizziness ▪ GI: N/V/D, dry mouth ▪ HEM: ***megaloblastic***

Note: Side/adverse effects: common in *italic;* serious in ***boldface italic.***

*Available in Canada only.

anemia (rare) ▪ INT: *photosensitivity, rash* ▪ MET: hyperkalemia ▪ Other: ***anaphylaxis.***

DRUG INTERACTIONS: Use c̄ lithium best avoided because of ↑ in lithium serum levels ▪ Use c̄ dig glycosides may ↑ their activity.

NURSING MANAGEMENT

ADMINISTRATION: Assess for hx of hypersensitivity ▪ Assess F/E balance; normal serum K^+ level: 3.5-5mEq/L; do *not* administer if hyperkalemic; notify physician ▪ Assess renal function; do *not* administer if impaired ▪ Administer pc ▪ Avoid exposure to moisture, light in storage ▪ Elderly may require ↓ dosage.

EVALUATION: Monitor F/E, hepatic, renal status ▪ Monitor VS, esp BP, pulse ▪ Monitor serum for ↑ BUN, creatinine, uric acid ▪ Assess for hyperkalemia; D/C drug, notify physician ▪ Monitor fluid retention (I&O, daily weight).

EDUCATION: Expect ↑ urine output; have bathroom facilities easily accessible ▪ May cause weakness, lethargy ▪ Take c̄ food/milk on waking, at same time each day, even if symptom free; take second dose (if ordered) after dinner ▪ Used to control, *not* cure, hypertension ▪ Notify physician of signs of hyperkalemia (weakness, tingling/numbness, irregular heartbeat) ▪ Avoid changing positions (lying/sitting/standing) rapidly ▪ Take as directed by physician; do *not* skip doses ▪ Avoid high-Na^+ foods (canned soups, lunch meats, cheese) ▪ Avoid high-K^+ foods (bananas, citrus juices, raisins) ▪ Check c̄ physician before using salt substitutes ▪ Maintain optimum weight ▪ Avoid exposure to direct sunlight, UV light (sunlamps); use sunscreen, protective clothing ▪ Check c̄ physician/pharmacist before taking OTC preparations ▪ Store in tightly closed, light-resistant container ▪ Keep scheduled appointments c̄ physician; have BP checked regularly ▪ Full drug effect may require several wks.

NOTES:

trihexyphenidyl hcl • (trye-hex-ee-fen-i-dill)

CATEGORY: *Antiparkinsonian agent:* anticholinergic Rx; Preg Cat NA

BRAND NAMES	DOSAGE FORMS
**Aparkane (ICN)*	Tablet: 2, 5mg
Artane (Lederle)	Elixir: 2mg/5ml SR capsule: 5mg Tablet: 2, 5mg
**Novohexidyl (Novopharm)*	Tablet: 2, 5mg
**Apo-Trihex (Apotex)*	Tablet: 2, 5mg

ACTION: Antiparkinsonian effect due to central anticholinergic inhibition of hyperactive cholinergic activity in striated fibers. **USE:** Adjunct in treatment of all forms of Parkinson disease ▪ Management of extrapyramidal symptoms (except tardive dyskinesia) induced by antipsychotic agents.

PHARMACOKINETICS

PO absorption	Onset	Peak	Duration	Excretion
Rapid	1h	2-3h	6-12h	Via urine as unchanged drug

CONTRAINDICATIONS: Hypersensitivity, glaucoma.

DOSAGE

Adult *PO* Usual maintenance dose 6-10mg/d divided. For drug-induced symptoms, 5-15 mg/d divided

SIDE/ADVERSE EFFECTS: EENT: blurred vision ▪ GI: dry mouth, dysphagia, constipation, N/V ▪ Other: allergic rxs (rare).

DRUG INTERACTIONS: Use c̄ antihistamines, phenothiazines, tricyclic antidepressants ↑ anticholinergic effects ▪ Amantadine can significantly ↑ anticholinergic effects.

NURSING MANAGEMENT

ADMINISTRATION: Assess for hx of hypersensitivity ▪ Administer in divided doses c̄ meals, or as a single AM/hs dose; administer SR capsules whole, q12h ▪ Avoid exposure to moisture in storage ▪ Avoid abrupt withdrawal ▪ Elderly may require ↓ dosage.

Note: Side/adverse effects: common in *italic;* serious in ***boldface italic.***

*Available in Canada only.

EVALUATION: Monitor GI, GU, CV status ▪ Assess for muscle weakness ▪ Observe for exaggerated anticholinergic effects ▪ Monitor VS ▪ Monitor I&O ▪ Monitor IOP ▪ Assess for tolerance to therapeutic dose.

EDUCATION: Drowsiness may occur; use caution in potentially hazardous activities ▪ Avoid use $\bar{c}$ alcohol, other CNS depressants ▪ Take $\bar{c}$ meals ▪ Avoid extremes in exercise, hot climates ▪ Take as ordered by physician; do *not* ↑ dose ▪ Store in tightly closed container ▪ Schedule periodic eye exams ▪ Use sugarless gum/hard candy to diminish dry mouth ▪ Take antacid/antidiarrheal preparations at least 1h before/after drug ▪ Wear sunglasses to ↓ discomfort from bright lights ▪ Avoid changing positions (lying/sitting/standing) rapidly ▪ Safety precautions $\bar{c}$ ↑ activity ▪ Women: avoid breastfeeding ▪ Full drug effect may require several ds.

NOTES:

trimethobenzamide hcl • (trye-meth-oh-ben-za-mide)

CATEGORY: *Antiemetic* Rx; Preg Cat NA

BRAND NAME

Tigan (SKB)

DOSAGE FORMS

Capsule: 100, 250mg
Injection (IM): 100mg/ml
Pediatric suppository: 100mg
Suppository: 200mg

ACTION: Antiemetic activity due to inhibition of chemoreceptor trigger zone in medulla. **USE:** Control of N/V.

PHARMACOKINETICS

Route	Onset	Duration	Excretion
PO	10-45m	3-4h	Via urine, feces as unchanged drug, metabolites
IM	15-40m	2-3h	

CONTRAINDICATIONS: Hypersensitivity, injection in children, suppositories in newborn infants, suppositories in pts hypersensitive to benzocaine.

DOSAGE

Pediatric *PO*	
30-90 lbs	100-200mg 3-4 times/d
Rectal	
<30lb	100mg 3-4 times/d
30-90lbs	100-200mg 3-4 times/d
Adult *PO*	250mg 3-5 times/d
IM	200mg 3-5 times/d
Rectal	200mg 3-5 times/d

SIDE/ADVERSE EFFECTS: CNS: ***Parkinsonlike symptoms, coma, convulsions,*** headache, drowsiness, dizziness, disorientation, mood depression ▪ EENT: blurred vision ▪ GI: diarrhea ▪ HEP: ***jaundice*** ▪ MS: muscle cramps, opisthotonos.

DRUG INTERACTIONS: Use c̄ CNS depressants can produce additive depression ▪ Use c̄ ototoxic drugs can mask their toxic effects ▪ Sequential use of antiemetic agents in pts recently given barbiturates, belladonna alkaloids, phenothiazines can result in opisthotonos, convulsions, coma, extrapyramidal symptoms.

Note: Side/adverse effects: common in *italic;* serious in ***boldface italic.*** *Available in Canada only.

NURSING MANAGEMENT

ADMINISTRATION: Assess for hx of hypersensitivity ▪ PO: take $\bar{c}$ H_2O; may empty capsule ▪ IM: administer via Z-track ▪ Do *not* administer IV ▪ Avoid exposure to light in storage ▪ Store suppositories in refrigerator.

EVALUATION: Monitor VS, esp BP ▪ Monitor F/E status ▪ Assess for potentiation of CNS depressants.

EDUCATION: Dizziness/drowsiness may occur; use caution in potentially hazardous activities ▪ Notify physician *immediately* of rash, lethargy, tremors; D/C drug ▪ Take 15-30m before activity that may precipitate vomiting ▪ Avoid use $\bar{c}$ alcohol, other CNS depressants ▪ Use sugarless gum/hard candy to diminish dry mouth ▪ *Not* used to prevent motion sickness ▪ Procedure for suppository insertion.

NOTES:

trimethoprim • (trye-meth-oh-prim)

CATEGORY: *Antiinfective*: urinary tract antimicrobial Rx; Preg Cat C

BRAND NAMES	DOSAGE FORMS
Proloprim (B-W)	Tablet: 100, 200mg
Trimpex (Roche)	Tablet: 100mg

ACTION: Bacteriostatic activity due to inhibition of folic acid synthesis. **USE:** Treatment of initial episodes of uncomplicated UTIs caused by susceptible strains of *Enterobacter* spp, *Escherichia coli, Klebsiella* spp, *Proteus mirabilis, Staphylococcus,* coagulase (-) organisms.

PHARMACOKINETICS

PO absorption	Peak	Half-life	Protein binding	Excretion
Rapid	1-4h	8-10h	44%	50%-60% via urine as unmetabolized drug (80%) in 24h

CONTRAINDICATIONS: Hypersensitivity, folate-deficient megaloblastic anemia.

DOSAGE

Adult *PO*	100mg q12h for 10d; use one-half dosage in pts c̄ creatinine clearance 15-30ml/m

SIDE/ADVERSE EFFECTS: GI: epigastric distress, N/V, glossitis ▪ HEM: ***thrombocytopenia,*** leukopenia, neutropenia, ***megaloblastic anemia,*** methemoglobinemia ▪ INT: *rash*, pruritus, ***exfoliative dermatitis*** ▪ MET: ↑ serum transaminase, creatinine, BUN.

DRUG INTERACTIONS: Avoid urinary acidifiers, which ↑ excretion of trimethoprim.

NURSING MANAGEMENT

ADMINISTRATION: Assess for hx of hypersensitivity ▪ Obtain C&S before therapy ▪ Assess renal function; may require ↓ dosage if impaired ▪ Administer 1h ac/2h pc (c̄ food if GI irritation occurs) ▪ Administer folic acid concurrently if megaloblastic anemia present ▪ Maintain hydration ▪ Avoid exposure to moisture in storage.

EVALUATION: Monitor hepatic, renal status ▪ Monitor VS, esp temperature ▪ Monitor CBC, UA ▪ Monitor I&O.

EDUCATION: Complete full course of therapy (usually 10d) even if symptoms subside ▪ Take on empty stomach $\bar{c}$ full glass of H_2O; if upset stomach occurs, take $\bar{c}$ food ▪ Take at equal intervals around clock to maintain blood levels ▪ Store in tightly closed, light-resistant container ▪ Discard unused, outdated preparations ▪ Maintain good personal hygiene (esp perineal, oral) ▪ ↑ Fluid intake (8-10 glasses/d) ▪ Notify physician of fever, sore throat, difficult breathing, rash, bruising/bleeding ▪ Women: avoid pregnancy, breastfeeding ▪ Do *not* give to infants or children.

NOTES:

valproic acid/valproate sodium ▲ • (val-proe-ic)

CATEGORY: *Anticonvulsant* Rx; Preg Cat D

BRAND NAME
Depakene (Abbott)

DOSAGE FORMS
Capsule: 250mg
Syrup▲: 250mg/5ml

ACTION: Anticonvulsant mechanism not determined; studies indicate valproic acid may ↑ brain levels of γ-aminobutyric acid (GABA), an inhibitory neurotransmitter. **USE:** Treatment of simple/complex absence seizures incl petit mal ▪ Adjunct in treatment of multiple seizure types incl absence seizures.

PHARMACOKINETICS

PO absorption	Peak	Half-life	Protein binding	Excretion
Rapid	1-4h	6-16h	90%	Via urine as unchanged drug, metabolites

CONTRAINDICATIONS: Hypersensitivity, hepatic disease, significant hepatic dysfunction.

DOSAGE

Pediatric/Adult *PO*	Initial dose 15mg/kg/d, ↑ at 1wk intervals by 5-10mg/kg/d until seizures controlled or adverse effects preclude further ↑; maximum daily dose 60mg/kg/d

SIDE/ADVERSE EFFECTS: CNS: sedation, ataxia, headache, nystagmus, diplopia, asterixis, dysarthria, dizziness, incoordination ▪ END: irregular menses, secondary amenorrhea, breast enlargement (rare), galactorrhea, abnormal thyroid tests ▪ GI: *N/V/D, gastric distress,* abdominal cramps, ***pancreatitis*** ▪ HEM: ***thrombocytopenia,*** leukopenia, eosinophilia ▪ HEP: dose-related ↑ AST, ALT, LDH; severe behavioral deterioration.

DRUG INTERACTIONS: Use c̄ CNS depressants can produce additive depression ▪ Use c̄ barbiturates may produce ↑ serum levels of barbiturates ▪ Use c̄ clonazepam may produce absence status ▪ Use c̄ drugs affecting coagulation best avoided ▪ Use c̄ phenytoin may produce breakthrough seizures.

NURSING MANAGEMENT

ADMINISTRATION: Assess for hx of hypersensitivity ▪ Assess hepatic function; do *not* administer if impaired ▪ Administer capsules whole; do *not* crush/chew ▪ Avoid abrupt withdrawal; D/C gradually; institute strict seizure precautions if drug abruptly withdrawn ▪ Avoid exposure to moisture, light in storage; do *not* refrigerate.

EVALUATION: Monitor hepatic, renal, cardiac, respiratory status ▪ Monitor occurrence/characteristics of seizures ▪ Monitor activity status (safety precautions) ▪ May produce false (+) urine ketones ▪ Therapeutic blood levels: 50-100μg/ml.

EDUCATION: Drowsiness may occur; use caution in potentially hazardous activities ▪ Avoid use c̄ alcohol, other CNS depressants ▪ Take as ordered by physician; do *not* ↑ dose ▪ Take c̄ food to ↓ GI distress; swallow capsules whole ▪ Dietary protein restrictions (hyperammonemia) ▪ Notify physician/dentist of use before treatment ▪ Notify physician *immediately* of bruising/bleeding ▪ Check c̄ physician/pharmacist before taking OTC preparations ▪ Store in tightly closed, light-resistant container ▪ Carry identification (MedicAlert) ▪ Do *not* omit daily dose.

NOTES:

vancomycin hcl • (van-koe-mye-sin)

CATEGORY: *Antibiotic*

Rx; Preg Cat C

BRAND NAMES	DOSAGE FORMS
Vancocin HCl (Lilly)	Capsule: 125, 250mg Powder for injection (IV): 500mg, 1g/vial Powder for PO solution: 1, 10g container
Vancoled (Lederle)	Powder for injection (IV): 500mg/vial

ACTION: Antibacterial activity due to inhibition of cell wall synthesis in susceptible organisms. The drug also affects cell membrane permeability and RNA synthesis.

USE: Treatment of severe infections due to susceptible methicillin-resistant strains of staphylococci ▪ Endocarditis caused by staphylococci, *Streptococcus* spp, and diphtheroids ▪ In combination c̄ an aminoglycoside for enterococcal endocarditis ▪ In combination c̄ rifampin for endocarditis ▪ Alternate in penicillin-allergic pts c̄ heart damage who require dental procedures ▪ Life-threatening infections that are resistant to less toxic antibiotics ▪ PO treatment (drug not absorbed) of staphylococcal enterocolitis and antibiotic-induced pseudomembranous colitis produced by *Clostridium difficile*.

PHARMACOKINETICS

IV peak	Half-life	Protein binding	Excretion
5m	4-6h	55%	80% of a single dose via urine after 24h as unchanged drug

CONTRAINDICATIONS: Hypersensitivity.

DOSAGE

IV: For normal renal function, c̄ each dose administered over a 60m period

Neonate	Initial dose of 15mg/kg, followed by 10mg/kg q12h for first week of life and q8h thereafter up to age of 1 month
Pediatric	40mg/kg/24h in divided doses
Adult	2g/d divided (500mg q6h or 1g q12h)

PO

Pediatric	40mg/kg/d in 3-4 divided doses for 7-10d. Do *not* exceed 2g/d
Adult	0.5-2g/d in 3-4 divided doses for 7-10d

NURSING MANAGEMENT

NOTES:

ADMINISTRATION: Assess for hx of hypersensitivity ▪ Obtain C&S before therapy ▪ Obtain pt weight for dose calculation ▪ Determine creatinine clearance before administration ▪ PO: used to treat local intestinal infections; reconstitute powder according to manufacturer's directions $\bar{c}$ distilled/deionized H_2O, stable for 14d (refrigerated) ▪ IV: administer via IV infusion only, over 60m period; prepare according to manufacturer's directions, stable for 96h (refrigerated) ▪ Maintain hydration ▪ Elderly may require ↓ dosage.

EVALUATION: Monitor VS, esp temperature ▪ Assess hearing (ototoxicity), UA (nephrotoxicity); notify physician ▪ Monitor CBC (leukopenia, neutropenia); notify physician ▪ Assess for "red neck" syndrome (hypotension, erythema of face, neck, upper body) ▪ IV: avoid extravasation; assess for pain, edema, redness at insertion site ▪ May ↑ BUN.

EDUCATION: Drowsiness may occur; use caution in potentially hazardous activities ▪ Notify nurse/physician *immediately* of hearing disturbances, difficult breathing, blood in urine ▪ May cause unpleasant taste.

vasopressin • (vay-soe-press-in)

CATEGORY: *Posterior pituitary hormone*: antidiuretic

Rx; Preg Cat NA

BRAND NAME
Pitressin (P-D)

DOSAGE FORMS
Injection (aqueous) (IM/SC): 20 pressor U/ml

ACTION: Vasopressin causes contraction of smooth muscle of GI tract, vascular beds; antidiuretic activity due to H_2O reabsorption in renal tubule. **USE:** Treatment of abdominal distention, diabetes insipidus ▪ Abdominal roentgenography.

PHARMACOKINETICS: Aqueous injection has duration of antidiuretic activity 2-8h, oil-based injection 48-72h.

CONTRAINDICATIONS: Hypersensitivity.

DOSAGE IM is preferred route

Adult

Abdominal distention	Usual post-op dose 5U initially, ↑ to 10U prn for subsequent administration IM/SC
Abdominal roentgenography	2 injections of 10U given 2h, 1/2 h, respectively, before procedure
Diabetes insipidus	5-10U repeated 2-3 times/d prn Aqueous injection: can be administration by nasal spray/on pledgets inserted into nose. Dosage must be individualized Oil injection: 0.3-1ml IM, repeat prn

SIDE/ADVERSE EFFECTS: CNS: tremor, vertigo, head pain, sweating ▪ GI: cramps, flatulence, N/V ▪ INT: urticaria ▪ RESP: bronchial constriction ▪ Other: ***anaphylaxis,*** pallor.

DRUG INTERACTIONS: Use c̄ chlorpropamide/clofibrate may enhance antidiuretic effect ▪ Use c̄ lithium, alcohol, demeclocycline may block antidiuretic effect.

NURSING MANAGEMENT

ADMINISTRATION: Assess for hx of hypersensitivity ▪ Assess bowel sounds, measure abdominal girth before administration ▪ Administer 1-2 glasses H_2O immediately after injection (↑ effectiveness).

EVALUATION: Monitor VS, esp BP ▪ Monitor F/E status (I&O, specific gravity, daily weight) esp in children ▪ Assess for H_2O intoxication (lethargy, confusion, headache) ▪ Assess for urinary retention, abdominal distention (use rectal tube to expel flatus) ▪ Monitor IV site closely; avoid extravasation.

EDUCATION: Notify physician of ↑ thirst, ↑ urination ▪ Rectal tube will be inserted to relieve gas/fullness in abdomen ▪ Avoid ingestion of concentrated fluids, excessive use of alcohol, acetaminophen (Tylenol) ▪ IM injection may be painful ▪ Procedure for specific gravity determination.

NOTES:

verapamil hcl • (ver-ap-a-mill)

CATEGORY: *Calcium blocker:* antianginal, antiarrhythmic, slow channel blocker Rx; Preg Cat C

BRAND NAMES	DOSAGE FORMS
Calan (Searle)	SR caplets: 120, 180, 240mg
	Tablet: 40, 80, 120mg
Isoptin (Knoll)	Injection (IV): 5mg/2ml
	Tablet: 40, 80, 120mg
**Isoptin Oral (Searle)*	Tablet: 80, 120mg
Veralan (Lederle)	SR capsule: 120, 180, 240mg

ACTION: Antianginal effect due to inhibition of extracellular calcium-ion transmembrane migration in cardiac, vascular smooth muscle via slow channel passageway, resulting in coronary dilation; ↑ myocardial oxygen supply, ↓ oxygen consumption. Antiarrhythmic effect due to sinus arrest in sick sinus syndrome; slowing of conduction, lengthening of refractory period in AV node. **USE:** Treatment of chronic stable, vasospastic, unstable angina pectoris (PO) ▪ Treatment of paroxysmal supraventricular tachycardia (IV) ▪ Prophylaxis of paroxysmal supraventricular tachycardia ▪ Temporary control of rapid ventricular rate in atrial flutter/atrial fibrillation (IV) ▪ Treatment of essential hypertension (SR only).

CONTRAINDICATIONS: Hypersensitivity, severe hypotension/cardiogenic shock, 2°/3° AV block, sick sinus syndrome (except c̄ pacemaker), CHF (unless 2° to supraventricular tachycardia amenable to verapamil IV), IV beta-adrenergic administration, atrial flutter c̄ hx of accessory bypass tracts (IV), severe left ventricular dysfunction (PO).

PHARMACOKINETICS

	PO absorption	Onset	Peak	Half-life	Protein binding	Excretion
PO	90%	30m	1-2h	2-3h	90%	70% via urine, 16% in feces in 5d as metabolites
IV	—	3-5m	5m	2-8h	90%	

Note: Side/adverse effects: common in *italic;* serious in ***boldface italic.***

*Available in Canada only.

DOSAGE

Pediatric *IV*	≤1y/o: 0.1-0.2mg/kg as bolus over 2m. Repeat dose may be given after 30m 1-15y/o: 0.1-0.3mg/kg as bolus over 2m. Do *not* exceed 5mg/dose. Repeat dose (not exceeding 10mg) may be given after 30m
Adult *PO*	Starting dose 80mg 3-4 times/d, c̄ daily range 240-480mg. Optimum dose range usually 320-480mg/d. Daily dose >480mg not currently established
IV	5-10mg as bolus over 2m. Repeat dose ≤10mg may be given after 30m
Geriatric *IV*	5-10mg as bolus over 3m. Repeat dose ≤10mg may be given after 30m

SIDE/ADVERSE EFFECTS: CNS: *dizziness*, headache, insomnia, confusion ▪ CV: *hypotension*, peripheral edema, ***AV block,*** bradycardia, CHF ▪ EENT: blurred vision ▪ GI: *constipation,* nausea ▪ GU: gynecomastia, spotty menstruation ▪ INT: alopecia ▪ MS: muscle cramps.

DRUG INTERACTIONS: Use c̄ dig may ↑ dig body levels ▪ Use c̄ disopyramide best avoided ▪ Use c̄ antihypertensives may ↑ hypotensive effects.

NURSING MANAGEMENT

ADMINISTRATION: Assess for hx of hypersensitivity, heart failure (use c̄ caution) ▪ Assess BP, heart rate; if apical pulse <60, hold dose, notify physician ▪ IV: cardiac monitor; administer IV, over 2m (3m for elderly); maintain supine position 1h after administration ▪ Avoid exposure to light, freezing ▪ Do *not* administer discolored/precipitated solutions ▪ Have emergency support equipment available ▪ Elderly may require ↓ dosage.

EVALUATION: Monitor VS, esp BP (IV: q5-10m), heart rate; I&O; hepatic, renal status ▪ Assess for CHF, notify physician ▪ Digitalized pts: assess for dig toxicity (bradycardia, anorexia, palpitations).

EDUCATION: Dizziness may occur; use caution in potentially hazardous activities ▪ Avoid changing positions rapidly ▪ Procedure for checking radial pulse ▪ If pulse slow (<60)/irregular, do *not* take dose, notify physician ▪ Avoid caffeine, alcohol ▪ Check c̄ physician/pharmacist before taking OTC preparations ▪ Take as ordered by physician; do *not* change dose ▪ Notify physician of difficult breathing, chest pain, swelling of hands or legs; D/C drug ▪ Keep appointments c̄ physician ▪ Continue to use SL nitroglycerin (if ordered) to relieve sudden chest pain or for prophylaxis before exertion.

vinblastine sulfate • (vin-blas-teen)

CATEGORY: *Antineoplastic* Rx; Preg Cat NA

BRAND NAMES	DOSAGE FORMS
Velban (Lilly)	Powder for injection (IV): 10mg vial
**Velbe (Lilly)*	Powder for injection (IV): 10mg vial

ACTION: Antineoplastic activity due to microtubular protein binding, resulting in mitotic arrest during metaphase; drug also interferes c̄ glutamic acid, aspartate metabolism, nucleic acid synthesis; vinblastine also exerts immunosuppressive activity. **USE:** Palliation of advanced carcinoma of testes, generalized Hodgkin's disease, histiocytic lymphoma, Kaposi's sarcoma, Letterer-Siwe disease, lymphocytic lymphoma, mycosis fungoides ▪ Breast cancer, choriocarcinoma unresponsive to other treatment.

PHARMACOKINETICS: Limited studies indicate rapid distribution from blood into body tissue; drug metabolized in liver, excreted via urine, feces.

CONTRAINDICATIONS: Leukopenia, bacterial infection.

DOSAGE: *(IV)* Leukopenic response to drug usually restricts administration to single weekly doses; recommended weekly schedule:

	Pediatric	Adult
Dose 1	2.5mg/m^2	3.7mg/m^2
Dose 2	3.75mg/m^2	5.5mg/m^2
Dose 3	5mg/m^2	7.4mg/m^2
Dose 4	6.25mg/m^2	9.25mg/m^2
Dose 5	7.5mg/m^2	11.1mg/m^2

Dose should not be ↑ after dose that ↓ WBC to 3000 cells/mm^3. Maintenance dose should be one increment lower than dose that will produce leukopenia count 3000. Do *not* administer weekly dose, even though 7d may have elapsed, until WBC ≥ 4000. Duration of maintenance varies c̄ disease, combination of drugs used.

SIDE/ADVERSE EFFECTS: CNS: numbness, peripheral neuritis, paresthesias, headache, loss of deep tendon reflexes, ***convulsions***, depression ▪ GI: N/V, anorexia, oral vesiculation, pharyngitis, ***rectal bleeding, peptic ulcer hemorrhage, hemorrhagic enterocolitis*** ▪ HEM:

Note: Side/adverse effects: common in *italic;* serious in ***boldface italic.***

*Available in Canada only.

leukopenia ▪ INT: local rxs (cellulitis, phlebitis, sloughing at IV site) ▪ Other: weakness, vesiculation of skin, pain at tumor site.

DRUG INTERACTIONS: Use of live vaccines contraindicated during therapy ▪ Radiation therapy, bone marrow depressants produce additive bone marrow depression.

NURSING MANAGEMENT

ADMINSTRATION: Check pt hx for recent course of radiation or antineoplastic agents; report to physician ▪ Assess hepatic function; ↓ dosage if impaired ▪ Avoid exposure to moisture, light in storage ▪ Avoid contact c̄ eyes during preparation ▪ Administer antiemetic before therapy ▪ Avoid IM injections during therapy ▪ Provide emotional support ▪ Reconstitute c̄ 10 ml NaCl injection; may administer IVPB, direct IV (over 1m); may refrigerate for 30d w/out loss of potency ▪ Rinse needle, syringe c̄ venous blood before withdrawal.

EVALUATION: Monitor VS (avoid rectal temperature) ▪ Monitor CBC throughout therapy; if WBC <4000, platelets <100,000/mm^3, do not administer ▪ Assess for infection, bleeding, anemia ▪ May produce ↑ serum uric acid level ▪ Monitor hepatic function ▪ Assess abdominal distention, bowel sounds; administer laxative as ordered for constipation ▪ Monitor IV site closely; avoid extravasation ▪ Assess hydration status (I&O, daily wieght) ▪ Assess for neurotoxicity, skin breakdown ▪ Assess for mental depression.

EDUCATION: Store in tightly closed, light-resistant container ▪ ↑ Fluid intake (8-10 glasses/d) ▪ Avoid exposure to infection ▪ Check c̄ physician before immunization (pt, family) ▪ Diet as tolerated; avoid spicy foods ▪ Maintain good oral hygiene; use soft-bristled toothbrush ▪ Notify physician of symptoms of bone marrow depression (fever, sore throat, bruising, bleeding, lethargy) ▪ Women: avoid breastfeeding ▪ Avoid exposure to direct sunlight, UV light (sunlamps); use sunscreen, protective clothing ▪ Encourage ventilation of feelings ▪ Use contraception if sexually active.

NOTES:

vincristine sulfate • (vin-kris-teen)

CATEGORY: *Antineoplastic*

Rx; Preg Cat NA

BRAND NAME
Oncovin (Lilly)

DOSAGE FORMS
Injection (IV): 1mg/ml

ACTION: Antineoplastic activity due to microtubular protein binding, resulting in mitotic arrest during metaphase. **USE:** Treatment of acute leukemia, esp pediatric lymphoblastic ▪ Treatment of Hodgkin's disease, lymphosarcoma, reticulum cell sarcoma, rhabdomyosarcoma, neuroblastoma, Wilms' tumor.

PHARMACOKINETICS: Limited studies indicate rapid distribution from blood into body tissue; drug metabolized in liver, exhibits high protein binding, long half-life; is excreted primarily via feces, c̄ some renal excretion.

CONTRAINDICATIONS: Demyelinating form of Charcot-Marie-Tooth disease.

DOSAGE

Pediatric *IV*	2mg/m^2 at weekly intervals
Adult *IV*	1.4mg/m^2 at weekly intervals

SIDE/ADVERSE EFFECTS: CNS: neuritic pain, sensory loss, paresthesia, slapping gait, loss of deep tendon reflexes, ***convulsions,*** footdrop, cranial nerve manifestations ▪ CV: hypertension ▪ EENT: photophobia, diplopia, transient cortical blindness ▪ GI: N/V, constipation, oral ulceration, cramps; paralytic ileus, esp in children ▪ HEM: anemia (rare), leukopenia ▪ INT: *alopecia* ▪ Other: syndrome attributed to inappropriate antidiuretic hormone secretion c̄ high degree of Na^+ excretion, jaw pain, bone pain, limb pain.

DRUG INTERACTIONS: Use of live vaccines best avoided during therapy ▪ Radiation therapy, bone marrow depressants produce additive bone marrow depression ▪ Use c̄ neurotoxic drugs produces additive neurotoxicity.

NURSING MANAGEMENT

ADMINISTRATION: Assess pt for hx for recent course of radiation/antineoplastic agents; report to physician ▪ Assess hepatic function; ⬇ dosage if impaired ▪ Avoid exposure to moisture, light in storage ▪ Reconstitute according to manufacturer's directions; may administer direct IV (over 1m) ▪ Avoid contact c̄ eyes during preparation ▪ Administer antiemetic before therapy ▪ Avoid IM injection during therapy ▪ Provide emotional support ▪ Rinse needle, syringe c̄ venous blood before withdrawal.

EVALUATION: Monitor VS (avoid rectal temperature) ▪ Monitor CBC throughout therapy; if WBC <4000, platelets <100,000/mm^3, do *not* administer ▪ Assess for infection, bleeding, anemia ▪ Monitor hepatic function ▪ Assess abdominal distention, bowel sounds; administer laxative as ordered for constipation ▪ Monitor IV site closely; avoid extravasation ▪ Assess hydration status (I&O, daily weight) ▪ Assess for mental depression, neurotoxicity (ataxia, ↓ LOC, tremors).

EDUCATION: Store in tightly closed, light-resistant container ▪ ↑ Fluid intake (8-10 glasses/d) ▪ Avoid exposure to infection ▪ Check c̄ physician before immunization (pt, family) ▪ Diet as tolerated; avoid spicy foods ▪ Maintain good oral hygiene; use soft-bristled toothbrush ▪ Notify physician of symptoms of bone marrow depression (fever, sore throat, bruising, bleeding, lethargy) ▪ Loss of hair may occur (reversible) ▪ Women: avoid breastfeeding ▪ Encourage ventilation of feelings ▪ Use contraception if sexually active.

NOTES:

warfarin sodium • (war-far-in)

CATEGORY: *Coumarin anticoagulant*

Rx; Preg Cat X

BRAND NAMES	DOSAGE FORMS
Coumadin (Du Pont)	Injection (IM/IV): 50mg/vial Tablet: 1, 2, 2.5, 5, 7.5, 10mg
Panwarfin (Abbott)	Tablet: 2, 2.5, 5, 7.5, 10mg
**Warfilone Sodium*	

ACTION: Coumarin anticoagulants inhibit synthesis of prothrombin (factor II), proconvertin (factor VII), Christmas factor (factor IX), Stuart-Prower factor (factor X) in liver by interfering c̄ action of vitamin K. **USE:** Adjunct in coronary occlusion ▪ Treatment of atrial fibrillation c̄ embolism ▪ Prophylaxis, treatment of venous thrombosis, pulmonary embolism.

CONTRAINDICATIONS: Hypersensitivity, subacute bacterial endocarditis, any bleeding/potential bleeding condition, pregnancy.

DOSAGE

Adult *PO* PT determines maintenance dose, usually 2-10mg/d

SIDE/ADVERSE EFFECTS: GI/GU: ***hemorrhage*** ▪ HEM: ***agranulocytosis,*** leukopenia, anemia ▪ HEP: hepatitis, jaundice ▪ INT: dermatitis, urticaria, alopecia ▪ Other: fever.

PHARMACOKINETICS

PO absorption	Peak	Duration	Half-life	Protein binding	Excretion
Almost complete	1-9h	36-72h	0.5-3d	98%	Mainly as metabolites via urine, bile

Note: Side/adverse effects: common in *italic;* serious in ***boldface italic.***

*Available in Canada only.

DRUG INTERACTIONS: List of drug interactions extremely long; main interactions that ↑ anticoagulant activity include enzyme ↓ of biotransformation, displacement from inactive protein storage sites, ↓ intestinal absorption of vitamin K, alteration of intestinal bacterial flora, alteration of platelet count/activity ▪ Main interaction that ↓ anticoagulant activity is enzyme induction of biotransformation ▪ Drugs that ↑ activity include anabolic steroids, broad-spectrum antibiotics, clofibrate, dextrothyroxine, disulfiram, oxyphenbutazone, phenylbutazone, salicylates ▪ Drugs that ↓ activity include barbiturates, cholestyramine, estrogens, glutethimide, PO contraceptives.

NURSING MANAGEMENT

ADMINISTRATION: Assess for hx of coumarin anticoagulant hypersensitivity ▪ PO: administer as single daily dose c̄ food ▪ Avoid abrupt withdrawal ▪ Avoid exposure to moisture in storage ▪ Regulate dosage according to PT ▪ Have vitamin K available ▪ Elderly may require ↓ dosage.

EVALUATION: Monitor hepatic, renal status ▪ Monitor PT; maintain at 1.5-2.5 times control value ▪ Monitor serum for ↑ ALT, AST, LDH ▪ Observe pt for signs of hemorrhage, incl abdominal/lumbar pain; treat c̄ vitamin K/whole blood.

EDUCATION: Notify physician *immediately* of unusual bleeding/bruising, blood detected in urine/stool ▪ Take c̄ food ▪ Follow dosage exactly as prescribed by physician ▪ Use electric razor/depilatory for hair removal ▪ Check c̄ physician/pharmacist before taking OTC preparations ▪ Avoid aspirin-containing products ▪ Avoid engaging in contact sports, other potentially injurious activities ▪ Do *not* change dietary habits in relation to daily intake of fat, green leafy vegetables, fish, vitamin K, alcoholic beverages ▪ Keep laboratory appointments as scheduled for PT determination ▪ Women: avoid pregnancy, breastfeeding; report menstrual flow ▪ Carry identification (MedicAlert) if receiving anticoagulant therapy ▪ Notify physician/dentist of anticoagulant use before treatment ▪ May turn urine red/brown ▪ Avoid changing brand-name preparations.

NOTES:

zalcitabine (dideoxycytidine)• (zal-sit-ah-been)

CATEGORY: *Antiviral:* synthetic pyrimidine nucleoside analog Rx; Preg Cat C

BRAND NAME
Hivid (Roche)

DOSAGE FORMS
Tablets: 0.375, 0.75mg

ACTION: Antiviral activity due to inhibition of viral DNA synthesis. **USE:** In combination c̄ zidovudine in adult pts c̄ advanced HIV infection c̄ significant clinical or immunologic deterioration (CD4 cell count ≤300/mm^3).

PHARMACOKINETICS

PO absorption	Peak	Half-life	Excretion
80%	0.8-1.6h	1-3h	70% single dose in 24h via urine

CONTRAINDICATIONS: Hypersensitivity.

DOSAGE

Adult *PO* 0.75mg + 200mg zidovudine q8h

SIDE/ADVERSE EFFECTS: CNS: headache, seizures, Bell's palsy, confusion, loss of mental acuity, nervousness, peripheral sensorimotor neuropathy of distal extremities (numbness, burning dysesthesia) ▪ CV: hypertension, rhythm irregularities, rare cases of ***cardiomyopathy/CHF*** ▪ EENT: abnormal vision and taste, ear blockage, tinnitus, xerophthalmia ▪ GI: esophageal/oral ulcers, N/V/D, dyspepsia, glossitis, rectal bleeding, dry mouth, ***pancreatitis*** ▪ GU: ***acute renal failure, toxic neuropathy,*** hyperuricemia, calculus ▪ HEM: anemia, leukopenia, ***thrombocytopenia*** ▪ HEP: jaundice, hepatitis, ***hepatocellular damage*** ▪ INT: acne, alopecia, bulbous eruptions, follicular rash ▪ MS: arthralgia, myalgia, gout ▪ Other: fever, ↓ weight, coughing, dypsnea, flulike symptoms, fever.

DRUG INTERACTIONS: Use c̄ didanosine best avoided ▪ Use c̄ peripheral neurotoxic, nephrotoxic, pancreatoxic drugs can result in additive toxicity.

NURSING MANAGEMENT

ADMINISTRATION: Assess for hx of hypersensitivity ▪ Administer 1h ac/2h pc ▪ Avoid exposure to light.

EVALUATION: Monitor VS, esp temperature ▪ Monitor hepatic, renal status ▪ Monitor WBC counts (anemia, granulocytopenia); repeated blood transfusions may be necessary.

EDUCATION: Take as ordered by physician at equal intervals around the clock to maintain blood levels; do *not* ↑ dose ▪ Do *not* share drug ▪ Women: avoid breast-feeding ▪ Used to control, *not* cure, HIV infections ▪ Notify physician of any change in health status ▪ Check $\bar{c}$ physician/pharmacist before taking OTC preparations ▪ Avoid sexual contact/blood donation (risk of HIV transmission) ▪ Keep scheduled appointments $\bar{c}$ physician/ for blood work.

NOTES:

zidovudine (azt)• (zye-doe-view-deen)

CATEGORY: *Antiviral*

Rx; Preg Cat C

BRAND NAME
Retrovir (B-W)

DOSAGE FORMS
Capsule: 100mg
IV infusion: 10mg/20ml
Syrup: 50mg/5ml

ACTION: Antiviral activity due to inhibition of viral replication in selected retroviruses incl human immunodeficiency virus (HIV/HTLV III), etiological agent of AIDS, ARC; drug is thymidine analogue that inhibits HIV reverse transcriptase enzymes, required for DNA synthesis. **USE:** Management (PO) of asymptomatic and symptomatic HIV infections in children >3mo/o and adults ▪ Management (IV) of selected adult symptomatic HIV infections & advanced ARC in pts c̄ confirmed *Pneumocystic carinii* pneumonia (PCP) or lymphocyte (T_4 cells) count <200/mm^3.

PHARMACOKINETICS

PO absorption	Peak	Half-life	Excretion
52%-75%	0.5-1.5h	0.78-1.93h	Via urine as metabolites (GAZT)

CONTRAINDICATIONS: Hypersensitivity that are life-threatening allergic rxs.

DOSAGE: Must be individualized (adjusted to the degree of anemia and/or granulocytopenia present)

Pediatric *PO* (3mo-12y/o)	Recommended starting dose 180mg/m^2 q6h (720mg/m^2/d). Do *not* exceed 200mg q6h
Adult *PO*	
Asymptomatic	100mg q4h while awake (500mg/d)
Symptomatic	Starting dose 200mg q4h (1200mg/d). Dosage may be ↓ to 100mg q4h (600mg/d) after 1mo
IV	1-2mg infused over 1h q4h (6 times/d)

SIDE/ADVERSE EFFECTS: CNS: anxiety, dizziness, insomnia, loss of mental acuity/confusion, nervousness, somnolence, vertigo ▪ CV: ECG abnormalities, vasodilation, ***phlebitis (IV)*** ▪ GI: anorexia, dyspepsia, abdominal pain, N/V/D, bleeding from gums/rectum, oral ulcers, HEM: ***anemia, granulocytopenia*** ▪ EENT: pharyngitis, sinusitis, hoarseness, rhinitis, amblyopia, hearing loss, photophobia ▪ GU: dysuria, polyuria, urinary frequency/hesitancy ▪ INT: acne, pruritus, urticaria ▪ MS: arthralgia, muscle spasms/tremor ▪ Other: chills, chest pains, lip edema.

DRUG INTERACTIONS: Use c̄ acetaminophen can ↑ incidence of granulocytopenia ▪ Use c̄ nephrotoxic drugs, cytotoxic drugs, or bone marrow depressants can result in additive toxicity ▪ Use c̄ probenecid may ↓ zidovudine renal excretion.

NURSING MANAGEMENT

ADMINISTRATION: Assess for hx of hypersensitivity ▪ Avoid administration of acetaminophen during therapy ▪ Avoid exposure to light.

EVALUATION: Monitor VS, esp temperature ▪ Monitor hepatic, renal status ▪ Monitor WBC counts (anemia, granulocytopenia); repeated blood transfusions may be necessary.

EDUCATION: Take as ordered by physician at equal intervals around clock to maintain blood levels; do *not* ↑ dose ▪ Do *not* share drug ▪ Women: avoid breastfeeding ▪ Used to control, *not* cure, HIV infections ▪ Notify physician of any change in health status ▪ Avoid concurrent use of acetaminophen (↑ toxicity) ▪ Check c̄ physician/pharmacist before taking OTC preparations ▪ Avoid sexual contact/blood donation (risk of HIV transmission) ▪ Keep scheduled appointments c̄ physician/for blood work.

NOTES:

DESCRIPTION: Large, varied group of drugs that can duplicate/mimic (sympathomimetic) effects of catecholamines, esp norepinephrine, at postganglionic adrenoreceptor in sympathetic nervous system; selected agents capable of central sympathomimetic activity ▪ Adrenoreceptors currently divided into alpha (α) receptors, which produce stimulatory responses, & beta (β) receptors, which usually produce inhibitory responses, except in heart, which are stimulatory. Furthermore, beta adrenoreceptors are subdivided into $beta_1$ receptors (heart) & $beta_2$ receptors (bronchi, GI tract, uterus). Recent investigations suggest that alpha adrenoreceptors can also be subdivided ($alpha_1$, $alpha_2$ receptors) ▪ Predominant alpha adrenergic agonist response is vasoconstriction, CNS stimulation. Beta adrenergic agonist response results in relaxation of bronchial, GI, uterine smooth muscle ($beta_2$ activity), cardiac stimulation ($beta_1$ activity).

DRUGS: Predominant adrenergic activity listed: α **Drugs**: amphetamine complex (*Biphetamine*), amphetamine, benzphetamine (*Didrex*), dextroamphetamine (*Dexedrine*), diethylpropion (*Tenuate, Tepanil*), fenfluramine (*Pondimin*), mazindol (*Mazanor*), methamphetamine (*Desoxyn*), methoxamine (*Vasoxyl*), naphazoline (*Privine*), oxymetazoline (*Afrin*), phendimetrazine (*Bontril, Plegine*), phenteramine (*Fastin, Ionamin*), phenylephrine (*Neo-Synephrine*), phenylpropanolamine (*Acutrim, Control, Dexatrim*), pseudoephedrine (*Sudafed*), tetrahydrozoline (*Visine*), xylometazoline (*Otrivin*) ▪ α-β **Drugs**: dipivefrin (*Propine*), ephedrine, epinephrine, ethylnorepinephrine (*Bronkephrine*), mephentermine (*Wyamine*), metaraminol (*Aramine*), norepinephrine (*Levophed*) ▪ β **Drugs:** isoproterenol (*Aerolone, Isuprel*), metaproterenol (*Alupent, Metaprel*), ritodrine (*Yutopar*) ▪ β_1 **Drugs:** dobutamine (*Dobutrex*), dopamine (*Intropin*) ▪ β_2 **Drugs:** albuterol (*Proventil, Ventolin*), bitolteroll (*Tornalate*), terbutaline (*Brethine, Bricanyl*).

MECHANISM OF ACTION: Sympathomimetics produce agonist effects by direct activity c̄ adrenoreceptor; by causing release of norepinephrine from storage vesicles in adrenergic neurons (indirect); combination of both mechanisms (mixed).

THERAPEUTIC USE: Anorexiant: Several current references separate this group from adrenergic drugs, esp amphetamine-like drugs: amphetamine complex, amphetamine sulfate, benzphetamine hcl, dextroamphetamine sulfate, diethylpropion, flenfluramine hcl, mazindol, phendimetrazine tartrate, phenmetrazine hcl, phenylpropanolamine hcl ▪ **Bronchodilator:** albuterol, albuterol sulfate, bitolterol mesylate, ephedrine & salts, epinephrine & salts, ethylnorepinephrine, isoetharine, isoproterenol hcl, isoproterenol sulfate, metaproterenol sulfate, terbutaline hcl ▪ **Nasal decongestant:** epinephrine hcl, ephedrine salts, naphazoline hcl, oxymetazoline hcl, phenylephrine hcl, phenylpropanolamine hcl, pseudoephedrine hcl, tetrahydrozoline hcl ▪ **Ophthalmic decongestant:** epinephrine hcl, naphazoline hcl, phenylephrine hcl, tetrahydrozoline hcl ▪ GLAUCOMA: (open angle): epinephrine hcl, dipivefrin ▪ MYDRIATRIC: epinephrine hcl, hydroxyamphetamine HBr, phenylephrine hcl ▪ SHOCK (inotropic/vasopressor activity): dobutamine, dopamine hcl, ephedrine sulfate, epinephrine hcl, isoproterenol hcl, mephentermine sulfate, metaraminol bitartrate, methoxamine hcl, norepinephrine bitartrate, phenylephrine hcl ▪ *See* individual drug cards for further information.

NURSING MANAGEMENT

ASSESS: Hx of catecholamine hypersensitivity ▪ Adequate renal function ▪ ABGs, lung sounds ▪ CAUTION: diabetes ▪ **ndx Therapeutic effects**: Ineffective airway clearance ▪ Ineffective breathing pattern ▪ ↓ Cardiac output ▪ High risk for injury ▪ Sleep pattern disturbance ▪ Altered tissue perfusion ▪ Altered patterns of urinary elimination. **PLAN:** Check preparation, dosage calculations c̄ another nurse ▪ Maintain IV access site, cardiac monitoring, hydration ▪ **Special considerations:** G: caution, ↓ dosage (↑ sensitivity) ▪ P: caution, ↓ dosage (↑ sensitivity) ▪ OB: avoid breastfeeding ▪ **Dietary management**: Avoid caffeine ▪ **Lab test evaluation:** ABGs, FBS (diabetics). **IMPLEMENT**: Utilize infusion control device for regulation ▪ Monitor VS closely ▪ Monitor I&O, lung sounds. **Patient Education**: Maintain fluid intake ▪ Avoid exposure to allergens, URI ▪ Report abnormal rxs to drug therapy (irregular, rapid heartbeat; difficult breathing). **EVALUATE**: **Observe for therapeutic effects:** ↑ BP ▪ ↑ Heart rate ▪ ↑ Force of cardiac contraction ▪ ↑ Air exchange.

DESCRIPTION: Group of diverse chemicals that block effects of catecholamines & alpha-adrenergics at postganglionic alpha adrenoreceptors in sympathetic nervous system.

DRUGS: Dihydroergotamine mesylate (*DHE 45*), ergoloid mesylates (*Gerimal, Hydergine*), ergotamine tartrate (*Ergostat*), methysergide maleate (*Sansert),* phenoxybenzamine hcl (*Dibenzyline*), phentolamine mesylate (*Regitine, *Rogitine hcl *Rogitine Mesylate*), tolazoline hcl (*Priscoline*).

MECHANISM OF ACTION: Agents exhibit varying degrees of competitive/noncompetitive alpha-adrenergic blocking activity; exhibit vasoconstrictor, oxytoxic, antiserotonin activity. Alpha-adrenergic blocking activity inhibits pressor effects of epinephrine on BP, opposes activity of norepinephrine.

THERAPEUTIC USE: Since introduction, these agents have been used for various conditions, esp hypertension, but poor clinical efficacy has ↓ usefulness for vascular headaches, maligant hypertension.

DOSAGE

Adult DHE	Vascular headache: 1mg IM. May be repeated twice at 1h intervals
Ergoloid	Symptomatic relief of senility: 1mg tid PO/SL
Ergotamine	Vascular headache: 1-2mg. May be repeated twice at 1/2h intervals
Methysergide	Vascular headache: 4-8mg/d PO
Phenoxybenzamine	Pheochromocytoma (hypertension): 10-40mg PO 2-3 times/d
Phentolamine	Pheochromocytoma (surgery & dx): 5mg IM/IV prn during surgery
Neonatal	
Tolazoline	Neonatal pulmonary hypertension: 1-2mg/kg IV followed by infusion of 1-2mg/kg/h

CONTRAINDICATIONS: Hypersensitivity, MI, coronary artery disease, peripheral vascular disease, pregnancy. *See* individual drug cards; specific contraindications vary.

SIDE/ADVERSE EFFECTS: CV: postural hypotension ▪ EENT: nasal stuffiness ▪ GI: gastric upset ▪ GU: oliguria, hematuria ▪ Other: ergotism (for ergot derivatives), N/V/D, cramps, drowsiness, dizziness, headache, mental confusion.

DRUG INTERACTIONS: Disulfiram-like reaction c̄ tolazoline, alcohol ▪ Phentolamine use in pediatric diabetics may ↑ antidiabetic effects ▪ Use of nonselective adrenergic agents c̄ phenoxybenzamine may produce hypotension, tachycardia.

NURSING MANAGEMENT

ASSESS: Hx of hypersensitivity ▪ BP ▪ Peripheral circulation ▪ CAUTION: coronary artery disease ▪ **ndx Therapeutic effects:** High risk for injury ▪ Altered tissue perfusion ▪ **Adverse effects:** Diarrhea ▪ High risk for fluid volume deficit ▪ High risk for injury ▪ Pain ▪ Altered tissue perfusion **PLAN:** Prevent postural hypotension ▪ **Special considerations:** G: caution (↑ hypotensive effects) ▪ P: caution (immature systems) ▪ OB: caution if pregnant, breastfeeding ▪ **Dietary management:** Avoid alcohol, high-Na^+ foods ▪ **Lab test evaluation**: Serum catecholamine, glucose. **IMPLEMENT:** Monitor BP ▪ Observe for hypotension ▪ Monitor peripheral circulation (skin color, temperature, pulses) ▪ Monitor CV, hepatic, renal status. **Patient education:** Avoid sudden position changes (postural hypotension) ▪ Comply c̄ prescribed drug regimen ▪ Avoid smoking, alcohol, constrictive clothing, extremely hot objects, OTC cough/cold/allergy preparations. **EVALUATE: Observe for therapeutic effects:** ↓ BP ▪ ↑ Peripheral circulation ▪ Relief of pain.

DESCRIPTION: Group of semisynthetic broad-spectrum, water-soluble, bactericidal antibiotics.

DRUGS: amikacin sulfate (*Amikin*), gentamicin sulfate (*Garamycin, *Cidomycin*), kanamycin sulfate (*Kantrex, *Anamid*), neomycin sulfate (*Mycifradin, Myciguent, *Neocin*), netilmicin sulfate (*Netromycin*), paromomycin sulfate (*Humatin*), streptomycin sulfate, tobramycin sulfate (*Nebcin, *Tobrex*).

MECHANISM OF ACTION: Bactericidal activity due to inhibition of ribosomal protein synthesis in susceptible organisms; neomycin limited to nonsystemic use because of high toxicity; paromomycin usually separated from group & classified c̄ amebicides.

THERAPEUTIC USE: Treatment of infections caused (combined spectrums) by susceptible strains ▪ The specific gram-negative spectrum does vary; selection of drug is based on the causative organism ▪ Treatment of tularemia, plague, TB (streptomycin) ▪ In combined therapy for enterococcal endocarditis ▪ Alternate for penicillin-resistant *Staphylococcus* infections ▪ In combination c̄ carbenicillin for treating stubborn *Pseudomonas* infections.

PHARMACOKINETICS

	IM peak	Half-life	Protein binding	Excretion
amikacin	1h	2h	0%-11%	92% unchanged in urine in 8h
gentamicin	1/2-1h	2-2 1/2h	0%-30%	70% unchanged in urine in 24h
kanamycin	1h	2-2 1/2h	—	50% unchanged in urine in 4h
netilmicin	1/2-1h	2-2 1/2h	0%-30%	80% unchanged in urine in 24h
streptomycin	1h	2-3h	35%	29%-89% unchanged in urine in 24h
tobramycin	1/2-1 1/2	2h	—	84% unchanged in urine in 8h

CONTRAINDICATIONS: Hypersensitivity, previous hx of serious aminoglycoside toxicity.

DOSAGE: Usual adult IM/IV range. Dosage must be ↓ in pts c̄ impaired renal function.

amikacin	15mg/kg/d in 2-3 doses. Do not exceed 1.5g/d
gentamicin	3-5mg/kg/d in 3-4 doses
kanamycin	7.5-15mg/kg/d in 2-3 doses
netilmicin	3-6.5mg/kg/d in 2-3 doses
streptomycin	1-4g/d
tobramycin	3-5mg/kg/d in 3 doses

SIDE/ADVERSE EFFECTS: EENT: ***ototoxicity*** ▪ GI: N/V ▪ GU: ***nephrotoxicity***, casts, proteinuria, ↑ BUN, ↑ NPN, serum creatinine ▪ HEM: anemia ▪ Other: arthralgia, convulsions, fever, hypotension (rare).

DRUG INTERACTIONS: Avoid use c̄ neurotoxic/ nephrotoxic drugs ▪ Dimenhydrinate can mask aminoglycoside toxicity ▪ Use c̄ succinylcholine, tubocurarine will ↑ their activity ▪ PO anticoagulant activity may ↑.

NURSING MANAGEMENT

ASSESS: Hx of hypersensitivity ▪ Baseline hearing status, renal function ▪ Peak, trough serum concentrations ▪ Pt weight for dose calculation ▪ CAUTION: renal failure ▪ **ndx Therapeutic effects:** High risk for altered body temperature ▪ High risk for infection ▪ Impaired skin/tissue integrity ▪ **Adverse effects:** Diarrhea ▪ High risk for fluid volume deficit, injury ▪ Sensory/perceptual alteration (auditory) ▪ High risk for impaired skin integrity ▪ Altered patterns of urinary elimination. **PLAN:** Maintain hydration ▪ Administer at equal intervals around clock to maintain blood levels ▪ **Special considerations:** G: caution, ↓ dosage (renal dysfunction) ▪ P: caution, ↓ dosage (prolonged half-life) ▪ OB: not recommended if pregnant; avoid if breastfeeding ▪ **Dietary management:** Encourage alkaline ash foods (UTI) ▪ **Lab test evaluation:** Peak, trough serum concentrations; BUN, serum creatinine. **IMPLEMENT:** Obtain C&S; check results ▪ Observe for signs of superinfection (diarrhea, URI, coated tongue) ▪ Monitor for hearing dysfunction, nephrotoxicity, neuromuscular blockade, respiratory paralysis. **PATIENT EDUCATION:** Report hearing, balance difficulties to physician at once ▪ ↑ Fluid intake (10-12 glasses/d) ▪ Notify physician of symptoms of allergic rx (fever, difficult breathing, rash, burning/stinging in eyes). **EVALUATE: Observe for therapeutic effect:** Resolution of infection.

DESCRIPTION: Group of antihypertensive drugs that inhibit ACE resulting in a hypotensive effect.

DRUGS: benazepril hcl (*Lotensin*), captopril (*Capoten*), enalapril maleate (*Vasotec*), enalaprilat (*Vasotec IV*), fosinopril sodium (*Monopril*), lisinopril (*Prinivil, Xestril*), quinapril hcl (*Accupril*), ramipril (*Altace*).

MECHANISM OF ACTION: Antihypertensive activity appears related to suppression of renin-angiotensin aldosterone system by competitive inhibition of ACE, which produces angiotensin II from angiotensin I, resulting in a ↓ of peripheral arterial resistance, ↓ in aldosterone secretion.

THERAPEUTIC USE: Treatment of hypertension as sole agent or in combination c̄ other antihypertensives. (Preg Cat C for 1st trimester, and Cat D for 2nd & 3rd trimesters).

CONTRAINDICATIONS: Hypersensitivity.

PHARMACOKINETICS

	PO absorption	Peak	Half-life	Protein binding	Excretion
benazepril	37%	0.5-1h	10-11h	96.7%	Via urine as metabolites
captopril	75%	1h	1-1.5h	25%-30%	95% via urine
enalapril	60%	1h	1.5h	NA	95% via urine in 24h
fosinopril	35%	3h	2-3h	95%	50% via urine, 50% via feces in 24h
lisinopril	25%	7h	6-7h	NA	98%-100% via urine in 24h
quinapril	60%	1h	2-3h	97%	96% via urine as metabolites
ramipril	50%-60%	1h	1h	73%	60% via urine, 40% via feces in 24h

DOSAGE: Adult *PO*

benazepril	20-40mg/d
captopril	50-100mg/d
enalapril	10-40mg/d
fosinopril	10mg/d
lisinopril	20-40mg/d
quinapril	10-80mg/d
ramipril	2.5-20mg/d

SIDE/ADVERSE EFFECTS: CNS: headache, dizziness, mood changes ▪ CV: hypotension, tachycardia, chest pain, palpitation, ***MI (rare), Raynaud's syndrome*** ▪ GI: V/D, pain, dyspepsia, gastroenteritis ▪ HEM: ***agranulocytosis***, anemia, *thrombocytosis*, neutropenia ▪ INT: rash, pruritus ▪ Other: loss of taste, proteinuria, hyperkalemia.

DRUG INTERACTIONS: Use c̄ aspirin, indomethacin, other NSAIAs may antagonize therapeutic response ▪ Use K^+-sparing diuretics c̄ caution due to hyperkalemia ▪ Concurrent use c̄ lithium can ↑ its toxicity.

NURSING MANAGEMENT

ASSESS: Hx of hypersensitivity ▪ BP ▪ Adequate renal function ▪ CAUTION: CV, hepatic, renal impairment ▪ **ndx Therapeutic effects**: ↓ Cardiac output ▪ Altered tissue perfusion ▪ **Adverse effects:** High risk for activity intolerance ▪ ↓ Cardiac output ▪ Fatigue ▪ High risk for injury ▪ Sensory/perceptual alterations ▪ High risk for impaired skin integrity. **PLAN**: Observe for edema in extremities ▪ Prevent postural hypotension ▪ **Special considerations:** G: caution, ↓ dosage (renal impairment) ▪ P: not recommended ▪ OB: avoid use if pregnant, breastfeeding ▪ **Dietary management**: Avoid high-Na^+/high-K^+ foods, alcohol; calorie restrictions ▪ **Lab test evaluation**: Electrolytes. **IMPLEMENT:** Monitor BP; observe for hypotension ▪ Monitor I&O, daily weight ▪ Monitor CV, hepatic, renal status. **Patient education:** Avoid sudden position changes (postural hypotension) ▪ Comply c̄ prescribed drug regimen ▪ Avoid smoking, alcohol, constrictive clothing, extremely hot objects, OTC cough/cold/allergy preparations ▪ Follow low-Na^+ diet ▪ Have BP checked regularly ▪ Keep appointments c̄ physician ▪ Carry medical identification (MedicAlert). **EVALUATE: Observe for therapeutic effect:** ↓ BP.

DESCRIPTION: Large group of OTC preparations available in assorted dosage preparations c̄ single/multiple antacid formulations; recent mass media advertisements stress Ca^{++}-containing formulas for osteoporosis, low-Na^{+}/Na^{+}-free preparations. Many preparations contain simethicone, which reduces gas, bloating.

DRUGS: Antacid chemicals used as sole agents or in combination c̄ other antacids include aluminum carbonate, aluminum hydroxide, aluminum phosphate, bismuth aluminate, calcium carbonate, dihydroxyaluminum aminoacetate, dihydroxyaluminum sodium carbonate, glycine, hydroxymagnesium aluminate, magaldrate, magnesium carbonate, magnesium hydroxide, magnesium oxide, magnesium trisilicate, sodium bicarbonate ▪ **Brand names:** *Alka-Seltzer, Alkets, ALternaGEL, Aludrox, *Alumag, Amphojel, Basaljel, Bisodol, Camalox, Chooz, Citrocarbonate, Discarbosil, Di-Gel, Equilet, Gaviscon, Gaviscon-2, Gelusil* preparations, *Maalox* preparations, *Magnatril, Milk of Magnesia, Mylanta, Mylanta-II, Nephrox, Noralac, Phosphaljel, Riopan* preparations, *Rolaids, Titralac, Tums, WinGel.*

MECHANISM OF ACTION: Chemical neutralization of rx.

THERAPEUTIC USE: Treatment of hyperacidity.

SIDE/ADVERSE EFFECTS: GI: diarrhea c̄ Mg preparations, esp Milk of Magnesia; constipation c̄ Al-, Ca- containing products ▪ MET: alkalosis (systemic products).

DRUG INTERACTIONS: Concurrent administration c̄ any drug *not* recommended because of poor PO absorption ▪ Contraindicated c̄ tetracycline therapy.

NURSING MANAGEMENT

ASSESS: GI, renal status ▪ Characteristics of discomfort ▪ CHF, hypertension, fluid retention (avoid Na^{+}-containing preparations) ▪ Renal impairment (avoid Mg^{++}-containing preparations) ▪ CAUTION: abdominal pain ▪ **ndx Therapeutic effects**: Pain ▪ **Adverse effects:** Constipation ▪ Diarrhea. **PLAN:** Avoid concurrent administration c̄ any drug; poor PO absorption results ▪ **Special considerations:** G: caution (⬇ GI motility; renal impairment) ▪ P: caution <6y/o (vague symptoms) ▪ OB: no reported pre-

*Available in Canada only.

cautions ▪ **Dietary management**: Avoid GI irritating foods ▪ **Lab test evaluation**: Serum electrolytes (long-term). **IMPLEMENT:** Shake PO suspensions well before pouring; follow c̄ H_2O to ensure reaching stomach ▪ Avoid concurrent drug administration, esp tetracycline & enteric-coated preparations ▪ Administer 1-3h pc & hs **PATIENT EDUCATION:** Comply c̄ prescribed dosage regimen ▪ Comply c̄ dietary restrictions ▪ Notify physician if GI distress persists or worsens (black, tarry stools; coffee-ground emesis). **EVALUATE: Observe for therapeutic effect:** ↓ GI distress.

DESCRIPTION: Antiarrhythmics (antidysrhythmics) are used to treat various cardiac arrhythmias.

DRUGS: Classified by pharmacologic/therapeutic drug categories, and effect produced on action potential of cardiac electrophysiology ▪ **Pharmacologic/therapeutic**: BETA BLOCKERS: acebutolol (*Sectral*), esmolol (*Brevibloc*), propranolol hcl (*Inderal*) ▪ CALCIUM BLOCKERS: verapammil hcl (*Calan, Isoptin*) ▪ CARDIAC GLYCOSIDES: digoxin (*Lanoxin*), digitoxin (*Crystodigin*) ▪ LOCAL ANESTHETICS/ DERIVATIVES: flecainide hcl (*Tambocor*), lidocaine hcl, mexiletine hcl (*Mexitil*), procainamide hcl (*Pronestyl*), propafenone hcl (*Rythmol*), tocainide hcl (*Tonocard*) ▪ QUINIDINE SALTS: quinidine gluconate (*Quinaglute*), quinidine polygalacturonate (*Cardioquin*), quinidine sulfate (*Quinidex*) ▪ MISCELLANEOUS: amiodarone hcl (*Cordarone*), bretylium tosylate (*Bretylol*) disopyramide (*Norpace*), moricizine hcl (*Ethmoxzine*) ▪ **Action potential:** Phase 0, rapid depolarization of ventricular cardiac tissue (QRS complex of ECG); phases 1, 2, 3, repolarization; phase 4, resting ▪ CLASS I DRUGS: (membrane stabilizing) depress phase 0: I—moricizine hcl (*Ethmozine*); IA—quinidine salts, disopyramide, procainamide; IB—lidocaine, mexiletine, tocainide; IC—flecainide, propafenone ▪ CLASS II DRUGS: beta adrenergic blockers, depress phase 4 depolarization: acebutolol, esmolol, propranolol hcl ▪ CLASS III DRUGS: prolong repolarization in phase 3: amiodarone hcl, bretylium tosylate ▪ CLASS IV DRUGS: calcium blockers, depress phase 4 depolarization, prolong repolarization of phases 1, 2: cardiac glycosides, verapamil hcl.

DOSAGE: Usual adult range

acebutolol *PO*	600-1200mg/d divided
amiodarone *PO*	800-1600mg/d divided
bretylium *IV*	5-10mg/kg
digitoxin *PO*	0.05-0.3mg/d
digoxin *PO*	0.125-0.5mg/d
disopyramide *PO*	400-800mg/d divided
esmolol *IV*	500µg/kg/m, then 50-100µg/kg/4m
flecainide *PO*	100-600mg/d divided
lidocaine *IV*	50-100mg c̅ 1-4mg/m maintenance
mexilitine *PO*	200mg q8h
moricizine *PO*	600-900mg/d divided
procainamide *PO*	0.5-1g q4-6h (atrial) 50mg/kg divided q3h then adjusted (ventricular)

propafenone *PO*	450-900mg/d divided
propranolol *PO*	10-30mg 3-4 times/d 180-240mg/d divided (MI prevention)
quinidine gluconate *PO*	324-648mg q8-12h
quinidine poly-galacturonate *PO*	275mg 3-4 times/d
quinidine sulfate *PO*	0.2-0.3g 3-4 times/d (premature atrial/ventricular contractions)
tocainide *PO*	1200-1800mg in 3 doses
verapamil *PO*	320-480mg/d divided

NURSING MANAGEMENT

ASSESS: Hx of hypersensitivity ▪ Apical pulse, BP, ECG ▪ Lung sounds ▪ Therapeutic blood level ▪ CAUTION: heart failure ▪ **ndx Therapeutic effects:** ↓ Cardiac output ▪ Altered tissue perfusion ▪ **Adverse effects:** High risk for activity intolerance ▪ ↓ Cardiac output ▪ Constipation ▪ Diarrhea ▪ High risk for fluid volume deficit ▪ Altered thought processes ▪ Impaired tissue integrity (oral mucous membrane) ▪ Altered patterns of urinary elimination. **PLAN:** Institute cardiac monitoring (IV, initial PO) ▪ Administer at equal intervals around clock to maintain blood levels ▪ **Special considerations:** G: caution, ↓ dosage (↓ metabolism; chronic illness) ▪ P: caution (immature systems) ▪ OB: caution if pregnant; breastfeeding not recommended ▪ **Dietary management:** Avoid caffeine, alcohol, Na^+-containing foods ▪ **Lab test evaluation:** Therapeutic blood levels. **IMPLEMENT:** Assess apical pulse for 1m ▪ Monitor F/E status (I&O, daily weight, peripheral edema). **PATIENT EDUCATION:** Procedure for checking radial pulse ▪ Comply c̄ prescribed dosage regimen ▪ Report abnormal rxs to physician (difficult breathing; rapid, irregular heart rate) ▪ Check c̄ physician/pharmacist before taking OTC preparations ▪ Keep appointments c̄ physician ▪ Carry identification (MedicAlert). **EVALUATE: Observe for therapeutic effects:** ↓ Cardiac arrhythmias ▪ Normal heart rate, rhythm.

DESCRIPTION: Large, diverse group of natural, semisynthetic & synthetic drugs that block effects of acetylcholine at postganglionic parasympathetic muscarinic receptors; also known as antimuscarinics, parasympatholytics. Natural drugs obtained from deadly nightshade plants, including *Atropa belladonna, Hyoscyamus* (henbane).

DRUGS: ▪ **Natural:** atropine sulfate, belladonna tincture/extract (**Belladenal, *Belladenal Spacetabs*), hyoscyamine (*Cystospaz*), hyoscyamine sulfate (*Anaspaz, Cystospaz-M, Levsin*), *hyoscine hydrobromide, scopolamine (*Transderm-Scop*), scopolamine hydrobromide (*Triptone*) ▪ **Semisynthetic:** homatropine hydrobromide *(*Isopto Homatropine)* ▪ **Synthetic:** anisotropine methylbromide, clidinium bromide (*Quarzan, Librax, Menrium*), dicyclomine hcl (*Bentyl, Byclomine*), glycopyrrolate (*Robinul*), hexocyclium methylsulfate, isopropamide iodide (*Darbid*), mepenzolate bromide (*Cantil*), methantheline bromide (*Banthine*), oxyphencyclimine hcl (*Daricon*), propantheline bromide (*Pro-Banthine*), tridihexethyl chloride (*Pathilon*).

MECHANISM OF ACTION: Anticholinergic activity due to competition c̄ acetylcholine for receptors at postganglionic fiber of parasympathetic nervous system, resulting in biliary dilation, bronchial dilation, cycloplegia, ↓ gastric secretion, ↓ GI motility, ↓ salivation, ↓ sweating, drying of mucous membranes, ↑ IOP, mydriasis, tachycardia, urinary retention.

THERAPEUTIC USE: Treat/manage/cause bradycardia, bronchial asthma (cholinergic mediated), cardiospasm, colitis, dilation of pupils, dysmenorrhea relief, enuresis control, GI spasm; inhibition of bronchial/gastric secretions, salivation, sweating; paralysis of accommodation, pylorospasm; secretion due to coryza, hay fever, rhinitis; spastic/rigid states due to CNS injury; ureteral colic, urinary frequency reduction.

CONTRAINDICATIONS: Adhesions, advanced hepatic/renal impairment, asthma, hiatal hernia associated c̄ reflux esophagitis, hypersensitivity, intestinal atony, myasthenia gravis, narrow-angle glaucoma, obstructive diseases of GI/urinary tract, severe ulcerative colitis.

DOSAGE: Usual adult *PO*

anisotropine	50mg tid
atropine	0.1-0.5mg q4-6h
belladonna extract	15mg 3-4 times/d
belladonna tincture	0.3-1ml 3-4 times/d
clidinium	2.5-5mg 3-4 times/d
dicyclomine	40mg 4 times/d
glycopyrrolate	1-2mg tid
homatropine	5-10mg tid
hyoscyamine	0.15-0.3mg qid
isopropamide	5mg q12h
methantheline	50-100mg q6h
methscopolamine	2.5-3mg qid
oxyphencyclimine	5-10mg bid
propantheline	15mg tid
scopolamine	0.4-0.8mg 3-4 times/d
tridihexethyl chloride	25-50mg 3-4 times/d

SIDE/ADVERSE EFFECTS: CNS: mental confusion ▪ CV: tachycardia ▪ EENT: blurred vision, cycloplegia, mydriasis ↓ ocular tension, photophobia ▪ GU: urinary retention ▪ GI: N/V, constipation ▪ Other: suppression of lactation/body secretions, rash.

DRUG INTERACTIONS: Use c̄ antihistamines, phenothiazines, tricyclic antidepressants produces ↑ anticholinergic effects ▪ MAO-I ↑ activity by ↓ anticholinergic biotransformation ▪ Use c̄ other drugs ↑ their GI absorption.

NURSING MANAGEMENT

ASSESS: Hx of hypersensitivity ▪ VS, esp heart rate, BP ▪ Urinary retention ▪ Bowel sounds, GI status ▪ CAUTION: hepatic/renal impairment, cardiopulmonary disease, GI/urinary tract obstruction ▪ **ndx Therapeutic effects:** ↓ Cardiac output ▪ Diarrhea ▪ Fluid volume deficit ▪ Impaired physical mobility. **Adverse effects:** ↓ Cardiac output ▪ Sensory/perceptual alterations (visual) ▪ Altered thought processes ▪ Impaired tissue integrity (oral mucous membrane) ▪ Urinary retention. **PLAN:** Check all dosages carefully ▪ **Special considerations:** G: caution, ↓ dosage (↑ sensitivity) ▪ P: not recommended ▪ OB: caution if pregnant; avoid breastfeeding ▪ **Dietary management:** ↑ Bulk-containing foods (constipation) ▪ **Lab test evaluation:** None specific. **IMPLEMENT:** Monitor VS, esp heart rate ▪ Observe for exaggerated anticholinergic effects ▪ Monitor I&O, GI function. **PATIENT EDUCATION:** Expect anticholinergic side effects (dry mouth, photophobia, constipation) ▪ Blurred vision may occur ▪ Protect eyes in sunlight ▪ Use sugarless gum/hard candy to diminish dry mouth ▪ Frequent oral hygiene is required ▪ Avoid OTC cough/cold/allergy preparations. **EVALUATE: Observe for therapeutic effect:** ↓ Parasympathetic activity.

DESCRIPTION: Anticonvulsants (antiepileptics) are composed of several chemically distinct groups of drugs that selectively depress CNS to prevent epileptic seizures w/out impairing consciousness. Epilepsy is not a specific disease, but assortment of convulsive symptoms, precipitated by abnormal focus of neuronal discharges that originates in brain, esp motor cortex ▪ Disease categorized by specific EEG patterns & clinical nature of seizures. Therapy must always be individualized to specific seizure patterns, because no anticonvulsant drug equally effective in treating various forms of epilepsy ▪ It is generally accepted that anticonvulsant drugs prevent seizures by acting on nonneuronal cells & therefore have some indirect effect on seizure center (eg, vascular blood supply) ▪ Acting to prevent hyperactive neuron discharge located in the epileptic seizure focus ▪ Acting to prevent seizure spread to normal neurons located near seizure focus.

DRUGS: ▪ **Barbiturates:** mephobarbital (*Mebaral*), phenobarbital (*Luminal*), primidone (*Mysoline*) ▪ **Benzodiazephine:** clonazepam (*Klonopin*), diazepam (*Valium*) ▪ **Hydantoins:** ethotoin (*Peganone*), mephenytoin (*Mesantoin*), phenytoin (*Dilantin*) ▪ **Oxazolidinediones:** paramethadione (*Paradione*), trimethadione (*Tridione*) ▪ **Succinimides:** ethosuximide (*Zarontin*), methsuximide (*Celontin*), phensuximide (*Milontin*) ▪ **Miscellaneous:** acetazolamide (*Diamox*), carbamazepine (*Tegretol*), divalproex sodium (*Depakote*), magnesium sulfate, valproic acid (*Depakene*).

THERAPEUTIC USE: Absence seizures: acetazolamide, clonazepam, oxazolidinediones, succinimides (esp ethosuximide), valproic acid ▪ **Generalized tonic-clonic/ focal seizures:** barbiturates (esp phenobarbital), carbamazepine, hydantoins (esp phenytoin) ▪ **Psychomotor:** carbamazepine, hydantoin, primidone ▪ **Status epilepticus:** diazepam, phenytoin ▪ **Miscellaneous:** (seizures associated c̄ preeclampsia, eclampsia, cerebral edema, glomerulonephritis): magnesium sulfate.

DOSAGE: Usual adult *PO* range

acetazolamide	375mg-1g/d
carbamazepine	800-1200mg/d
clonazepam	0.1-0.2mg/kg/d
diazepam	2-10mg 2-4 times/d

divalproex sodium	15-60mg/kg/d
ethosuximide	0.5-1.5g/d
ethotoin	2-3g/d in 4-6 divided doses
magnesium sulfate	1-5g prn *IM*
mephenytoin	0.2-0.6g/d
mephobarbital	400-600mg/d
methsuximide	0.3-1.2g/d
paramethadione	300-600mg 3-4 times/d
phenobarbital	50-100mg 2-3 times/d
phensuximide	1-3g/d
phenytoin	300-600mg/d
primidone	250-500mg 3-4 times/d
trimethadione	300-600mg 3-4 times/d
valproic acid	15-60mg/kg/d

NURSING MANAGEMENT

ASSESS: Hx of hypersensitivity ▪ Neurologic status ▪ Seizure activity characteristics ▪ Therapeutic blood levels ▪ CAUTION: hepatic, hemopoietic, renal impairment ▪ **ndx Therapeutic effects:** High risk for injury ▪ Sensory/perceptual alterations ▪ **Adverse effects:** High risk for injury ▪ Sensory/perceptual alterations (visual) ▪ High risk for impaired skin integrity ▪ Altered thought processes ▪ Impaired tissue integrity. **PLAN:** Institute seizure precautions ▪ Maintain safety precautions ▪ Administer at equal intervals around clock to maintain blood levels ▪ **Special considerations:** G: caution, ↓ dosage (↓ metabolism) ▪ P: caution (check dosage forms carefully) ▪ OB: caution if pregnant; avoid breastfeeding ▪ **Dietary management:** Avoid alcohol ▪ **Lab test evaluation**: Therapeutic blood levels. **IMPLEMENT:** Monitor VS ▪ PO: administer c̄ food to ↓ GI irritation ▪ Avoid mixing parenteral dosage forms c̄ other IV preparations ▪ Avoid abrupt withdrawal ▪ Monitor neurologic status, incl seizure characteristics. **PATIENT EDUCATION:** Comply c̄ prescribed therapy; take at equal intervals, do *not* omit doses ▪ Avoid use c̄ alcohol ▪ Take safety precautions c̄ hazardous activity ▪ Frequent oral hygiene is required (phenytoin) ▪ Keep scheduled appointments c̄ physician/for blood work ▪ Carry medical identification (MedicAlert). **EVALUATE: Observe for therapeutic effect:** ↓ /Absent seizure activity.

DESCRIPTION: Diverse group of drugs classified as H_1 or H_2 blockers; term "antihistamine" usually reserved for H_1 blockers (H_1 receptor antagonists); H_2 blockers (H_2 receptor antagonists) are newer, smaller group, used for GI disorders.

DRUGS: ▪ **H_1 blockers:** astemizole (*Hismanal*), azatadine maleate (*Optimine*), brompheniramine maleate (*Dimetane*), chlorpheniramine maleate (*Chlor-Trimeton, *Chlorphen, *Novopheniram*), clemastine fumarate (*Tavist*), cyproheptadine hcl (*Periactin, *Vimicon*), dexchlorpheniramine maleate (*Polaramine*), diphenhydramine hcl (**Allerdryl, Benadryl*), doxylamine succinate (*Unisom Sleep-Aid*), loratadine (*Claritin*), methdilazine (*Tacaryl, *Dilosyn*), promethazine hcl (**Histanil, Phenergan, *Rhinaris*), terfenadine (*Seldane*), trimeprazine tartrate (*Panectyl, Temaril*), tripelennamine hcl (*PBZ, *Pyribenzamine hcl*), triprolidine hcl (*Actidil*) ▪ **H_2 blockers:** cimetidine (*Tagamet, *Novocimetine, Peptol*), cimetidine hcl (*Tagamet hcl*), famotidine (*Pepcid*), nizatidine (*Azid*), ranitidine hcl (*Zantac*).

MECHANISM OF ACTION: H_1 antihistamines antagonize effects of histamine by selectively/competitively occupying H_1 histamine receptors on peripheral effector cells. H_2 antagonists inhibit effects of histamine by selectively/competitively occupying H_2 histamine receptors on parietal cells.

THERAPEUTIC USE: H_1 blockers: Allergies: all medications listed ▪ Motion sickness; buclizine, cyclizine, dimenhydrinate, diphenhydramine, meclizine, promethazine ▪ Parkinsonism: diphenhydramine ▪ Sleep: diphenhydramine, doxylamine ▪ Vertigo: buclizine, dimenhydrinate, meclizine.

CONTRAINDICATIONS: Hypersensitivity, neonates, nursing mothers, lower respiratory tract symptoms (incl asthma).

DOSAGE: Adult *PO*

astemizole	10mg once/d
azatadine	1-2mg bid
brompheniramine	4-8mg 3-4 times/d
chlorpheniramine	4mg q4-6h
clemastine	1.34-2.68mg 1-3 times/d
cyproheptadine	4mg 3-4 times/d
dexchlorpheniramine	2mg 3-4 times/d

diphenhydramine	25-50mg 3/4 times/d
doxylamine	25mg hs
loratadine	10mg once/d ac
methdilazine	8mg 2-4 times/d
promethazine	12.5-25mg tid
terfenadine	60mg bid
trimeprazine	2.5mg qid
tripelennamine	25-50mg q4-6d
triprolidine	2.5mg q4-6h

SIDE/ADVERSE EFFECTS: CNS: *drowsiness*, dizziness, fatigue, euphoria, paresthesias ▪ CV: hypotension, palpitations, tachycardia, extrasystole ▪ EENT: blurred vision, nasal stuffiness ▪ GI: N/V, anorexia ▪ HEM: ***agranulocytosis, hemolytic anemia, thrombocytopenia*** ▪ RESP: wheezing, thickening of bronchial secretions ▪ Other: anticholinergic effects.

DRUG INTERACTIONS: Use c̄ anticholinergics or CNS depressants produces additive effects ▪ MAO-I can intensify anticholinergic effects of antihistamines.

NURSING MANAGEMENT
ASSESS: Hx of hypersensitivity ▪ Allergy symptoms ▪ Lung sounds ▪ CAUTION: GI, cardiac, hepatic impairment; pregnancy, lactation ▪ **ndx Therapeutic effects**: Ineffective airway clearance ▪ Anxiety ▪ Ineffective breathing pattern ▪ High risk for fluid volume deficit ▪ High risk for injury ▪ Impaired skin integrity ▪ **Adverse effects:** High risk for activity intolerance ▪ Sensory/perceptual alterations (visual) ▪ High risk for impaired skin integrity ▪ Impaired tissue integrity (oral mucous membrane) ▪ Altered patterns of urinary elimination. **PLAN:** Maintain hydration ▪ **Special considerations:** G: caution, ↓ dosage (↑ sensitivity; chronic illness) ▪ P: caution, ↓ dosage (paradoxic rx) ▪ OB: caution if pregnant; avoid breastfeeding ▪ **Dietary management**: Avoid alcohol ▪ **Lab test evaluation**: CBC (c̄ prolonged therapy). **IMPLEMENT:** Administer PO forms c̄ meals ▪ Monitor VS, esp BP ▪ Monitor activity status ▪ Monitor children for paradoxic rxs (CNS stimulation). **PATIENT EDUCATION:** Drowsiness, dizziness may occur ▪ Avoid potentially hazardous activity ▪ Take PO forms c̄ meals ▪ ↑ Fluid intake ▪ Avoid CNS depressants, incl alcohol ▪ Use sugarless gum/hard candy to diminish dry mouth. **EVALUATE: Observe for therapeutic effects:** ↓ Cold/ allergy symptoms.

DESCRIPTION: Drugs used in treatment of essential (1°), malignant (2°) hypertension; antihypertensives are large category of therapeutic drugs that exhibit various hypotensive pharmacologic mechanisms.

DRUGS: Alteration of catecholamine synthesis: Hypotensive mechanism that ↓ catecholamine synthesis (metyrosine) or produces synthesis of alpha-methyl norepinephrine (methyldopa), which stimulates central inhibitory alpha adrenergic receptors: methyldopa (*Aldomet*), methyldopate hcl (*Aldomet*), metyrosine (*Demser*) ▪ **Alpha adrenergic activity:** Hypotensive effect probably due to central alpha adrenergic activity c̄ $alpha_1$ or $alpha_2$ receptors: clonidine hcl (*Catapres*), doxazosin mesylate (*Cardura*), guanabenz acetate (*Sytensin*), guanfacine (*Tenex*), terazosin hcl (*Hytrin*) ▪ **Angiotensin inhibition:** Inhibition of angiotensin-converting enzyme blocks conversion of angiotensin I to angiotensin II, resulting in hypotensive effect: benazepril (*Lotensin*), captopril (*Capoten*), enalapril maleate (*Vasotec*), fosinopril (*Monopril*), lisinopril (*Prinivil, Zestril*), quinapril hcl (*Accupril*), ramipril (*Altace*) ▪ **Beta adrenergic blockage:** Exact antihypertensive mechanism not determined: acebutolol hcl (*Sectral),* atenolol (*Tenormin*), betaxolol hcl (*Kerlone*), carteolol (*Cartrol*), labetatol (*Normodyne, Trandate* [alpha-beta blocker]), metoprolol tartrate (*Lopressor*), nadolol *(Corgard*), penbutolol (*Levatol*), pindolol (*Visken*), propranolol hcl (*Inderal*), timolol maleate (*Blocadren*) ▪ **Calcium blockers:** Amlodipine (*Norvasac*), diltiazem (*Cardizem*—only SR dosage forms), felodipine *(Plendil*), isradipine (*DynaCirc),* nicardipine (*Cardene*), nifedipine (*Procardia*—only SR dosage formed), verapamil (*Calan, Isoptin, Verelan*—only SR dosage forms) ▪ **Direct vasodilators:** diazoxide (*Hyperstat IV*), hydralazine hcl (*Apresoline*), minoxidil (*Loniten*), prazosin hcl (*Minipress*), sodium nitroprusside (*Nipride, Nitropress*) ▪ **Ganglionic blockers:** Produce hypotensive effect by blocking autonomic ganglia transmission; primarily used in treatment of malignant hypertension (mecamylamine hcl [*Inversine*]), hypertensive emergencies (trimethaphan camsylate [*Arfonad*]) ▪ **MAO-Is:** Exact antihypertensive mechanism not determined: pargyline hcl (*Eutony*) ▪ **Norepinephrine depletors:** Hypotensive effect probably due to slow depletion of norepinephrine in adrenergic fibers, esp in vascular smooth muscle: deserpidine, guanadrel monosulfate (*Hylorel*), guanethidine sulfate (*Ismelin Sulfate*), *Rauwolfia serpentina (Raudixin)*, rescinnamine (*Moderil*), reserpine (*Serpalan, Serpasil*) ▪ **Diuretics:** amiloride hcl (*Midamor*), bendroflumethiazide (*Naturetin*), bumetanide (*Bumex*), chlorothiazide (*Diachlor, Diuril*), chlorthalidone (*Hygroton, Thalitone*), ethacrynic acid (*Edecrin*), furosemide (*Lasix*), hydrochlorothiazide (*Esidrix, Hydrodiuril, Thiuretic*), hydroflumethiazide (*Diucardin, Saluron*), indapamide (*Lozol*), methyclothiazide (*Aquatensen, Enduron*), metolazone (*Diulo*), polythiazide (*Renese*), quinethazone (*Hydromox*), spironolactone (*Aldactone*), triamterene (*Dyrenium*), trichlormethiazide (*Metahydrin, Naqua*) ▪ **Miscellaneous:** nitroglycerin IV (*Nitrobid, Nitrol IV, Nitrostat IV, Tridil*), phenoxybenzamine hcl (*Dibenzyline* [malignant hypertension]).

DOSAGE: Adult *PO**

deserpidine	0.25-1mg/d
doxazosin	1-16mg/d
guanadrel	20-75mg/d
mecamylamine	2.5-25mg/d
metyroxine	1-4g/d
rauwolfia	50-300mg/d
rescinnamine	0.25-0.5mg/d
terazosin	1-5mg/d

*Consult category cards or individual drug card for other doses.

NURSING MANAGEMENT

ASSESS: Hx of hypersensitivity ▪ BP ▪ Adequate renal function ▪ CAUTION: CV, hepatic, renal impairment ▪ **ndx Therapeutic effects:** ↓ Cardiac output ▪ Altered tissue perfusion ▪ **Adverse effects:** High risk for activity intolerance ▪ ↓ Cardiac output ▪ Fatigue ▪ High risk for injury ▪ Sensory/perceptual alterations ▪ Sexual dysfunction ▪ High risk for impaired skin integrity. **PLAN:** Observe extremities for edema ▪ Prevent postural hypotension ▪ **Special considerations:** G: caution (↑ hypotensive effects; chronic illness) ▪ P: caution (immature systems) ▪ OB: caution if pregnant, breastfeeding ▪ **Dietary management:** Avoid high-Na^+ foods, alcohol; calorie restrictions ▪ **Lab test evaluation:** Electrolytes. **IMPLEMENT:** Monitor BP; observe for hypotension ▪ Monitor I&O, daily weight ▪ Monitor CV, hepatic, renal status. **PATIENT EDUCATION:** Avoid sudden position changes (postural hypotension) ▪ Comply c̄ prescribed drug regimen ▪ Avoid smoking, alcohol, constrictive clothing, extremely hot objects, OTC cough/cold/allergy preparations ▪ Follow low-Na^+ diet ▪ Have BP checked regularly ▪ Keep appointments c̄ physician ▪ Carry identification (MedicAlert). **EVALUATE: Observe for therapeutic effect:** ↓ BP.

DESCRIPTION: Large group of highly reactive cytotoxic cycle phase nonspecific agents that have polyfunctional alkylating properties; main alkylating effect on DNA, resulting in disruption of DNA replication; many alkylating agents also interfere c̄ RNA transcription.

DRUGS: busulfan *(Myleran),* carboplatin *(Paraplatin),* carmustine *(BiCNU),* chlorambucil *(Leukeran),* cisplatin (Platinol), cyclophosphamide *(Cyoxan, Neosar, *Procytox),* decarbazine *(*DTIC, DTIC-Dome),* ifosfamide *(Ifex),* lomustine *(*CCNU, CeeNU),* mechlorethamine *(Mustargen),* melphalan *(Alkeran),* pipobroman *(Vercyte),* streptozocin *(Zanosar),* thiotepa, uracil mustard.

MECHANISM OF ACTION: These agents add alkyl groups (alkylation) to DNA in exchange for hydrogen ions; resulting alkylation interferes c̄ DNA replication, RNA transcription, which is usually cytoxic, most lethal type of alkylation produces crosslinking of DNA strands. Alkylating agents not specific in cytoxic effects, & interact c̄ rapidly dividing normal body cells; therefore they are highly toxic agents c̄ array of significant adverse effects, esp bone marrow & immune suppression.

THERAPEUTIC USE: Treatment of various neoplasms as sole agent, or in combination antineoplastic chemotherapy, usually preferred because it produces greater results, ↑ remissions in many types of carcinomas.

CONTRAINDICATIONS: Hypersensitivity, pts who exhibit unacceptable toxic effect from previous chemotherapy/radiation.

SIDE/ADVERSE EFFECTS: GI: N/D, oral ulcers, hemorrhagic colitis ▪ GU: cystitis, hemorrhagic cystitis, fibrosis, amenorrhea ▪ HEM: ***bone marrow depression*** resulting in anemia, leukopenia, neutropenia, pancytopenia, ***thrombocytopenia*** ▪ HEP: ***hepatotoxicity*** ▪ INT: alopecia, pigmentation ▪ Other: **2°** ***malignancies, pulmonary fibrosis.***

DRUG INTERACTIONS: Vaccinations c̄ live vaccines contraindicated during therapy ▪ Use c̄ steroids produces addictive immunosuppressant activity ▪ Radiation therapy, other myelosuppressive drugs produce additive bone marrow depression.

Note: Side/adverse effects: common in *italic;* serious in ***boldface italic.***

*Available in Canada only.

NURSING MANAGEMENT

ASSESS: Hx of previous radiation, antineoplastic therapy ▪ Infection, bleeding, anemia ▪ CAUTION: bone marrow depression, acute infection, sexually active females ▪ **ndx Therapeutic effects:** Impaired tissue integrity ▪ **Adverse effects:** High risk for activity intolerance ▪ Diarrhea ▪ Fatigue ▪ High risk for fluid volume deficit ▪ High risk for infection ▪ Altered nutrition: less than body requirement ▪ Impaired tissue integrity (oral mucous membrane). **PLAN:** Maintain optimum hydration ▪ Adminsiter antiemetic as ordered ▪ Display hopeful approach ▪ Encourage ventilation of feelings ▪ **Special considerations:** G: caution, ↓ dosage (↑ sensitivity) ▪ P: caution (immature systems) ▪ OB: avoid use if pregnant, breastfeeding ▪ **Dietary management:** Avoid spicy foods, institute methods to stimulate appetite ▪ **Lab test evaluation:** CBC, platelets, serum uric acid. **IMPLEMENT:** Force fluids ▪ Observe for infection, bleeding, anemia ▪ Monitor hepatic, renal function ▪ IV: check site closely, avoid extravasation ▪ Observe for gout symptoms (↑ serum uric acid) ▪ Monitor I&O, daily weight ▪ Provide emotional support. **PATIENT EDUCATION:** Comply $\bar{c}$ prescribed dosage regimen ▪ ↑ Fluid intake (10-12 glasses/d) ▪ Avoid exposure to infection ▪ Diet as tolerated; avoid spicy foods ▪ Maintain good oral hygiene; use soft-bristled toothbrush ▪ Notify physician of symptoms of bone marrow depression (fever, sore throat, bruising, bleeding, lethargy) ▪ Side effects are reversible ▪ Take measures to conserve energy ▪ Use contraceptives if sexually active ▪ Check $\bar{c}$ physician before immunization ▪ Keep scheduled appointments $\bar{c}$ physician/for blood work. **EVALUATE: Observe for therapeutic effects:** ↓ Proliferation of malignant cells ▪ Regression of tumor.

DESCRIPTION: Small, diverse group of cytotoxic drugs that are chemical analogs of folic acid, nucleic acid purines, or pyrimidines; produce antineoplastic effects by interfering c̄ various cellular metabolic pathways.

DRUGS: Folic acid antagonists: Inhibit metabolism of folic acid by blocking enzyme dihydrofolate reductase: methotrexate (amethopterin MTX), (Folex PFS, Rheumatrex Dose Pack) ▪ **Purine antagonists:** Antineoplastic activity due to inhibition of purine pathways, ultimately resulting in DNA, RNA synthesis inhibition: fludarabine phosphate (Fludara), mercaptopurine *(Purinethol),* thioguanine ▪ **Pyrimidine antagonists:** Inhibit DNA, RNA synthesis by interfering c̄ pyrimidine metabolic pathways: cytarabine *(Cytosar-U),* floxuridine *(FUDR),* fluorouracil (5FU) *(Adrucil).*

NURSING MANAGEMENT

ASSESS: Hx of previous radiation, antineoplastic therapy ▪ Infection, bleeding, anemia ▪ CAUTION: bone marrow depression, acute infection, sexually active females ▪ **ndx Therapeutic effects:** Impaired tissue integrity ▪ **Adverse effects:** High risk for activity intolerance ▪ Diarrhea ▪ Fatigue ▪ High risk for fluid volume deficit ▪ High risk for infection ▪ Altered nutrition: less that body requirement ▪ Impaired tissue integrity (oral mucous membrane). **PLAN:** Maintain optimum hydration ▪ Administer antiemetic as ordered ▪ Display hopeful approach ▪ Encourage ventilation of feelings ▪ **Special considerations:** G: caution, ↓ dosage (↑ sensitivity) ▪ P: caution (immature systems) ▪ OB: avoid use if pregnant, breastfeeding ▪ **Dietary management:** Avoid spicy foods, institute methods to stimulate appetite ▪ **Lab test evaluation:** CBC, platelets, serum uric acid. **IMPLEMENT:** Force fluids ▪ Observe for infection, bleeding, anemia ▪ Monitor hepatic, renal function ▪ IV: check site closely, avoid extravasation ▪ Observe for gout symptoms (↑ serum uric acid) ▪ Monitor I&O, daily weight ▪ Provide emotional support. **PATIENT EDUCATION:** Comply c̄ prescribed dosage regimen ▪ ↑ Fluid intake (10-12 glasses/d) ▪ Avoid exposure to infection ▪ Diet as tolerated; avoid spicy foods ▪ Maintain good oral hygiene; use soft-bristled toothbrush ▪ Notify physician of symptoms of bone marrow depression (fever, sore throat, bruising, bleeding, lethargy) ▪ Side effects are reversible ▪ Take measure to conserve energy ▪ Use contraceptives if sexually active ▪

Check $\bar{c}$ physician before immunization ▪ Keep scheduled appointments $\bar{c}$ physician/for blood work. **EVALUATE: Observe for therapeutic effects:** ↓ Proliferation of malignant cells ▪ Regression of tumor.

DESCRIPTION: Symptoms of Parkinson disease primarily due to imbalance between central dopaminergic & cholinergic mechanisms; pathophysiology of disorder due to tissue degeneration w/in basal ganglia of brain, resulting in low concentrations of dopamine, esp in corpus striatum, substantia nigra; cholinergic transmission becomes hyperactive, intensifying symptoms ▪ Dopamine has inhibitory effect in nigrostriatal system, acetylcholine produces excitatory effects; drug therapy must either restore dopamine levels or antagonize hyperactive cholinergic activity. Until recently, classic treatment for disorder included anticholinergic drugs that could penetrate blood-brain barrier to ↓ cholinergic activity. Most effective treatment currently available is dopamine replacement therapy c̄ levodopa (biologic precursor of dopamine); levodopa enters brain after administration, is converted into dopamine by enzyme dopa decarboxylase. Dopamine cannot be used because it does not penetrate blood-brain barrier. Centrally acting direct/indirect dopaminergics also used ▪ Activity of levodopa can be augmented by concurrent use of carbidopa (dopa decarboxylase enzyme inhibitor that cannot enter brain), which inhibits peripheral dopa decarboxylase activity, & therefore more levodopa available to cross blood-brain barrier.

DRUGS: ▪ **Anticholinergic drugs**: benztropine mesylate (*Cogentin*), biperiden hcl (*Akineton*), procyclidine hcl (*Kemadrin*), trihexyphenidyl hcl (*Artane*) ▪ **Antihistamines** (c̄ anticholinergic activity): diphenhydramine hcl (*Benadryl*), ethopropazine hcl (*Parisdol*) ▪ **Dopaminergic agents:** REPLACEMENT: carbidopa (*Lodosyn*), levodopa (*Dopar, Larodopa*), levodopa-carbidopa (*Sinemet 10/100, 25/100,, 25/250*) ▪ DIRECT ACTING: (on dopamine receptors); bromocriptine mesylate (*Parlodel*), pergolide mesylate (*Permax*), selegiline (*Elderpryl*) ▪ INDIRECT ACTING: (may block dopamine reuptake/cause its release): amantadine hcl (*Symmetrel*).

DOSAGE: Usual adult *PO*

amantadine	100-400mg/d divided
benztropine	1-2mg/d c̄ range of 0.5-6mg/d
biperidine	2mg 3-4 times/d
bromocriptine	Maximum of 100mg/d divided
carbidopa	Maximum of 200mg/d in combination c̄ levodopa
diphenhydramine	25-50mg 3-4 times/d
ethopropazine	100-600mg/d divided
pergolide	Maximum of 5mg/d in combination c̄ levodopa-carbidopa
procyclidine	2.5-5mg tid

selegiline	5mg bid in combination c̄ levodopa-carbidopa
trihexphenidyl	6-10mg/d divided

NURSING MANAGEMENT

ASSESS: Hx of hypersensitivity ▪ BP ▪ Parkinson & extrapyramidal symptoms ▪ GI, renal status ▪ CAUTION: cardiac dysfunction, prostatic hypertrophy ▪ **ndx Therapeutic effects**: High risk for aspiration ▪ High risk for injury ▪ Impaired physical mobility ▪ Self-care deficit ▪ Impaired swallowing ▪ **Adverse effects:** High risk for activity intolerance ▪ High risk for fluid volume deficit ▪ Impaired physical mobility ▪ Sensory/perceptual alterations ▪ High risk for impaired skin integrity ▪ Altered thought processes ▪ Altered tissue perfusion. **PLAN:** Avoid abrupt withdrawal ▪ Assess for therapeutic dose tolerance ▪ Prevent postural hypotension ▪ **Special considerations:** G: caution, ↓ dosage (↓ tolerance, ↑ CNS sensitivity, ↑ fractures) ▪ P: not recommended ▪ OB: avoid use if pregnant, breastfeeding ▪ **Dietary management:** Avoid alcohol ▪ **Lab test evaluation:** CBC, H&H, serum creatinine. **IMPLEMENT:** Administer c̄ food to ↓ GI irritation ▪ Monitor VS, esp BP ▪ Monitor activity status (safety precautions) ▪ Observe for visual problems ▪ Monitor bowel function, I&O, IOP ▪ Observe for exaggerated anticholinergic effects ▪ Assess for muscle weakness ▪ Monitor GI, GU, CV status. **PATIENT EDUCATION:** Comply c̄ prescribed drug therapy ▪ Full drug effects may take several mos ▪ Avoid use of alcohol ▪ Use sugarless gum/hard candy to diminish dry mouth ▪ Frequent oral hygiene necessary ▪ Protect eyes in sunlight ▪ Use safety precautions c̄ ambulation, hazardous activity ▪ Avoid sudden position changes (postural hypotension) ▪ Avoid extremes in exercise, climate ▪ Check c̄ physician/pharmacist before taking OTC preparations. **EVALUATE: Observe for therapeutic effect:** ↑ Neuromuscular function.

DESCRIPTION: Group of antibiotics & synthetic antiinfective agents classified into first-line (primary), second-line (secondary) and third-line (tertiary)† drugs according to their antimycobacterial activity, efficacy, & potential adverse & toxic effects.

DRUGS: **First line:** ethambutol (*Myambutal*), isoniazid (*Laniazide, Nydrazid*), rifampin (*Rifadin, Rimactane*) ▪ **Second line:** pyrazinamide, streptomycin ▪ **Third line:** aminosalicyclate sodium (*PAS*), capreomycin (*Capastat*), cycloserine (*Seromycin*), ethionamide (*Trecator-SC*), kanamycin (*Kantrex*) ▪ **Combinations:** isoniazid/rifampin (*Rifamate,* 150mg/300mg; *Rimactane/INH,* 300mg/300mg).

MECHANISM OF ACTION

aminosalicylate sodium	Tuberculostatic—inhibits folic acid synthesis
capreomycin	Tuberculostatic—unknown mechanism
cycloserine	Tuberculocidal/static‡—inhibits cell wall synthesis
ethambutol	Tuberculostatic—inhibits RNA synthesis
ethionamide	Tuberculocidal/static‡—inhibits peptide synthesis
kanamycin	Tuberculocidal—inhibits protein synthesis
isoniazid	Tuberculocidal/static‡—inhibits transaminase activity
pyrazinamide	Tuberculocidal/static‡—unknown mechanism
rifampin	Tuberculocidal/static‡—inhibits DNA dependent RNA polymerase activity
streptomycin	Tuberculocidal—inhibits protein synthesis

Note: Side/adverse effects: common in *italic;* serious in ***boldface italic.***

*Available in Canada only.

† Many references only utilize first- & second-line classifications.

‡Depends on concentration of drug at site of infection & susceptibility of tubercular bacilli.

PHARMACOKINETICS

	PO absorption	Peak	Half-life	Excretion
aminosalicylate	Well	3-4h	1h	77% metabolites via urine in 24h
capreomycin	IM	1-2h	4-6h	57% unchanged via urine in 24h
cycloserine	70%-90%	3-4h	10h	60%-70% unchanged via urine in 24h
ethambutol	75%-80%	2-4h	3.3h	50% unchanged via urine in 24h
ethionamide	80%	3h	3h	95% unchanged via urine in 24h
isoniazid	Well	1-2h	1-4h	50%-70% unchanged via urine in 24h
kanamycin	IM	1h	2-2.5h	50% unchanged via urine in 24h
pyrazinamide	Well	2h	9-10h	70% unchanged via urine in 24h
rifampin	Well	2-4h	3h	60% unchanged via urine in 24h
streptomycin	IM	1h	2-3h	29%-89% unchanged via urine in 24h

THERAPEUTIC USES: Treatment of TB or prophylaxis. The effectiveness of antimycobacterial therapy is dependent on type of infection, adequate dosing, sufficient treatment period(s), & effective drug combinations when required (usually retreatment). Effective combinations include isoniazid/rifamprin; isoniazid/ethambutol; and isoniazid/ethambutol, streptomycin.

DOSAGE/ADVERSE EFFECTS

Drug	Usual adult dose	Adverse effects
aminosalicylate	10-12g/d	GI disturbances, hepatotoxicity
capreomycin	15mg/kg/d IM	Ototoxicity, nephrotoxicity
cycloserine	500-750mg/d	Psychotic behavior, seizures
ethambutol	15mg/kg as single dose	Optic toxicity
ethionamide	750-1000mg/d	GI disturbances, hepatotoxicity
isoniazid		Hepatitis; peripheral neuropathy
prophylaxis	300mg once/d	
active TB	5-10mg/kg once/d	
kanamycin	0.5-1g/d IM	Hepatotoxicity, ototoxicity, nephrotoxicity
pyrazinamide	15-30mg/kg once/d	Hepatotoxicity, hyperuricemia
rifamprin	600mg once/d	Hematologic, hepatotoxicity
streptomycin	1g IM once/d	Hepatotoxicity, ototoxicity, nephrotoxicity

NURSING MANAGEMENT

ASSESS: Hx of hypersensitivity (incl ethionamide, pyrazinamide, niacin) ▪ Hepatic function (↓ dose if impaired) ▪ Visual disturbances (ocular toxicity) ▪ CAUTION: hepatic impairment. **ndx Therapeutic effects**: Ineffective airway clearance ▪ High risk for altered body temperature ▪ Ineffective breathing pattern ▪ High risk for infection ▪ Impaired gas exchange ▪ **Adverse effects:** High risk for activity intolerance ▪ High risk for injury ▪ Sensory/perceptual alterations (visual) ▪ High risk for impaired skin integrity ▪ Altered thought processes ▪ Impaired tissue integrity. **PLAN:** Administer at equal intervals around clock to maintain blood levels ▪ Maintain hydration ▪ Have IV pyridoxine (vitamin B_6) available for OD ▪ **Special considerations:** G: caution, ↓ dosage (hepatotoxicity; renal impairment) ▪ P: caution if <5y/o (immature systems) ▪ OB: avoid use if pregnant, caution if breastfeeding ▪ **Dietary management**: Avoid alcohol, tyramine-containing (aged, fermented) foods; vitamin B_6 supplements (neurotoxicity) ▪ **Lab test evaluation**: Serum uric acid, AST, ALT; use Clinistix/Tes-Tape for urine glucose. **IMPLEMENT:** Obtain C&S; check results ▪ Monitor VS, esp temperature, BP ▪ Monitor hepatic, renal status. **PATIENT EDUCATION:** Comply $\bar{c}$ prescribed drug regimen ▪ Avoid sudden position changes ▪ Keep appointments for eye exams/$\bar{c}$ physician ▪ Notify physician *immediately* of visual problems, tingling/numbness of hands/feet, jaundice, lethargy, dark urine ▪ Safety precautions $\bar{c}$ ↑ activity ▪ Full drug effects may require several wks of therapy. **EVALUATE: Observe for therapeutic effect:** Resolution of tubercular infection.

DESCRIPTION: Group of drugs c̄ a limited antiviral spectrum; chemically most of these agents are synthetic purine or pyrimidine nucleosides.

DRUGS: acyclovir (*Zovirax*), amantadine (*Symmetrel*), didanosine (*Videx*), foscarnet (*Foxcavir*), ganciclovir (*Cytovene*), idoxuridine (*Herplex, Stoxil*), ribavirin (*Virazole*), trifluridine (*Viroptic*), vidarabine (*Vira*-A), zalcitabine (*Hivid*), zidovudine (*Retrovir*).

Mechanism of Action: *Purine* nucleoside analogs acyclovir, didanosine, ganciclovir, vidarabine, *pyrimidine* nucleoside analogs, idoxuridine, trifluridine, zalcitabine, zidovudine & pyrophosphate foscarnet interfere c̄ DNA synthesis, which results in inhibition of viral replication. Amantadine hcl inhibits cellular viral penetration and viral release. The mechanism for vibavirin is unknown.

Therapeutic Use: acyclovir: initial & recurrent cutaneous mucosal HSV-1, HSV-2 infection, herpes zoster (shingles), amantadine: prevention/treatment of influenza-A, didanosine: alternate for advanced HIV infection, foscarnet: cytomegalovirus (CMV) retinitis in AIDS pts, ganciclovir: cytomegalovirus (CMV) retinitis in AIDS pts, idoxuridine: HSV keratitis, trifluridine: HSV-1 & HSV-2 keratoconjunctivitis, recurrent epithelial keratitis, vidarabine: HSV encephalitis, neonatal HSV infection, herpes zoster (shingles), HSV-1 & HSV-2 keratoconjunctivitis, recurrent epithelial keratitis, zalcitabine: In combination c̄ zidovudine for advanced HIV infection, zidovudine: asymptomatic, symptomatic HIV infection.

DOSAGE †: Usual adult dose

amantadine	100mg bid or 200mg once/d
ganciclovir	Induction dose 5mg/kg IV at a constant rate q12h for 14-21d; maintenance dose 5mg/kg IV over 1h/d or 6mg/kg/d for 5d qwk
idoxuridine	1 gtt qh to infected eye during day, q2h at night
ribavirin	Aerosol treatment c̄ SPAG-2 for 12-18h/d c̄ drug concentration of 20mg/ml in drug reservoir of the unit. Average aerosol concentration for 12h period is 190µg/L of air
trifluridine	1gtt q2h to affected eye

Note: Side/adverse effects: common in *italic;* serious in ***boldface italic.***

*Available in Canada only.

† For remaining doses consult individual drug cards.

vidarabine	*IV*, 15mg/kg/d for 10d for HSV infections, 20mg/kg/d for 5d for shingles *Ocular*, 1/2 inch of ointment in lower conjunctival sac 5 times/d at 3h intervals

NURSING MANAGEMENT

ASSESS: Hx of hypersensitivity ▪ Hepatic, renal function ▪ Signs of toxicity (CNS, neurotoxicity) ▪ Therapeutic drug level ▪ CAUTION: hepatic, renal impairment. **ndx Therapeutic effects**: High risk for infection ▪ Impaired skin integrity ▪ **Adverse effects:** High risk for activity intolerance ▪ ↓ Cardiac output ▪ High risk for injury ▪ Sensory/perceptual alterations ▪ High risk for impaired skin integrity ▪ Altered thought processes ▪ Impaired tissue integrity. **plan**: Administer at equal intervals around clock to maintain blood levels ▪ Maintain hydration. **Special considerations:** G: caution (renal impairment) ▪ P: avoid use if <3mos (↑ sensitivity) ▪ OB: avoid use if pregnant, breastfeeding. **Dietary management**: None specific. **Lab test evaluation**: BUN, serum creatinine (IV); therapeutic drug levels. **IMPLEMENT:** Monitor VS ▪ Monitor F/E, hepatic, renal status ▪ Topical: use glove to prevent herpes transmission. **PATIENT EDUCATION:** Comply c̄ prescribed drug regimen ▪ Safety precautions c̄ hazardous activity ▪ ↑ Fluid intake (8-10 glasses/d) ▪ Procedure for topical/ophthalmic preparations ▪ Use condoms if sexually active ▪ Information on herpes (symptoms, hygiene, transmission). **evaluate: Observe for therapeutic effects:** Prevention/resolution of viral infection.

DESCRIPTION: Group of CNS depressant drugs that are chemical derivatives of barbituric acid; exhibit similar pharmacologic activity; classified according to onset, duration of activity.

DRUGS: Ultrashort: methohexital sodium (*Brevital Sodium*), thiamylal sodium (*Surital*), thiopental sodium (*Pentothal*) ▪ **Short:** pentobarbital (*Nembutal, *Nova-Recal, *Pentagen*), pentobarbital sodium (*Nembutal Sodium*), secobarbital (*Seconal*), secobarbital sodium (*Seconal Sodium*) ▪ **Intermediate:** amobarbital (*Amytal, *Isabec*), amobarbital sodium (*Amytal Sodium*), aprobarbital (*Alurate*), butabarbital sodium (*Butisol Sodium*) ▪ **Long:** mephobarbital (*Mebaral*), phenobarbital (*Luminal*), phenobarbital sodium (*Luminal Sodium*).

MECHANISM OF ACTION: Barbiturates act primarily on brainstem reticular formation to produce dose-related sedative, hypnotic effects. In high doses, barbiturates can produce surgical anesthesia (ultrashort) ▪ Capable of raising convulsive threshold; selective barbiturates used for epileptic seizure prophylaxis ▪ Barbiturates are scheduled drugs because of potential for misuse/addiction.

THERAPEUTIC USE: Ultrashort: anesthesia induction, surgical procedures, convulsive states, narcoanalysis, narcosynthesis ▪ **Short:** sedation, hypnotic, acute convulsive states ▪ **Intermediate**: sedation, hypnotic, acute convulsive states ▪ **Long:** sedation, hypnotic, convulsive prophylaxis.

CONTRAINDICATIONS: Hypersensitivity, severe liver/respiratory impairment, porphyria, addiction.

DOSAGE: *PO* (daily ranges)

	Convulsive	Hypnotic	Sedation
amobarbital	—	65-200mg	50-400mg
aprobarbital	—	40-160mg	120mg
butabarbital	—	50-100mg	45-120mg
mephobarbital	400-600mg	—	90-400mg
pentobarbital	—	100mg	40-160mg
phenobarbital	100-300mg	100-320mg	30-120mg
secobarbital	—	100-200mg	40-120mg

SIDE/ADVERSE EFFECTS: CNS: *drowsiness, lethargy, hangover,* headache, dizziness, paradoxical restless-

Note: Side/adverse effects: common in *italic;* serious in ***boldface italic.***

*Available in Canada only.

ness/excitement ▪ GI: N/V ▪ INT: morbilliform rash, ***Stevens-Johnson syndrome***, urticaria ▪ Other: asthma, ***angioneurotic edema.***

DRUG INTERACTIONS: Use c̄ alcohol, antihistamines, benzodiazepines, methotrimeprazine, narcotics, tranquilizers produces ↑ depressant effects ▪ Barbiturates are enzyme inducers; can ↓ effects of PO anticoagulants, other drugs ▪ MAO-I ↑ barbiturate activity ▪ Barbiturates ↓ PO absorption of griseofulvin.

NURSING MANAGEMENT

ASSESS: Hx of hypersensitivity ▪ Recent CNS depressant administration (hold drug) ▪ Respiratory status; do *not* administer if <12/m ▪ Therapeutic blood levels ▪ Signs of dependence ▪ Actual swallowing of PO forms ▪ CAUTION: hepatic, renal, respiratory impairment ▪ **ndx Therapeutic effects**: Anxiety ▪ Ineffective individual coping ▪ Sleep pattern disturbance ▪ **Adverse effects:** High risk for activity intolerance ▪ Ineffective breathing pattern ▪ Constipation ▪ Diarrhea ▪ High risk for fluid volume deficit ▪ High risk for injury ▪ Impaired physical mobility ▪ High risk for impaired skin integrity ▪ Altered thought processes. **PLAN:** Have emergency support measures available ▪ Avoid abrupt withdrawal ▪ Assess for tolerance of therapeutic dose ▪ Maintain safety precautions (raise bedrails, bed in low position, call bell) ▪ **Special considerations:** G: caution (paradoxic rxs) ▪ P: caution (paradoxic rxs), premies (↑ CNS sensitivity) ▪ OB: avoid use if pregnant, breastfeeding ▪ **Dietary management**: Avoid alcohol ▪ **Lab test evaluation**: PT (anticoagulants), therapeutic blood levels. **IMPLEMENT:** Monitor VS, esp c̄ parenteral doses ▪ Check for signs of dependence ▪ Monitor occurrence/characteristics of seizure activity ▪ Monitor activity status (safety precautions) ▪ Assess for paradoxic rxs (CNS stimulation) esp in elderly ▪ Check for depression; suicide precautions prn. **PATIENT EDUCATION:** Comply c̄ prescribed drug regimen; indiscriminate use may lead to dependence ▪ Store properly (do *not* keep at bedside) ▪ Avoid alcohol/CNS depressants ▪ Use safety precautions c̄ ambulation, hazardous activity ▪ Avoid smoking after administration ▪ Use relaxation techniques, sleep-producers (reading, warm milk, soft music). **EVALUATE: Observe for therapeutic effects:** ↓ Anxiety ▪ ↓ Insomnia ▪ ↓ convulsive episodes ▪ ↑ Induction of anesthesia (ultra-short acting).

DESCRIPTION: Large group of anxiolytic agents that are chemical congeners of original prototype drug chlordiazepoxide.

DRUGS: alprazolam (*Xanax*), chlordiazepoxide (*Libritabs*), chlordiazepoxide hcl (**Apo-Chlorax, Librium, *Medilium, *Novopoxide, *Solium*), clonazepam (*Klonopin, *Rivotril*), clorazepate dipotassium (*Tranxene*), diazepam (*Valium*), estazolam (*ProSom*), flurazepam (*Dalmane, *Novoflupam*), halazepam (*Paxipam*), lorazepam (*Activan*), oxazepam (**Ox-Pam, Serax, *Zapex*), prazepam (*Centrax*), quazepam (*Doral*), temazepam (*Restoril*), triazolam (*Halcion*).

MECHANISM OF ACTION: Anxiolytic activity appears related to depression of CNS at brainstem formation, limbic systems. Benzodiazepines also depress polysynaptic reflex arcs in spinal cord, which may result in mild skeletal relaxation. They exhibit sedative, appetite-stimulating, weak analgesic, varying degrees of anticonvulsant activity.

THERAPEUTIC USE: Alcoholism: chlordiazepoxide, clorazepate, diazepam, oxazepam ▪ **Anxiety**: alprazolam, chlordiazepoxide, clorazepate dipotassium, diazepam, halazepam, lorazepam, oxazepam ▪ **Convulsive states:** clonazepam, clorazepate, diazepam ▪ **Hypnotic:** flurazepam, temazepam, triazolam ▪ **Muscle spasms:** diazepam.

CONTRAINDICATIONS: Hypersensitivity, narrow-angle glaucoma.

DOSAGE: Adult *PO*

alprazolam	0.25-0.5mg tid
chlordiazepoxide	5-25mg 3/4 times/d
clonazepam	Up to 20mg/d divided
clorazepate dipotassium	15-60mg/d divided
diazepam	2-10mg 3-4 times/d
estazolam	1-2mg hs
flurazepam	15-30mg hs
halazepam	20-40mg 3-4 times/d
lorazepam	2-6mg/d divided
oxazepam	10-30mg 3-4 times/d
prazepam	20-60/mg divided
quazepam	7.5-15mg hs
temazepam	15-30mg hs
triazolam	0.25-0.5mg hs

SIDE/ADVERSE EFFECTS: CNS: *drowsiness, fatigue, ataxia,* headache ▪ GI: N/V ▪ GU: urinary retention ▪ HEM: neutropenia (rare) ▪ INT: rash, urticaria, pruritus ▪ PSYCH: paradoxical anxiety, depression, hallucinations, hyperexcited states.

OVERDOSE TREATMENT: Administer competitive antagonist flumazenil (*Mazicon*). Initial dose of 0.2mg IV over 15s. Subsequent doses if required must be individualized/be prepared for possible seizures.

DRUG INTERACTIONS: Use c̄ other CNS depressants produces additive effects ▪ Use c̄ MAO-I, disulfiram can produce serious toxic effects due to ↓ metabolism of benzodiazepines ▪ Smoking can ↓ effects of benzodiazepines.

NURSING MANAGEMENT

ASSESS: Hx of hypersensitivity ▪ Recent CNS depressant administration (hold drug) ▪ Respiratory status ▪ Signs of dependence ▪ Pt sleep patterns ▪ CAUTION: hepatic, renal, respiratory impairment ▪ **ndx Therapeutic effects**: Anxiety ▪ Ineffective individual coping ▪ Impaired physical mobility ▪ Sleep pattern disturbance ▪ **Adverse effects:** High risk for activity intolerance ▪ Ineffective breathing pattern ▪ Constipation ▪ Diarrhea ▪ High risk for fluid volume deficit ▪ High risk for injury ▪ Impaired physical mobility ▪ High risk for impaired skin integrity ▪ Altered thought processes. **PLAN:** Have emergency support measures available ▪ Avoid abrupt withdrawal ▪ Assess for tolerance to therapeutic dose ▪ Maintain safety precautions (↑ bedrails, bed in low position, call bell) ▪ **Special considerations:** G: caution, ↓ dosage (↑ CNS sensitivity) ▪ P: caution, ↓ dosage (↑ sensitivity) ▪ OB: not recommended if pregnant, breastfeeding ▪ **Dietary management**: Avoid alcohol ▪ **Lab test evaluation**: CBC (long-term), serum creatinine. **IMPLEMENT:** Monitor VS, esp c̄ parenteral doses ▪ Check for signs of dependence ▪ Monitor occurrence/characteristics of seizure activity ▪ Monitor activity status (safety precautions) ▪ Assess for paradoxic rxs (CNS stimulation), esp in elderly ▪ Check for depression; suicide precautions prn. **PATIENT EDUCATION:** Comply c̄ prescribed drug regimen; indiscriminate use may lead to dependence ▪ Store properly (do *not* keep at bedside) ▪ Avoid alcohol, other CNS depressants ▪ Use safety precautions c̄ ambulation, hazardous activity ▪ Avoid smoking after administration ▪ Use relaxation techniques, sleep-producers (reading, warm milk, soft music). **EVALUATE: Observe for therapeutic effects:** ↓ Anxiety ▪ ↓ Insomnia.

DESCRIPTION: Nonselective (β_1, β_2) & selective β_1 agents that block normal agonist response at beta adrenergic receptors in sympathetic nervous system; labetalol also exhibits alpha blockage.

DRUGS: Nonselective blockers: carteolol (*Cartrol*), labetalol (*Normodyne, Trandate*), nadolol (*Corgard*), penbutolol (*Levatol*), pindolol (*Visken*), propranolol (*Inderal*), sotalol hcl (*Betapace*), timolol (*Blocadren*) ▪ **Selective blockers:** acebutolol (*Sectral*), atenolol (*Tenormin*), betaxolol hcl (*Kerlone*), metoprolol (*Lopressor*) ▪ **Topical:** betaxolol (*Betopic 0.25, 0.5%*), levobunolol (*Betagan 0.5%*), metipranolol (*Opti Pranolol 0.3%*), timolol (*Timoptic 0.25, 0.5%*).

MECHANISM OF ACTION: Beta blockers competitively prevent access of catecholamine neurotransmitters at beta receptors in sympathetic nervous system. Nonselective agents block both β_1-, β_2-adrenergic receptors, whereas selective agents only block β_1-receptors, primarily located in cardiac tissue; selective β_1-blockers also inhibit β_2-receptors in high doses. β_2-receptors mainly located in bronchial, vascular smooth muscle ▪ β_1-Adrenoreceptor blockage produces ↓ heart rate, ↓ cardiac output, ↓ conduction velocity at SA & AV nodes, myocardial automaticity, contractility; ↓ myocardial O_2 consumption, ↑ cardiac volume, quinidine-like membrane-stabilizing effect.

THERAPEUTIC USE: Antianginal: nadolol, propranolol ▪ **Antiarrhythmic:** acebutolol, propranolol, sotalol ▪ **Antihypertensive:** acebutolol, atenolol, betaxolol, carteolol, labetalol, metoprolol, nadolol, penbutolol, pindolol, propranolol, timolol ▪ **MI**: metoprolol, propranolol, timolol ▪ **Migraine:** propranolol ▪ Topical treatment of glaucoma (usual dose one gtt 1-2 times/d).

CONTRAINDICATIONS: Hypersensitivity, bronchial asthma (nonselective blockers), heart block, cardiac failure, cardiogenic shock.

DOSAGE

acebutolol	400-1200mg/d
atenolol	50-100mg/d
betaxolol	10-20mg/d
carteolol	2.5-10mg/
labetalol	200-800mg/d
metoprolol	100-450mg/d

nadolol	80-640mg/d
penbutolol	20mg/d
pindolol	10-60mg/d
propranolol	30-650mg/d
sotalol	160-320mg/d
timolol	20-60mg/d

SIDE/ADVERSE EFFECTS: CNS: dizziness, mental depression, fatigue, hallucinations ▪ CV: bradycardia, CHF, hypotension, peripheral vascular insufficiency, exacerbation of AV block ▪ EENT: visual disturbances; dry mouth, eyes ▪ GI: N/V/D, cramps, constipation, ischemic colitis ▪ GU: impotence ▪ HEM: **agranulocytosis**, thrombocytopenic purpura ▪ INT: rash, pruritus, alopecia ▪ MS: joint pain ▪ RESP: bronchospasm.

DRUG INTERACTIONS: Use c̄ reserpine, other catecholamine-depleting drugs can result in serious adrenergic blockage ▪ Nonselective beta adrenergics antagonize therapeutic effects.

NURSING MANAGEMENT

ASSESS: Hx of hypersensitivity ▪ BP, apical pulse, respiratory distress ▪ CAUTION: hepatic, respiratory impairment, diabetics ▪ **ndx Therapeutic effects**: ↓ Cardiac output ▪ Pain ▪ Altered tissue perfusion ▪ **Adverse effects:** High risk for activity intolerance ▪ Ineffective breathing pattern ▪ ↓ Cardiac output ▪ Diarrhea ▪ Fatigue ▪ High risk for fluid volume deficit ▪ Self-esteem disturbance ▪ Sensory/perceptual alterations ▪ Sexual dysfunction ▪ Altered thought processes ▪ Altered tissue perfusion. **plan:** Prevent postural hypotension ▪ Institute cardiac monitoring (IV) ▪ **Special considerations:** G: caution, ↓ dosage (↓ metabolism, ↑ sensitivity) ▪ P: not recommended ▪ OB: caution if pregnant, breastfeeding ▪ **Dietary management**: Avoid high-Na^+ foods, alcohol; do *not* abstain from food for >12 hr (diabetics) ▪ **Lab test evaluation**: FBS (diabetics). **implement:** Assess apical pulse: if <60/m hold drug ▪ Monitor BP; observe for hypotension ▪ Monitor I&O, daily weight ▪ Monitor blood glucose in diabetics (hypoglycemia). **patient education:** Avoid sudden position changes (postural hypotension) ▪ Comply c̄ prescribed drug regimen ▪ Avoid smoking, alcohol, constrictive clothing, extremely hot objects, OTC cough/cold/allergy preparations ▪ Follow low-Na^+ diet ▪ Check for leg/foot swelling ▪ Check c̄ physician/pharmacist before taking OTC preparations ▪ Have BP checked regularly ▪ Keep appointments c̄ physician ▪ Carry identification (MedicAlert). **evaluate: Observe for therapeutic effects:** ↓ BP ▪ Normal sinus rhythm.

DESCRIPTION: Small group of drugs used in treatment of angina, arrhythmias; also called calcium antagonists, slow channel blockers, calcium channel blocking agents.

DRUGS: amlodipine (*Norvac*), bepridil (*Vascor*), diltiazem hcl (*Cardizem*), felodipine (*Plendil*), isradipine (*DynaCirc*), nicardipine hcl (*Cardene*), nifedipine (*Procardia*), nimodipine (*Nimotop*), verapamil hcl (*Calan, Isoptin, Verelan*).

MECHANISM OF ACTION: Antianginal effect due to inhibition of extracellular calcium-ion transmembrane migration in cardiac, vascular smooth muscle via slow channel pathway, resulting in coronary dilation; in addition, ↑ myocardial O_2 supply, ↓ O_2 consumption. Antiarrhythmic effect of verapamil due to effect on SA node, prolongation of AV refractory period.

PHARMACOKINETICS

	Absorption		Onset	Peak	Half-life	Protein binding	Excretion
amlodipine	PO	NA	NA	6-12h	30-50h	93%	Via urine
bepridil	PO	100%	1h	2-3h	24h	99%	Via urine
diltiazem	PO	80%	30m	2-3h	3.5-9h	70%-85%	Via urine
felodipine	PO	100%	2-5h	2-5h	11-16h	99%	Via urine
isradipine	PO	90%-95%	20m	1.5h	1.5-8h	95%	Via urine
nicardipine	PO	100%	20m	0.5-2h	2-4h	>95%	Via urine & feces
nifedipine	PO	90%	20m	30m	2h	92%-98%	Via urine
nimodipine	PO	NA	NA	1h	1-2h	95%	Via urine
verapamil	PO	90%	30m	1-2h	2-8h	90%	Via urine
	IV	—	3-5m	5m	2-8h	90%	Via urine

THERAPEUTIC USE: Treatment of vasospastic angina: amlodipine, diltiazem, nifedipine, verapamil ▪ **Chronic stable angina:** amlodipine, bepridil, diltiazem, nicardipine, nifedipine, verapamil ▪ **Hypertension:** amlodipine, diltiazem (only SR dosage forms), felodipine, isradipine, nicardipine, nifedipine (only SR dosage forms), verapamil (only SR dosage forms) ▪ **Arrhythmias:** verapamil (control of rapid ventricular rate in atrial flutter/fibrillation and prophylaxis of repetitive paroxysmal supraventricular tachycardia) ▪ **Spasm of subarachnoid hemorrhage:** nimodipine.

DOSAGE: Usual adult dosage range

amlodipine *PO*	5-10mg once/d
bepridil *PO*	200-400mg/d
diltiazem *PO*	180-240mg divided, 3-4 times/d
felodipine *PO*	5-10mg/d
isradipine *PO*	5-20mg/d divided
nicardipine *PO*	20-40mg tid
nifedipine *PO*	10-20mg tid
nimodipine *PO*	60mg q4h for 21 d
verapamil *PO*	320-480mg divided
IV	5-10mg bolus over 2m

NURSING MANAGEMENT

ASSESS: Hx of hypersensitivity ▪ Apical pulse, BP, ECG ▪ Lung sounds ▪ CAUTION: hepatic disease, heart failure ▪ **ndx Therapeutic effects**: ↓ Cardiac output ▪ Pain ▪ Altered tissue perfusion ▪ **Adverse effects:** High risk for activity intolerance ▪ Anxiety ▪ Ineffective breathing patterns ▪ ↓ Cardiac output ▪ Constipation ▪ Fluid volume excess ▪ Pain. **plan:** Prevent postural hypotension ▪ Institute cardiac monitoring (IV, initial PO) ▪ Administer at equal intervals around clock to maintain blood levels ▪ **Special considerations:** G: caution, ↓ dosage (renal impairment, prolonged half-life) ▪ P: caution, ↓ dosage (↑ hemodynamic effect) ▪ OB: caution if pregnant, breastfeeding not recommended ▪ **Dietary management**: Avoid caffeine, alcohol, high-Na^+ foods ▪ **Lab test evaluation**: Serum digoxin levels (digitalized pts). **implement:** Assess apical pulse for 1m ▪ Monitor F/E status (I&O, daily weight, peripheral edema). **patient education:** Procedure for checking radial pulse ▪ Comply c̄ prescribed drug therapy ▪ Take safety precautions c̄ ambulation, hazardous activity ▪ Report abnormal rxs to physician (chest pain; difficult breathing; rapid, irregular heart rate) ▪ Avoid sudden position changes (postural hypotension) ▪ Check c̄ physician/pharmacist before taking OTC preparations ▪ Keep appointments c̄ physician. **EVALUATE: Observe for therapeutic effects:** ↓ Cardiac arrhythmias ▪ Normal heart rate, rhythm ▪ ↓ BP.

DESCRIPTION: Obtained from dried leaves of *Digitalis lanata* (Grecian foxglove), which yields digoxin; *D. purpurea* (purple foxglove) yields powdered digitalis leaf, digitoxin. Amrinone lactate (synthetic) often listed c̄ dig drugs.

DRUGS: amrinone lactate (*Inocor*), digitoxin (*Crystodigin*), digoxin (*Lanoxicaps, Lanoxin, *Novodigoxin*).

MECHANISM OF ACTION: Produces dramatic changes in cardiac contractility (inotropic), electrophysiologic activity; + inotropic effect due to membrane electrolyte transport system (Na^+-K^+ pump) changes; Ca^{++}-dependent cardiac contractile mechanism altered because more intracellular Ca^{++} ions available to cardiac myofibrils. Digitalization in CHF produces positive inotropic effect w/out corresponding ↑ O_2 consumption, ↑ stroke volume, ↓ coronary circulation ▪ ↓ Heart rate, conductivity in AV node, bundle of His ▪ ↓ Diastolic heart size, venous blood pressure, vein engorgement ▪ Prolonged atrial, ventricular refractory periods ▪ Diuresis c̄ ↓ edema, palliation of exertional/paroxysmal nocturnal dyspnea, cough, cyanosis.

THERAPEUTIC USE: Glycosides have same clinical efficacy, PO route preferred, digitoxin indicated in pts c̄ renal impairment ▪ Treatment of congestive heart failure (CHF) ▪ Treatment of supraventricular arrhythmias incl atrial flutter/fibrillation, sinus tachycardia due to CHF ▪ Use in cardiogenic shock controversial.

CONTRAINDICATIONS: Hypersensitivity, ventricular tachycardia, toxic effects.

DOSAGE: Adult: Usual dig; usual maintenance

amrinone *IV*	0.75mg/kg (direct); 5-10μg/kg/m
digitoxin *PO/IV*	1.2mg/24h; 0.15mg/d
digoxin *PO/IV*	1-1.5mg/24h; 0.125-0.5mg/d

SIDE/ADVERSE EFFECTS: CNS: apathy, fatigue, headache, psychosis ▪ CV: bradycardia, arrhythmias ▪ GI: *N/V*, anorexia, diarrhea ▪ EENT: blurred/yellow vision ▪ Other: estrogen-like effects (long-term use).

DRUG INTERACTIONS: Acetazolamide, amphotericin B, chlorthalidone, ethacrynic acid, furosemide, laxatives, thiazides ↑ dig toxicity by inducing hypokalemia ▪

Note: Side/adverse effects: common in *italic;* serious in ***boldface italic.***

*Available in Canada only.

Parenteral Ca administration can produce serious arrhythmias ▪ Barbiturates, hydantoins, phenylbutazone may ↓ dig activity by enzyme induction ▪ Ion-exchange resins inhibit PO dig absorption ▪ Quinidine ↑ dig, digitoxin levels.

NURSING MANAGEMENT

ASSESS: Hx of hypersensitivity ▪ Apical pulse ▪ Lung sounds ▪ Renal function ▪ Therapeutic blood levels ▪ CAUTION: renal impairment, ventricular arrhythmias ▪ **ndx Therapeutic effects:** ↓ Cardiac output ▪ Altered tissue perfusion ▪ **Adverse effects:** High risk for activity intolerance ▪ ↓ Cardiac output ▪ High risk for fluid volume deficit ▪ Altered nutrition: less than body requirements ▪ Sensory/perceptual alterations (visual) ▪ Altered tissue perfusion. **PLAN:** Institute cardiac monitoring (IV) ▪ Identify exact dig preparation, dosage form ▪ **Special considerations:** G: caution (hepatic, renal impairment) ▪ P: caution, may require ↑ dosage to achieve effect ▪ OB: caution if pregnant, breastfeeding ▪ **Dietary management:** ↑ K^+, ↓ Na^+ ▪ **Lab test evaluation:** Electrolytes (K^+, Ca^{++}, Mg^{++}) therapeutic blood levels. **Implement:** Assess apical pulse for 1m (hold dose if <60) ▪ Monitor VS, esp heart rate, BP ▪ Monitor F/E status (I&O, daily weight, peripheral edema) ▪ Check for toxicity before administering each dose (N/V, bradycardia, arrhythmias). **Patient education:** Procedure for checking radial pulse ▪ Comply c̄ prescribed drug therapy ▪ Report signs of toxicity to physician (loss of appetite, N/D, visual problems, irregular heartbeat) ▪ Follow low-Na^+, high-K^+ diet ▪ Check for leg/foot swelling ▪ Keep appointments c̄ physician. **Evaluate: Observe for therapeutic effects:** ↑ Cardiac output ▪ ↑ Urinary output ▪ ↓ Dyspnea.

OVERDOSE MANAGEMENT: Toxic dose 3/5 (60%) > therapeutic dose ▪ Principal symptoms: visual, conduction disturbances (arrhythmias) ▪ Treatment: adult—KCl 3-6g divided; pediatric—1-1.5mEq/kg divided ▪ Digoxin immune Fab (ovine) indicated in life-threatening OD; administered by IV infusion over 30m; bolus IV dose recommended in imminent cardiac arrest. Dosage variable; follow manufacturer's recommendation.

DESCRIPTION: Large diverse group of β-lactam antibiotics that are semisynthetic, H_2O soluble, broad spectrum, bactericidal against array of microbes; chemically related to penicillins ▪ Divided into 1st-, 2nd-, 3rd-generation cephalosporins, on basis of bacterial spectrum of drugs, not chronological development ▪ Cefoxitin, cefotetan (cephamycin antibiotics), usually classified c̄ cephalosporins.

MECHANISM OF ACTION: Bactericidal activity due to inhibition of mucopeptide cell wall synthesis in susceptible organisms.

DRUGS: First generation: Active against gram-positive bacteria, selected gram-negative organisms: cefadroxil (*Duricef, Ultracef*), cefazolin sodium (*Ancef, Kefzol*), cephalexin (*Keflex*), cephalothin (*Keflin*), cephapirin (*Cefadyl*), cephradine (*Anspor, Velosef*) ▪ **Second generation:** Similar spectrum of organisms susceptible to 1st-generation drugs but more active against greater variety of gram-negative organisms: cefaclor (*Ceclor*), cefamandole naftate (*Mandol*), cefmetazole (*Zefazone*), cefametazole sodium (*Zefazone*), cefonicid sodium (*Monocid*), ceforanide (*Precef*), cefoxitin sodium (*Mefoxin*), cefrozil (*Cefzil*), cefroxime proxitil (*Vantin*), cefuroxime sodium (*Kefurox, Zinacef*) ▪ **Third generation:** Less active against gram-positive organisms, expanded spectrum against gram-negative bacteria: cefixime (*Suprax*), cefoperazone sodium (*Cefobid*), cefotaxime sodium (*Claforan*), cefotetan disodium (*Cefotan*), ceftazidime (*Fortaz, Tazicef, Tazidime*), ceftizoxime (*Cefizox*), ceftriaxone sodium (*Rocephin*), moxalactam disodium (*Moxam*).

CAUTIONS: Coagulation irregularities can occur c̄ cefamandole, cefoperazone, moxalactam; observe for signs of hemorrhage ▪ Overgrowth of nonsusceptible organisms, pseudomembranous colitis can occur c̄ broad-spectrum antibiotics.

NURSING MANAGEMENT

ASSESS: Hx of hypersensitivity (incl penicillin) ▪ VS, hepatic, renal function ▪ CAUTION: hepatic, renal impairment ▪ **ndx Therapeutic effects**: High risk for altered body temperature ▪ High risk for infection ▪ **Adverse effects:** Diarrhea ▪ High risk for fluid volume deficit ▪ High risk for injury ▪ High risk for impaired skin integrity. **plan:** Administer at equal intervals around clock to maintain blood levels ▪ Maintain hydration ▪ **Special considerations:** G: caution, ↓ dosage (renal impairment, ↑ superinfection, coagulopathy) ▪ P: caution, ↓ dosage (prolonged half-life) ▪ OB: caution if pregnant, breastfeeding ▪ **Dietary management**: Avoid alcohol ▪ **Lab test evaluation**: CBC; use Clinistix/Tes-Tape for urine glucose. **Implement:** Obtain C&S; check results ▪ Observe for signs of superinfection (diarrhea, URI, coated tongue) ▪ Administer on empty stomach. **Patient education:** Comply $\bar{c}$ prescribed drug therapy ▪ ↑ Fluid intake (8-10 glasses/d) ▪ Take on empty stomach ▪ Diarrhea may occur ▪ Notify physician of symptoms of allergic rx (fever, difficult breathing, rash). **Evaluate: Observe for therapeutic effect:** Resolution of infection.

DESCRIPTION: The adrenal gland is regulated by the pituitary gland & is divided into cortex and medulla ▪ Cortex produces glucocorticoids (glucosteroids) & mineralocorticoids (mineralosteroids) ▪ Glucosteroids regulate metabolism of carbohydrates, lipids, proteins, to lesser extent minerals; potent inhibitors of inflammatory process, immune response; other significant effects incl ↓ number of circulating eosinophils, lymphocytes ▪ Glucosteroids are not curative agents, but used for potent antiinflammatory, immune suppressive activity in various pathophysiological conditions. Prolonged administration of natural/synthetic steroids produces fluid & salt retention, suppression of hypothalamus, pituitary, adrenal glands. Synthetic glucosteroids are preferred because of lower salt & fluid retention properties ▪ Mineralosteroids regulate electrolyte metabolism, water balance; used in maintenance treatment of Addison disease in conjunction c̄ glucosteroids ▪ In addition to corticosteroids is small group of adrenal inhibitors consisting of aminoglutetethimide, trilostane; used in treatment of Cushing syndrome.

DRUGS: Glucosteroids: beclomethasone dipropionate (*Beclovent, Vanceril*), betamethasone (*Celestone*), cortisone acetate (*Cortone Acetate*), dexamethasone (*Decadron*), dexamethasone acetate (*Decadron-LA*), dexamethasone sodium phosphate (*Decadron Phosphate*), fludrocortisone acetate (*Florinef*), hydrocortisone (*Cortef*), hydrocortisone acetate (*Hydrocortone Acetate*), hydrocortisone cypionate (*Cortef Suspension*), hydrocortisone sodium phosphate (*Hydrocortisone Phosphate, Solu-Cortef*), methylprednisolone (*Medrol*), methylprednisolone acetate (*Depro-Medrol*), methylprednisolone sodium succinate (*A-methaPred, SoluMedrol*), prednisolone (*Delta-Cortef*), prednisolone acetate (*Key-Pred*), prednisolone sodium phosphate (*Hydeltrasol*), prednisolone terbutate (*Hydelta-T.B.A.*), prednisone (*Deltasone, Meticorten, Orasone*), triamcinolone (*Aristocort, Kenacort*), triamcinolone acetonide (*Kenalog-10*), triamcinolone diacetate (*Aristocort Syrup, Kenacort Diacetate Syrup*), triamcinolone hexacetonide (*Aristopan*) ▪ **Mineralosteroids:** fliudrocortisone acetate (*Florinef Acetate*) ▪ **Adrenal inhibitors:** aminoglutethimide, trilostane (*Modrastane*).

NURSING MANAGEMENT

ASSESS: Hx of hypersensitivity ▪ Adrenal insufficiency (lethargy, N/V, hypotension, confusion) ▪ CAUTION: infection, long-term therapy ▪ **ndx Therapeutic effects**: Activity intolerance ▪ Ineffective airway clearance ▪ High risk for injury ▪ Impaired physical mobility ▪ Pain ▪ Impaired tissue integrity ▪ **Adverse effects:** Fluid volume excess ▪ High risk for infection ▪ Impaired physical mobility ▪ Altered nutrition: less than body requirement ▪ Self-esteem disturbance ▪ Sensory/perceptual alterations (visual) ▪ High risk for impaired skin integrity ▪ Impaired tissue perfusion. **plan:** Maintain hydration ▪ Administer in AM ▪ **Special considerations:** G: caution (↓ metabolism, chronic illness) ▪ P: caution (↓ bone growth) ▪ OB: caution if pregnant; avoid breastfeeding ▪ **Dietary management**: ↑ K^+, protein; ↓ Na^+ ▪ Avoid black licorice ▪ **Lab test evaluation**: Electrolytes; blood/urine glucose (diabetics). **Implement:** Monitor VS, esp BP ▪ Monitor F/E status (I&O, daily weight, peripheral edema) ▪ PO: administer c̄ food to ↓ GI irritation ▪ Avoid abrupt withdrawal. **Patient education:** Comply c̄ prescribed drug therapy; take c̄ food/milk in AM ▪ Check c̄ physician before vaccinations ▪ Avoid exposure to infection ▪ Notify physician of black/tarry stools, slow wound healing, blurred vision, bruising/bleeding, emotional changes ▪ Keep scheduled appointments c̄ physician ▪ Body image changes may occur c̄ prolonged use (reversible) ▪ Carry identification (MedicAlert). **Evaluate: Observe for therapeutic effects:** ↓ Inflammation ▪ ↓ Immune response.

DESCRIPTION: Small group of drugs that promote diuresis, electrolyte excretion; bumetanide, furosemide are sulfonamide-like; ethacrynic acid is not.

DRUGS: bumetanide (*Bumex*), ethacrynate sodium (*Sodium Edecrin*), ethacrynic acid (*Edecrin*), furosemide (**Furoside, Lasix, *Neo-Renal, *Uritol*).

MECHANISM OF ACTION: Promote excretion of H_2O, Na^+, Cl^-, other electrolytes (esp K^+) by inhibiting tubular reabsorption, esp in medullary, cortical portions of ascending limb of loop of Henle ▪ Antihypertensive activity due to ↓ peripheral vascular resistance.

THERAPEUTIC USE: Treatment of edema due to CHF, renal, hepatic dysfunction ▪ Treatment of hypertension (furosemide) ▪ Short-term management of ascites due to malignancy, idiopathic edema, lymphedema, pediatric congenital heart disease, nephrotic syndrome (ethacrynate sodium, ethacrynic acid).

CONTRAINDICATIONS: Hypersensitivity, anuria, severe electrolyte imbalance, hepatic coma, watery diarrhea during treatment, nursing mothers (ethacrynic acid or ethacrynate).

PHARMACOKINETICS: *See* individual drug cards.

DOSAGE: Adult

bumetanide *PO*	0.5-2mg/d to maximum 10mg
ethacrynic acid *PO*	50-300mg/d
furosemide *PO*	20-80mg/d to maximum 600mg for refractory cases
ethacrynate sodium *IV*	50mg or 0.5-1mg/kg

SIDE/ADVERSE EFFECTS: CNS: dizziness, headache, encephalopathy in preexisting liver disease (bumetamide only) ▪ CV: hypotension ▪ EENT: blurred vision, hearing loss, tinnitus ▪ GI: N/V, abdominal pain, watery diarrhea, bleeding (ethacrynic acid only) ▪ HEM: anemia, **thrombocytopenia, aplastic anemia** (rare; furosemide only), neutropenia, Henoch-Schonlein purpura (ethacrynic acid only) ▪ INT: rash, urticaria, **exfoliative dermatitis, erythema multiforme** (furosemide only) ▪ MS: muscle cramps, arthritic pain (bumetanide only).

Note: Side/adverse effects: common in *italic;* serious in ***boldface italic.***

*Available in Canada only.

DRUG INTERACTIONS: Use c̄ neurotoxic drugs incl aminoglycosides, capreomycin, chloroquine, oxyphenbutazone, phenylbutazone, vancomycin, viomycin can result in significant toxicity ▪ Induced hypokalemia, ↑ dig toxicity ▪ Avoid use c̄ nephrotoxic drugs, lithium, probenecid, indomethacin ▪ Antihypertensives may require dosage adjustments ▪ Use c̄ corticosteroids can produce severe hypokalemia.

NURSING MANAGEMENT

ASSESS: Hx of hypersensitivity (incl sulfonamides) ▪ Adequate renal function ▪ Serum K^+ (normal level: 3.5-5mEq/L) ▪ Hydration status ▪ CAUTION: ascites, renal failure, gout, diabetes ▪ **ndx Therapeutic effects**: Fluid volume excess ▪ Altered tissue perfusion ▪ **Adverse effects:** High risk for activity intolerance ▪ Ineffective breathing pattern ▪ ↓ Cardiac output ▪ Diarrhea ▪ ↑ High risk for ↑ fluid volume deficit ▪ Sensory/perceptual alterations (auditory, visual) ▪ High risk for impaired skin integrity ▪ Altered patterns of urinary elimination. **plan:** Maintain hydration ▪ **Special considerations:** G: caution, ↓ dosage (↑ sensitivity) ▪ P: caution (↑ electrolyte imbalance) ▪ OB: caution if pregnant, breastfeeding not recommended ▪ **Dietary management**: ↑ K^+, ↓ Na^+ ▪ **Lab test evaluation**: Electrolytes, FBS, BUN, serum uric acid. **IMPLEMENT:** Administer on awakening ▪ Monitor BP, K^+, I&O, daily weight, edema, lung sounds, skin turgor/mucous membranes ▪ Observe for changes in hearing & visual acuity. **PATIENT EDUCATION:** Expect ↑ urine output; have bathroom facilities close ▪ Eat foods high in K^+; avoid black licorice, high-Na^+ foods ▪ Take on arising qd ▪ Watch for signs of hypokalemia (muscle cramps, lethargy, anorexia), hyponatremia (thirst, dry mouth, drowsiness). **EVALUATE: Observe for therapeutic effects:** ↑ Urine output ▪ ↓ Edema ▪ ↓ BP.

DESCRIPTION: Large group of diuretic-antihypertensive agents that are sulfonamide-like chemical derivatives of benzothiadiazine.

DRUGS: ▪ **Thiazide diuretics:** bendroflumethiazide (*Naturetin*), benzthiazide (*Exna*), chlorothiazide (*Diachlor, Diuril*), hydrochlorothiazide (**Diuchlor H, Esidrix, Hydro*DIURIL, **Nefrol, *Neo-Codema, Oretic, Thiuretic, *Urozide*), hydroflumethiazide (*Diurcardin, Saluron*), methyclothiazide (*Aquatensen, Enduron*), polythiazixde (*Renese*), trichlormethiazide (*Metahydrin, Naqua*) ▪ **Thiazide-like diuretics:** chlorthalidone (*Hygroton, Thalitone, *Uridon*), indapamide **Lozide, Lozol*), metolazone (*Diulo, Zaroxolyn*), quinethazone (**Aquamox, Hydromox*).

MECHANISM OF ACTION: Thiazides promote excretion of H_2O, Na^+, Cl^- by inhibiting reabsorption of Na^+, primarily in ascending loop of Henle & in early distal tubule of nephron; enhance excretion of K^+, bicarbonate, other ions w/out significantly altering pH of urine; lower peripheral vascular resistance, resulting in significant antihypertensive activity; exhibit similar clinical efficacy.

PHARMACOKINETICS: *See* individual drug cards.

THERAPEUTIC USE: Treatment of hypertension as sole agent/in combination c̄ other antihypertensives ▪ Treatment of edema due to renal dysfunction ▪ Adjunct in treating edema due to CHF, hepatic cirrhosis, corticosteroid/estrogen therapy.

CONTRAINDICATIONS: Hypersensitivity due to any thiazide, other sulfonamide-derivative drug; anuria.

DOSAGE: Usual adult range *PO*

bendroflumethiazide	2.5-15mg/d
benzthiazide	50-200mg/d
chlorothiazide	0.5-2g/d
chlorthalidone	50-100mg/d; 100mg qod
hydrochlorothiazide	50-200mg/d
hydroflumethiazide	50-200mg/d
indapamide	2.5-5mg/d
methyclothiazide	2.5-10mg/d
metolazone	2.5-10mg/d
polythiazide	2-4mg/d
quinethazone	50-100mg/d
trichlormethiazide	2-4mg/d

SIDE/ADVERSE EFFECTS: CNS: *dizziness*, vertigo, paresthesia, headache ▪ EENT: blurred vision, xanthopsia ▪ GI: anorexia, N/V/D, jaundice ▪ HEM: **agranulocytosis, aplastic anemia,** leukopenia, **thrombocytopenia** ▪ INT: purpura, urticaria, photosensitivity ▪ MET: hypokalemia, glycosuria, hyperglycemia, hyperuricemia, hypochloremic alkalosis ▪ MS: *fatigue, leg cramps* ▪ RESP: respiratory distress ▪ Other: necrotizing angiitis.

DRUG INTERACTIONS: ↑ Dig toxicity due to hypokalemia ▪ Use c̄ corticosteroids ↑ hypokalemia ▪ Antidiabetic agents may require dose adjustments ▪ Use c̄ diazoxide can produce significant diabetogenic effects.

NURSING MANAGEMENT

ASSESS: Hx of hypersensitivity (incl sulfonamides) ▪ Adequate renal function ▪ Serum K^+ (normal level: 3.5-5mEq/L) ▪ Hydration status ▪ CAUTION: ascites, renal failure, gout, diabetes ▪ **ndx Therapeutic effects**: Fluid volume excess ▪ Altered tissue perfusion ▪ **Adverse effects:** High risk for activity intolerance ▪ Ineffective breathing pattern ▪ ↓ Cardiac output ▪ Diarrhea ▪ High risk for fluid volume deficit ▪ Sensory/perceptual alterations (visual) ▪ High risk for impaired skin integrity ▪ Altered patterns of urinary elimination. **plan:** Maintain hydration ▪ **Special considerations:** G: caution, ↓ dosage (↑ sensitivity) ▪ P: caution (↑ electrolyte imbalance) ▪ OB: caution if pregnant; breastfeeding not recommended ▪ **Dietary management**: ↑ K^+, ↓ Na^+ ▪ **Lab test evaluation**: Electrolytes, FBS, BUN, serum uric acid. **IMPLEMENT:** Administer on awakening ▪ Monitor BP, K^+, I&O, daily weight, edema, lung sounds, skin turgor/mucous membranes ▪ Observe for changes in hearing & visual acuity. **PATIENT EDUCATION:** Expect ↑ urine output; have bathroom facilities close ▪ Eat foods high in K^+; avoid black licorice, high-Na^+ foods ▪ Take on arising qd ▪ Watch for signs of hypokalemia (muscle cramps, lethargy, anorexia), hyponatremia (thirst, dry mouth, drowsiness). **EVALUATE: Observe for therapeutic effects:** ↑ Urine output ▪ ↓ Edema ▪ ↓ BP.

DESCRIPTION: Small protein endocrine hormone secreted by pancreatic beta cells; required for proper metabolism of glucose. Deficiency of endogenous insulin results in diabetes mellitus, a serious metabolic disease. Treatment of diabetes currently is with insulin obtained from beef/pork pancreas extraction & from recombinant DNA strains of bacteria (*Escherichia coli*), which produce human insulin; human insulin can also be made semisynthetically from pork insulin ▪ Exogenous insulin is presently modified according to onset, peak, and duration of activity into six separate insulin preparations. This manipulation of insulin activity is required to help satisfy various metabolic demands for insulin in pts c̄ diabetes. Further modification possible by mixing compatible insulin preparations before administration.

Insulin preparations composed of insulin extracted from animal pancreas contain trace amounts of proinsulin, a protein prohormone that can cause allergic reactions in a very small percentage of diabetics. ▪ FDA regulations state that all insulin preparations must not exceed more than 25 ppm proinsulin. Insulin products labeled purified must not exceed 10 ppm proinsulin; all other preparations no more than 20 ppm proinsulin ▪ Insulin products usually contain 40U or 100U/ml.

PREPARATIONS: Insulin injection (regular): *Humulin BR* (human); *Humulin R* (human); *Iletin I* (beef-pork); *Iletin II* (purified beef or purified pork); *Insulin Regular* (pork or purified pork); *Novolin R* (human); *Velosulin* (purified pork); *Velosulin Human* ▪ **Insulin suspension, isophane (NPH):** *Humulin N* (human); *Iletin I, NPH* (beef-pork); *Iletin II, NPH* (purified beef or purified pork); *Insulatard NPH Human; Insulatard NPH* (purified pork); *Insulin, NPH* (beef); *Insulin, NPH* (purified pork); *Novolin N* (human) ▪ **Insulin suspension, protamine & zinc (PZI):** *Protamine, Zinc & Iletin I* (beef-pork); *Protamine, Zinc & Iletin II* (purified beef or purified pork); **Insulin zinc suspension (lente):** *Humulin L* (human); *Iletin I, Lente* (beef-pork); *Iletin II, Lente* (purified beef or purified pork); *Insulin, Lente* (beef); *Insulin, Lente* (purified pork); *Novolin L* (human) ▪ **Insulin suspension, extended (ultralente):** *Humulin U* (human); *Iletin I, Ultralente* (beef-pork); *Insulin, Ultralente* (beef or purified pork) ▪ **Insulin suspension, prompt (semilente):** *Iletin I, Semilente* (beef-pork); *Insulin, Semilente* (beef or purified pork) ▪ **Other:** *Humulin 70/30* (human), *Mixtard, Mixtard Human, Novolin 70/30* (30% regular and 70% isophane insulin).

MECHANISM OF ACTION: Insulin required for transport of monosaccharides, amino acids, through cell membrane of insulin-sensitive cells, incl skeletal muscle, cardiac muscle, mammary glands, anterior pituitary, aorta, lens of eye ▪ Pork insulin differs from human insulin in one amino acid (alanine [P] for threonine [H]) of 51 amino acids in insulin molecule; therefore they are extremely similar. Beef insulin differs in three amino acids, is less similar to human insulin.

THERAPEUTIC USE: Management of diabetic coma (regular insulin), diabetes mellitus (all insulins).

CONTRAINDICATIONS: Hypersensitivity.

DOSAGE: Must be individualized.

SIDE/ADVERSE EFFECTS: ***Hypoglycemia*** due to overdosage, insulin resistance, localized urticarial lesions (usually disappear), atrophy of subcutaneous fat, hypersensitivity rxs incl ***anaphylactic shock***, angioneurotic edema, urticaria.

PHARMACOKINETICS

	Onset	Peak	Duration
Rapid			
Insulin injection	0.5h	2.5-5h	8h
Prompt insulin zinc suspension	1-5h	5-10h	16h
Extended "intermediate acting"			
Insulin zinc suspension	2.5h	7-15h	24h
Isophane insulin suspension	1.5h	4-12h	24h
Extended "long acting"			
Extended insulin zinc suspension	4-8h	10-30h	36h
Protamine-zinc-insulin suspension	4-8h	14-24h	36h
Mixtard (etc.)	0.5h	4-8h	24h

DRUG INTERACTIONS: Use c̄ chlorthalidone, corticosteroids, diazoxide, epinephrine, ethacrynic acid, furosemide, glucagon, phenytoin, thiazides, thyroid hormones will antagonize hypoglycemic effects of insulin ▪ Use c̄ alcohol, anabolic steroids, guanethidine, MAO-I, propranolol, salicylates will intensity hypoglycemic effects of insulin.

NURSING MANAGEMENT

ASSESS: Hx of hypersensitivity ▪ Hypo/hyperglycemic rxs ▪ Hepatic, renal function ▪ CAUTION: hypoglycemia, CV, hepatic, renal impairment ▪ **ndx Therapeutic effects**: High risk for altered nutrition: less than body requirements ▪ **Adverse effects:** High risk for infection ▪ High risk for injury ▪ High risk for impaired skin integrity. **PLAN:** Obtain proper equipment (appropriate insulin syringe c̄ 25-gauge needle) ▪ Check solution for discoloration/precipitation; do *not* use ▪ Check calculation/preparation (strength/type) c̄ another nurse ▪ Administer single AM dose before breakfast ▪ Assess pt need to change dosage in relation to exercise, stress, appetite ▪ **Special considerations:** None (individualized dosage) ▪ **Dietary management**: Avoid alcohol; ADA diet (↓ carbohydrate, ↓ fat); calorie restrictions ▪ **Lab test evaluation**: FBS, urine glucose/ketones. **IMPLEMENT:** Monitor FBS; blood/urine glucose/ketones ac & hs or as ordered ▪ Administer single AM dose before breakfast ▪ IV: administer REGULAR insulin only ▪ Monitor for hypo/hyperglycemic rxs. **PATIENT EDUCATION:** Comply c̄ prescribed therapy ▪ Follow special diet (↓ carbohydrate, ↓ fat) ▪ Proper storage (refrigerate), preparation (roll between palms; do *not* shake) ▪ Procedure for SC administration (rotate sites) ▪ Mixing insulins: draw clear (regular) into syringe before cloudy (NPH suspension) ▪ Signs of hypo/hyperglycemia ▪ Procedure for blood/urine, glucose/ketone testing ▪ Keep medical appointments/for blood work ▪ Avoid alcohol ▪ Carry identification (MedicAlert) ▪ Procedure for hypoglycemia rx (always carry sugar source) ▪ Long-term therapy; used to control, *not* cure diabetes ▪ Avoid changing brand name preparations/equipment ▪ Report infection. **EVALUATE: Observe for therapeutic effects:** ↓ Blood sugar ▪ ↓ Hyperglycemia.

DESCRIPTION: Small group of drugs that inhibit activity of monoamine oxidase enzyme system.

DRUGS: isocarboxazid (*Marplan*), phenelzine (*Nardil*), tranylcypromine (*Parnate*).

MECHANISM OF ACTION: Antidepressant activity appears related to inhibition of MAO enzyme system, resulting in ↑ levels of epinephrine, norepinephrine, serotonin at adrenergic neuron storage sites ▪ pargyline has hypotensive activity by an unknown mechanism.

PHARMACOKINETICS: Not available.

THERAPEUTIC USE: Treatment of depression not responsive to other drugs ▪ Moderate/severe hypertension (pargyline) ▪ Investigational treatment of panic disorder syndromes (phenelzine).

CONTRAINDICATIONS: Hypersensitivity; cerebrovascular defects, CV disorders, pheochromocytoma; in combination c̄ benzodiazepines, adrenergics, tyramine-rich foods, narcotics, hypotensive agents; severe liver & renal impairment; geriatric pts.

DOSAGE: Adult

Isocarboxazid *PO*	Initial dose 30mg/d, maintenance dose 10-20mg/d
Phenelzine	Initial dose 45-90mg/d, maintenance dose 15mg/d or qod
Tranylcypromine	Initial dose 20mg/d, usual maintenance dose 10-20mg/d

SIDE/ADVERSE EFFECTS: CNS: restlessness, insomnia, drowsiness, dizziness, headache ▪ CV: tachycardia, edema, palpitations, postural hypotension ▪ EENT: blurred vision ▪ GI: anorexia, dry mouth, N/D, abdominal cramps ▪ GU: impotence ▪ HEP: ↑ Serum AST, ALT, bilirubin; hepatitis ▪ INT: skin rash.

DRUG INTERACTIONS: Serious/fatal results can occur c̄ adrenergics, benzodiazepines, narcotics, tricyclic antidepressants.

NURSING MANAGEMENT

ASSESS: Hx of hypersensitivity ▪ BP ▪ Signs of hypertensive crisis (tachycardia, stiff neck, chest pain) ▪ CAUTION: hepatic, renal impairment ▪ **ndx Therapeutic effects:**

Ineffective individual coping ▪ Self-esteem disturbance ▪ High risk for self-directed violence ▪ **Adverse effects:** High risk for activity intolerance ▪ ↓ Cardiac output ▪ Diarrhea ▪ Fuid volume excess ▪ High risk for injury ▪ Pain ▪ Sensory/perceptual alterations ▪ Sexual dysfunction ▪ High risk for impaired skin integrity. **PLAN:** Prevent postural hypotension ▪ Avoid abrupt withdrawal ▪ Institute suicide precautions ▪ Ensure drug ingestion ▪ **Special considerations:** G: not recommended ▪ P: not recommended ▪ OB: caution if pregnant, breastfeeding ▪ **Dietary management:** Avoid alcohol, caffeine, tyramine-containing foods ▪ **Lab test evaluation:** CBC. **IMPLEMENT:** Monitor BP ▪ Suicide precaution prn ▪ Monitor hepatic, renal status. **PATIENT EDUCATION:** Comply c̄ prescribed drug regimen ▪ Avoid sudden position changes (postural hypotension) ▪ Use safety precautions c̄ hazardous activity ▪ Full drug effects may require several wks of therapy ▪ Use sugarless gum/hard candy to diminish dry mouth ▪ Check c̄ physician before taking OTC preparations ▪ Avoid alcohol, caffeine, tyramine-containing foods ▪ Symptoms of hypertensive crisis ▪ Carry identification (MedicAlert). **EVALUATE: Observe for therapeutic effects:** ↓ Depression ▪ Mood elevation.

DESCRIPTION: Narcotics are natural opiate agonists, semisynthetic opiate agonists, or synthetic opiates (agonist opiates, agonist-antagonist opiates) ▪ Excellent analgesics; exhibit phenomenon of tolerance; have varying abuse/addiction potentials; most are schedule drugs.

DRUGS: Natural opiates: codeine phosphate (C-II), codeine sulfate (C-II), morphine sulfate (C-II), opium preparations—deodorized tincture of opium (C-II), opium alkaloids (C-II; *Pantopon*), paregoric (C-III) ▪ **Semisynthetic:** hydromorphone hcl (C-II; *Dilaudid*), oxymorphone hcl (C-II; *Numorphan*) ▪ **Synthetic opiates**—AGONIST: fentanyl citrate (C-II; *Sublimaze*), levorphanol tartrate (C-II; *Levo-Dromoran*), meperidine hcl (C-II; *Demerol*), methadone hcl (C-II; *Dolophine*), oxycodone hcl (C-II), sufentanil citrate (C-II; *Sufenta*) ▪ AGONIST-ANTAGONIST: buprenorphine hcl (C-V; *Buprenex*), butorphanol tartrate (*Stadol*), dezocine (*Dalgan*), nalbuphine hcl (*Nubain*), pentazocine (C-IV; *Talwin*).

MECHANISM OF ACTION: Analgesic activity probably due to interference c̄ pain impulses at subcortical level of brain. Narcotics significantly alter psychological response to pain, suppress anxiety/apprehension by producing euphoria.

PHARMACOKINETICS: *See* individual drug cards.

THERAPEUTIC USE: Relief of severe pain ▪ Sedation/hypnosis when pain present ▪ Preanesthetic sedation; post-op analgesia (obstetric); support of anesthesia ▪ Antitussive, antidiarrheal.

CONTRAINDICATIONS: Hypersensitivity.

DOSAGE: Adult

buprenorphine *IM/IV*	0.3mg q6h
butorphanol *IM*	2mg q3-4h
codeine *PO*	15-60mg q4-6h
dezocine *IV/Epidural intrathecal*	2-10mg/70g
fentanyl *IM*	0.5-0.1mg pre-op
hydromorphone	2mg q4-6h
levorphanol *PO/SC*	2mg
meperidine *PO/IM/SC*	50-150mg q3-4h
methadone *IM/SC*	2.5-10mg
morphine *SC*	10-15mg q4h
nalbuphine *IM/IV/SC*	10-20mg
oxycodone *PO*	5mg q6h
oxymorphone *IM/SC*	1-1.5mg

pantopon *PO*	2-4mg q4-6h
pentazocine *IM/IV/SC*	30mg q3-4h
sufentanil *IV*	0.5-1μg/kg; 2-8μg/kg initially

SIDE/ADVERSE EFFECTS: CNS: *lightheadedness, dizziness, sedation, sweating,* euphoria, disorientation, transient hallucination, weakness ▪ CV: hypotension, palpitation; flushing of face, phlebitis after IV injection ▪ GI: dry mouth, constipation, anorexia, biliary tract spasm ▪ UG: urinary retention, ureteral spasm ▪ INT: pruritus, urticaria ▪ RESP: respiratory depression, apnea.

DRUG INTERACTIONS: Use c̄ alcohol, antihistamines, barbiturates, benzodiazepines, methotrimeprazine, phenothiazines, other CNS depressants can produce additive effects ▪ Use c̄ tricyclic antidepressants can produce respiratory depression ▪ Meperidine contraindicated c̄ MAO-I ▪ Methadone maintenance may produce withdrawal symptoms c̄ opiate agonist-antagonist drugs.

NURSING MANAGEMENT

ASSESS: Hx of opioid hypersensitivity ▪ Respirations; do *not* administer if <12/m ▪ Pain characteristics ▪ Signs of dependence ▪ Signs of OD (coma, pinpoint pupils, respiratory depression); have naloxone hcl (Narcan) available ▪ Bowel function, abdominal distension ▪ Renal function, urinary retention ▪ CAUTION: recent CNS depressant administration; hepatic, renal, respiratory impairment; craniocerebral trauma ▪ **ndx Therapeutic effects**: Pain ▪ **Adverse effects:** High risk for activity intolerance ▪ Ineffective breathing pattern ▪ Constipation ▪ High risk for injury ▪ Sensory/perceptual alterations (visual) ▪ High risk for impaired skin integrity ▪ Altered thought processes ▪ Altered tissue perfusion ▪ Altered patterns of urinary elimination. **plan:** Have emergency support measures available ▪ Administer *before* pain becomes severe ▪ Maintain safety precautions (↑ bedrails, bed in low position, call bell) ▪ Maintain hydration ▪ Store under double lock/key; document use accurately ▪ **Special considerations:** G: caution, ↓ dosage (↑ sensitivity) ▪ P: caution (↑ sensitivity) ▪ OB: caution if pregnant, breastfeeding ▪ **Dietary management**: Avoid alcohol; ↑ bulk-containing foods (constipation) ▪ **Lab test evaluation**: None specific. **IMPLEMENT:** Monitor VS, respirations, circulatory function ▪ Monitor activity status (safety precautions) ▪ Check for potentiation of CNS depressant effect. **PATIENT EDUCATION:** Comply c̄ prescribed drug regimen; indiscriminate use may lead to dependence ▪ Avoid alcohol, CNS depressants ▪ Use safety precautions c̄ ambulation, hazardous activity ▪ Avoid smoking after administration ▪ Avoid sudden position changes (postural hypotension) ▪ ↑ Fluids, dietary bulk. **EVALUATE: Observe for therapeutic effect: ↓** Pain.

DESCRIPTION: Large, chemically diverse group of drugs that produce main pharmacologic effects by inhibiting synthesis, release of prostaglandins. Chemically divided into salicylates, propionic acid derivatives, fenamates, indoles, oxicams, pyrazolines; several references classify these agents as prostaglandin inhibitors rather than NSAIAs ▪ Prostaglandins are naturally occurring fatty acid derivatives of prostanoic acid; possess potent physiologic activity; exhibit wide tissue distribution $\bar{c}$ high concentrations in seminal fluid; are synthesized locally (by enzyme system prostaglandin synthetase), where they act as local tissue hormones; affect CV, GI, reproductive, respiratory smooth muscle; play role in blood platelet aggregation, inflammatory response, pain sensation, fever.

DRUGS: ▪ **Salicylates:** aspirin (*ASA, Ecotrin*), choline magnesium trisalicylate (*Trilisate*), choline salicylate (*Arthropan*), diflunisal (*Dolobid*), magnesium salicylate, salsalate (*Disalcid*), sodium salicylate (*Uracel 5*) ▪ **Propionic acid derivatives:** fenoprofen calcium (*Nalfon*), flurbiprofen (*Ansaid*), ibuprofen (*Advil, Haltran, Nuprin, Motrin*), ketoprofen (*Orudis*), naproxen (*Anaprox, Naprosyn*), oxaprozin (*Daypro*) ▪ **Fenamates:** meclofenamate (*Meclomen*), mefanamic acid (*Ponstel*) ▪ **Indoles:** etodalac (*Lodine*), indomethacin (*Indocin*), sulindac (*Clinoril*) ▪ **Oxicams:** piroxicam (*Feldene*) ▪ **Pyrazolines:** oxyphenbutazone, phenylbutazone (*Azolid, Butazolidin*) ▪ **Other:** diclofenac (*Voltaren*), ketorolac tromethamine (*Toradol*), nabumetone (*Relafen*), tolmetin (*Tolectin*).

DOSAGE: Usual adult dose ranges *PO*

aspirin	
choline magnesium trisalicylate	325-6000mg/d
choline salicylate	1500-3000mg/d
diclofenac	870-5220mg/d
diflunisal	100-200mg/d
etodolac	250-2500mg/d
fenoprofen	200-1200mg/d
flurbiprofen	300-3200mg/d
ibuprofen	50-300mg/d
indomethacin	200-3200mg/d
ketoprofen	25-200mg/d
ketorolac	25-300mg/d
magnesium salicylate	10-60mg/d
meclofenamate	325-4800mg/d
mefenamic acid	50-400mg/d
nabumetone	250-1250mg/d
naproxen	500-2000mg/d
oxaprozin	250-1250mg/d
phenylbutazone	600-1800mg/d

piroxicam	100-2400mg/d
salsalate	10-20mg/d
sodium salicylate	500-3000mg/d
sulindac	325-3900mg/d
tolmetin sodium	150-400mg/d
	200-2000mg/d

NURSING MANAGEMENT

ASSESS: Hx of hypersensitivity ▪ Pain characteristics ▪ Bleeding, esp c̄ anticoagulant therapy ▪ CAUTION: GI bleeding/bleeding disorders; CV, hepatic, renal impairment ▪ **ndx Therapeutic effects**: Impaired physical mobility ▪ Pain. **Adverse effects:** High risk for activity intolerance ▪ Constipation ▪ High risk for fluid volume deficit ▪ Fluid volume excess ▪ High risk for injury ▪ Sensory/perceptual alterations (visual) ▪ High risk for impaired skin integrity ▪ Altered tissue perfusion ▪ Altered patterns of urinary elimination. **plan:** Observe for edema in extremities ▪ Evaluate vision, hearing ▪ Avoid use c̄ aspirin ▪ **Special considerations:** G: caution (↑ sensitivity; renal impairment) ▪ P: avoid use (Reye's syndrome) ▪ OB: avoid use if pregnant, breastfeeding ▪ **Dietary management**: Avoid alcohol, GI-irritating foods ▪ **Lab test evaluation**: Blood glucose levels ↓ (diabetics). **IMPLEMENT:** Administer c̄ food to ↓ GI irritation; encourage upright position for 15-30m ▪ Monitor F/E status (I&O, daily weight, peripheral edema) ▪ Check for bleeding; D/C drug, notify physician. **PATIENT EDUCATION:** Comply c̄ prescribed drug regimen ▪ Notify physician *immediately* of bleeding, rash, flu-like symptoms, swelling of feet/legs, GI distress, jaundice, ↓ urine output, visual disturbances ▪ Take c̄ food/milk ▪ Check c̄ physician/pharmacist before using OTC preparations ▪ Avoid alcohol ▪ Use safety precautions c̄ hazardous activity (drowsiness, dizziness, visual disturbance). **EVALUATE: Observe for therapeutic effects:** ↓ Pain ▪ ↓ Inflammation.

DESCRIPTION: An array of estrogen-progestin combination products ("the pill") or progestin preparations ("mini-pill") ▪ Estrogenic agent may be ethinyl estradiol or menstranol; progestational agent may be ethynodiol diacetate, levonogestrol, nogestrol, norethindrone, norethindrone acetate, or norethynodrel ▪ Combinations may be low-, intermediate-, or high-dose ratio preparations.

FORMULATIONS: Estrogen-progestin combination products: ***Monophasic:*** Fixed estrogen-progestin dosage ratio for qd of cycle in 21d or 28d dosage formulations: Brevicon, Demulen, Enovid, Enovid-E, Genora, Levlen, Loestrin, Loestrin-FE, Lo/Ovral, Modicon, Nelova, Nordette, Norinyl, Norlestrin, Ortho-Novum, Ovcon, Ovral, Ovulen. ***Biphasic:*** Fixed estrogen dose c̄ low progestin dose 1st 10d, higher progestin dose rest of cycle in 21d or 28d dosage formulations: Nelova 10/11, Ortho-Novum 10/11-21, Ortho-Novum 10/11-28. ***Triphasic:*** Three different estrogen/progestin dose ratios, administered sequentially during cycle in 21d or 28d dosage formulations: Ortho-Novum 7/7/7, Tri-Levlen, Tri-Norinyl, Triphasil ▪ ***Progestin products:*** norethindrone (*Micronor, Nor-QD*), norgestrel (*Ovrette*).

MECHANISM OF ACTION: Prevent ovulation by inhibiting release of gonadotropins & by ↑ uterine mucous viscosity, which ↓ sperm movement, egg penetration (fertilization), possibility of zygote (fertilized egg) implantation.

PHARMACOKINETICS: Good absorption patterns, wide tissue distribution, high protein binding, variable half-lives; excretion via feces/urine primarily as conjugated metabolites.

THERAPEUTIC USE: Prevention of pregnancy ▪ Treatment of endometriosis, hypermenorrhea; to produce cyclic withdrawal bleeding (high-dose combination formulations).

CONTRAINDICATIONS: Known/suspected pregnancy; present/past thrombophlebotic disorders; known/suspected breast cancer, estrogen neoplasia; undiagnosed abnormal genital bleeding; cerebrovascular coronary artery disease; benign/malignant liver tumors associated c̄ estrogen-containing products.

DOSAGE: Monophasic combinations: Dosage starts on 5th day of cycle or on 1st Sunday after menstruation starts; 1 tablet/d from day 5 to day 24/25 of cycle ▪ **Biphasic combinations:** Dosage starts on 1st day of cycle if Sunday or on 1st Sunday after menstruation starts; 1 tablet/d (in correct sequence) for 21/28 days, depending on product ▪ **Triphasic combinations:** Dosage starts on 1st day of cycle if Sunday or on 1st Sunday after menstruation starts; 1 tablet/d (in correct sequence) for 21 days.

SIDE/ADVERSE EFFECTS: CNS: migraine, mental depression ▪ CV: ***cerebral hemorrhage/thrombosis, coronary thrombosis, arterial thromboembolism, mesenteric thrombosis, pulmonary embolism,*** Raynaud disease, ***thrombosis,*** optic neuritis, corneal curvature changes ▪ GI: N/V, bloating, colitis, cramps ▪ GU: breakthrough bleeding, spotting, amenorrhea, dysmenorrhea, vaginal candidiasis, cervical erosion, ↑ size of uterine leiomyomas ▪ HEP: liver tumors, cholestatic jaundice ▪ INT: rash, melasma ▪ Other: congenital anomalies; breast enlargement, tenderness, secretions; weight changes; ↓ tolerance to CHO; prolactin-secreting pituitary tumors.

DRUG INTERACTIONS: Use c̄ nicotine (smoking) ↑ risk of MI, stroke, hypertension, thromboembolism, visual disturbances, liver tumor, gallbladder disease, teratogenic fetal effects ▪ Drugs that ↓ effectiveness of PO contraceptives incl ampicillin, analgesics, antihistamines, barbiturates, chloramphenicol, griseofulvin, isoniazid, migraine preparations, neomycin, nitrofurantoin, penicillin V, phenytoin, primidone, rifampin, sulfonamides, tetracyclines, tranquilizers ▪ PO contraceptives can ↓ therapeutic effects of anticonvulsants, beta blockers, guanethidine, hypnotics, hypoglycemic agents, PO anticoagulants, theophylline, tranquilizers, tricyclic antidepressants, vitamins.

NURSING MANAGEMENT

ASSESS: Hx of estrogen/progestin hypersensitivity ▪ Pregnancy; do *not* administer, notify physician ▪ CAUTION: thrombophlebotic disorders, coronary artery disease, hepatic impairment ▪ **ndx Therapeutic effects**: Sexual dysfunction ▪ **Adverse effects:** High risk for fluid volume deficit ▪ Fuid volume excess ▪ Pain ▪ High risk for impaired skin integrity ▪ Impaired tissue perfusion.

PLAN: Administer *exactly* as scheduled ▪ **Special considerations:** G: caution (chronic illness) ▪ P: avoid use (immature systems) ▪ OB: caution if pregnant, breast-feeding ▪ **Dietary management**: Avoid caffeine, high-Na^+ foods ▪ **Lab test evaluation**: FBS; hepatic, thyroid function tests. **IMPLEMENT:** Administer c̄ food/milk to ↓ GI irritation ▪ Monitor for thromboembolic phenomena; notify physician. **PATIENT EDUCATION:** Use second method of birth control during 1st m after starting & for 3 mo after D/C birth control pills ▪ Take *exactly* as scheduled c̄ food/milk ▪ Notify physician *immediately* of unusual bleeding, severe headache, difficult breathing, changes in vision/coordination, chest/leg pain ▪ Avoid smoking ▪ Keep appointments c̄ physician ▪ Describe administration of specific product, review package insert c̄ pt ▪ Instruct pt on procedure for missed dose: 1st day ▪ Take as soon as remembered; if not until 2nd day, take 2; continue regular dose schedule; use 2nd method of birth control until end of cycle; notify physician; 3rd day D/C drug, use another method of birth control; notify physician *immediately*. **EVALUATE: Observe for therapeutic effect:** Prevention of pregnancy.

DESCRIPTION: Oral hypoglycemic sulfonylurea derivatives.

DRUGS: ▪ **First-generation sulfonylureas:** acetohexamide (*Dymelor*), chlorpropamide (*Diabinese, *Novo-propamide*), tolazamide (*Tolinase*), tolbutamide (*Orinase*) ▪ **Second-generation sulfonylureas:** glipizide (*Glucotrol*), glyburide (*DiaBeta, Glynase PresTab, Micronase*).

MECHANISM OF ACTION: Antidiabetic activity due to stimulation of insulin release from functioning beta cells of pancreas; second-generation sulfonylureas have not demonstrated clear advantage over first-generation drugs.

THERAPEUTIC USE: Management of type 2 (non-insulin-dependent) diabetes that cannot be controlled by diet alone.

CONTRAINDICATIONS: Hypersensitivity; diabetic ketoacidosis c̄, w/out coma.

DOSAGE: Usual adult PO range

acetohexamide	250mg-1.5g/d
chlorpropamide	100-500mg/d
glipizide	2.5-40mg/d
glyburide	1.25-20mg/d
tolazamide	100mg-1g/d
tolbutamide	0.25-2g/d

PHARMACOKINETICS

	PO absorption	Peak	Duration	Half-life	Excretion
acetohexamide	Rapid	3h	12-24h	1.3h	80% via urine in 24h
chlorpropamide	Rapid	2-4h	Up to 24h	36h	80%-90% via urine in 96h
glipizide	Rapid	1-3h	Up to 24h	2-4h	90% as metabolites in urine
glyburide	Rapid	2-4h	Up to 24h	10h	50% via urine, 50% via bile
tolazamide	Slow	2-6h	10h	7h	85% via urine
tolbutamide	Rapid	3-5h	6-12h	4-7h	75% via urine

Note: Side/adverse effects: common in *italic;* serious in ***boldface italic.***

*Available in Canada only.

SIDE/ADVERSE EFFECTS: GI: *nausea, epigastric fullness,* heartburn ▪ HEM: ***aplastic anemia, agranulocytosis,*** leukopenia, ***hemolytic anemia,*** pancytopenia, ***thrombocytopenia*** ▪ INT: erythremia, morbilliform/maculopapular eruptions, photosensitivity ▪ MET: hypoglycemia.

DRUG INTERACTIONS: Use c̄ alcohol, MAO-I, phenylbutazones, beta blockers can significantly ↑ hypoglycemic effects ▪ Use c̄ anabolic steroids, chloramphenicol, guanethidine, PO anticoagulants, probenecid, salicylates, sulfinpyrazone, sulfonamides ↑ hypoglycemic effects ▪ Use c̄ adrenergics, corticosteroids, phenytoin, thiazides, thyroid preparations ↓ hypoglycemic effects.

NURSING MANAGEMENT

ASSESS: Hx of hypersensitivity ▪ Hypo/hyperglycemic rxs ▪ Hepatic, renal function ▪ CAUTION: hypoglycemia, CV, hepatic, renal impairment ▪ **ndx Therapeutic effects:** High risk for altered nutrition: less than body requirements ▪ **Adverse effects:** High risk for infection ▪ High risk for injury ▪ High risk for impaired skin integrity. **PLAN:** Administer as single AM dose c̄ breakfast, divided doses c̄ meals ▪ Assess pt need to change dosage in relation to exercise, stress, appetite ▪ **Special considerations:** G: caution, ↓ dosage (↑ sensitivity) ▪ P: not recommended (use insulin) ▪ OB: caution if pregnant (use insulin) ▪ **Dietary management:** Avoid alcohol; ADA diet (↓ carbohydrate, ↓ fat); calorie restrictions ▪ **Lab test evaluation:** FBS, urine glucose/ketones. **IMPLEMENT:** Monitor FBS; blood/urine glucose/ketones ac & hs or as ordered ▪ Administer single AM dose c̄ breakfast, divided doses c̄ meals ▪ Monitor for hypo/hyperglycemic rxs. **PATIENT EDUCATION:** Comply c̄ prescribed therapy ▪ Follow special diet (↓ carbohydrate, ↓ fat) ▪ Proper storage ▪ Signs of hypo/hyperglycemia ▪ Procedure for blood/urine, glucose/ketone testing ▪ Keep scheduled appointments ▪ Avoid alcohol ▪ Procedure for hypoglycemia rx (always carry sugar source) ▪ Carry identification (MedicAlert) ▪ Report infection. **EVALUATE: Observe for therapeutic effect:** ↓ Hyperglycemic manifestations.

DESCRIPTION: Amino: Bactericidal, acid-stable, penicillinase-labile, penicillin derivatives ▪ **Penicillinase resistant:** Bactericidal, acid-stable (except methicillin) penicillinase-stable penicillin derivatives.

DRUGS: Amino: amoxicillin (*Amoxil, *Apo-Amoxi, Biomox, *Novomoxin, Polymox, Trimox, Wymox*), ampicillin (*Amcil, *Ampicin, *Ampilean, *Apo-Ampi, *Novoampicillin, *Penbriten, Polycillin, Principen, Omnipen, Totacillin*), bacampicillin (**Penglobe, Spectrobid*) ▪ **Penicillinase resistant:** cloxacillin (**Apo-Cloxi, *Bactopen, Cloxapen, *Novocloxin, *Orbenin, Tegopen*), dicloxacillin (*Dynapen, Dycill, Pathocil*), methicillin (*Staphcillin*), nafcillin (*Nafcil, Nallpen, Unipen*), oxacillin (*Bactocill, Prostaphlin*).

MECHANISM OF ACTION: Bactericidal activity due to inhibition of mucopeptide cell wall synthesis in susceptible organisms.

THERAPEUTIC USE: Amino: Spectrum similar to penicillin G/V but more effective against wider variety of gram-negative bacteria. Use should be limited to organisms that are not sensitive to penicillin G/V. Bacampicillin changed to ampicillin in body. Treatment of infections caused by susceptible strains of *Escherichia coli, Haemophilus influenzae, Neisseria meningitidis, Proteus mirabilis, Salmonella* spp, *Shigella* spp, *Neisseria* gonorrhoeae ▪ Treatment of subacute bacterial endocarditis, enterococcal infections ▪ Ampicillin drug of choice for treating typhoid fever (*Salmonella typhi*) resistant to chloramphenicol ▪ **Penicillinase resistant:** Indicated in treatment of infections due to penicillinase-producing staphylococci ▪ Resistance to any penicillinase-stable penicillin should be interpreted as resistance to all ▪ Cross-resistance c̄ cephalosporins occurs frequently.

CONTRAINDICATIONS: Hypersensitivity to any penicillin.

DOSAGE: Adult

amoxicillin, ampicillin, cyclacillin *PO*	250-500mg qid
bacampicillin *PO*	400-800mg bid
cloxacillin *PO*	250-500mg or more q6h
dicloxacillin *PO*	125-500mg or more q6h

methicillin *IM*	1g q4-6h
IV	1g q6h
nafcillin *PO*	250mg-1g q4-6h
IM	500mg q4-6h
IV	500mg-1g 4-6h
oxacillin *PO*	250-500mg or more q4-6h
IM/IV	250mg-1g or more q4-6h

SIDE/ADVERSE EFFECTS: CNS: neuropathy usually associated c̄ high parenteral doses ▪ CV: edema ▪ GI: PO incl *N/V/D, epigastric distress*, black hairy tongue, flatulence, smell/taste disturbances ▪ GU: ***interstitial nephritis*** (rare) usually associated c̄ methicillin ▪ HEM: anemia, eosinophilia, leukopenia, neutropenia, ***thrombocytopenia*** ▪ HEP: ↑ Serum levels of AST, ALT, LDH ▪ INT: maculopapular rashes (most frequent), ***erythema multiforme, exfoliative dermatitis*** (infrequent), rash, pruritus, urticaria ▪ MS: arthralgia ▪ Other: *local irritation at injection site*, fever, ***anaphylaxis***, laryngeal edema.

DRUG INTERACTIONS: Do *not* use PO dosage forms c̄ antacids, antidiarrheal suspensions, ion-exchange resins ▪ Use c̄ bacteriostatic antibiotics can result in antibiotic antagonism ▪ Avoid concurrent use of bacampicillin, disulfiram ▪ PO anticoagulant therapy may require dose adjustments esp c̄ amino pencillins.

NURSING MANAGEMENT

ASSESS: Hx of hypersensitivity (incl cephalosporins) ▪ Hepatic, renal function ▪ CAUTION: hepatic, renal impairment ▪ **ndx Therapeutic effects:** High risk for altered body temperature ▪ High risk for infection ▪ **Adverse effects:** Diarrhea ▪ High risk for fluid volume deficit ▪ High risk for injury ▪ High risk for impaired skin integrity. **PLAN:** Administer at equal intervals around clock to maintain blood levels ▪ Maintain hydration ▪ **Special considerations:** G: caution, ↓ dosage (renal impairment, ↑ superinfection) ▪ P: caution (↑ sensitivity) ▪ OB: caution if pregnant, breastfeeding ▪ **Dietary management:** None specific ▪ **Lab test evaluation:** CBC. **IMPLEMENT:** Obtain C&S, check results ▪ Observe for signs of superinfection (diarrhea, URI, coated tongue) ▪ Administer on empty stomach. **PATIENT EDUCATION:** Comply with prescribed drug therapy ▪ ↑ Fluid intake (8-10 glasses/d) ▪ Take on empty stomach ▪ Diarrhea may occur ▪ Notify physician of symptoms of allergic rx (fever, difficult breathing, rash). **EVALUATE: Observe for therapeutic effect:** Resolution of infection.

DESCRIPTION: Group of semisynthetic penicillins that exhibit ↑ spectrum against gram-negative organisms that is vastly superior to penicillin G/V and greater than the amino penicillins.

DRUGS: carbenicillin indanyl sodium (*Geocillin*), mezlocillin (*Mezlin*), piperacillin (*Pipracil*), ticarcillin (*Ticar*).

MECHANISM OF ACTION: Bactericidal activity due to inhibition of mucopeptide cell wall synthesis in susceptible organisms.

PHARMACOKINETICS: *See* individual drug cards.

THERAPEUTIC USE: Individual gram-negative spectrum varies. The combined spectrum incl *Acinetobacter* spp, *Bacteroides* spp, *Enterobacter* spp, *Escherichia coli, Haemophilus influenzae, Klebsiella* spp, *Neisseria* spp, *Peptococcus* spp, *Peptostreptococcus* spp, *Proteus* spp, *Pseudomonas aeruginosa, Providencia rettgeri, Serratia* spp, *Streptococcus faecalis, Streptococcus pneumoniae* ▪ Treatment of bacterial septicemia; bone/joint, gynecologic, intraabdominal, respiratory, skin, UTIs caused by susceptible microorganisms ▪ Initial treatment of mixed infections before identification of causative organism ▪ In combination c̄ aminoglycoside for treatment of stubborn gram(−) infections, esp *Pseudomonas.*

CONTRAINDICATIONS: Hypersensitivity to any penicillin.

DOSAGE: All extended-spectrum penicillins but carbenicillin indanyl sodium administered parenterally.

carbenicillin indanyl disodium	382mg PO qid
mezlocillin	100-300mg/kg/d divided
piperacillin	125-300mg/kg/d divided
ticarcillin	150-300mg/kg/d divided

SIDE/ADVERSE/EFFECTS: GI: N/V/D, flatulence, smell/taste disturbances ▪ HEM: anemia, eosinophilia, leukopenia, neutropenia, ***thrombocytopenia*** ▪ HEP: ↑ Serum AST, ALT, LDH ▪ INT: rash, pruritus, urticaria ▪ MS: arthralgia, neuromuscular hyperirritability ▪ Other: *discomfort at site of injection, esp c̄ continuous administration;* ***anaphylaxis.***

DRUG INTERACTIONS: Use of bacteriostatic antibiotics c̄ any penicillin can lead to antibiotic antagonism ▪ PO anticoagulant therapy may require dose adjustment.

NURSING MANAGEMENT

ASSESS: Hx of hypersensitivity (incl cephalosporins) ▪ Hepatic, renal function ▪ CAUTION: hepatic, renal impairment ▪ **ndx: Therapeutic effects:** High risk for altered body temperature ▪ High risk for infection ▪ **Adverse effects:** Diarrhea ▪ High risk for fluid volume deficit ▪ High risk for injury ▪ High risk for impaired skin integrity. **PLAN:** Administer at equal intervals around clock to maintain blood levels ▪ Maintain hydration ▪ **Special considerations:** G: caution, ↓ dosage (renal impairment, ↑ superinfection) ▪ P: caution (↑ sensitivity) ▪ OB: caution if pregnant, breastfeeding ▪ **Dietary management:** None specific ▪ **Lab test evaluation:** CBC. **IMPLEMENT:** Obtain C&S; check results ▪ Observe for signs of superinfection (diarrhea, URI, coated tongue) ▪ Administer on empty stomach. **PATIENT EDUCATION:** Comply c̄ prescribed drug therapy ▪ ↑ Fluid intake (8-10 glasses/d) ▪ Take on empty stomach ▪ Diarrhea may occur ▪ Notify physician of symptoms of allergic rx (fever, difficult breathing, rash). **EVALUATE: Observe for therapeutic effect:** Resolution of infection.

DESCRIPTION: Large group of antipsychotic (neuroleptic) agents that are chemical derivatives of phenothiazine ring. Several phenothiazine-like antipsychotic agents are chemically different but clinically similar.

DRUGS: acetophenazine maleate (*Tindal*), chlorpromazine (**Chlor-Promanyl, *Largactil, *Novochlorpromazine, Thorazine* suppositories), chlorpromazine hcl (*Thorazine*), fluphenazine decanoate (**Moditen, Prolixin Decanoate*), fluphenazine enanthate (*Prolixin, Enanthate*), fluphenazine hcl (*Permitil, Prolixin*), mesoridazine besylate (*Serentil*), perphenazine (**Apo-Perphenazine, Trilafon*), prochlorperazine (*Compazine* suppositories, **Stemetil*), prochlorperazine edisylate (*Compazine* injection, syrup; **Stemetil*), prochlorperazine maleate (*Compazine*), promazine hcl (**Promanyl, Sparine*), thioridazine (**Apo-Thioridazine, Mellaril-S, *Novoridazine, *PMS Thioridazine*), trifluoperazine hcl (*Stelazine*), triflupromazine hcl (*Vesprin*) ▪ Other antipsychotics: chlorprothixene (*Taractan*), chlorprothixene hcl (*Taractan* injection), chlorprothixene lactate (*Taractan* concentrate), haloperidol (*Haldol*), haloperidol lactate (*Haldol* concentrate, IM), loxapine hcl (**Loxapac, Loxitane-C* concentrate, IM), loxapine succinate (*Loxitane*), molindone hcl (*Moban*), thiothixene (*Navane*), thiothixene hcl (*Navane* concentrate IM).

MECHANISM OF ACTION: Antipsychotic activity appears associated c̄ ↓ neural transmissions in central dopamine-dependent pathways. These agents block postsynaptic dopamine receptors in limbic system, basal ganglia, resulting in tranquilizing effect in psychotic pts ▪ Various phenothiazines, other antipsychotic agents do not differ significantly in antipsychotic efficacy, but exhibit significant differences in adverse effects, potency ▪ Agents also possess anti-alpha adrenergic, anticholinergic activity; varying degrees of antiemetic activity; antihistamine, antiserotonin, sedative, ganglionic blocking activity.

PHARMACOKINETICS: *See* individual drug cards.

THERAPEUTIC USE: Treatment of psychotic states ▪ Antiemetics (eg, chlorpromazine) ▪ Treatment of intractable hiccups, intermittent porphyria (chlorpromazine).

CONTRAINDICATIONS: Hypersensitivity, comatose states, bone marrow depression, presence of large amounts of CNS depressants.

DOSAGE: Adult *PO*. Usual antipsychotic range

acetophenazine	40-600mg/d
chlorpromazine	30-1000mg/d
chlorprothixene	75-600mg/d
fluphenazine	0.5-20mg/d
haloperidol	2-100mg/d
loxapine	20-100mg/d
mesoridazine	100-400mg/d
molindone	20-225mg/d
perphenazine	6-100mg/d
prochlorperazine	15-150mg/d
promazine	40-1200mg/d
thioridazine	200-800mg/d
thiothixene	6-30mg/d
trifluoperazine	5-40mg/d
triflupromazine	30-150mg/d

SIDE/ADVERSE EFFECTS: CNS: drowsiness, extrapyramidal rxs, tardive dyskinesia ▪ CV: postural hypotension, tachycardia, ECG changes in Q&T waves ▪ EENT: blurred vision, corneal/lenticular changes, epithelial keratopathy, pigmentary retinopathy, nasal congestion ▪ END: lactation/moderate breast enlargement in women ▪ HEM: ***agranulocytosis,*** eosinophilia, leukopenia, ***hemolytic anemia,*** thrombocytopenic purpura ▪ HEP: cholestatic jaundice ▪ INT: urticaria, photosensitivity, ***exfoliative dermatitis,*** skin pigmentation (rare) ▪ PSYCH: adverse behavioral changes incl catatonic-like states ▪ Other: fever, hyperpyrexia, neuroleptic malignant syndrome, hypothermia.

DRUG INTERACTIONS: Aluminum-magnesium antacid preparations ↓ absorption ▪ Use c̄ narcotics, barbiturates, other CNS depressants ↑ CNS depression ▪ Guanethidine, other related antihypertensive effects antagonized.

NURSING MANAGEMENT

ASSESS: Hx of hypersensitivity ▪ BP ▪ Extrapyramidal rxs (spasm, trembling, shuffling gait) ▪ CAUTION: hepatic disease, seizure disorder, myasthenia gravis, Parkinson disease ▪ **ndx: Therapeutic effects:** Defensive coping ▪ Ineffective individual coping ▪ Altered thought processes ▪ **Adverse effects:** High risk for activity intolerance ▪ High risk for altered body temperature ▪ ↓ Cardiac output ▪ Hypothermia ▪ High risk for injury ▪ Impaired physical mobility ▪ Sensory/perceptual alterations (visual) ▪ High risk for impaired skin integrity. **PLAN:** Prevent postural hypotension ▪ Avoid skin contact c̄ liquid forms (contact dermatitis) ▪ Position vomiting pt to avoid aspiration ▪ Avoid abrupt withdrawal ▪ Maintain hydration ▪ **Special considerations:** G: caution, ↓ dosage (↑ sensitivity) ▪ P: caution, avoid use if <6 mos ▪ OB: caution if pregnant; avoid breastfeeding ▪ **Dietary management:** Avoid alcohol ▪ ↑ Bulk-containing foods (constipation) ▪ **Lab test evaluation:** CBC. **IMPLEMENT:** Assess VS, esp BP ▪ Monitor hepatic, ophthalmic, renal status ▪ Monitor fluid retention (I&O, daily weight), constipation ▪ Assess for extrapyramidal rx ▪ Seizure precautions in pts c̄ hx of convulsive disorders ▪ Long-term therapy: assess for jaundice, agranulocytosis. **PATIENT EDUCATION:** Avoid sudden position changes (postural hypotension) ▪ Use safety precautions c̄ hazardous activity ▪ Comply c̄ prescribed drug regimen ▪ Avoid use of alcohol, other CNS depressants ▪ Use sugarless gum/hard candy to diminish dry mouth ▪ Constipation may occur; ↑ fluids, bulk-containing foods ▪ May turn urine pink/red/brown ▪ Full drug effects may take several wks ▪ Avoid temperature extremes ▪ Avoid direct sunlight/UV light (photosensitivity) ▪ Notify physician of fever, sore throat, bruising/bleeding, tics/spasms, trembling, shuffling gait. **EVALUATE: Observe for therapeutic effect:** ↓ Psychotic manifestations.

DESCRIPTION: Chemical derivatives of salicylic acid that exhibit wide array of pharmacologic activity incl topical, systemic applications.

DRUGS: ▪ **Systemic salicylates:** aspirin (*ASA, Ecotrin*), systemic choline magnesium trisalicylate (*Trilisate*), choline salicylate (*Arthropan*), diflunisal (*Dolobid, *Trilisate*), magnesium salicylate (*Doan's Pills, Magan*), osalazine sodium (*Dipentum*), salsalate (*Disalcid, Mono-Gesic*), sodium salicylate (*Uracel 5, *S-60*), sodium thiosalicylate (*Tusal*) ▪ **Topical salicylates:** salicylic acid (**Keralyt Gel, *Salingel*), methyl salicylate, triethanolamine salicylate (*Aspercreme, Exocaine, *Royflex*).

MECHANISM OF ACTION: Analgesic/antiinflammatory effect may be due to effect on prostaglandin synthesis. Antipyresis due to effect on thermoregulatory areas in hypothalamus, resulting in dilation of peripheral blood vessels, marked sweating. Antithrombotic effect due to inhibition of platelet aggregation (limited to aspirin). Salicylates may interfere c̄ synthesis of hepatic coagulation factors.

THERAPEUTIC USE: Analgesic for mild-moderate pain ▪ Antipyretic ▪ Rheumatoid arthritis, osteoarthritis, other arthritic diseases ▪ Symptomatic treatment of rheumatic fever ▪ Prophylaxis (aspirin) of thrombotic diseases, esp coronary artery disease ▪ Remission of ulcerative colitis in pts intolerant to sulfasalazine (osalazine sodium) ▪

PHARMACOKINETICS

	Absorption						
	PO	Rectal	Peak	Duration	Half-life	Protein binding	Excretion
aspirin	80%-100%	70%-100%	15m-2h	4-6h	15-30m	90%	98% in urine as metabolites
diflunisal	98%-100%	—	2-3h	8-12h	8-12h	99%	90% in urine as metabolites
osalazine	2.4%	—	1h	NA	0.9h	99%	>90% urine, feces as metabolites
salsalate	98%-100%	—	2-4h	3-6h	1h	—	98% in urine as metabolites

Note: Side/adverse effects: common in *italic;* serious in ***boldface italic.***

*Available in Canada only.

Topical salicylates are used as rubefacients (heat producing on skin) except for salicyclic acid (antifungal & keratolytic).

CONTRAINDICATIONS: Hypersensitivity, active ulcers, magnesium salicylate c̄ advanced renal impairment.

DOSAGE: Adult *PO*

aspirin	325-650mg 4-6 times/d
choline magnesium trisalicylate	150-300mg/d
choline salicylate	870mg 5-8 times/d
diflunisal	250-500mg q8-12h
magnesium salicylate	325-650mg 3-4 times/d
olsalazine sodium	500mg bid
salsalate	500mg 4-6 times/d
sodium salicylate	325-600mg q4h

SIDE/ADVERSE EFFECTS: CNS: tinnitus (use in febrile pediatric pts c̄ selected virus infections may induce Reye syndrome) ▪ GI: epigastric distress, nausea, ***bleeding, ulcers*** ▪ HEM: hypothrombinemia ▪ HEP: ↑ AST, ALT.

DRUG INTERACTIONS: Use c̄ other ulcerogenic drugs best avoided ▪ Salicylates ↑ effects of PO anticoagulants, antidiabetics ▪ Use c̄ alcohol ↑ GI bleeding ▪ Salicylates ↓ PO absorption, uricosuric effects of indomethacin, other NSAIAs ▪ Use c̄ antacids ↓ salicylate PO absorption.

NURSING MANAGEMENT

ASSESS: Hx of hypersensitivity ▪ GI irritation ▪ Bleeding ▪ Toxicity (CNS disturbances, tinnitus, hyperventilation) ▪ Pain characteristics ▪ CAUTION: active ulcers, renal impairment ▪ **ndx: Therapeutic effects:** High risk for altered body temperature ▪ Impaired physical mobility ▪ Pain ▪ Altered tissue perfusion ▪ **Adverse effects:** High risk for injury ▪ Pain ▪ Sensory/perceptual alterations (auditory) ▪ Altered tissue perfusion. **PLAN:** Avoid concurrent administration c̄ large amounts of antacids ▪ **Special considerations:** G: caution (↑ sensitivity; renal impairment) ▪ P: avoid use (Reye's syndrome) ▪ OB: avoid use if pregnant, breastfeeding ▪ **Dietary management:** Avoid GI irritating foods ▪ **Lab test evaluation:** ↓ Blood glucose levels (diabetics). **IMPLEMENT:** Administer c̄ food to ↓ GI irritation ▪ Check for bleeding; D/C drug, notify physician ▪ Monitor VS, esp temperature. **PATIENT EDUCATION:** Comply c̄ prescribed drug regimen ▪ Take c̄ food/milk ▪ Notify physician immediately of bleeding, rash, hearing disturbances ▪ Check c̄ physician/pharmacist before taking OTC products. **EVALUATE: Observe for therapeutic effects:** ↓ Fever ▪ ↓ Pain ▪ ↓ Inflammation ▪ ↓ Clot formation.

DESCRIPTION: Bacteriostatic sulfonamide derivatives of *p*-aminobenzene sulfonamide (sulfanilamide).

DRUGS: sulfacytine (*Renoquid*), sulfadiazine, sulfamethizole (*Thiosulfil, Forte*), sulfamethoxazole (**Apo-Sulfamethoxazole, Gantanol)*, sulfapyridine, sulfasalazine (*Azulfidine*), sulfisoxazole (**Apo-Sulfisoxazole, Gantrisin, *Novosoxazole*), trisulfapyrimidines.

MECHANISM OF ACTION: Bacteriostatic activity due to inhibition of folic acid synthesis in susceptible microorganisms.

PHARMACOKINETICS: *See* individual drug cards.

THERAPEUTIC USE: Antibacterial: SYSTEMIC: sulfacytine, sulfadiazine, sulfamethizole, sulfamethoxazole, sulfisoxazole, trisulfapyrimidines ▪ GI TRACT: sulfasalazine ▪ **Dermatitis herpetiformis:** sulfapyridine ▪ **Nocardiosis:** sulfadiazine, sulfisoxazole, sulfamethoxazole, trisulfapyrimidines.

CONTRAINDICATIONS: Hypersensitivity, pregnancy at term, nursing mothers, infant <2mo (except in treatment of congenital toxoplasmosis), urinary acidifiers.

DOSAGE FORMS: Adult *PO*

sulfacytine	500mg loading dose followed by 250mg qid
sulfadiazine	2-4g loading dose followed by 1g q4-6h
sulfamethizole	0.5-1g 3/4 times/d
sulfamethoxazole	2g loading dose followed by 1g 2-3 times/d
sulfapyridine	500mg qid until improvement. ↓ dose by 500mg every 3d until symptom-free maintenance achieved
sulfasalazine	3-4g/d divided. Maintenance dose 2g
sulfisoxazole	2-4g loading dose followed by 4-8g/d in 4-6 doses
trisulfapyrimidines	2-4g loading dose followed by 2-4g/d in 3-6 doses

SIDE/ADVERSE EFFECTS: CNS: headache, peripheral neuritis, depression, ataxia, ***convulsions*** ▪ GI: N/V/D, anorexia, abdominal pain, ***pancreatitis***, stomatitis ▪ GU: ***crystalluria, toxic nephrosis*** ▪ HEM: ***agranulocytosis, aplastic anemia, hemolytic anemia, thrombocytopenia***, purpura, methemoglobinemia, hypoprothrombinemia, leukopenia ▪ INT: maculopapular/bullous eruptions, ***Stevens-Johnson syndrome, epidermal necrolysis, exfoliative dermatitis***, urticaria, photosensitivity ▪ MS: arthralgia ▪ Other: serum sickness, allergic myocarditis, periorbital edema.

DRUG INTERACTIONS: Avoid *p*-aminobenzoic preparations during therapy ▪ Use c̄ PO anticoagulant may require dosage adjustment due to ↓ vitamin K synthesis in gut ▪ Sulfonamides can enhance activity of PO hypoglycemics, methotrexate.

NURSING MANAGEMENT

ASSESS: Hx of hypersensitivity (incl furosemide, thiazide diuretics) ▪ Hepatic, renal function ▪ CAUTION: hepatic, renal impairment ▪ **ndx Therapeutic effects**: High risk for altered body temperature ▪ High risk for infection ▪ **Adverse effects:** Diarrhea ▪ High risk for fluid volume deficit ▪ High risk for injury ▪ High risk for impaired skin integrity ▪ Altered patterns of urinary elimination. **PLAN:** Administer at equal intervals around clock to maintain blood levels ▪ Maintain hydration ▪ **Special considerations:** G: caution (hepatic, renal impairment) ▪ P: caution; avoid use if <2mos ▪ OB: caution if pregnant, breastfeeding ▪ **Dietary management**: Avoid urinary acidifiers (crystalluria) ▪ **Lab test evaluation**: CBC, UA. **IMPLEMENT:** Obtain C&S; check results ▪ Observe for signs of superinfection (diarrhea, URI, coated tongue) ▪ Administer on an empty stomach. **PATIENT EDUCATION:** Comply c̄ prescribed drug therapy ▪ ↑ Fluid intake (8-10 glasses/d) ▪ Take on empty stomach ▪ Diarrhea may occur ▪ Avoid exposure to UV light ▪ Notify physician of fever, sore throat, difficult breathing, rash, bruising/bleeding. **EVALUATE: Observe for therapeutic effect:** Resolution of infection.

DESCRIPTION: Broad-spectrum bacteriostatic antibiotics obtained semisynthetically or from natural *Streptomyces* spp fermentation.

DRUGS: demeclocycline hcl (*Declomycin*), doxycycline hyclate (*Vibramycin*), minocycline hcl (*Minocin*), oxytetracycline hcl (*Terramycin*), tetracycline hcl (**Achromycin, Achromycin V, *Apo-tetra, *Medicycline, *Neo-Tetrine, *Novetetra, Sumycin, *Tetracyn*).

MECHANISM OF ACTION: Bacteriostatic effect due to inhibition of ribosomal protein synthesis in susceptible microorganisms.

THERAPEUTIC USE: Drug(s) of choice for *Chlamydia*: lymphogranuloma venereum; psittacosis; nonspecific endocervical, rectal, urethral infections ▪ *Mycoplasma: Mycoplasma* pneumonia ▪ *Rickettsia*: Q fever, rickettsialpox, Rocky Mountain spotted fever, scrub typhus, typhus ▪ Drug(s) of choice for acne control, balantidiasis, brucellosis, chancroid, cholera, granuloma inguinale, shigellosis, spirochetal relapsing fever ▪ Alternative in penicillin allergy (esp for gonorrhea, syphilis), infections where bacteriologic testing indicates good pathogen susceptibility.

PHARMACOKINETICS

	PO absorption					
	No food	Food	Half-life	Protein binding	MIC	Excretion
demeclocycline	60%-80%	10%-30%	10-16h	35%-85%	4μg/ml	Renal, feces
doxycycline	90%-100%	70%-80%	14-24h	30%-90%	4μg/ml	Renal, feces
minocycline	90%-100%	70%-80%	11-26h	55%-80%	4μg/ml	Renal, feces
oxytetracycline	60%-80%	10%-30%	6-10h	20%-40%	4μg/ml	Renal, feces
tetracycline	60%-80%	10%-30%	6-12h	20%-65%	4μg/ml	Renal, feces

CONTRAINDICATIONS: Hypersensitivity to any tetracycline; pregnancy, nursing mothers, neonates, children <8 yrs.

DOSAGE: Adult *PO*

Doxycycline, minocycline	50-100mg bid
Demeclocycline	150mg qid
Oxytetracycline, tetracycline	250mg qid

SIDE/ADVERSE EFFECTS: GI: *gastric upset, diarrhea,* bleeding, enterocolitis ▪ GU: dose-related ↑ BUN ▪ HEM: ***hemolytic anemia, thrombocytopenia*** ▪ INT: *Monilia overgrowth,* maculopapular rash, ***exacerbation of SLE,*** photosensitivity ▪ MS: reversible bulging fontanel in neonates, fetal skeletal retardation, tooth discoloration (<8y/o).

DRUG INTERACTIONS: Antacids, antidiarrheals, dairy products ↓ PO absorption ▪ Use c̄ methoxyflurane may produce nephrotoxicity ▪ PO anticoagulant activity may ↑ due to ↓ intestinal vitamin K synthesis ▪ Tetracyclines antagonize effects of bactericidal antibiotics.

NURSING MANAGEMENT

ASSESS: Hx of hypersensitivity ▪ Hepatic, renal function ▪ CAUTION: hepatic, renal impairment ▪ **ndx Therapeutic effects**: High risk for altered body temperature ▪ High risk for infection ▪ **Adverse effects:** Diarrhea ▪ High risk for fluid volume deficit ▪ High risk for injury ▪ High risk for impaired skin integrity. **PLAN:** Administer at equal intervals around clock to maintain blood levels ▪ Maintain hydration ▪ **Special considerations:** G: caution (renal impairment) ▪ P: avoid use if <8y/o (permanent tooth discoloration; ↓ bone growth) ▪ OB: avoid use if pregnant, breastfeeding ▪ **Dietary management**: Avoid taking c̄ dairy products, antacids, antidiarrheals ▪ **Lab test evaluation:** CBC. **IMPLEMENT:** Obtain C&S; check results ▪ Observe for signs of superinfection (diarrhea, URI, coated tongue) ▪ Administer on empty stomach ▪ Check for ↑ PO anticoagulant activity ▪ Monitor for phlebitis c̄ IV use. **PATIENT EDUCATION:** Comply c̄ prescribed therapy ▪ Take on empty stomach ▪ Diarrhea may occur ▪ Avoid exposure to UV light ▪ Avoid use c̄ dairy products, antacids. **EVALUATE: Observe for therapeutic effect:** Resolution of infection.

DESCRIPTION: Natural, synthetic thyroid agents.

DRUGS: Natural preparations: Thyroid: obtained from fresh desiccated domesticated animal thyroid glands; active thyroid hormones levothyroxine (T_4), liothyronine (T_3), l-triiodothyroxine present in natural states, ratio ▪ **Synthetically produced preparations:** levothyroxine sodium (T_4; *Levothroid, Synthroid*), liothyronine sodium (T_3; *Cytomel*), liotrix (*Thyrolar, Euthroid*): combination of synthetic microcrystalline T_4 sodium, T_3 sodium in various specific amounts, as indicated by the label of the preparation.

MECHANISM OF ACTION: Thyroid hormones regulate general body metabolism by controlling cellular oxidative process; influence growth; tissue differentiation, maturation.

THERAPEUTIC USE: Treatment of hypothyroidism ▪ Suppression of pituitary TSH in prevention/treatment of various types of goiters (T_3) ▪ Diagnostic T_3 suppression test for hyperthyroidism (T_3).

CONTRAINDICATIONS: Thyrotoxicosis, uncorrected adrenocortical deficiency, acute MI.

DOSAGE: Must be individualized to approximate deficient thyroid activity; normal protein-bound iodine values 4-8 μg/dl; values <4μg suggest hypothyroidism, need for supplemental thyroid therapy.

Adult *PO* maintenance dose

levothyroxine	50-200μg/d
liothyronine	25-100μg/d
liotrix	Based on thyroid equivalent (30-180mg thyroid)
thyroid	65-200mg/d

SIDE/ADVERSE EFFECTS: CNS: headache, insomnia, nervousness, tremors ▪ CV: angina, ***cardiac arrhythmias,*** palpitations, tachycardia ▪ GI: diarrhea ▪ Other: intolerance to heat; sweating, weight loss.

DRUG INTERACTIONS: Use c̄ epinephrine in coronary disease may induce coronary insufficiency ▪ Use c̄ PO anticoagulants ↑ their activity, requires lower anticoagulant doses ▪ Use c̄ cholestyramine ↓ PO absorption of thyroid preparations ▪ Use in diabetic pts may require ↑ dosage of hypoglycemic agents.

NURSING MANAGEMENT

ASSESS: Hx of hypersensitivity ▪ Heart rate ▪ Signs of toxicity (nervous, chest pain, rapid/irregular heartbeat) ▪ CAUTION: CV impairment ▪ **ndx Therapeutic effects:** Altered nutrition: less than body requirements ▪ **Adverse effects:** High risk for anxiety ▪ ↓ Cardiac output ▪ Diarrhea ▪ Fatigue ▪ Pain ▪ Altered thought processes ▪ Altered tissue perfusion. **PLAN:** Administer daily dose before breakfast ▪ **Special considerations:** G: caution, ↓ dosage (↓ metabolism) ▪ P: temporary alopecia may occur ▪ OB: caution if pregnant, breastfeeding ▪ **Dietary management:** Avoid high-iodine foods (soybean, cabbage, shellfish) ▪ **Lab test evaluation:** Thyroid function tests (T_3, T_4, TSH); blood glucose (diabetics). **IMPLEMENT:** Monitor VS, esp heart rate ▪ Observe for signs of OD (chest pain, fever, nervousness, rapid heartbeat) ▪ Monitor thyroid function tests; evaluate pt use of iodine-containing substances before exam ▪ Diabetics: closely monitor blood glucose level (hyperglycemia). **PATIENT EDUCATION:** Comply $\bar{c}$ prescribed drug regimen ▪ Procedure for checking radial pulse; take pulse on arising qd, notify physician if irregular, D/C drug ▪ Notify physician/dentist of use before treatment ▪ Avoid high-iodine foods ▪ Keep scheduled appointments for lab work/$\bar{c}$ physician ▪ Do *not* change brand name preparations ▪ Avoid alcohol ▪ Notify physician *immediately* of breathing, chest pain, rapid/irregular heart beat; DC drug ▪ Check $\bar{c}$ physician/pharmacist before taking OTC products. **EVALUATE: Observe for therapeutic effects:** ↑ Metabolic rate ▪ ↓ Manifestations of hypothyroidism.

DESCRIPTION: Immunizing biologicals that produce acquired active artificial immunity against selected viral and bacterial diseases ▪ Toxoids are antigenic preparations of G^+ bacterial exotoxins that are detoxified c̄ formaldehyde and /or heat. Highly antigenic, and cannot revert back to a toxic form. Stimulate specific antitoxin antibodies that neutralize tissue, destroying bacterial exotoxins. Immunity is effective and long lasting. Available preparations include Diphtheria, Tetanus, and a combination c̄ Pertussis vaccine (DPT) ▪ *Vaccines* induce the immune system to produce immunity (humoral or cell-mediated) against specific microorganisms. Vaccine-induced immunity varies c̄ the specific vaccine utilized and ranges from poor to excellent. Classic vaccines contain the actual pathogen (except smallpox, cowpox), which is either living, attenuated (weakened), or inactivated (killed). The attenuating and/or killing agent is usually formaldehyde or heat. Attenuation is also accomplished by the repeated passage through some animal or tissue. Live vaccines produce greater and longer lasting immunity than inactivated vaccines.

Newer vaccines utilize some extract or synthetic extract (genetic engineering) of the pathogen rather than the actual microbe. Since the microbe is not present in the vaccine, they are really viral, or bacterial, antigenic preparations. Hepatitis B and influenza vaccine contain either the natural or synthetic viral surface antigens of the virus. In addition, influenza vaccine may contain the whole virus or the split virus particle. Meningitis (meningococcal), *Haemophilus*, and pneumococcal vaccines contain selected bacterial capsular polysaccharides that are extracted from the respective microbes.

PREPARATIONS: Toxoids: Diphtheria toxoid adsorbed, diphtheria and tetanus toxoid adsorbed, tetanus toxoid fluid, tetanus toxoid adsorbed, diphtheria, and tetanus toxoids and pertussis vaccine—DPT ▪ **Vaccines:** *Bacterial:* BCG vaccine, cholera vaccine, *Haemophilus b* conjugate vaccine, meningitis vaccine, plague vaccine, pneumococcal vaccine polyvalent ▪ **Viral:** hepatitis b vaccine, influenza vaccine, measles vaccine live, measles and rubella vaccine live, measles, mumps, and rubella vaccine live, mumps vaccine live, polio virus vaccine inactivated-Salk, polio virus vaccine live-Sabin, rabies vaccine, rubella vaccine live, rubella and mumps vaccine live, yellow fever vaccine. In addition, the Centers for Disease Control (CDC) provides an assortment of rare vaccines including smallpox.

THERAPEUTIC USE: Production of active artificial immunity to infectious diseases.

CONTRAINDICATIONS: Hypersensitivity, tuberculin-positive individuals (BCG), immune deficiencies or immunosuppressive therapy (esp for live vaccines), acute febrile infections, pt age and/or pregnancy for selected vaccines.

PEDIATRIC IMMUNIZATION SCHEDULES

diphtheria toxoid	*IM*	2, 4, 6, 18 mo; 4-6 yr
measles vaccine	*SC*	≥12 mo
mumps vaccine	*SC*	≥12 mo
pertussis vaccine	*IM*	2, 4, 6, 18 mo; 4-6 yr
rubella vaccine	*SC*	≥12 mo
tetanus toxoid	*IM*	2, 4, 6, 18 mo; 4-6 yr
oral polio vaccine		2, 4, 6, 18 mo; 4-6 yr

DRUG INTERACTIONS: Use c̄ immunosuppressive drugs will antagonize effects (immunity) and may induce serious infections c̄ live or attenuated vaccines.

NURSING MANAGEMENT

ASSESS: Hx of hypersensitivity to any component of the vaccine ▪ Injection site for redness, edema, pain ▪ CAUTION: immunocompromised pts ▪ **ndx Therapeutic effects**: High risk for infection ▪ **Adverse effects:** High risk for injury ▪ High risk for impaired skin integrity ▪ Impaired tissue integrity. **PLAN:** Have epinephrine (1:1000), oxygen, support equipment available for anaphylaxis ▪ Document immunization for pt; notify when repeat vaccine/booster is needed ▪ **Special considerations:** G: caution (chronic illness) ▪ P: caution (immature systems) ▪ OB: avoid use if pregnant, breastfeeding ▪ **Dietary management and Lab test evaluation:** None specific. **IMPLEMENT:** Parenteral: administer IM via deltoid muscle or SC as directed; do *not* administer IV; rotate sites ▪ TOPV: may be mixed c̄ H_2O, milk, syrup or placed on bread, sugar cube ▪ Monitor for hypersensitivity rxs (difficult breathing, chest pain, pruritus) ▪ Assess for discomfort following injection; provide comfort measures as needed. **PATIENT EDUCATION:** Notify physician/nurse of chest pain, difficult breathing, any unusual rx to immunization ▪ Comfort measures postimmunization (analgesics, moist heat to injection site). **EVALUATE: Observe for therapeutic effect:** Prevention of specific disease.

DESCRIPTION: Large group of antidepressants chemically similar to phenothiazines.

DRUGS: amitriptyline hcl (**Apo-Amitriptylline, Elavil, Endep, Enovil, *Levate, *Meravil, *Novotriptyn*), amoxapine (*Asendin*), clomipramine hcl (*Anafranil*), clozapine (*Clozaril*), desipramine hcl (*Norpramin, Pertofrane*), doxepin hcl (*Sinequan*), imipramine hcl (**Apo-Imipramine, *Impril, Janimine, *Novopramine, Tofranil*), imipramine pamoate (*Tofranil-PM*), maprotiline hcl (*Ludiomil*), nortriptyline hcl (*Aventyl*), protriptyline hcl (*Vivactil, *Triptil*), trimipramine maleate (*Surmontil*).

MECHANISM OF ACTION: Antidepressant activity appears related to inhibition of norepinephrine reuptake in central adrenergic neurons after its release. They affect serotonin, possess strong anticholinergic activity, produce varying degrees of sedation.

PHARMACOKINETICS: *See* individual drug cards.

THERAPEUTIC USE: Treatment of endogenous depression ▪ Imipramine: adjunct for treating enuresis (children >6y/o).

CONTRAINDICATIONS: Hypersensitivity, MAO-I therapy, MI (acute recovery period). ▪ Doxepin: glaucoma, urinary retention.

DOSAGE: Adult *PO*

amitriptyline	75-150mg/d
amoxapine	150-300mg/d
clomipramine	25-250mg/d
clozapine	25-900mg/d
doxepin	75-100mg/d
imipramine hcl	75-200mg/d
imipramine pamoate	75-200mg/d
maprotiline	75-225mg/d
nortriptyline	25-100mg/d
protriptyline	15-60mg/d
trimipramine	75-200mg/d

SIDE/ADVERSE EFFECTS: CNS: drowsiness, dizziness, headache, incoordination, tremors, extrapyramidal symptoms, paresthesia (extremities), insomnia ▪ CV: ***arrhythmias,*** MI, stroke, ***heart block,*** postural hypotension ▪ EENT: tinnitus ▪ END: gynecomastia, testicular swelling, galactorrhea, breast enlargement (women) ▪ GI: anorexia, N/V/D, stomatitis, cramps, black hairy tongue, dry mouth, constipation ▪ GU: urinary hesitancy ▪ HEM: ***agranulocytosis,*** eosinophilia, ***thrombocytopenia*** ▪ HEP: cholestatic jaundice ▪ INT: skin rash, photosensitivity, alopecia ▪ PSYCH: disorientation, delusions, hallucinations, exacerbation of psychosis, confusion ▪ Other: parotid swelling.

DRUG INTERACTIONS: Significant depressant effects c̄ alcohol ▪ Anticholinergics, chlorpromazine produce ↑ atropine-like effects; paralytic ileus could occur ▪ Significant ↑ activity c̄ epinephrine, levarterenol, other adrenergic agents ▪ Significant antagonism of effects of reserpine, clonidine, guanethidine-type antihypertensives.

NURSING MANAGEMENT

ASSESS: Hx of hypersensitivity ▪ BP ▪ CAUTION: hepatic, renal impairment ▪ **ndx Therapeutic effects**: Ineffective individual coping ▪ Self-esteem disturbance ▪ High risk for violence: self-directed ▪ **Adverse effects:** High risk for activity intolerance ▪ ↓ Cardiac output ▪ Diarrhea ▪ High risk for fluid volume deficit ▪ High risk for injury ▪ Impaired physical mobility ▪ Sensory/perceptual alterations ▪ Sexual dysfunction ▪ High risk for impaired skin integrity. **PLAN:** Prevent postural hypotension ▪ Heavy smokers may require ↑ dosage ▪ Avoid abrupt withdrawal ▪ Institute suicide precautions ▪ Ensure drug ingestion ▪ **Special considerations:** G: caution (↑ sensitivity) ▪ P: not recommended ▪ OB: avoid use if pregnant, breastfeeding ▪ **Dietary management:** Avoid alcohol ▪ **Lab test evaluation:** CBC. **IMPLEMENT:** Monitor BP ▪ Suicide precaution prn ▪ Monitor hepatic, renal status. **PATIENT EDUCATION:** Comply c̄ prescribed drug regimen ▪ Avoid sudden position changes (postural hypotension) ▪ Use safety precautions c̄ hazardous activity ▪ Full drug effects may take several wks ▪ Use sugarless gum/hard candy to diminish dry mouth ▪ Check c̄ physician before taking OTC preparations ▪ Avoid alcohol ▪ Carry identification (MedicAlert). **EVALUATE: Observe for therapeutic effects:** ↓ Depression ▪ Mood elevation.

Product	Use	Adult Dose*
Accutrim	Diet control	1 tab in AM
Acid Mantle Creme	Skin irritations	Use several x/d
Actifed	Allergy/decongestant	1 tab 4-6h
Afrin	Nasal decongestant	Spray 2-3 x in AM & PM
Agoral	Laxative emulsion	1/2-1 T hs
Alophen	Laxative	1-3 tab hs
Allerest (maximum strength)	Allergy/decongestant	2 tab q4h (maximum strength)
Amsec	Asthma	1 cap q6h
Anbesol	Topical oral analgesic	Apply to affected area
ARM	Allergy/decongestant	1 cap q4h
Ascriptin A/D	Extra buffered analgesic	2-3 capl qid
Benylin Decongestant	Allergy/decongestant	2 t q4h
Benylin Expectorant	Allergy/expectorant	2-4 t q4h
Bronkaid	Asthma/congestion	1 tab q4h
Bronkolixir	Asthma/congestion	2 t q3-4h
Bronitin	Asthma/congestion	1 tab q4h
Cama	Buffered analgesic	2 tab q6h
Campho-Phenique	Cold sores/skin lesions	Apply directly 3-4x/d
Cheracol-D	Antitussive/expectorant	2 t q4h
Cheracol Plus	Antitussive/expectorant/decongestant	1 T q4h
Citrucel	Bulk laxative	1 T $\bar{c}$ 8 oz H_2O 1-3x/d
Contac	Antihistamine/decongestant	1 cap q12h
Coricidin	Analgesic/antihistamine	2 tab q4h

Tab, tablet; *capl*, caplet; *caps*, capsule.

Coricidin-D	Analgesic/antihistamine/decongestant	2 tab q4h
Correctol	Laxative	1-2 tab/d in AM or PM
Cruex	Topical antifungal	Apply in AM & PM
Debrox	Cerumen removal	5-10 drops bid in ear
Delfen	Contraceptive foam	Use before coitus
Desenex	Antifungal	Apply in AM & PM
Dialose	Stool softener/laxative	1-2 tab in AM & hs
Dialose Plus	Softener/stimulant laxative	1 tab prn
Dimetapp	Antihistamine/decongestant	1 extentab q12h
Donnagel	Diarrhea	2 T/tab after each BM
Dristan Cold	Antihistamine/analgesic/decongestant	2 tab q4h
Drixoral	Antihistamine/decongestant	1 SA tab q12h
Dulcolax	Laxative	2-3 tab/1 suppository once/d
Emetrol	Nausea	1-2 T q15m prn
Emko	Contraceptive foam	Use before coitus
Ex-Lax Chewables	Laxative	1-2 tab hs
Feosol	Iron supplement	3-4 tab pc & hs
Fiberall	Bulk laxative	1-3 wafers/d $\bar{c}$ 8oz H_2O
Geritol Complete	Multivitamin $\bar{c}$ minerals	1 tab/d pc
Gly-Oxide	Oral oxygen producing antiseptic	Apply directly into mouth
Gyne-Lotrimin	Vaginal antifungal	Apply cream/ointment to vagina
Gynol II	Diaphragm contraceptive jelly	Apply to diaphragm before coitus
Haley's MO	Laxative emulsion	1-2 T at hs & AM
Halotussin	Expectorant	1-2 t q4h
Halotussin DM	Antitussive/expectorant	1-2 t q6h
Imodium A-D	Diarrhea	4 t/2capl after 1st BM
Isoclor	Antihistamine/decongestant	1 cap q12h
Kasof	Stool softener/laxative	1 cap/d

Koromax	Contraceptive jelly	Use before coitus
Kwell	Lice/scabies	Apply cream/lotion to affected area
Lotrimin AF	Topical antifungal	Apply cream/lotion/solution bid
Maltsupex	Laxative	12-64g $\bar{c}$ adequate fluid
Metamucil	Bulk laxative	1 packet 1-3 x/d $\bar{c}$ 8 oz H_2O
Micatin	Topical antifungal	Apply in AM & PM
Midol	Menstrual discomfort	2 capl q4h
Momentum	Backache analgesic combination	2 capl qid
Monistat 7	Vaginal antifungal	1 applicatorful/suppository/d
Naldecon DX	Antitussive/decongestant/expectorant	2 t q4h
Neoloid	Laxative emulsion	2-4 T/d
Novahistine	Antihistamine/decongestant	2 t q4h
Novahistine DMX	Antihistamine/antitussive/decongestant	2 t q4h
NP-27	Topical antifungal	Apply 2x/d
Nytol	Sleep aid	1-2 tab hs
Ornex	Analgesic/decongestant	2 capl q4h
Pamprin	Menstrual discomfort	2 capl/tab q3-4h
Percogesic	Analgesic combination	1-2 tab q4h
Peri-Colace	Softener/stimulant laxative	1-2 cap/T hs
Phazyme	Flatulence	1 tab qid
Polysporin	Topical antibiotic combination	Apply 1-3x/d
Primatene	Asthma	1-2 tab stat, then 1 q4h prn
Pyrroxate	Analgesic/antihistamine/decongestant	1 cap q4h
Robitussin	Expectorant	2-4 t q4h

Tab, tablet; *capl*, caplet; *caps*, capsule.

Robitussin-CF	Antitussive/expectorant/decongestant	2 t q4h
Robitussin-DM	Antitussive/expectorant	2 t q4h
Robitussin-PE	Antitussive/expectorant	2 t q4h
Robitussin Max Cough	Antitussive	2 t q6-8h
Robitussin Night Relief	Analgesic/antitussive/expectorant/decongestant	1 fl oz hs
Ryna	Antihistamine/decongestant	1 t q6h
Semecid	Contraceptive insert	Insert 1 before coitus
Senokot	Laxative	1-2 t/2-4 tab bid
Serutan	Bulk laxative	1-3 t on food $\bar{c}$ H_2O 1-3x/d
Sleep-Eze 3	Sleep aid	2 tab hs
Sinarest	Analgesic/antihistamine/decongestant	2 tab q4h
Sominex	Sleep aid	1 capl/2 tabs hs
Sudafed	Decongestant	2 tab q4-6h
Syllact	Bulk laxative	1 t $\bar{c}$ H_2O 1-3 x/d
Syllamalt	Bulk/stimulant laxative	1-2 t $\bar{c}$ H_2O 1-3 x/d
Tedral	Asthma combination	1-2 tab q4h/1 SA tab q12h
Tinactin	Topical antifungal	Apply all forms in AM & PM
Ting	Topical antifungal	Apply all forms in AM & PM
Triaminic	Antihistamine/decongestant	2 t q4h
Triaminic-DM	Antihistamine/decongestant	2 t q4h
Triaminic Expectorant	Expectorant/decongestant	2 t q4h
Triaminicin	Analgesic/antihistamine/decongestant	1 tab q4h
Trichotine	Vaginal douche	Dilute before use
Unisom	Sleep aid	1 tab hs
Vagisec	Vaginal douche	Dilute before use
Vanquish	Buffered analgesic combination	2 capl q4h
Zonite	Vaginal douche	Dilute before use

APPENDIX: Syringe compatibility chart

Key
C = compatible
I = incompatible
Blank spaces indicate either no data, insufficient data, or conflicting data.

	Aminophylline	Atropine	Calcium gluconate	Diazepam	Diphenhydramine	Epinephrine	Hydroxyzine	Meperidine	Metoclopramide	Morphine	Nalbuphine	Pentazocine	Pentobarbital	Phenobarbital	Procainamide	Prochlorperazine	Promethazine	Scopolamine	Secobarbital	Verapamil
Aminophylline	*		C	I	C	I	I	I		I		I	C	I	C	I	I			C
Atropine		*		I	C	I	C	C	C	C	C	C	C			C	C	C		
Calcium gluconate	C		*	I	C	I									C				I	C
Diazepam	I	I	I	*	I	I	I	I	I	I	I	I	I	I	I	I	I	I	I	I
Diphenhydramine	C	C	C	I	*			C		C			I	I	C	C	C	C		
Epinephrine	I	I	I	I		*									I					
Hydroxyzine	I	C		I			*	C	C	C	C	C	I	I		C	C	C		
Meperidine	I	C		I	C		C	*	C	I		C	I	I		C	C	C		
Metoclopramide		C		I			C	C	*	C		C						C		
Morphine	I	C		I	C		C	I	C	*		C		I		I		C		
Nalbuphine		C		I			C				*						I	C		
Pentazocine	I	C		I			C	C	C	C		*	I	I			C	C		
Pentobarbital	C	C		I	I		I	I				I	*			I	I	C		
Phenobarbital	I			I	I		I	I		I		I		*		I				
Procainamide	C		C	I	C	I									*					C
Prochlorperazine	I	C		I	C		C	C		I			I	I		*		C		
Promethazine	I	C		I	C		C	C	C		I	C	I				*	C		
Scopolamine		C		I	C		C	C	C	C	C	C	C			C	C	*	I	
Secobarbital			I	I														I	*	
Verapamil	C		C	I											C					*

No distinction was made between compatible or temporarily compatible mixtures because drugs mixed in a syringe or infusion bottle should be used *immediately*. Furthermore, it is the responsibility of the "mixer" to ascertain by close observation that the mixture is compatible before administration. Therefore any compatibility chart is not absolute and the final authority is the dispenser of the mixture.

A

B

C

D

H

I

M

Q

R

S

U

V

NO POSTAGE
NECESSARY
IF MAILED
IN THE
UNITED STATES

BUSINESS REPLY MAIL

FIRST CLASS MAIL PERMIT NO. 135 ST. LOUIS, MO

POSTAGE WILL BE PAID BY ADDRESSEE

ATTN: PAT NEWMAN
MOSBY
11830 WESTLINE INDUSTRIAL DRIVE
P.O. BOX 46908
ST. LOUIS, MO 63146-9934

Drug:

CATEGORY: Preg Cat:

DOSAGE FORMS

DOSAGE:

ACTION/USE:

SIDE/ADVERSE EFFECTS:

PHARMACOKINETICS:

DRUG INTERACTIONS:

CONTRAINDICATIONS:

NURSING MANAGEMENT

NOTES:

ADMINISTRATION:

EVALUATION:

EDUCATION:

OVERDOSE MANAGEMENT:

Drug:

CATEGORY: Preg Cat:

DOSAGE FORMS

DOSAGE:

ACTION/USE:

SIDE/ADVERSE EFFECTS:

PHARMACOKINETICS:

DRUG INTERACTIONS:

CONTRAINDICATIONS:

NURSING MANAGEMENT
ADMINISTRATION:

NOTES:

EVALUATION:

EDUCATION:

OVERDOSE MANAGEMENT:

Drug:

CATEGORY: Preg Cat:

DOSAGE FORMS **DOSAGE:**

ACTION/USE:

SIDE/ADVERSE EFFECTS:

PHARMACOKINETICS:

DRUG INTERACTIONS:

CONTRAINDICATIONS:

NURSING MANAGEMENT
ADMINISTRATION:

NOTES:

EVALUATION:

EDUCATION:

OVERDOSE MANAGEMENT:

Drug:

CATEGORY: Preg Cat:

DOSAGE FORMS

DOSAGE:

ACTION/USE:

SIDE/ADVERSE EFFECTS:

PHARMACOKINETICS:

DRUG INTERACTIONS:

CONTRAINDICATIONS:

NURSING MANAGEMENT
ADMINISTRATION:

NOTES:

EVALUATION:

EDUCATION:

OVERDOSE MANAGEMENT: